Pharmaceutics

The Science of Dosage Form Design

Commissioning Editor: Ellen Green
Project Development Manager: Janice Urquhart
Project Manager: Nancy Arnott
Designer: Sarah Russell
Illustrated by: Chartwell Illustrators

Pharmaceutics

The Science of Dosage Form Design

Edited by

Michael E. Aulton BPharm PhD FAAPS MRPharmS
Professor of Pharmaceutical Technology,
School of Pharmacy,
De Montfort University,
Leicester, UK

SECOND EDITION

CHURCHILL
LIVINGSTONE

EDINBURGH LONDON NEW YORK OXFORD PHILADELPHIA ST LOUIS SYDNEY TORONTO 2002

CHURCHILL LIVINGSTONE
An imprint of Elsevier Limited

First published 1988
Second edition 2002

Standard Edition ISBN 0 443 05517 3
 Reprinted 2002, 2003 (twice), 2004, 2005 (twice)

International Student Edition ISBN 0 443 05550 5
 Reprinted 2002, 2003 (twice), 2004 (twice), 2005 (twice)

British Library Cataloguing in Publication Data
A catalogue record for this book is available from the British Library

Library of Congress Cataloging in Publication Data
A catalog record for this book is available from the Library of Congress

Notice
Medical knowledge is constantly changing. Standard safety precautions must be followed, but as new research and clinical experience broaden our knowledge, changes in treatment and drug therapy may become necessary or appropriate. Readers are advised to check the most current product information provided by the manufacturer of each drug to be administered to verify the recommended dose, the method and duration of administration, and contraindications. It is the responsibility of the practitioner, relying on experience and knowledge of the patient, to determine dosages and the best treatment for each individual patient. Neither the Publisher nor the editors/contributor assumes any liability for any injury and/or damage to persons or property arising from this publication.

The Publisher

ELSEVIER
your source for books, journals and multimedia in the health sciences
www.elsevierhealth.com

Working together to grow
libraries in developing countries

www.elsevier.com | www.bookaid.org | www.sabre.org

ELSEVIER   BOOK AID International   Sabre Foundation

The
Publisher's
policy is to use
**paper manufactured
from sustainable forests**

Printed in Spain

Preface

This is the second edition of *Pharmaceutics: the science of dosage form design*; the first edition was published in 1988. The pedigree of the book is actually much older than that. It was originally known as *Tutorial Pharmacy* and edited by John Cooper and Colin Gunn, and later by Sidney Carter.

The philosophy of this second edition remains unchanged, i.e. it is designed and written intentionally for newcomers to the design of dosage forms – other expert texts can take you into much more detail in each of the subject areas once you have mastered these basics. The subject matter of the book remains essentially the same, but the detail has been changed significantly because pharmaceutics has changed. Since the last edition there have been changes in both the concept and the content of pharmaceutics. These developments are reflected in this new edition.

The structure of the content of this edition has changed somewhat to reflect modern thinking and current university curricula. More importantly, every chapter has received attention and has been updated appropriately. Some of the basic science remains virtually unchanged (and will always remain so) but other areas, particularly biopharmaceutics, some areas of drug delivery and our understanding of the significance of the solid state, have changed enormously since the last edition. The current and future use of biotechnology products has also been reflected in this new edition.

The involvement of a wide range of authors continues in this edition, each an accepted expert in the field on which they have written and, just as importantly, each has experience and the ability to impart that information to undergraduate pharmaceutical scientists and those practitioners new to the subject. Many authors from the first edition remain, as they are still world leaders in their field. Others (who were either unable to contribute to the second edition, have retired or, sadly, died) have been replaced by a new generation of experts. The new authorship reflects modern knowledge and thinking in pharmaceutics.

I wish you well in your studies if you are an undergraduate or with your career if you are working in industry or the hospital service. I sincerely hope that this book helps you with your understanding of pharmaceutics – the science of dosage form design.

M E A   Leicester

Acknowledgements

The editor wishes to take this opportunity to thank the following who have assisted with the preparation of this text:

Mr Sidney Carter, who edited this book's predecessor, *Cooper and Gunn's Tutorial Pharmacy,* for passing on to me the opportunity to edit the first edition of this textbook. His invaluable experience and guidance aided me throughout the preparation of that edition and those principles are carried forward to this new edition.

I am extremely indebted to the authors for the work and time that they put into their texts, often under pressure from numerous other commitments, and from me. Modern life has few spare moments and so the time that they spent in contributing so knowledgeably and professionally to this text is warmly appreciated.

The many secretaries and artists who assisted the authors in the preparation of their work.

My wife Christine, for typing and other secretarial assistance, and help in a million other ways which enabled me to spend time on this edition of the book.

Ellen Green and Janice Urquhart of Churchill Livingstone, for their special expertise and assistance in the preparation of this second edition.

The many academic and industrial pharmaceutical scientists who helped during the design of the contents of this edition to ensure that it corresponds as closely as possible with modern practice and with the curricula of current pharmacy and pharmaceutical science courses.

Those publishing companies who have given their permission to reproduce material in this edition.

Michael E. Aulton

Contributors

Göran Alderborn PhD
Professor in Pharmaceutical Technology,
Department of Pharmacy, Uppsala University,
Sweden

Marianne Ashford BSc PhD MRPharmS
Manager, Preformulation & Biopharmaceutics,
AstraZeneca, Alderley Park, Cheshire, UK

David Attwood BPharm PhD DSc C Chem FRSC
Reader, School of Pharmacy and Pharmaceutical
Sciences, University of Manchester, Manchester, UK

Michael E. Aulton BPharm PhD FAAPS MRPharmS
Professor of Pharmaceutical Technology, School of
Pharmacy, De Montfort University, Leicester, UK

Brian W. Barry
BSc PhD DSc FRPharmS CChem FRSC
Professor of Pharmaceutical Technology, University
of Bradford, Bradford, UK

Michael R. Billany BSc MRPharmS
Principal Lecturer in Formulation Science,
De Montfort University, Leicester, UK

Graham Buckton BPharm PhD DSc FRPharmS FRSC
Professor of Pharmaceutics, School of Pharmacy,
University of London, London, UK

John H. Collett PhD DSc FRPhamS
Reader, University of Manchester, Manchester, UK

Daan J. A. Crommelin PhD
Scientific director, Utrecht Institute for
Pharmaceutical Sciences, Utrecht, The Netherlands

Dixie A. Dean
BPharm FRPharmS FFS FInstPkg DBA FIPSA
Former Head of Quality Control, Package Division
and Head of Packaging Research Laboratory, Boots
Ltd; Former Head of Packaging Development and
Devices, Deputy Group Head – Pharmacy, Fisons
Pharmaceuticals

John T. Fell BSc PhD MRPharmS
Senior Lecturer, School of Pharmacy and
Pharmaceutical Sciences, University of Manchester,
Manchester, UK

Josephine Ferdinando BSc MSc PhD
Head of Formulation, Pharmaceutical Research
Europe, RP Scherer Ltd, Swindon, UK

Geoff W. Hanlon BSc PhD MRPharmS
Reader in Pharmaceutical Microbiology, School of
Pharmacy and Biomolecular Sciences, University of
Brighton, Brighton, UK

Norman A. Hodges BPharm MRPharmS PhD
Principal Lecturer in Pharmaceutical Microbiology,
University of Brighton, Brighton, UK

John E. Hogan BPharm PhD MRPS
Manager of Pharmaceutical Technology, Central
Research, Pfizer Europe, Sandwich, UK

Keith G. Hutchison BSc(Pharm) PhD
Vice President of Research and Development, R. P.
Scherer, Swindon, UK

Brian E. Jones BPharm MPharm FRPharmS
Shonogi Qualicaps, SA, Alcobendas (Madrid),
Spain

Chris Marriott PhD DSc FRPharmS CChem FRSC
Professor of Pharmaceutics, King's College
London, London, UK

Albert Mekking BSc MSc
Manager, Clinical Production, OctoPlus BV,
Leiden, The Netherlands

R. Christian Moreton
BPharm MSc PhD MRPharmS MInstPkg
Vice President Research and Development,
Genpharm Inc., Etobicoke, Ontario, Canada

Malcolm S. Parker BSc MSc PhD FRPharmS
Formerly Dean of the Faculty of Health, University
of Brighton, Brighton, UK

The late **Stuart G. Proudfoot**
BPharm PhD MRPharmS
Formerly Principal Lecturer in Pharmaceutics,
School of Pharmacy, De Montfort University,
Leicester, UK

W. John Pugh BPharm PhD MRPharmS
Lecturer in Pharmaceutical Chemistry, Welsh
School of Pharmacy, Cardiff University, Cardiff,
UK

John N. Staniforth BSc PhD
Professor of Pharmaceutics, Department of
Pharmacy and Pharmacology, University of Bath,
Bath, UK

Malcolm P. Summers BSc(Pharm) PhD MRPharmS
Unit Manager, Abridged Licensing Medicines
Control Agency, London

Kevin M. G. Taylor BPharm PhD MRPharmS
Senior Lecturer in Pharmaceutics, School of
Pharmacy, University of London, London, UK

Peter M. Taylor PhD BSc(Hons)
Senior Lecturer in Pharmaceutics, School of
Pharmacy and Pharmaceutical Sciences, De
Montfort University, Leicester, UK

Josef J. Tukker PhD
Associate Professor of Pharmaceutics, Utrech
Institute for Pharmaceutical Sciences, University of
Utrecht, The Netherlands

Andrew M. Twitchell BSc(Pharm) PhD MRPharmS
Principal Lecturer in Pharmaceutical Technology,
School of Pharmacy, De Montfort University,
Leicester, UK

Ewoud van Winden PhD
Director, Regulon S.A., Athens, Greece

James I. Wells
BSc(Pharm) MSc PhD MRPharmS MInstPkg
Senior Lecturer (Industrial Pharmacy), Liverpool
John Moores University, Liverpool, UK

Peter York BSc (Pharm) PhD FRPharmS FRSC
Professor of Physical Pharmaceutics, Drug Delivery
Group, School of Pharmacy, University of
Bradford, Bradford, UK

Contents

What is 'Pharmaceutics'?

One of the earliest impressions that many new pharmacy and pharmaceutical science students have of their chosen subject is the large number of long and sometimes unusual-sounding names that are used to describe the various subject areas within pharmacy. The aim of this section is to explain to the reader what is meant by the term 'pharmaceutics', how it has been interpreted for the purpose of this book, and how pharmaceutics fits into the overall scheme of pharmaceutical science. It will also lead the reader through the organization of this book and explain why an understanding of the material contained in its chapters is important in the design of modern drug delivery systems.

The word pharmaceutics is used in pharmacy and pharmaceutical science to encompass many subject areas, which are all associated with the steps to which a drug is subjected towards the end of its development – i.e. it is the stages that follow its discovery or synthesis, its isolation and purification, and testing for advantageous pharmacological effects and the absence of serious toxicological problems. Put at its most simplistic, pharmaceutics converts a drug into a medicine. Pharmaceutics, and therefore this book, is concerned with the scientific and technological aspects of the design and manufacture of dosage forms.

Pharmaceutics is arguably the most diverse of all the subject areas in pharmaceutical science and encompasses:

- an understanding of the basic physical chemistry necessary for the efficient design of dosage forms (physical pharmaceutics)
- the design and formulation of medicines (dosage form design),
- the manufacture of these medicines on both a small (compounding) and a large (pharmaceutical technology) scale;
- the cultivation, avoidance and elimination of microorganisms in medicines (microbiology).

Medicines are drug delivery systems. That is, they are a means of administering drugs to the body in a safe, efficient, reproducible and convenient manner. The first chapter in the book introduces, in a general way, the considerations that must be made so that this conversion of drug to medicine can take place. It emphasizes the fact that medicines are rarely drugs alone, but require additives to make them into dosage forms and this in turn introduces the concept of formulation. The chapter explains that there are three major considerations in the design of dosage forms:

1. The physicochemical properties of the drug itself,
2. Biopharmaceutical considerations, such as how the route of administration of a dosage form affects the rate and extent of drug absorption into the body, and
3. Therapeutic considerations of the disease state to be treated, which in turn decide the most suitable type of dosage form, possible routes of administration and the most suitable duration of action and dose frequency for the drug in question.

This first chapter is an excellent introduction to the book as a whole and the perfect justification for the need to understand the subject matter of this text. New readers are encouraged to read this chapter thoroughly and carefully so they can grasp the basics before delving into the later, more detailed information.

Part 1 of this book describes some of the more important physicochemical knowledge that it is necessary to have in order to study and understand the design and preparation of dosage forms. The chapters have been designed to give the reader an insight into those scientific and physicochemical principles that are important to the formulation scientist. They are not intended as a substitute for a thorough understanding of physical chemistry, and many specific, more detailed, texts are available with this information.

For many reasons, which are discussed in the book, the vast majority of dosage forms are administered orally in the form of solid products such as tablets and capsules. This means that one of the most important stages in drug administration is the dissolution of solid particles to form a solution in the gastrointestinal tract. This means that the formulation scientist must have a knowledge of both liquid and solid materials, and particularly the properties of drugs in solution and the factors influencing drug dissolution from solid particles. Once solutions are formed, the reader must understand the properties of solutions and these are discussed next. The reader will see later in the book how drug release and absorption are strongly dependent on solution properties, such as solute dissociation and diffusion, and flow properties. A knowledge of these subjects is useful in solving certain problems relating to the properties of fluids and the performance of solutions and semisolids as dosage forms in their own right.

The properties of interfaces are described next. These are important to an understanding of adsorption on to solid surfaces as involved in the dissolution of solid particles and the study of disperse systems such as colloids, suspensions and emulsions. The scientific background to such systems is also discussed.

Before finalizing on a possible dosage form there must be a clear understanding of the stability of drug(s) and other additives in the formulation with respect to the reasons why and the rates at which they degrade. There must be an awareness of the means of inhibiting decomposition and increasing the shelf-life of a product. These points are discussed.

The subject known as preformulation is considered next. This is a consideration of the steps that need to be considered before formulation itself can begin. Preformulation involves a full understanding of the physicochemical properties of drug molecules and excipients and how they interact in dosage forms. Thus a grasp of this knowledge early on is of great use to the formulation scientist and teaches many scientific principles on which future dosage form design is dependent. The results of tests carried out at this stage of development can give a much clearer indication of the possible dosage forms for a new drug candidate.

Part Two of the book collects together those aspects of pharmaceutics associated with powdered materials. By far the majority of drugs are solid

powders, and unfortunately most of these have numerous adverse properties that must be overcome during the design of medicines to enable their satisfactory manufacture and subsequent performance in dosage forms.

The book therefore explains the concept of the solid state and how the internal and surface properties of solids are important and need to be characterized. This is followed by an explanation of the more macroscopic properties of powders that influence their performance during the design and manufacture of dosage forms – particle size and its measurement, size reduction, and size separation of powders from those of other sizes. There follows an explanation of the many problems associated with the mixing and flow of powders. In high-speed tablet and capsule production, for example, powders must contain a satisfactory mix of all the ingredients and achieve fast and uniform powder flow. For convenience, the mixing of liquids and semi-solids is also discussed here as the basic theory is the same.

Even with this fundamental knowledge it is not possible to begin to design a dosage form without having an understanding of how drugs are absorbed into the body, the various routes that can be used for this purpose, and the fate of the drugs once they enter the body and reach their site(s) of action. This book concentrates on the preparation, administration, release and absorption of drugs, but stops short at the cellular level and leaves to other texts the detail of how drugs enter individual cells, how they act, how they are metabolized and how they are eliminated. These cellular considerations are not within the remit of this book.

The terms bioavailability and biopharmaceutics are defined and explained in Part Three. The factors influencing the bioavailability of a drug and methods of its assessment are described. This is followed by a consideration of the manner in which the frequency of administration of a drug and the rate at which it is released affect its level in the blood at any given time. Part Three then goes on to discuss actual drug delivery systems which are available to modify and control the rate and extent of the release of drugs from dosage forms.

In Part Four, the book discusses the design of dosage forms and their manufacture It covers their formulation, the rate and extent of drug release from them, their advantages and disadvantages as a dosage form, and the way in which they are manufactured on a large scale in industry.

Dosage forms suitable for the administration of drugs through almost every possible body orifice and external surface is discussed, as well as a consideration of novel or future drug delivery systems that will be necessary for tomorrow's biotechnology products.

This part ends with a consideration of the pack into which the medicine is put. The pack and any possible interactions between it and the drug or medicine it contains are so vitally linked that the pack must not be considered as an afterthought. Packaging considerations should be uppermost in the minds of the formulators as soon as they receive the drug powder on which to work. The technology of packaging and filling of products is also discussed.

Following this in Part Five, techniques associated with the microbiological aspects of medicine development and production are discussed. These are necessary in industry to eliminate microorganisms from the product both before and during manufacture. Microbiology is a very wide-ranging subject. This book concentrates only on those aspects that are directly relevant to the design, production and distribution of dosage forms. This mainly involves avoiding (asepsis) and eliminating (sterilization) their presence (contamination) in medicines, and preventing the growth of any microorganism that might enter the product during storage and use (preservation). Techniques for testing that these intentions have been achieved are also described.

At this point the pharmaceutical technologist passes the product on to another aspect of pharmacy – the interface with the patient, i.e. dispensing and pharmacy practice. These disciplines are dealt with in the companion volume *Pharmaceutical Practice*, (1998), 2nd edition eds A J Winfield and R M E Richards (Churchill Livingstone).

1

The design of dosage forms

Peter York

PRINCIPLES OF DOSAGE FORM DESIGN

Drugs are rarely administered as pure chemical substances alone and are almost always given as formulated preparations or medicines. These can vary from relatively simple solutions to complex drug delivery systems through the use of appropriate additives or excipients in the formulations. The excipients provide varied and specialized pharmaceutical functions. It is the formulation additives that, among other things, solubilize, suspend, thicken, preserve, emulsify, modify dissolution, improve the compressibility and flavour drug substances to form various preparations or dosage forms.

The principal objective of dosage form design is to achieve a predictable therapeutic response to a drug included in a formulation which is capable of large-scale manufacture with reproducible product quality. To ensure product quality, numerous features are required: chemical and physical stability, suitable preservation against microbial contamination if appropriate, uniformity of dose of drug, acceptability to users including both prescriber and patient, as well as suitable packaging and labelling. Ideally, dosage forms should also be independent of patient to patient variation, although in practice this is difficult to achieve. However, recent developments that rely on the specific metabolic activity of individual patients, or implants that respond, for example, to externally applied sound or magnetic fields to trigger a drug delivery function, are beginning to accommodate this requirement.

Consideration should be given to differences in bioavailability between apparently similar formulations, and the possible causes for this. In recent years increasing attention has therefore been directed towards eliminating variation in bioavailability characteristics, particularly for chemically equivalent products, as it is now recognized that formulation

1

factors can influence their therapeutic performance. To optimize the bioavailability of drug substances it is often necessary to carefully select the most appropriate chemical form of the drug. For example, such selection should address solubility requirements, drug particle size and physical form, and consider appropriate additives and manufacturing aids coupled to selecting the most appropriate administration route(s) and dosage form(s). Suitable manufacturing processes and packaging are also required.

There are numerous dosage forms into which a drug substance can be incorporated for the convenient and efficacious treatment of a disease. Dosage forms can be designed for administration by alternative delivery routes to maximize therapeutic response. Preparations can be taken orally or injected, as well as being applied to the skin or inhaled, and Table 1.1 lists the range of dosage forms that can be used to deliver drugs by the various administration routes. However, it is necessary to relate the drug substance to the clinical indication being treated before the correct combination of drug and dosage form can be made, as each disease or illness often requires a specific type of drug therapy. In addition, factors governing the choice of administration route and the specific requirements of that route which affect drug absorption need to be taken into account when designing dosage forms.

Many drugs are formulated into several dosage forms of varying strengths, each having selected phar-

maceutical characteristics suitable for a specific application. One such drug is the glucocorticoid prednisolone, used in the suppression of inflammatory and allergic disorders. Through the use of different chemical forms and formulation additives a range of effective anti-inflammatory preparations are available, including tablet, enteric-coated tablet, injections, eye drops and enema. The extremely low aqueous solubility of the base prednisolone and acetate salt makes these forms useful in tablet and slowly absorbed intramuscular suspension injection forms, whereas the soluble sodium phosphate salt enables a soluble tablet form, and solutions for eye and ear drops, enema and intravenous injection to be prepared. The analgesic paracetamol is also available in a range of dosage forms and strengths to meet specific needs of the user, including tablets, dispersible tablets, paediatric soluble tablets, paediatric oral solution, sugar-free oral solution, oral suspension, double-strength oral suspension and suppositories.

It is therefore apparent that before a drug substance can be successfully formulated into a dosage form many factors must be considered. These can be broadly grouped into three categories:

1. Biopharmaceutical considerations, including factors affecting the absorption of the drug substance from different administration routes;
2. Drug factors, such as the physical and chemical properties of the drug substance;
3. Therapeutic considerations, including consideration of the clinical indication to be treated and patient factors.

High-quality and efficacious medicines will be formulated and prepared only when all these factors are considered and related to each other. This is the underlying principle of dosage form design.

BIOPHARMACEUTICAL ASPECTS OF DOSAGE FORM DESIGN

Biopharmaceutics can be regarded as the study of the relationship between the physical, chemical and biological sciences applied to drugs, dosage forms and drug action. Clearly, understanding the principles of this subject is important in dosage form design, particularly with regard to drug absorption, as well as drug distribution, metabolism and excretion. In general, a drug substance must be in solution form before it can be absorbed via the absorbing membranes and epithelia of the skin, gastrointestinal tract and lungs into body fluids. Drugs are absorbed in two

Table 1.1 Dosage forms available for different administration routes

Administration route	Dosage forms
Oral	Solutions, syrups, suspensions, emulsions, gels, powders, granules, capsules, tablets
Rectal	Suppositories, ointments, creams, powders, solutions
Topical	Ointments, creams, pastes, lotions, gels, solutions, topical aerosols
Parenteral	Injections (solution, suspension, emulsion forms), implants, irrigation and dialysis solutions
Respiratory	Aerosols (solution, suspension, emulsion, powder forms) inhalations, sprays, gases
Nasal	Solutions, inhalations
Eye	Solutions, ointments, creams
Ear	Solutions, suspensions, ointments creams

general ways, by passive diffusion and by specialized transport mechanisms. In passive diffusion, which is thought to control the absorption of most drugs, the process is driven by the concentration gradient that exists across the cellular barrier, with drug molecules passing from regions of high to those of low concentration. Lipid solubility and the degree of ionization of the drug at the absorbing site influence the rate of diffusion. Several specialized transport mechanisms are postulated, including active and facilitated transport. Once absorbed, the drug can exert a therapeutic effect either locally or at a site of action remote from that of administration. In the latter case the drug has to be transported in body fluids (Fig. 1.1).

When the drug is administered from dosage forms designed to deliver via the buccal, respiratory, rectal, intramuscular or subcutaneous routes, it passes directly into the blood-stream from absorbing tissues, but the intravenous route is the most direct of all. When delivered by the oral route the onset of drug action will be delayed because of the required transit time in the gastrointestinal tract, the absorption process and hepatoenteric blood circulation features.

The physical form of the oral dosage form will also influence absorption rate and onset of action, with solutions acting faster than suspensions, which in turn generally act faster than capsules and tablets. Dosage forms can thus be listed in order of time of onset of therapeutic effect (Table 1.2). However, all drugs, irre-

Table 1.2 Variation in time of onset of action for different dosage forms	
Time of onset of action	Dosage forms
Seconds	i.v. injections
Minutes	i.m. and s.c. injections, buccal tablets, aerosols, gases
Minutes to hours	Short-term depot injections, solutions, suspensions, powders, granules, capsules, tablets, modified-release tablets
Several hours	Enteric-coated formulations
Days	Depot injections, implants
Varies	Topical preparations

Fig. 1.1   Pathways a drug may take following the administration of a dosage form by different route.

spective of their delivery route, remain foreign substances to the human body, and distribution, metabolic and elimination processes commence immediately following absorption until the drug is eliminated from the body via the urine, faeces, saliva, skin or lungs in either unchanged or metabolized form.

Routes of drug administration

The absorption pattern of drugs varies considerably between individual substances as well as between the different administration routes. Dosage forms are designed to provide the drug in a suitable form for absorption from each selected route of administration. The following discussion considers briefly the routes of drug administration, and although dosage forms are mentioned this is intended only as an introduction, as they will be dealt with in greater detail in other parts of this book.

Oral route

The oral route is the one most frequently used for drug administration. Oral dosage forms are usually intended for systemic effects resulting from drug absorption through the various epithelia and mucosa of the gastrointestinal tract. A few drugs, however, are intended to dissolve in the mouth for rapid absorption, or for local effect in the tract, either because of the poor absorption by this route or because of their low aqueous solubility. Compared with other routes, the oral route is the simplest, most convenient and safest means of drug administration. Disadvantages, however, include the relatively slow onset of action, the possibilities of irregular absorption and the destruction of certain drugs by the enzymes and secretions of the gastrointestinal tract. For example, insulin-containing preparations are inactivated by the action of stomach fluids.

Several specific features relating to drug absorption from the gastrointestinal tract can be emphasized in the context of routes of administration. Changes in drug solubility can result from reactions with other materials present in the gastrointestinal tract, as for example the interference of absorption of tetracyclines through the formation of insoluble complexes with calcium, which can be available from foodstuffs or formulation additives. Gastric emptying time is an important factor for effective drug absorption from the intestine. Slow gastric emptying can be detrimental to drugs inactivated by the gastric juices, or slow down the absorption of drugs that are more effectively absorbed from the intestine. In addition, because environmental pH can influence the ionization and

lipid solubility of drugs, the pH change that occurs along the gastrointestinal tract, from about 1 in the stomach to approximately 7 or 8 in the large intestine, is important to both degree and site of drug absorption. As membranes are more permeable to unionized rather than ionized forms, and as most drugs are weak acids or bases, it can be shown that weak acids, being largely unionized, are well absorbed from the stomach. In the small intestine (pH about 6.5), with its extremely large absorbing surface, both weak acids and weak bases are well absorbed.

The most popular oral dosage forms are tablets, capsules, suspensions, solutions and emulsions. Tablets are prepared by compression and contain drugs and formulation additives, which are included for specific functions, such as disintegrants which promote tablet break-up into granules and powder particles in the gastrointestinal tract, thereby facilitating drug dissolution and absorption. Tablets are often coated, either to provide a protection against environmental factors for drug stability purposes or to mask unpleasant drug taste, as well as to protect drugs from the acid conditions of the stomach (enteric coating). Increasing use is being made of modified-release tablet products, such as fast-dissolving systems and controlled, delayed or sustained-release formulations. The benefits of controlled-release tablet formulations, achieved for example by the use of polymeric-based tablet cores or coating membranes, include reduced frequency of drug-related side-effects and the maintenance of steady drug-plasma levels for extended periods. These factors are important when medications are delivered for chronic conditions, or where constant levels are required to achieve optimal efficacy, as in treating angina and hypertension.

Capsules are solid dosage forms containing drug and usually appropriate filler(s), enclosed in a hard or soft gelatin shell. As with tablets, uniformity of dose can be readily achieved and various sizes, shapes and colours of shell are commercially available. The gelatin shell readily ruptures and dissolves following oral administration, and in most cases the drug is released from a capsule faster than from a tablet. Recently, renewed interest has been shown in filling semisolid and microemulsion formulations into hard gelatin capsules to provide rapidly dispersing dosage forms for poorly soluble drugs.

Suspensions, which contain finely divided drugs suspended in a suitable vehicle, are a useful means of administering large amounts of drugs that would be inconvenient if taken in tablet or capsule form. They are also useful for patients who experience difficulty in swallowing tablets and capsules, and for paediatric use. Whereas dissolution of drugs is required prior to absorption following administration, fine particles with a large surface area are presented to dissolving fluids, which facilitate dissolution in the gastrointestinal tract, absorption, and hence the onset of drug action. Not all oral suspensions are formulated for systemic effects however, and several, for example kaolin and morphine mixture, are designed for local effects in the gastrointestinal tract. On the other hand, solutions, including formulations such as syrups and linctuses, are absorbed more rapidly than solid dosage forms or suspensions, as drug dissolution is not required.

Rectal route

Drugs given rectally in solution, suppository or emulsion form are generally administered for local rather than systemic effects. Suppositories are solid forms intended for introduction into body cavities (usually rectal, but also vaginal and urethral), where they melt, releasing the drug, and the choice of suppository base or drug carrier can greatly influence the degree and rate of drug release. This route of administration is indicated for drugs that are inactivated by the gastrointestinal fluids when given orally, or when the oral route is precluded, as for example when a patient is vomiting or unconscious. Drugs administered rectally also enter the systemic circulation without passing through the liver, an advantage for drugs that are significantly inactivated by the liver following oral absorption. However, the rectal route is inconvenient and drug absorption is often irregular and difficult to predict.

Parenteral route

A drug administered parenterally is one injected via a hollow needle into the body at various sites and to varying depths. The three main parenteral routes are subcutaneous (s.c.), intramuscular (i.m.) and intravenous (i.v.). Other routes, such as intracardiac and intrathecal, are used less frequently. The parenteral route is preferred when rapid absorption is essential, as in emergency situations or when patients are unconscious or unable to accept oral medication, and in cases when drugs are destroyed or inactivated or poorly absorbed following oral administration. Absorption after parenteral drug delivery is rapid and, in general, blood levels attained are more predictable than those achieved by oral dosage forms.

Injectable preparations are usually sterile solutions or suspensions of drugs in water or other suitable physiologically acceptable vehicles. As previously mentioned, drugs in solution are rapidly absorbed and so injection suspensions are slower acting than solutions. In addition, because body fluids are aqueous, by using drugs suspended in oily vehicles a preparation exhibiting slower absorption characteristics can be formulated to provide a depot preparation, providing a reservoir of drug which is slowly released into the systemic circulation. Such preparations are administered by intramuscular injection deep into skeletal muscles (e.g. several penicillin-containing injections). Alternatively, depot preparations can be achieved by subcutaneous implants or pellets, which are compressed or moulded discs of drug placed in loose subcutaneous tissue under the outer layers of the skin. Such systems include solid microspheres, polymeric biodegradable polymeric microspheres (e.g. polylactide co-glycollic acid homo- and copolymers) containing proteins or peptides (e.g. human growth hormone and leuprolide). More generally, subcutaneous injections are aqueous solutions or suspensions that allow the drug to be placed in the immediate vicinity of blood capillaries. The drug then diffuses into the capillaries. The inclusion of vasoconstrictors or vasodilators in subcutaneous injections will clearly influence blood flow through the capillaries, thereby modifying the capacity for absorption. This principle is often used in the administration of local anaesthetics with the vasoconstrictor adrenaline, which delays drug absorption. Conversely, improved drug absorption can result when vasodilators are included. Intravenous administration involves the injection of sterile aqueous solutions directly into a vein at an appropriate rate. Volumes delivered can range from a few millilitres, as in emergency treatment or for hypnotics, up to litre quantities, as in replacement fluid treatment or nutrient feeding.

Given the generally negative patient acceptance of this important route of drug delivery, primarily associated with pain and inconvenience, recent developments have focused on 'needle-free' injection systems which propel drugs in aqueous solution or powder form at high velocity directly through the external layers of the skin.

Topical route

Drugs are applied topically, that is to the skin, mainly for local action. Although this route can also be used for systemic drug delivery, percutaneous absorption is often poor and erratic, although several transdermal patches delivering drug for systemic distribution are available (e.g. glyceryl trinitrate patches for the prophylaxis and treatment of angina). Drugs applied to the skin for local effect include antiseptics, antifungals, anti-inflammatory agents, as well as skin emollients for protective effects.

Pharmaceutical topical formulations – ointments, creams and pastes – are composed of drug in a suitable semisolid base which is either hydrophobic or hydrophilic in character. The bases play an important role in determining the character of drug release from the formulation. Ointments are hydrophobic, oleaginous-based dosage forms, whereas creams are semisolid emulsions. Pastes contain more solids than ointments and thus are stiffer in consistency. For topical application in liquid form other than solution, lotions – suspensions of solids in aqueous solution – or emulsions are used. More recently, interest in transdermal electrotransport systems has grown. Here a low electrical potential maintained across the skin can improve drug transport.

The application of drugs to other topical surfaces, such as the eye, ear and nose, is common and ointments, creams, suspensions and solutions are utilized. Ophthalmic preparations are required, among other features, to be sterile. Nasal dosage forms include solutions or suspensions delivered by drops or fine aerosol from a spray. Ear formulations in general are viscous to prolong contact with affected areas.

Respiratory route

The lungs provide an excellent surface for absorption when the drug is delivered in gaseous, aerosol mist or ultrafine solid particle form. For drug presented in an aerosol or solid form, particle size largely determines the extent to which they penetrate the alveolar region, the zone of rapid absorption. Particles in the region 0.5–1 μm diameter reach the alveolar sacs. Particles outside this range are either exhaled or deposited upon larger bronchial airways. This delivery route has been found particularly useful for the treatment of asthmatic problems, using both powder aerosols (e.g. sodium cromoglycate) and metered aerosols containing the drug in liquefied inert propellant (e.g. salbutamol sulphate aerosol). Importantly, this delivery route is being increasingly recognized as a means of administering the therapeutic agents emerging from biotechnology, such as peptides and proteins.

DRUG FACTORS IN DOSAGE FORM DESIGN

Each type of dosage form requires careful study of the physical and chemical properties of drug sub-

stances to achieve a stable, effective product. These properties, such as dissolution, crystal size and polymorphic form, solid-state stability and drug – additive interactions, can have profound effects on the physiological availability and physical and chemical stability of the drug. By combining such data with those from pharmacological and biochemical studies, the most suitable drug form and additives can be selected for the formulation of chosen dosage forms. Although comprehensive property evaluation will not be required for all types of formulations, those properties that are recognized as important in dosage form design and processing are listed in Table 1.3, together with the stresses to which the formulation might be exposed during processing and manipulation into dosage forms, as well as the procedures involved. Variations in physicochemical properties, occurring for example between batches of the same material or resulting from alternative treatment procedures, can modify formulation requirements as well as processing and dosage form performance. For instance, the fine milling of poorly soluble drug substances can modify their wetting and dissolution characteristics, properties that are important during granulation and product performance, respectively. Careful evaluation of these properties and understanding of the effects of these stresses upon these parameters is therefore important in dosage form design and processing, as well as in product performance.

Particle size and surface area

Particle size reduction results in an increase in the specific surface (i.e. surface area per unit weight) of powders. Drug dissolution rate, absorption rate, dosage form content uniformity and stability are all dependent to varying degrees on particle size, size distribution and interactions of solid surfaces. In many cases, for both drugs and additives particle size reduction is required to achieve the desired physiochemical characteristics.

It is now generally recognized that poorly aqueous-soluble drugs showing a dissolution rate-limiting step in the absorption process will be more readily bioavailable when administered in a finely subdivided form with larger surface than as a coarse material. Examples include griseofulvin, tolbutamide, indomethacin, spironolactone and nifedipine. The fine material, often in micrometre or submicrometre (nanometre) form with large specific surface, dissolves at a faster rate, which can lead to improved drug absorption by passive diffusion. On the other hand, with formulated nitrofurantoin preparations an

Table 1.3 Properties of drug substances important in dosage form design and potential stresses occurring during processes, with range of manufacturing procedures

Properties	Processing stresses	Manufacturing procedures
Particle size, surface area	Pressure	Precipitation
Solubility	Mechanical	Filtration
Dissolution	Radiation	Emulsification
Partition coefficient	Exposure to liquids	Milling
Ionization constant	Exposure to gases and liquid vapours	Mixing
Crystal properties, polymorphism	Temperature	Granulation
Stability		Drying
Organoleptic		Compression
(Other properties)		Autoclaving
		Crystallization
		Handling
		Storage
		Transport

optimal particle size of 150 μm reduces gastrointestinal distress while still permitting sufficient urinary excretion of this urinary antibacterial agent.

Rates of drug dissolution can be adversely affected, however, by unsuitable choice of formulation additives, even though solids of appropriate particle size are used. Tableting lubricant powders, for example, can impart hydrophobicity to a formulation and inhibit drug dissolution. Fine powders can also increase air adsorption or static charge, leading to wetting or agglomeration problems. Micronizing drug powders can lead to polymorphic and surface energy changes which cause reduced chemical stability. Drug particle size also influences content uniformity in solid dosage forms, particularly for low-dose formulations. It is important in such cases to have as many particles as possible per dose to minimize potency variation between dosage units. Other dosage forms are also affected by particle size, including suspensions (for controlling flow properties and particle interactions), inhalation aerosols (for optimal penetration of drug particles to absorbing mucosa) and topical formulations (for freedom from grittiness).

Solubility

All drugs, by whatever route they are administered, must exhibit at least limited aqueous solubility for therapeutic efficiency. Thus relatively insoluble compounds can exhibit erratic or incomplete absorption, and it might be appropriate to use more soluble salt or other chemical derivatives. Alternatively, micronizing, complexation or solid dispersion techniques might be employed. Solubility, and especially degree of saturation in the vehicle, can also be important in the absorption of drugs already in solution in liquid dosage forms, as precipitation in the gastrointestinal tract can occur and bioavailability be modified.

The solubilities of acidic or basic compounds are pH dependent and can be altered by forming salt forms with different salts exhibiting different equilibrium solubilities. However, the solubility of a salt of a strong acid is less affected by changes in pH than is the solubility of a salt of a weak acid. In the latter case, when pH is lower the salt hydrolyses to an extent dependent on pH and pK_a, resulting in decreased solubility. Reduced solubility can also occur for slightly soluble salts of drugs through the common ion effect. If one of the ions involved is added as a different, more water-soluble salt, the solubility product can be exceeded and a portion of the drug precipitates.

Dissolution

As mentioned above, for a drug to be absorbed it must first be dissolved in the fluid at the site of absorption. For example, an orally administered drug in tablet form is not absorbed until drug particles are dissolved or solubilized by the fluids at some point along the gastrointestinal tract, depending on the pH–solubility profile of the drug substance. Dissolution describes the process by which the drug particles dissolve.

During dissolution, the drug molecules in the surface layer dissolve, leading to a saturated solution around the particles that forms the diffusion layer. Dissolved drug molecules then pass throughout the dissolving fluid to contact absorbing mucosa, and are absorbed. Replenishment of diffusing drug molecules in the diffusion layer is achieved by further drug dissolution, and the absorption process continues. If dissolution is fast, or the drug is delivered and remains in solution form, the rate of absorption is primarily dependent upon its ability to transverse the absorbing membrane. If, however, drug dissolution is slow owing to its physicochemical properties or formulation factors, then dissolution may be the rate-limiting step in absorption and influence drug bioavailability. The dissolution of a drug is described in a simplified manner by the Noyes–Whitney equation:

$$\frac{dm}{dt} = kA(C_S - C)$$

where $\frac{dm}{dt}$ is the dissolution rate, k is the dissolution rate constant, A is the surface area of dissolving solid, and C_S is the concentration of drug in the dissolution medium at time t. The equation reveals that dissolution rate can be raised by increasing the surface area (reducing particle size) of the drug, by increasing the solubility of the drug in the diffusing layer and by increasing k, which incorporates the drug diffusion coefficient and diffusion layer thickness. During the early phases of dissolution $C_S > C$, and if the surface area A and experimental conditions are kept constant, then k can be determined for compacts containing drug alone. The constant k is now termed the intrinsic dissolution rate constant, and is a characteristic of each solid drug compound in a given solvent under fixed hydrodynamic conditions.

Drugs with k values below 0.1 mg^{-1} cm^{-2} usually exhibit dissolution rate-limiting absorption. Particulate dissolution can also be examined where an effort is made to control A, and formulation effects can be studied.

Dissolution rate data, when combined with solubility, partition coefficient and pK_a, provide an insight to the formulator into the potential in vivo absorption characteristics of a drug. However, in vitro tests only have significance when they are related to in vivo results. Once such a relationship has been established, in vitro dissolution tests can be used as a predictor of in vivo behaviour. The impor-

tance of dissolution testing has been widely recognized by official compendia, as well as drug registration authorities, with the inclusion of dissolution specifications using standardized testing procedures for a range of preparations.

Partition coefficient and pK_a

As pointed out above, for relatively insoluble compounds the dissolution rate is often the rate-determining step in the overall absorption process. Alternatively, for soluble compounds the rate of permeation across biological membranes is the rate-determining step. Whereas dissolution rate can be changed by modifying the physicochemical properties of the drug and/or by altering the formulation composition, the permeation rate is dependent upon the size, relative aqueous and lipid solubility and ionic charge of drug molecules, factors that can be altered through molecular modifications. The absorbing membrane acts as a lipophilic barrier to the passage of drugs which is related to the lipophilic nature of the drug molecule. The partition coefficient, for example between oil and water, is a measure of lipophilic character.

The majority of drugs are weak acids or bases and, depending on their pH, exist in an ionized or unionized form. Membranes of absorbing mucosa are more permeable to unionized forms of drugs than to ionized species, because of the greater lipid solubility of the unionized forms and the highly charged nature of the cell membrane, which results in the binding or repelling of the ionized drug, thereby decreasing penetration. Therefore, the dominating factors that influence the absorption of weak acids and bases are the pH at the site of absorption and the lipid solubility of the unionized species. These factors, together with the Henderson–Hasselbalch equations for calculating the proportions of ionized and unionized species at a particular pH, constitute the pH-partition theory for drug absorption. However, these factors do not describe completely the process of absorption, as certain compounds with low partition coefficients and/or which are highly ionized over the entire physiological pH range show good bioavailability, and therefore other factors are clearly involved.

Crystal properties: polymorphism

Practically all drug substances are handled in powder form at some stage during manufacture into dosage forms. However, for those substances composed of, or containing, powders or compressed powders in the finished product, the crystal properties and solid-state form of the drug must be carefully considered. It is well recognized that drug substances can be amorphous (i.e. without regular molecular lattice arrangements), crystalline, anhydrous, at various degrees of hydration or solvated with other entrapped solvent molecules, as well as varying in crystal hardness, shape and size. In addition, many drug substances can exist in more than one form, with different molecular packing arrangements in the crystal lattice. This property is termed polymorphism, and different polymorphs may be prepared by manipulating the conditions of particle formation during crystallization, such as solvent, temperature and rate of cooling. It is known that only one form of a pure drug substance is stable at a given temperature and pressure, with the other forms, termed metastable, converting at different rates of the stable crystalline form. The different polymorphs vary in physical properties such as dissolution and solid-state stability, as well as processing behaviour in terms of powder flow and compaction during tableting in some cases.

These different crystalline forms can be of considerable importance in relation to the ease or difficulty of formulation and as regards stability and biological activity. As might be expected, higher dissolution rates are obtained for metastable polymorphic forms; for example, the metastable form of chlortetracyline hydrochloride exhibits improved rate and extent of bioavailability. In some cases, amorphous forms are more active than crystalline forms.

The polypeptide hormone insulin, widely used in the regulation of carbohydrate, fat and protein metabolism, also demonstrates how differing degrees of activity can result from the use of different crystalline forms of the same agent. In the presence of acetate buffer, zinc combines with insulin to form an extremely insoluble complex of the proteinaceous hormone. This complex is an amorphous precipitate or crystalline product, depending on environmental pH. The amorphous form, containing particles of no uniform shape and smaller than 2 μm, is absorbed following i.m. or s.c. injection and has a short duration of action, whereas the crystalline product, consisting of 10–40 micrometre-sized rhombohedral crystals, is more slowly absorbed and has a longer duration of action. Insulin preparations that are intermediate in duration of action are prepared by taking physical mixtures of these two products.

Polymorphic transitions can also occur during milling, granulating, drying and compressing operations (e.g. transitions during milling for digoxin and spironolactone). Granulation can result in solvate

formation or, during drying, a solvated or hydrated molecule may be lost to form an anhydrous material. Consequently, the formulator must be aware of these potential transformations, which can result in undesirable modified product performance even though routine chemical analyses may not reveal any changes. Reversion from metastable forms, if used, to the stable form may also occur during the lifetime of the product. In suspensions this may be accompanied by changes in the consistency of the preparation which affect its shelf life and stability. Such changes can often be prevented by the inclusion of additives, such as hydrocolloids and surface-active agents.

Stability

The chemical aspects of formulation generally centre around the chemical stability of the drug and its compatibility with the other formulation ingredients. In addition it should be emphasised that the packaging of the dosage form is an important contributing factor to product stability and must be an integral part of stability testing programmes. Only a brief summary is given at this point. It has been mentioned previously that one of the principles of dosage form design is to ensure that the chemical integrity of drug substances is maintained during the usable life of the product. At the same time, chemical changes involving additive and any physical modifications to the product must be carefully monitored to optimize formulation stability.

In general, drug substances decompose as a result of the effects of heat, oxygen, light and moisture. For example, esters such as aspirin and procaine are susceptible to solvolytic breakdown, whereas oxidative decomposition occurs for substances such as ascorbic acid. Drugs can be classified according to their sensitivity to breakdown:

1. Stable under all conditions (e.g. kaolin)
2. Stable if handled correctly (e.g. aspirin)
3. Moderately stable even with special handling (e.g. vitamins)
4. Very unstable (e.g. certain antibiotics in solution form).

Although the mechanisms of solid-state degradation are complex and often difficult to analyse, a full understanding is not a prerequisite in the design of a suitable formulation containing solids. For example, in cases where drug substances are sensitive to hydrolysis, precautions such as minimum exposure to moisture during preparation, low moisture content specifications in the final product, and moisture resistant packaging can be used. For oxygen-sensitive drugs antioxidants can be included in the formulation and, as with light-sensitive materials, suitable packaging can reduce or eliminate the problem. For drugs administered in liquid form, the stability in solution as well as the effects of pH over the gastrointestinal pH range of 1–8 should be understood. Buffers may be required to control the pH of the preparation to improve stability, or where liquid dosage forms are sensitive to microbial attack, preservatives are required. In these formulations, and indeed in all dosage forms incorporating additives, it is also important to ensure that the components, which may include additional drug substances as in multivitamin preparations, do not produce chemical interactions themselves. Interactions between drug(s) and added excipients, such as antioxidants, preservatives, suspending agents, colourants, tablet lubricants and packaging materials, do occur and must be checked for during formulation. Over recent years data from thermal analysis techniques, particularly differential scanning calorimetry (DSC), when critically examined have been found useful in rapid screening for possible drug-additive and drug–drug interactions. For example, using DSC it has been demonstrated that the widely used tableting lubricant magnesium stearate interacts with aspirin and should be avoided in formulations containing this drug.

Organoleptic properties

Modern medicines require that pharmaceutical dosage forms are acceptable to the patient. Unfortunately, many drug substances in use today are unpalatable and unattractive in their natural state and dosage forms containing such drugs, particularly oral preparations, may require the addition of approved flavours and/or colours.

The use of flavours applies primarily to liquid dosage forms intended for oral administration. Available as concentrated extracts, solutions, adsorbed on to powders or microencapsulated, flavours are usually composed of mixtures of natural and synthetic materials. The taste buds of the tongue respond quickly to bitter, sweet, salt or acid elements of a flavour. In addition, unpleasant taste can be overcome by using water-insoluble derivatives of drugs which have little or no taste. An example is the use of amitriptyline pamoate. In such approaches other factors, such as bioavailability, must remain unchanged. If an insoluble derivative is unavailable or cannot be used, a flavour or perfume can be used. Alternatively, unpleasant drugs can be administered in capsules or prepared as coated particles, or tablets may be easily swallowed avoiding the taste buds.

The selection of flavour depends upon several factors, but particularly on the taste of the drug substance. Certain flavours are more effective at masking various taste elements: for example, citrus flavours are frequently used to combat sour or acid-tasting drugs. The solubility and stability of the flavour in the vehicle are also important. The age of the intended patient should also be considered, as children, for example, prefer sweet tastes, as well as the psychological links between colours and flavours (e.g. yellow is associated with lemon flavour). Sweetening agents may also be required to mask bitter tastes. Sucrose continues to be used, but alternatives such as sodium saccharin, which is 200–700 times sweeter depending on concentration, are available. Sorbitol is recommended for diabetic preparations.

Colours are employed to standardize or improve an existing drug colour, to mask a colour change or complement a flavour. Although colours are obtained both from natural sources (e.g. carotenoids) and synthesized (e.g. amaranth), the majority used are synthetically produced. Dyes may be aqueous (e.g. amaranth) or oil soluble (e.g. Sudan IV) or insoluble in both (e.g. aluminium lakes). Insoluble colours are known as pigments. Lakes (which are generally water-insoluble calcium or aluminium complexes of water-soluble dyes) are particularly useful in tablets and tablet coatings because of their greater stability to light than corresponding dyes, which also vary in their stability to pH and reducing agents. However, in recent years the inclusion of colours in formulations has become extremely complex because of the banning of many traditionally used colours in many countries. (A useful summary on colours is given in Martindale, *The Extra Pharmacopoeia*).

Other drug properties

At the same time as ensuring that dosage forms are chemically and physically stable and are therapeutically efficacious, it is also relevant to establish that the selected formulation is capable of efficient and, in most cases, large-scale manufacture. In addition to those properties previously discussed, such as particle size and crystal form, other characteristics, such as hygroscopicity, flowability and compressibility, are particularly valuable when preparing solid dosage forms where the drugs constitute a large percentage of the formulation. Hygroscopic drugs can require low-moisture manufacturing environments and need to avoid water during preparation. Poorly flowing formulations may require the addition of flow agents (e.g. fumed silica). Studies of the compressibility of drug substances are frequently undertaken using instrumented tablet machines in formulation laboratories to examine the tableting potential of the material, in order to foresee any potential problems during compaction, such as lamination or sticking which may require modification to the formulation or processing conditions.

THERAPEUTIC CONSIDERATIONS IN DOSAGE FORM DESIGN

The nature of the clinical indication, disease or illness against which the drug is intended is an important factor when selecting the range of dosage forms to be prepared. Factors such as the need for systemic or local therapy, the duration of action required and whether the drug will be used in emergency situations, need to be considered. In the vast majority of cases a single drug substance is prepared into a number of dosage forms to satisfy both the particular preferences of the patient or physician and the specific needs of a certain clinical situation. For example, many asthmatic patients use inhalation aerosols from which the drug is rapidly absorbed into the systematic circulation following deep inhalation for rapid emergency relief, and oral products for chronic therapy.

Patients requiring urgent relief from angina pectoris, a coronary circulatory problem, place tablets of nitroglycerin sublingually for rapid drug absorption from the buccal cavity. Thus, although systemic effects are generally obtained following oral and parenteral drug administration, other routes can be employed as the drug and the situation demand. Local effects are generally restricted to dosage forms applied directly, such as those applied to the skin, ear, eye and throat. Some drugs may be well absorbed by one route and not another, and must therefore be considered individually.

The age of the patient also plays a role in defining the types of dosage forms made available. Infants generally prefer liquid dosage forms, usually solutions and mixtures, given orally. Also, with a liquid preparation the amount of drug administered can be readily adjusted by dilution to give the required dose for the particular patient, taking weight, age and patient's condition into account. Children can have difficulty in swallowing solid dosage forms, and for this reason many oral preparations are prepared as pleasantly flavoured syrups or mixtures. Adults generally prefer solid dosage forms, primarily because of their convenience. However, alternative liquid preparations are usually available for those unable to take tablets and capsules.

Interest has grown recently in the design of formulations that deliver drugs to specific 'targets' in the body, for example the use of liposomes and nanoparticles, as well as providing drugs over longer periods of time at controlled rates. Alternative technologies for preparing particles with required properties – crystal engineering – provide new opportunities. Supercritical fluid processing using carbon dioxide as a solvent or antisolvent is one such method, allowing fine-tuning of crystal properties and particle design and fabrication. Undoubtedly these new technologies and others, as well as sophisticated formulations, will be required to deal with peptide and protein drugs, the advent of gene therapy and the need to deliver such labile macromolecules to specific cells in the body. Interest is also likely to be directed to individual patient requirements, such as age, weight and physiological and metabolic factors, features that can influence drug absorption and bioavailability.

SUMMARY

This chapter has demonstrated that the formulation of drugs into dosage forms requires the interpretation and application of a wide range of information from several study areas. Although the physical and chemical properties of drugs and additives need to be understood, the factors influencing drug absorption and the requirements of the disease to be treated also have to be taken into account when identifying potential delivery routes. The formulation and associated preparation of dosage forms demand the highest standards, with careful examination, analysis and evaluation of wide-ranging information by pharmaceutical scientists to achieve the objective of creating high-quality and efficacious dosage forms.

BIBLIOGRAPHY

Amidon, G.L., Lennernas, H., Shah, V.P., Crison, J.R. (1995). A theoretical basis for a biopharmaceutical drug classification: the correlation of in vitro drug product dissolution and bioavailability. *Pharmaceutical Research*, **12**, 413–420.

Martindale, W. (1999) *The Extra Pharmacopoeia*, Royal Pharmaceutical Society of Great Britain, London.

Modern Pharmaceutics, 3rd edn. (1999) (Eds Banker, G.S., Rhodes, C.T.) Marcel Dekker.

Pharmaceutical Dosage Forms and Drug Delivery Systems, 7th edn. (1999) (Eds Ansel, H.C., Allen, L.V., Popovitch, N.G.) Lippincott Williams & Wilkins, Philadelphia.

Physical Pharmacy: Physical Chemical Principles in the Pharmaceutical Sciences, 4th edn. (1993) Martin A.N. and Bustamanta, P. Lea and Febiger, Philadelphia.

Physicochemical Principles of Pharmacy, 3rd edn. (1998) Florence, A.T. and Attwood, D., Macmillan, Basingstoke.

Shekunov, B. Yu., York, P. (2000) Crystallization processes in pharmaceutical technology and drug delivery design. *Journal of Crystal Growth*, **211**, 122–136.

Solid State Chemistry of Drugs, 2nd edn. (1999) Byrn, S.R., Pfeiffer, R.R., Stowell, J.G., SSCI Inc., West Lafayette.

SCIENTIFIC PRINCIPLES OF DOSAGE FORM DESIGN

2

Dissolution and solubility

Michael Aulton

Solutions are encountered extremely frequently in pharmaceutical development, either as a dosage form in their own right or as a clinical trials material. Equally importantly, almost all drugs function in solution in the body. This book therefore starts with a description of the formation of solutions and a consideration of their properties.

This chapter discusses the principles underlying the formation of solutions from solute and solvent and the factors that affect the rate and extent of the dissolution process. It will discuss this process particularly in the context of a solid dissolving in a liquid, as this is the situation most likely to be encountered during the formation of a drug solution, either during manufacturing or during drug delivery.

Further properties of solutions are discussed in the subsequent chapters in Part One of this book. Because of the number of principles and properties that need to be considered, the contents of each of these chapters should only be regarded as introductions to the various topics. The student is therefore encouraged to refer to the bibliography at the end of each chapter in order to augment the present contents. The textbook written by Florence and Attwood (1998) is particularly recommended because of the large number of pharmaceutical examples that are used to aid an understanding of physicochemical principles.

DEFINITION OF TERMS

This chapter begins by clarifying a number of terms relevant to the formation and concentration of solutions

Solution, solubility

A *solution* may be defined as a mixture of two or more components that form a single phase which is homogeneous down to the molecular level. The component that determines the phase of the solution is termed the *solvent* and usually constitutes the largest proportion of the system. The other components are termed *solutes*, and these are dispersed as molecules or ions throughout the solvent, i.e. they are said to be *dissolved* in the solvent.

The transfer of molecules or ions from a solid state into solution is known as *dissolution*. The *extent* to which the dissolution proceeds under a given set of experimental conditions is referred to as the *solubility* of the solute in the solvent. Thus, the solubility of a substance is the *amount* of it that passes into solution when *equilibrium* is established between the solution and excess (undissolved) substance. The solution that is obtained under these conditions is said to be *saturated*.

Because the above definitions are general ones they may be applied to all types of solution involving any of the three states of matter (gas, liquid, solid) dissolved in any of the three states of matter. However, when the two components forming a solution are either both gases or both liquids it is more usual to talk in terms of *miscibility* rather than solubility.

One point to emphasize at this stage is that the rate of solution (dissolution) and amount which can be dissolved (solubility) are not the same and are not necessarily related, although in practice high drug solubility is usually associated with a high dissolution rate.

Expressions of concentration

Quantity per quantity

Concentrations are often expressed simply as the weight or volume of solute that is contained in a given weight or volume of the solution. The majority of solutions encountered in pharmaceutical practice consist of solids dissolved in liquids. Consequently, concentration is expressed most commonly by the weight of solute contained in a given volume of solution. Although the SI unit is kg m^{-3} the terms that are used in practice are based on more convenient or appropriate weights and volumes. For example, in the case of a solution with a concentration of 1 kg m^{-3} the strength may be denoted by any one of the following concentration terms, depending on the circumstances:

$$1 \text{ g L}^{-1}, 0.1 \text{ g per } 100 \text{ mL}, 1 \text{ mg mL}^{-1},$$
$$5 \text{ mg in } 5 \text{ mL, or } 1 \text{ } \mu g \text{ } \mu L^{-1}.$$

Percentage

Pharmaceutical scientists have a preference for quoting concentrations in percentages. The concentration of a solution of a solid in a liquid is given by:

$$\text{concentration in \% w / v} = \frac{\text{weight of solute}}{\text{volume of solution}} \times 100$$

Equivalent percentages based on weight and volume ratios (% v/w,% v/v and % w/w expressions) can also be used for solutions of liquids in liquids and solutions of gases in liquids.

It should be realized that if concentration is expressed in terms of weight of solute in a given volume of solution, then changes in volume caused by temperature fluctuations will alter the concentration.

Parts

Pharmacopoeias express some concentrations in terms of the number of 'parts' of solute dissolved in a stated number of 'parts' of solution. The use of this method to describe the strength of a solution of a solid in a liquid implies that a given number of parts by volume (mL) of solution contain a certain number of parts by weight (g) of solid. In the case of solutions of liquids in liquids, parts by volume of solute in parts by volume of solution are intended, whereas with solutions of gases in liquids parts by weight of gas in parts by weight of solution are implied.

Molarity

This is the number of moles of solute contained in 1 dm^3 (or, more commonly in pharmaceutical science, 1 litre) of solution. Thus, solutions of equal molarity contain the same number of solute molecules in a given volume of solution. The unit of molarity is mol L^{-1} (equivalent to 10^3 mol m^{-3} if converted to the strict SI unit).

Molality

This is the number of moles of solute divided by the mass of the solvent, i.e. its SI unit is mol kg^{-1}. Although it is less likely to be encountered in pharmaceutical science than the other terms it does offer a more precise description of concentration because it is unaffected by temperature.

Mole fraction

This is often used in theoretical considerations and is defined as the number of moles of solute divided by the total number of moles of solute and solvent, i.e.:

$$\text{mole fraction of solute } \left(x_1\right) = \frac{n_1}{n_1 + n_2} \quad (2.1)$$

where n_1 and n_2 are the numbers of moles of solute and solvent, respectively.

Milliequivalents and normal solutions

The concentrations of solutes in body fluids and in solutions used as replacements for those fluids are usually expressed in terms of the number of milli-moles (1 millimole = one thousandth of a mole) in a litre of solution. In the case of electrolytes, however, these concentrations may still be expressed in terms of milliequivalents per litre. A milliequivalent (mEq) of an ion is, in fact, one thousandth of the gram equivalent of the ion, which is in turn the ionic weight expressed in grams divided by the valency of the ion. Alternatively,

$$1 \text{ mEq} = \frac{\text{ionic weight in mg}}{\text{valency}}$$

A knowledge of the concept of chemical equivalents is also required in order to understand the use of 'normality' as a means of expressing the concentration of solutions, because a normal solution, i.e. concentration = 1 N, is one that contains the equivalent weight of the solute, expressed in grams, in 1 litre of solution. It was thought that this term would disappear on the introduction of SI units, but it is still encountered in some volumetric assay procedures.

THE PROCESS OF DISSOLUTION

States of matter

The kinetic theory of matter indicates that in condensed phases the thermal motions of molecules are reduced sufficiently so that intermolecular forces of attraction result in the formation of coherent masses of molecules, unlike the situation in gaseous phases, where the molecules move independently within the confines of the container. In solid condensed phases the thermal motion of molecules (or ions) is virtually restricted to vibrations about mean positions and the components tend to form three-dimensional arrangements or crystal lattices (see Chapter 9), in which the intercomponent forces are best satisfied and the potential energy of the system is minimized. In liquid condensed systems the thermal motions of molecules are greater than those in solids but less than those in gases. The structure of liquids is therefore intermediate between that of solids and that of gases. Thus, although the molecules can move within the confines of the liquid phase boundaries small groups of them tend to form regular arrangements in a transient manner. In addition, liquids are thought to contain a small amount of so-called 'free volume' in the form of 'holes' which, at a given instant, are not occupied by the solvent molecules themselves (discussed further in Chapter 3).

When a substance dissolves in a liquid the increase in volume of the latter is less than would be expected.

The process of dissolution may therefore be considered to involve the relocation of a solute molecule from an environment where it is surrounded by other identical molecules, with which it forms intermolecular attractions, into a cavity in a liquid, where it is surrounded by non-identical molecules, with which it may interact to different degrees.

Energy changes

In order for this process to occur spontaneously at a constant pressure the accompanying change in free energy, or Gibbs free energy (ΔG), must be negative. The free energy (G) is a measure of the energy available to the system to perform work. Its value decreases during a spontaneously occurring process until an equilibrium position is reached when no more energy can be made available, i.e. $\Delta G = 0$ at equilibrium.

This change in free energy is defined by the generally applicable thermodynamic equation:

$$\Delta G = \Delta H - T\Delta S \qquad (2.2)$$

where ΔH, which is known as the change in the enthalpy of the system, is the amount of heat absorbed or evolved as the system changes its thermodynamic state, i.e. in this case when dissolution occurs T is the thermodynamic temperature and ΔS is the change in the so-called entropy, which is a measure of the degree of disorder or randomness in the system.

The entropy change (ΔS) is usually positive for any process, such as dissolution, that involves mixing of two or more components. In an ideal solution there is, by definition, no net change in the intermolecular forces experienced by either solute or solvent when dissolution occurs. In such circumstances $\Delta H = 0$. Thus, the free energy change ΔG during the formation of an ideal solution is dictated solely by the term $T\Delta S$.

In most real systems dissolution is accompanied by a change in the intermolecular forces experienced by the solute and the solvent before and after the event. A change in enthalpy will therefore accompany dissolution in such systems. Equation 2.2 indicates that the likelihood of dissolution will depend on the sign of ΔH and, if this sign is positive, on the value of ΔH relative to that of $T\Delta S$. In other words, it follows from Eqn 2.2 that as $T\Delta S$ is usually positive then dissolution will occur if ΔH is either negative, zero or very slightly positive (i.e. it must be less than the value of $T\Delta S$).

The overall change in enthalpy of dissolution ΔH can be regarded as being made up of the change resulting from the removal of a solute molecule from its original environment plus that resulting from its new location in the solvent. For example, in the case of a crystalline solid dissolving in a liquid these contributions can be described by Eqn 2.3:

$$\Delta H = \Delta H_{cl} + \Delta H_{solv} \qquad (2.3)$$

where the change in crystal lattice enthalpy (ΔH_{cl}) is the heat absorbed when the molecules (or ions) of the crystalline solute are separated by an infinite distance against the effects of their intermolecular attractive forces. The enthalpy of solvation (ΔH_{solv}) is the heat absorbed when the solute molecules are immersed in the solvent.

ΔH_{cl} is always positive and ΔH_{solv} is most commonly negative. Thus, in most cases $\Delta H_{cl} > \Delta H_{solv}$, so that ΔH is also positive. In these cases heat is absorbed when dissolution occurs and the process is usually defined as an endothermic one. In some systems, where marked affinity between solute and solvent occurs, the negative ΔH_{solv} is so great that it exceeds the positive ΔH_{cl}. The overall enthalpy change then becomes negative, so that heat is evolved and the process is an exothermic one.

DISSOLUTION RATES OF SOLIDS IN LIQUIDS

Dissolution mechanisms

The dissolution of a solid in a liquid may be regarded as being composed of two consecutive stages.

1. First is an interfacial reaction that results in the liberation of solute molecules from the solid phase. This involves a phase change, so that molecules of solid become molecules of solute in the solvent in which the crystal is dissolving. The solution in contact with the solid will be saturated (because it is in direct contact with undissolved solid). Its concentration will be C_S, a saturated solution.
2. After this, the solute molecules must migrate through the boundary layers surrounding the crystal to the bulk of the solution, at which time its concentration will be C. This step involves the transport of these molecules away from the solid–liquid interface into the bulk of the liquid phase under the influence of diffusion or convection. Boundary layers are static or slow-moving layers of liquid that surround all wetted solid surfaces (see Chapter 4 for further details).

Mass transfer takes place more slowly through these static or slow-moving layers, which inhibit the movement of solute molecules from the surface of the solid to the bulk of the solution. The concentration of the solution in the boundary layers changes therefore from being saturated (C_S) at the crystal surface to being equal to that of the bulk of the solution (C) at its outermost limit.

These stages are illustrated in Figure 2.1.

Like any reaction that involves consecutive stages, the overall rate of dissolution will depend on whichever of these steps is the slowest (the rate-determining or rate-limiting step). In dissolution the interfacial step ((1) above) is virtually instantaneous and so the rate of dissolution will be determined by the rate of the slower step ((2) above), of diffusion of dissolved solute across the static boundary layer of liquid that exists at a solid–liquid interface.

The rate of diffusion will obey Fick's law of diffusion, i.e. the rate of change in concentration of dissolved material with time is directly proportional to the concentration difference between the two sides of the diffusion layer, i.e.,

$$\frac{dC}{dt} \propto \Delta C \qquad (2.4)$$

or

$$\frac{dC}{dt} = k\Delta C \qquad (2.5)$$

where the constant k is the rate constant (s^{-1}).

In the present context ΔC is the difference in concentration of solution at the solid surface (C_1) and the bulk of the solution (C_2). At equilibrium, the solution in contact with the solid (C_1) will be saturated (concentration = C_S), as discussed above.

If the concentration of the bulk (C_2) is greater than this, the solution is referred to as supersaturated and the movement of solid molecules will be in the direction of bulk to surface (as during crystallization), and if C_2 is less than saturated the molecules will move from the solid to the bulk (as during dissolution).

An equation known as the Noyes–Whitney equation was developed to define the dissolution from a single spherical particle. The rate of mass transfer of solute molecules or ions through a static diffusion layer (dm/dt) is directly proportional to the area available for molecular or ionic migration (A), the concentration difference (ΔC) across the boundary layer, and is inversely proportional to the thickness of the boundary layer (h). This relationship is shown in Eqn 2.6, or in a modified form in Eqn 2.7.

$$\frac{dm}{dt} = \frac{k_1 A \Delta C}{h} \qquad (2.6)$$

$$\frac{dm}{dt} = \frac{k_1 A (C_S - C)}{h} \qquad (2.7)$$

where the constant k_1 is known as the **diffusion coefficient**, D, and has the units of m^2/s.

If the solute is removed from the dissolution medium by some process at a faster rate than it passes into solution, then the term ($C_S - C$) in Eqn 2.7 may be approximated to C_S. Alternatively, if the volume of the dissolution medium is so large that C is not allowed to exceed 10% of the value of C_S, then the same approximation may be made in particular. In either of these circumstances dissolution is said to occur under 'sink' conditions, and Eqn 2.7 may be simplified to

$$\frac{dm}{dt} = \frac{DAC_S}{h} \qquad (2.8)$$

It should be realised that such 'sink' conditions may arise in vivo when a drug is absorbed from its solution in the gastrointestinal fluids at a faster rate than it dissolves in those fluids from a solid dosage form such as a tablet.

If solute is allowed to accumulate in the dissolution medium to such an extent that the above approximation is no longer valid, i.e. when $C > C_S/10$, then 'non-sink' conditions are said to be in operation. When $C = C_S$ it is obvious from Eqn 2.7 that the overall dissolution rate will be zero, as the dissolution medium is saturated with solute.

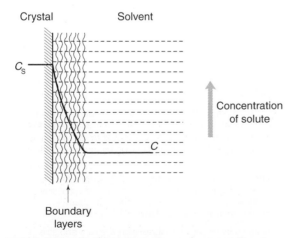

Fig. 2.1 Diagram of boundary layers and concentration change surrounding a dissolving particle.

Summary of factors affecting dissolution rates

These factors may be derived from a consideration of the terms that appear in the Noyes–Whitney equation (Eqn 2.7) and a knowledge of the factors that in turn affect these terms. Most of the effects of these factors are included in the summary given in Table 2.1. It should be borne in mind that pharmacists are often concerned with the rate of dissolution of a drug from a formulated product such as a tablet or a capsule, as well as with the dissolution rates of pure solids. Later chapters in this book should be consulted for information on the influence of formulation factors on the rates of release of drugs into solution from various dosage forms.

Intrinsic dissolution rate

Because the rate of dissolution is dependent on so many factors, it is advantageous to have a measure of the rate of dissolution which is independent of rate of agitation, area of solute available etc. In the latter case this will change greatly in a conventional tablet formulation, as the tablet breaks up into granules and then into primary powder particles as it comes into contact with water.

Table 2.1   Factors affecting in vitro dissolution rates of solids in liquids

Term in Noyes–Whitney equation	Affected by	Comments
A, surface area of undissolved solid	Size of solid particles	$A \propto 1/$particle size. Particle size will change during dissolution process, because large particles will become smaller and small particles will eventually disappear. Compacted masses of solid may also disintegrate into smaller particles
	Dispersibility of powdered solid in dissolution medium	If particles tend to form coherent masses in the dissolution medium then the surface area available for dissolution is reduced. This effect may be overcome by the addition of a wetting agent
	Porosity of solid particles	Pores must be large enough to allow access of dissolution medium and outward diffusion of dissolved solute molecules
C_S solubility of solid in dissolution medium.	Temperature	Dissolution may be an exothermic or an endothermic process
	Nature of dissolution medium	See previous comments on solubility parameters, cosolvents and pH.
	Molecular structure of solute	See previous comments on sodium salts of weak acids and esterification
	Crystalline form of solid	See previous comments on polymorphism and solvation
	Presence of other compounds	See previous comments on common ion effect, complex formation and solubilizing agents
C, concentration of solute in solution at time t	Volume of dissolution medium	If volume is small C will approach C_S if volume is large C may be negligible with respect to C_S i.e. apparent 'sink' conditions will operate
	Any process that removes dissolved solute from the dissolution medium	For example, adsorption on to an insoluble adsorbent, partition into a second liquid that is immiscible with the dissolution medium, removal of solute by dialysis or by continuous replacement of solution by fresh dissolution medium
k, dissolution rate constant	Thickness of boundary layer	Affected by degree of agitation, which depends, in turn, on speed of stirring or shaking, shape, size and position of stirrer, volume of dissolution medium, shape and size of container, viscosity of dissolution medium
	Diffusion coefficient of solute in the dissolution medium	Affected by viscosity of dissolution medium and size of diffusing molecules.

This is known as the intrinsic dissolution rate (IDR), which is the rate of mass transfer per area of dissolving surface and typically has the units of mg cm^{-2} min^{-1}. IDR should be independent of boundary layer thickness and volume of solvent (if sink conditions are assumed). Thus:

$$IDR = k_1 C_S \qquad (2.9)$$

Thus IDR measures the intrinsic properties of the drug only as a function of the dissolution medium, e.g. its pH, ionic strength, counter ions etc). Techniques for measuring IDR are discussed briefly below and in more detail in Chapter 8.

Measurement of dissolution rates

Many methods have been described in the literature, particularly in relation to the determination of the rate of release of drugs into solution from tablet and capsule formulations, because such release may have an important effect on the therapeutic efficiency of these dosage forms (see Chapters 17, 27, 29 and 30). Attempts have been made to classify the methods for determining dissolution rates. These classifications are based mainly on whether or not the mixing processes that take place in the various methods occur by natural convection arising from density gradients produced in the dissolution medium, or by forced convection brought about by stirring or shaking the system. The following brief descriptions are given as examples of the more commonly used methods that are illustrated in Figure 2.2.

Beaker method

The methodology of Levy and Hayes forms the basis of this technique. In their initial work they used a $400 cm^3$ beaker containing $250 dm^3$ of dissolution medium, which was agitated by means of a three-bladed polyethylene stirrer with a diameter of 50 mm. The stirrer was immersed to a depth of 27 mm into the dissolution medium and rotated at 60 rpm. Tablets were dropped into the beaker and samples of the liquid were removed at known times, filtered and assayed.

Flask–stirrer method

This is similar to the previous method except that a round-bottomed flask is used instead of a beaker. The use of a round-bottomed container helps to avoid the problems that may arise from the formation of 'mounds' of particles in different positions on the flat bottom of a beaker.

Rotating basket method

This method is described in most pharmacopoeias for the determination of the dissolution rates of drugs from tablets and capsules. Details of the apparatus and methods of operation are given in these official compendia. Basically these methods involve placing the tablet or capsule inside a stainless steel wire basket, which is rotated at a fixed speed while immersed in the dissolution medium, which is contained in a wide-mouthed cylindrical vessel, the bottom of which is either flat or spherical. Samples of the dissolution medium are removed at specified times, filtered and assayed.

Paddle method

This is another official method. The dissolution vessel described in the rotating basket method, i.e. the cylindrical vessel with the spherical bottom, is also used in this method. Agitation is provided by a rotating paddle and the dosage form is allowed to sink to the bottom of the dissolution vessel before agitation is commenced.

Rotating and static disc methods

In these methods the compound that is to be assessed for rate of dissolution is compressed into a non-disintegrating disc which is mounted in a holder so that only one face of the disc is exposed. The holder and disc are immersed in the dissolution medium and either held in a fixed position (static disc method) or rotated at a given speed (rotating disc method). Samples of the dissolution medium are removed after known times, filtered and assayed.

In both methods it is assumed that the surface area from which dissolution can occur remains constant. Under these conditions the amount of substance dissolved per unit time and unit surface area can be determined. This is the *intrinsic dissolution rate* and should be distinguished from the measurement obtained from the previously described methods. In these latter methods the surface area of the drug that is available for dissolution changes considerably during the course of the determination because the dosage form usually disintegrates into many smaller particles, and the size of these particles then decreases as dissolution proceeds. As these changes are not usually monitored the dissolution rate is measured in terms of the total amount of drug dissolved per unit time.

It should be appreciated from a consideration of the comments made in Table 2.1 that not only will different dissolution rate methods yield different

(a) Beaker method

(b) Flask-stirrer method

(c) Rotating basket method

(d) Paddle method

(e) Rotating disc method
Static disc method

Fig. 2.2   Methods of measuring dissolution rates.

results, but also changes in the experimental variables in a given method are likely to lead to changes in the results. This latter point is particularly important, as dissolution rate tests are usually performed in a comparative manner to determine, for example, the difference between two polymorphic forms of the same compound, or between the rates of release of a drug from two formulations. Thus, standardization of the experimental methodology is essential if such comparisons are to be meaningful.

Finally, it should also be realized that although the majority of dissolution testing is concerned with pure drugs or with conventional tablet or capsule formulations, knowledge of the rates of drug release from other types of dosage form is also important. Reference should be made therefore to later chapters in this book for information on the dissolution methods applied to these other dosage forms.

SOLUBILITY

The solution produced when equilibrium is established between undissolved and dissolved solute in a dissolution process is termed a **saturated solution**. The amount of substance that passes into solution in order to establish the equilibrium at constant temperature and pressure and so produce a saturated solution is known as the **solubility** of the substance. It is possible to obtain supersaturated solutions but these are unstable and the excess solute tends to precipitate readily.

Methods of expressing solubility

Solubilities may be expressed by means of any of the variety of concentration terms that are defined at the beginning of this chapter. They are expressed most commonly, however, in terms of the maximum mass or volume of solute that will dissolve in a given mass or volume of solvent at a particular temperature.

Pharmacopoeias give information on the approximate solubilities of official substances in terms of the number of parts by volume of solvent required to dissolve one part by weight of a solid, or one part by volume of a liquid. Unless otherwise specified, these solubilities apply at a temperature of 20°C. They also use the expression 'parts' in defining the approximate solubilities that correspond to descriptive terms such as 'freely soluble' and 'sparingly soluble'.

Prediction of solubility

Probably the most sought-after information about solutions in formulation problems is 'what is the best?' or 'what is the worst?' solvent for a given solute. Theoretical prediction of precise solubilities is an involved and occasionally unsuccessful operation, but from a knowledge of the structure and properties of solute and solvent an educated guess can be made. This is best expressed in subjective terms, such as 'very soluble' or 'sparingly soluble'. Often (particularly in pre- or early formulation) this is all the information that the formulator requires. The

Table 2.2	Descriptive solubilities
Description	Approximate weight of solvent (g) necessary to dissolve 1 g of solute
Very soluble	< 1
Freely soluble	Between 1 and 10
Soluble	Between 10 and 30
Sparingly soluble	Between 30 and 100
Slightly soluble	Between 100 and 1000
Very slightly soluble	Between 1000 and 10 000
Practically insoluble	> 10 000

interrelationships between such terms and approximate solubilities are shown in Table 2.2.

Speculation on what is likely to be a good solvent is usually based on the 'like dissolves like' principle, that is, a solute dissolves best in a solvent with similar chemical properties. The concept traditionally follows two rules:

1. Polar solutes dissolve in polar solvents.
2. Non-polar solutes dissolve in non-polar solvents.

In the context of solubility, a **polar molecule** has a dipole moment. Chemical groups that confer polarity to their parent molecules are known as **polar groups**.

To rationalize the above rules, consider the forces of attraction between solute and solvent molecules. If the solvent is A and the solute B and the forces of attraction are represented by A–A, B–B and A–B, one of three conditions will arise:

1. If A–A >> A–B, i.e. the affinity of a solvent molecule for its own kind is markedly greater than its affinity for a solute molecule, the solvent molecules will be attracted to each other and form aggregations from which the solute is excluded. As an example, benzene is almost completely insoluble in water. Attraction between water molecules is very strong, so that water exists as aggregates, which have a similar form to ice, floating in a matrix of free molecules. It may be visualized as 'icebergs' floating in a 'sea' of free water molecules. Molecules are continually moving from sea to icebergs and from icebergs to sea. The attraction between benzene molecules arises from weak van der Waals forces, so that although very little energy is required to disperse benzene molecules, discrete benzene molecules are unable to penetrate the closely bound water aggregates.

2. If B–B >> A–A, the solvent will not be able to break the binding forces between solute molecules and disperse them. This situation would apply if you tried to dissolve sodium chloride in benzene. The sodium chloride crystal is held together by strong electrovalent forces which cannot be broken by benzene. A conducting solvent, such as water, would be required to overcome the attraction between solute molecules.
3. If A–B > A–A or B–B, or the three forces are of the same order, the solute will disperse and form a solution.

The above is a simplified overview of the situation. The rest of this chapter will attempt to explain the basic physicochemical properties of solutions that lead to such observations.

Physicochemical prediction of solubility

Similar types of intermolecular force may contribute to solute–solvent, solute–solute and solvent–solvent interactions. The attractive forces exerted between polar molecules are much stronger, however, than those that exist between polar and non-polar molecules, or between non-polar molecules themselves. Consequently, a polar solute will dissolve to a greater extent in a polar solvent, where the strength of the solute–solvent interaction will be comparable to that between solute molecules, than in a non-polar solvent, where the solute–solvent interaction will be relatively weak. In addition, the forces of attraction between the molecules of a polar solvent will be too great to facilitate the separation of these molecules by the insertion of a non-polar solute between them, because the solute–solvent forces will again be relatively weak. Thus, solvents for non-polar solutes tend to be restricted to non-polar liquids.

The above considerations are often expressed very generally as 'like dissolves like', i.e. a polar substance will dissolve in a polar solvent and a non-polar substance will dissolve in a non-polar solvent. Such a generalization should be treated with caution, because the intermolecular forces involved in the process of dissolution are influenced by factors that are not obvious from a consideration of the overall polarity of a molecule. For example, the possibility of intermolecular hydrogen-bond formation between solute and solvent may be more significant than polarity.

Solubility parameter Attempts have been made to define a parameter that indicates the ability of a liquid to act as a solvent. The most satisfactory approach is based on the concept that the solvent power of a liquid is influenced by its intermolecular cohesive forces and that the strength of these forces can be expressed in terms of a solubility parameter. The initially introduced parameters, which are concerned with the behaviour of non-polar, non-interacting liquids, are referred to as Hildebrand solubility parameters. Although these provide good quantitative predictions of the behaviour of a small number of hydrocarbons, they only provide a broad qualitative description of the behaviours of most liquids because of the influence of factors such as hydrogen-bond formation and ionization. The concept has been extended, however, by the introduction of partial solubility parameters, e.g. Hansen parameters and interaction parameters, that have improved the quantitative treatment of systems in which polar effects and interactions occur.

Solubility parameters, in conjunction with the electrostatic properties of liquids, e.g. dielectric constant and dipole moment, have often been linked by empirical or semiempirical relationships either to these parameters or to solvent properties. Studies on solubility parameters are sometimes reported in the pharmaceutical literature. The use of dielectric constants as indicators of solvent power has also received attention, but deviations from the behaviour predicted by such methods may occur.

Mixtures of liquids are often used as solvents. If the two liquids have similar chemical structures, e.g. benzene and toluene, then neither tends to associate in the presence of the other, and the solvent properties of a 50:50 mixture would be a mean of those of each pure liquid. If the liquids have dissimilar structures, e.g. water and propanol, then the molecules of one of them tend to associate with each other and so form regions of high concentration within the mixture. The solvent properties of this type of system are not so simply related to its composition as in the previous case.

Solubility of solids in liquids

Solutions of solids in liquids are the most common type encountered in pharmaceutical practice. The pharmacist should therefore be aware of the general method of determining the solubility of a solid in a liquid and the various precautions that should be taken during such determinations.

Determination of the solubility of a solid in a liquid

The following points should be observed in all solubility determinations:

1. The solvent and the solute must be pure.

2. A saturated solution must be obtained before any solution is removed for analysis.
3. The method of separating a sample of saturated solution from undissolved solute must be satisfactory.
4. The method of analysing the solution must be reliable.
5. Temperature must be adequately controlled.

A saturated solution is obtained either by stirring excess powdered solute with solvent for several hours at the required temperature until equilibrium has been attained, or by warming the solvent with an excess of the solute and allowing the mixture to cool to the required temperature. It is essential that some undissolved solid should be present at the completion of this stage in order to ensure that the solution is saturated.

A sample of the saturated solution is obtained for analysis by separating it from the undissolved solid. Filtration is usually used, but precautions should be taken to ensure that:

1. it is carried out at the temperature of the solubility determination, in order to prevent any change in the equilibrium between dissolved and undissolved solute; and
2. loss of a volatile component does not occur.

The filtration process has been simplified by the introduction of membrane filters that can be used in conjunction with conventional syringes fitted with suitable inline adapters.

The amount of solute contained in the sample of saturated solution may be determined by a variety of methods, e.g. gravimetric or volumetric analysis, electrical conductivity measurements, ultraviolet (UV) spectrophotometry and chromatographic methods. The selection of an appropriate method is affected by the natures of the solute and the solvent and by the concentration of the solution.

Factors affecting the solubility of solids in liquids

Knowledge of these factors, which are discussed below together with their practical applications, is an important aspect of the pharmacist's expertise. Additional information, which shows how some of these factors may be used to improve the solubilities and bioavailabilities of drugs, is given in Chapters 21 and 17, respectively.

Temperature Earlier discussion centred on Eqn 2.2 shows that the free energy change (ΔG) that accompanies dissolution is dependent on the value and sign of the change in enthalpy (ΔH). The addi-

tional comments that referred to Eqn 2.3 indicate that when ΔH is positive the dissolution process is usually an endothermic one, i.e. heat is normally absorbed when dissolution occurs. If this type of system is heated it will tend to react in a way that will nullify the constraint imposed upon it, e.g. the rise in temperature. This tendency is an example of Le Chatelier's principle. Thus, a rise in temperature will lead to an increase in the solubility of a solid with a positive heat of solution. Conversely, in the case of the less commonly occurring systems that exhibit exothermic dissolution, an increase in temperature will give rise to a decrease in solubility.

Plots of solubility versus temperature, which are referred to as *solubility curves*, are often used to describe the effect of temperature on a given system. Some examples are shown in Figure 2.3. Most of the curves are continuous; however, abrupt changes in slope may be observed with some systems if a change in the nature of the dissolving solid occurs at a specific transition temperature. For example, sodium sulphate exist as the decahydrate $Na_2SO_4,10H_2O$ up to 32.5°C, and its dissolution in water is an endothermic process. Its solubility therefore increases with rise in temperature until 32.5°C is reached. Above this temperature the solid is converted into the anhydrous form Na_2SO_4, and the dissolution of this compound is an exothermic process. The solubility therefore exhibits a change from a positive to a negative slope as the temperature exceeds the transition value.

Fig. 2.3 Solubility curves for various substances in water

Molecular structure of solute It should be appreciated from the previous comments on the prediction of solubility that the natures of the solute and the solvent will be of paramount importance in determining the solubility of a solid in a liquid. It should also be realized that even a small change in the molecular structure of a compound can have a marked effect on its solubility in a given liquid. For example, the introduction of a hydrophilic hydroxyl group can produce a large improvement in water solubility, as evidenced by the more than 100-fold difference in the solubilities of phenol and benzene.

In addition, the conversion of a weak acid to its sodium salt leads to a much greater degree of ionic dissociation of the compound when it dissolves in water. The overall interaction between solute and solvent is markedly increased and the solubility consequently rises. A specific example of this effect is provided by a comparison of the aqueous solubilities of salicylic acid and its sodium salt, which are 1:550 and 1:1, respectively.

The reduction in aqueous solubility of a parent drug by its esterification may also be cited as an example of the effects of changes in the chemical structure of the solute. Such a reduction in solubility may provide a suitable method for:

1. masking the taste of a parent drug, e.g. chloramphenicol palmitate is used in paediatric suspensions rather than the more soluble and very bitter chloramphenicol base;
2. protecting the parent drug from excessive degradation in the gut, e.g. erythromycin propionate is less soluble and consequently less readily degraded than erythromycin;
3. increasing the ease of absorption of drugs from the gastrointestinal tract, e.g. erythromycin propionate is also more readily absorbed than erythromycin.

Nature of solvent: cosolvents The importance of the nature of the solvent has already been discussed in terms of the statement 'like dissolves like', and in relation to solubility parameters. In addition, the point has been made that mixtures of solvents may be employed. Such mixtures are often used in pharmaceutical practice to obtain aqueous-based systems that contain solutes in excess of their solubilities in pure water. This is achieved by using cosolvents such as ethanol or propylene glycol, which are miscible with water and which act as better solvents for the solute in question. For example, the aqueous solubility of metronidazole is about 100 mg in 10 mL. Chien (1984) has shown, however, that the solubility of this drug can be increased exponentially by the incorporation of one or more water-miscible cosolvents, so that a solution containing 500 mg in 10 mL and suitable for parenteral administration in the treatment of anaerobic infection, can be obtained.

Crystal characteristics: polymorphism and solvation The value of the term ΔH_{cl} in Eqn 2.3 is determined by the strength of the interactions between adjacent molecules (or ions) in a crystal lattice. These interactions will depend on the relative positions and orientations of the molecules in the crystal. When the conditions under which crystallization is allowed to occur are varied, some substances produce crystals in which the constituent molecules are aligned in different ways with respect to one another in the lattice structure. These different crystalline forms of the same substance, which are known as ***polymorphs***, consequently possess different lattice energies, and this difference is reflected by changes in other properties; for example, the polymorphic form with the lowest free energy will be the most stable and possess the highest melting point. Other less stable (or metastable) forms will tend to transform into the most stable one at rates that depend on the energy differences between the metastable and the stable forms. Polymorphs are explained more fully in Chapter 9.

The effect of polymorphism on solubility is particularly important from a pharmaceutical point of view, because it provides a means of increasing the solubility of a crystalline material and hence its rate of dissolution by using a metastable polymorph.

Although the more soluble polymorphs are metastable and will convert to the stable form the rate of such conversion is often slow enough for the metastable form to be regarded as being sufficiently stable from a pharmaceutical point of view. The degree of conversion should obviously be monitored during storage of the drug product to ensure that its efficacy is not altered significantly. In addition, conversion to the less soluble and most stable polymorph may contribute to the growth of crystals in suspension formulations.

Many drugs exhibit polymorphism, e.g. steroids, barbiturates and sulphonamides. Examples of the importance of polymorphism with respect to the bioavailabilities of drugs and to the occurrence of crystal growth in suspensions are given in Chapters 17 and 23, respectively.

The absence of crystalline structure that is usually associated with a so-called ***amorphous*** powder (see Chapter 9) may also lead to an increase in the solubility of a drug compared to that of its crystalline form.

In addition to the effect of polymorphism the lattice structures of crystalline materials may be altered by the incorporation of molecules of the solvent from which crystallization occurred. The resultant solids are called **solvates**; the phenomenon is referred to correctly as **solvation** and sometimes incorrectly and confusingly as **pseudopolymorphism**. The alteration in crystal structure that accompanies solvation will affect ΔH_{cl} so that the solubilities of solvated and unsolvated crystals will differ.

If water is the solvating molecule, i.e. if a **hydrate** is formed, then the interaction between the substance and water that occurs in the crystal phase reduces the amount of energy liberated when the solid hydrate dissolves in water. Consequently, hydrated crystals tend to exhibit a lower aqueous solubility than their unhydrated forms. This decrease in solubility can lead to precipitation of drugs from solutions.

In contrast to the effect of hydrate formation, the aqueous solubilities of other, i.e. non-aqueous, solvates are often greater than those of the unsolvated forms. Examples of the effects of solvation and the attendant changes in solubilities of drugs on their bioavailabilities are given in Chapter 17.

Particle size of the solid The changes in interfacial free energy that accompany the dissolution of particles of varying sizes cause the solubility of a substance to increase with decreasing particle size, as indicated by Eqn 2.10:

$$\log \frac{S}{S_o} = \frac{2\gamma M}{2.303RT\rho r} \qquad (2.10)$$

where S is the solubility of small particles of radius r, S_o is the normal solubility (i.e. of a solid consisting of fairly large particles), γ is the interfacial energy, M is the molecular weight of the solid, ρ is the density of the bulk solid, R is the gas constant and T is the thermodynamic temperature.

This effect may be significant in the storage of pharmaceutical suspensions, as the smaller particles in such a suspension will be more soluble than the larger ones. As the small particles disappear, the overall solubility of the suspended drug will decrease and the larger particles will grow. The occurrence of crystal growth by this mechanism is of particular importance in the storage of suspensions intended for injection (Winfield and Richards, 1998).

The increase in solubility with decrease in particle size ceases when the particles have a very small radius, and any further decrease in size causes a decrease in solubility. It has been postulated that this change arises from the presence of an electrical charge on the particles and that the effect of this charge becomes more important as the size of the particles decreases.

pH If the pH of a solution of either a weakly acidic drug or a salt of such a drug is reduced then the proportion of unionized acid molecules in the solution increases. Precipitation may therefore occur because the solubility of the unionized species is less than that of the ionized form. Conversely, in the case of solutions of weakly basic drugs or their salts precipitation is favoured by an increase in pH. Such precipitation is an example of one type of chemical incompatibility that may be encountered in the formulation of liquid medicines.

This relationship between pH and the solubility of ionized solutes is extremely important with respect to the ionization of weakly acidic and basic drugs as they pass through the gastrointestinal tract and experience pH changes between about 1 and 8. This will affect the degree of ionization of the drug molecules, which in turn influences their solubility and their ability to be absorbed. This aspect is discussed in some detail, elsewhere in this book and the reader is referred to Chapters 3 and 17 in particular.

The relationship between pH and the solubility and pK_a value of an acidic drug is given by Eqn 2.11, which is a modification of the Henderson–Hasselbalch equation (Eqn 3.12):

$$pH = pK_a + \log \frac{S - S_u}{S_o} \qquad (2.11)$$

where S is the overall solubility of the drug and S_u is the solubility of its unionized form, i.e. $S = S_o +$ solubility of ionized form (S_I). If the pH of the solution is known then Eqn 2.11 may be used to calculate the solubility of an acidic drug at that pH. Alternatively, the equation allows determination of the minimum pH that must be maintained in order to prevent precipitation from a solution of known concentration.

In the case of basic drugs the corresponding relationship is given by Eqn 2.12:

$$pH = pK_a + \log \frac{S_u}{S - S_u} \qquad (2.12)$$

Common ion effect The equilibrium in a saturated solution of a sparingly soluble salt in contact with undissolved solid may be represented by:

$$AB \Leftrightarrow A^+ + B^-$$
$$\text{(solid)} \quad \text{(ions)} \qquad (2.13)$$

From the Law of Mass Action the equilibrium constant K for this reversible reaction is given by Eqn 2.14:

$$K = \frac{[A^+][B^-]}{[AB]} \qquad (2.14)$$

where the square brackets signify concentrations of the respective components. As the concentration of a solid may be regarded as being constant, then

$$K_S' = [A^+][B^-] \qquad (2.15)$$

where K_S' is a constant which is known as the **solubility product** of compound AB.

If each molecule of the salt contains more than one ion of each type, e.g. $A_x^+B_y^-$, then in the definition of the solubility product the concentration of each ion is expressed to the appropriate power, i.e.:

$$K_S' = [A^+]^x [B^-]^y$$

These equations for the solubility product are only applicable to solutions of sparingly soluble salts.

If K_S' is exceeded by the product of the concentration of the ions, i.e. $[A^+][B^-]$, then the equilibrium shown above, (Eqn 2.13) moves towards the left in order to restore the equilibrium, and solid AB is precipitated. The product $[A^+][B^-]$ will be increased by the addition of more A^+ ions produced by the dissociation of another compound, e.g. $AX \rightarrow A^+ + X^-$, where A^+ is the common ion. Solid AB will be precipitated and the solubility of this compound is therefore decreased. This is known as the **common ion effect**. The addition of common B^- ions would have the same effect.

The precipitating effect of common ions is, in fact, less than that predicted from Eqn 2.15. The reason for this is explained below.

Effect of indifferent electrolytes on the solubility product
The solubility of a sparingly soluble electrolyte may be increased by the addition of a second electrolyte that does not possess ions common to the first, i.e. a different electrolyte.

The definition of the solubility product of a sparingly soluble electrolyte in terms of the concentration of ions produced at equilibrium, as indicated by Eqn 2.15, is only an approximation from the more exact thermodynamic relationship expressed by Eqn 2.16:

$$K_S = a_A^+ a_B^- \qquad (2.16)$$

where K_S' is the solubility product of compound AB and a_A^+ and a_B^- are known as the activities of the respective ions. The activity of a particular ion may be regarded as its 'effective concentration'. In general this has a lower value than the actual concentration, because some ions produced by dissociation of the electrolyte are strongly associated with oppositely charged ions and do not contribute so effectively as completely unallocated ions to the properties of the system. At infinite dilution the wide separation of ions prevents any interionic association, and the molar concentration (c_{A+}) and activity (a_{A+}) of a given ion (A^+) are then equal, i.e.:

$$a_{A+} = c_A \text{ or } \frac{a_{A+}}{c_{A+}} = 1$$

As the concentration increases, the effects of interionic association are no longer negligible and the ratio of activity to molar concentration becomes less than unity i.e.:

$$a_{A+} = \frac{f_{A+}}{c_{A+}}$$

or

$$a_{A+} = c_{A+} \cdot f_{A+}$$

where f_{A+} is known as the activity coefficient of A^+. If concentrations and activity coefficients are used instead of activities in Eqn 2.16, then

$$K_S = (cA^+ \cdot cB^-)(fA^+ \cdot fB^-)$$

The product of the concentrations, i.e. $(c_{A+} \cdot c_{B-})$, will be a constant (K_S') as shown by Eqn 2.15, and $(f_{A+} \cdot f_{B-})$ may be equated to f_{A+B-}, where f_{A+B-} is the mean activity coefficient of the salt AB, i.e.

$$K_S = K_S' f_{A+B-} \qquad (2.17)$$

Because f_{A+B-} varies with the overall concentration of ions present in solution (the ionic strength), and as K_S is a constant, it follows that K_S' must also vary with the ionic strength of the solution in an inverse manner to the variation of f_{A+B-}. Thus, in a system containing a sparingly soluble electrolyte without a common ion, the ionic strength will have an appreciable value and the mean activity coefficient f_{A+B-} will be less than 1.

From Eqn 2.17 it will be seen that K_S' will therefore be greater than K_S. In fact, the concentration solubility product K_S' will become larger and larger as the ionic strength of the solution increases. The solubility of AB will therefore increase as the concentration of added electrolyte increases.

This argument also accounts for the fact that if no allowance is made for the variation in activity with ionic strength of the medium, the precipitating effect of common ions is less than that predicted from the Law of Mass Action.

Effect of non-electrolytes on the solubility of electrolytes
The solubility of electrolytes depends on the dissociation of dissolved molecules into ions. The ease of this dissociation is affected by the dielectric constant of the solvent, which is a measure of the polar nature of the solvent. Liquids with a high dielectric constant (e.g. water) are able to reduce the attractive forces

that operate between oppositely charged ions produced by dissociation of an electrolyte.

If a water-soluble non-electrolyte such as alcohol is added to an aqueous solution of a sparingly soluble electrolyte, the solubility of the latter is decreased because the alcohol lowers the dielectric constant of the solvent and ionic dissociation of the electrolyte becomes more difficult.

Effect of electrolytes on the solubility of non-electrolytes Non-electrolytes do not dissociate into ions in aqueous solution, and in dilute solution the dissolved species therefore consists of single molecules. Their solubility in water depends on the formation of weak intermolecular bonds (hydrogen bonds) between their molecules and those of water. The presence of a very soluble electrolyte (e.g. ammonium sulphate), the ions of which have a marked affinity for water, will reduce the solubility of a non-electrolyte by competing for the aqueous solvent and breaking the intermolecular bonds between the non-electrolyte and the water. This effect is important in the precipitation of proteins.

Complex formation The apparent solubility of a solute in a particular liquid may be increased or decreased by the addition of a third substance which forms an intermolecular complex with the solute. The solubility of the complex will determine the apparent change in the solubility of the original solute. Use is made of complex formation as an aid to solubility in the preparation of solution of mercuric iodide (HgI_2). The latter is not very soluble in water but is soluble in aqueous solutions of potassium iodide because of the formation of a water-soluble complex, $K_2(HgI_4)$.

Solubilizing agents These agents are capable of forming large aggregates or micelles in solution when their concentrations exceed certain values. In aqueous solution the centre of these aggregates resembles a separate organic phase and organic solutes may be taken up by the aggregates, thus producing an apparent increase in their solubilities in water. This phenomenon is known as **solubilization**. A similar phenomenon occurs in organic solvents containing dissolved solubilizing agents, because the centre of the aggregates in these systems constitutes a more polar region than the bulk of the organic solvent. If polar solutes are taken up into these regions their apparent solubilities in the organic solvents are increased.

Solubility of gases in liquids

The amount of gas that will dissolve in a liquid is determined by the natures of the two components and by temperature and pressure.

Provided that no reaction occurs between the gas and liquid then the effect of pressure is indicated by Henry's law, which states that at constant temperature the solubility of a gas in a liquid is directly proportional to the pressure of the gas above the liquid. The law may be expressed by Eqn 2.18:

$$w = kp \qquad (2.18)$$

where w is the mass of gas dissolved by unit volume of solvent at an equilibrium pressure p and k is a proportionality constant. Although Henry's law is most applicable at high temperatures and low pressures, when solubility is low it provides a satisfactory description of the behaviour of most systems at normal temperatures and reasonable pressures, unless solubility is very high or reaction occurs. Equation 2.18 also applies to the solubility of each gas in a solution of several gases in the same liquid, provided that p represents the partial pressure of a particular gas.

The solubility of most gases in liquids decreases as the temperature rises. This provides a means of removing dissolved gases. For example, water for injections free from either carbon dioxide or air may be prepared by boiling water with minimal exposure to air and preventing the access of air during cooling. The presence of electrolytes may also decrease the solubility of a gas in water by a 'salting out' process, which is caused by the marked attraction exerted between electrolyte and water.

Solubility of liquids in liquids

The components of an ideal solution are miscible in all proportions. Such complete miscibility is also observed in some real binary systems, e.g. ethanol and water, under normal conditions. However, if one of the components tends to self-associate because the attractions between its own molecules are greater than those between its molecules and those of the other component, i.e. if a positive deviation from Raoult's law occurs, the miscibility of the components may be reduced. The extent of the reduction depends on the strength of the self-association and, therefore, on the degree of deviation from Raoult's law. Thus, partial miscibility may be observed in some systems, whereas virtual immiscibility may be exhibited when the self-association is very strong and the positive deviation from Raoult's law is great.

In cases where partial miscibility occurs under normal conditions the degree of miscibility is usually dependent on the temperature. This dependency is indicated by the **phase rule**, introduced by J. Willard Gibbs, which is expressed quantitatively by Eqn 2.19:

$$F = C - P + 2 \qquad (2.19)$$

where P and C are the numbers of phases and components in the system, respectively, and F is the number of degrees of freedom, i.e. the number of variable conditions such as temperature, pressure and composition that must be stated in order to define completely the state of the system at equilibrium.

The overall effect of temperature variation on the degree of miscibility in these systems is usually described by means of phase diagrams, which are graphs of temperature versus composition at constant pressure. For convenience of discussion of their phase diagrams the partially miscible systems may be divided into the following types.

Systems showing an increase in miscibility with rise in temperature

A positive deviation from Raoult's law arises from a difference in the cohesive forces that exist between the molecules of each component in a liquid mixture. This difference becomes more marked as the temperature decreases, and the positive deviation may then result in a decrease in miscibility sufficient to cause the separation of the mixture into two phases. Each phase consists of a saturated solution of one component in the other liquid. Such mutually saturated solutions are known as *conjugate solutions*.

The equilibria that occur in mixtures of partially miscible liquids may be followed either by shaking the two liquids together at constant temperature and analysing samples from each phase after equilibrium has been attained, or by observing the temperature at which known proportions of the two liquids, contained in sealed glass ampoules, become miscible, as shown by the disappearance of turbidity.

Systems showing a decrease in miscibility with rise in temperature

A few mixtures, which probably involve compound formation, exhibit a lower critical solution temperature (CST), e.g. triethylamine plus water, paraldehyde plus water. The formation of a compound produces a negative deviation from Raoult's law, and miscibility therefore increases as the temperature falls, as shown in Figure 2.4.

The effect of temperature on miscibility is of use in the preparation of paraldehyde enemas, which usually consist of a solution of paraldehyde in normal saline. Cooling the mixture during prepara-

Fig. 2.4 Temperature–composition diagram for the triethylamine–water system (at 101 325 kPa, standard atmospheric pressure).

tion allows more rapid solution, and storage of the enema in a cool place is recommended.

Systems showing upper and lower critical solution temperatures

The decrease in miscibility with increase in temperature in systems having a lower CST is not indefinite. Above a certain temperature, positive deviations from Raoult's law become important and miscibility starts to increase again with further rises in temperature. This behaviour produces a closed-phase diagram, as shown in Figure 2.5, which represents the nicotine–water system.

Fig. 2.5 Temperature–composition diagram for the nicotine–water system (at 101 325 kPa; standard atmospheric pressure).

In some mixtures where an upper and lower CST are expected, these points are not actually observed, as a phase change by one of the components occurs before the relevant CST is reached. For example, the ether–water system would be expected to exhibit a lower CST, but water freezes before the temperature is reached.

The effects of added substances on critical solution temperatures

It has already been stated that a CST is an invariant point at constant pressure. These temperatures are very sensitive to impurities or added substances. In general, the effects of additives may be summarized by Table 2.3.

The increase in miscibility of two liquids caused by the addition of a third substance is referred to as blending.

The use of propylene glycol as a blending agent, which improves the miscibility of volatile oils and water, can be explained in terms of a ternary phase diagram. This is a triangular plot which indicates the effects of changes in the relative proportions of the three components at constant temperature and pressure, and it is a good example of the interpretation and use of such phase diagrams.

Distribution of solutes between immiscible liquids

Partition coefficients

If a substance which is soluble in both components of a mixture of immiscible liquids is dissolved in such a mixture, then, when equilibrium is attained at constant temperature, it is found that the solute is distributed between the two liquids in such a way that the ratio of the activities of the substance in each liquid is a constant. This is known as the Nernst distribution law, which can be expressed by Eqn 2.20:

$$\frac{a_A}{a_B} = \text{constant} \tag{2.20}$$

where a_A and a_B are the activities of the solute in solvents A and B, respectively. When the solutions are dilute, or when the solute behaves ideally, the activities may be replaced by concentrations (C_A and C_B):

$$\frac{C_A}{C_B} = K \tag{2.21}$$

where the constant K is known as the **distribution coefficient** or **partition coefficient**. In the case of sparingly soluble substances K is approximately equal to the ratio of the solubilities (S_A and S_B) of the solute in each liquid, i.e.:

$$\frac{S_A}{S_B} = K \tag{2.22}$$

In most other systems, however, deviation from ideal behaviour invalidates Eqn 2.22. For example, if the solute exists as monomers in solvent A and as dimers in solvent B, the distribution coefficient is given by Eqn 2.23, in which the square root of the concentration of the dimeric form is used:

$$K = \frac{C_A}{\sqrt{C_B}} \tag{2.23}$$

If the dissociation into ions occurs in the aqueous layer, B, of a mixture of immiscible liquids, then the degree of dissociation (α) should be taken into account, as indicated by Eqn 2.24:

$$K = \frac{C_A}{C_B(1-\alpha)}. \tag{2.24}$$

The solvents in which the concentrations of the solute are expressed should be indicated when partition coefficients are quoted. For example, a partition coefficient of 2 for a solute distributed between oil and water may also be expressed as a partition coefficient between water and oil of 0.5. This can be represented as $K^{oil}_{water} = 2$ and $K^{water}_{oil} = 0.5$. The abbreviation K^o_w is often used for the former.

Table 2.3 The effects of additives on critical solution temperature (CST)

Type of CST	Solubility of additive in each component	Effect on CST	Effect on miscibility
Upper	Approx. equally soluble in both components	Lowered	Increased
Upper	Readily soluble in one component but not in other	Raised	Decreased
Lower	Approx. equally soluble in both components	Raised	Increased
Lower	Readily soluble in one component but not in other	Lowered	Decreased

Solubility of solids in solids

If two solids are either melted together and then cooled or dissolved in a suitable solvent, which is then removed by evaporation, the solid that is redeposited from the melt or the solution will either be a one-phase solid solution or a two-phase eutectic mixture.

In a solid solution, as in other types of solution, the molecules of one component (the solute) are dispersed molecularly throughout the other component (the solvent). Complete miscibility of two solid components is only achieved if:

1. the molecular size of the solute is the same as that of the solvent, so that a molecule of the former can be substituted for one of the latter in its crystal lattice structure; or
2. the solute molecules are much smaller than the solvent molecules, so that the former can be accommodated in the spaces of the solvent lattice structure.

These two types of solvent mechanism are referred to as substitution and interstitial effects, respectively. As these criteria are only satisfied in relatively few systems, partial miscibility of solids is more commonly observed. Thus, dilute solutions of solids in solids may be encountered in systems of pharmaceutical interest, for example when the solvent is a polymeric material with large spaces between its intertwined molecules that can accommodate solute molecules.

Unlike a solution, a simple eutectic consists of an intimate mixture of the two microcrystalline components in a fixed composition. However, both solid solutions and eutectics provide a means of dispersing a relatively water-insoluble drug in a very fine form, i.e. as molecules or microcrystalline particles, respectively, throughout a water-soluble solid. When the latter carrier solid is dissolved away the molecules or small crystals of insoluble drug may dissolve more rapidly than a conventional powder because the contact area between drug and water is increased. The rate of dissolution and, consequently, the bioavailabilities of poorly soluble drugs may therefore be improved by the use of solid solutions or eutectics.

REFERENCES

Chien, Y.W. (1984) *J. Parenteral Sci. Tech.*, **38**, 32–36.

Noyes, A.A. and Whitney, W.R. (1897). *J. Am. Chem. Soc.*, **19**, 930.

Winfield, A.J. and Richards, R.M.E. (1998) *Pharmaceutical Practice*, 2nd edn., Churchill Livingstone, Edinburgh.

BIBLIOGRAPHY

Barton, A.F.M. (1983) *Handbook of Solubility Parameters and other Cohesion Parameters*. CRC Press Inc., Boca Raton, Florida.

Beerbower, A., Wu, P.L. and Martin, A. (1984), *J. Pharm. Sci.*, **73**, 179–188.

British Pharmacopoeia (latest edition), HMSO. London.

Florence, A.T. and Attwood, D. (1998) *Physicochemical Principles of Pharmacy*, 3rd edn, Macmillan, London.

Pharmaceutical Handbook, 3rd edn (1999) (Ed. A. Wade). Pharmaceutical Press, London.

Rowlinson, J.S. and Swinton, F.L. (1982) *Liquids and Liquid Mixtures*, 3rd edn, Butterworths, London.

United States Pharmacopeia and National Formulary (latest edition) United States Pharmacopeial Convention Inc., Rockville, MD.

3

Properties of solutions

Michael Aulton

INTRODUCTION

The main aim of this chapter is to provide information on certain principles that relate to the applications of solutions in pharmaceutical science. It deals mainly with the physicochemical properties of solutions that are important with respect to pharmaceutical systems. These aspects are covered in sufficient detail to introduce the pharmaceutical scientist to these properties. Much is published elsewhere in far greater detail and any reader requiring this additional information is referred to the bibliography at the end of the chapter.

TYPES OF SOLUTION

Solutions may be classified according to the physical states (i.e. gas, solid or liquid) of the solute(s) and the solvent. Although a variety of different types can exist, solutions of pharmaceutical interest virtually all possess liquid solvents. In addition, the solutes are predominantly solid substances. Consequently, most of the comments made in this chapter are made with solutions of solids in liquids in mind. However, appropriate comments on other types, e.g. gases in liquids, liquids in liquids and solids in solids, are also included.

Vapour pressures of solids, liquids and solutions

An understanding of many of the properties of solutions requires an appreciation of the concept of an ideal solution and its use as a reference system, to which the behaviours of real (non-ideal) solutions can be compared. This concept is itself based on a consideration of vapour pressure. The present section is therefore included as an introduction to the later discussions on ideal and non-ideal solutions.

The kinetic theory of matter indicates that the thermal motion of molecules of a substance in its gaseous state is more than adequate to overcome the attractive forces that exist between the molecules. Thus, the molecules will undergo a completely random movement within the confines of the container. The situation is reversed, however, when the temperature is lowered sufficiently so that a condensed phase is formed. Thus, the thermal motions of the molecules are now insufficient to overcome completely the intermolecular attractive forces and some degree of order in the relative arrangement of molecules occurs. If the intermolecular forces are so strong that a high degree of order, which is hardly influenced by thermal motions, is brought about then the substance is usually in the solid state.

In the liquid condensed state the relative influences of thermal motion and intermolecular attractive forces are intermediate between those in the gaseous and the solid states. Thus, the effects of interactions between the permanent and induced dipoles, i.e. the so-called van der Waals forces of attraction, lead to some degree of coherence between the molecules of liquids. Consequently, unlike gases, liquids occupy a definite volume with a surface, and although there is evidence of structure within liquids such structure is much less apparent than in solids.

Although solids and liquids are condensed systems with cohering molecules, some of the surface molecules in these systems will occasionally acquire sufficient energy to overcome the attractive forces exerted by adjacent molecules. They can therefore escape from the surface to form a vapour phase. If temperature is maintained constant, equilibrium will eventually be established between the vapour and the condensed phases, and the pressure exerted by the vapour at equilibrium is referred to as the *vapour pressure* of the substance.

All condensed systems have the inherent ability to give rise to a vapour pressure. However, the vapour pressures exerted by solids are usually much lower than those exerted by liquids, because the intermolecular forces in solids are stronger than those in liquids. Thus, the escaping tendency for surface molecules is higher in liquids. Consequently, surface loss of vapour from liquids by the process of evaporation is more common than surface loss of vapour from solids via sublimation.

In the case of a liquid solvent containing a dissolved solute, molecules of both solvent and solute may show a tendency to escape from the surface and so contribute to the vapour pressure. The relative tendencies to escape will depend on the relative numbers of the different molecules in the surface of the solution. It will also depend on the relative strengths of the attractive forces between adjacent solvent molecules on the one hand and between solute and solvent molecules on the other. Therefore, as the intermolecular forces between solid solutes and liquid solvents tend to be relatively strong, such solute molecules do not generally escape from the surface of a solution and contribute to the vapour pressure. In other words, the solute is generally non-volatile and the vapour pressure arises solely from the dynamic equilibrium that is set up between the rates of evaporation and condensation of solvent molecules contained in the solution. In a mixture of miscible liquids, i.e. a liquid in liquid solution, the molecules of both components are likely to evaporate and contribute to the overall vapour pressure exerted by the solution.

Ideal solutions: Raoult's law

The concept of an ideal solution has been introduced to provide a model system that can be used as a standard against which real or non-ideal solutions can be compared. In the model it is assumed that the strengths of all intermolecular forces are identical. Thus solvent–solvent, solute–solvent and solute–solute interactions are the same and are equal, in fact, to the strength of the intermolecular interactions in either the pure solvent or the pure solute. Because of this equality, the relative tendencies of solute and solvent molecules to escape from the surface of the solution will be determined only by their relative numbers in the surface.

Because a solution is homogeneous by definition, the relative number of these surface molecules will be the same as the relative number in the whole of the solution. The latter can be expressed conveniently by the mole fractions of the components because, for a binary solution (one with two components), $x_1 + x_2 = 1$, where x_1 and x_2 are the mole fractions of the solute and the solvent, respectively. Thus, the total vapour pressure (P) exerted by such a binary solution is given by Eqn 3.1:

$$P = p_1 + p_2 = p^0_1 x_1 + p^0_2 x_2 \qquad (3.1)$$

where p_1 and p_2 are the partial vapour pressures exerted above the solution by solute and solvent, respectively, and p^0_1 and p^0_2 are the vapour pressures exerted by pure solute and pure solvent, respectively.

If the total vapour pressure of the solution is described by Eqn 3.1, then Raoult's law is obeyed by the system. Raoult's law states that the partial vapour pressure exerted by a volatile component in a solution at a given temperature is equal to the vapour pressure of the pure component at the same temperature, multiplied by its mole fraction in the solution, i.e.:

$$p_1 = p_1^0 x_1 \qquad (3.2)$$

One of the consequences of the preceding comments is that an ideal solution may be defined as one that obeys Raoult's law. In addition, ideal behaviour should be expected to be exhibited only by real systems comprised of chemically similar components, because it is only in such systems that the condition of equal intermolecular forces between components (as assumed in the ideal model) is likely to be satisfied. Consequently, Raoult's law is obeyed over an appreciable concentration range by relatively few systems in reality.

Mixtures of benzene + toluene, n-hexane + n-heptane and ethyl bromide + ethyl iodide are commonly mentioned systems that exhibit ideal behaviour, but a more pharmaceutically interesting example is provided by binary mixtures of fluorinated hydrocarbons. These latter mixtures are currently still used as propellants in therapeutic aerosols, although their usage is being phased out. Their approximation to ideal behaviour allows Eqn 3.1 to be used to calculate the total pressure exerted by a given mixture of propellants.

Real or non-ideal solutions

The majority of real solutions do not exhibit ideal behaviour because solute–solute, solute–solvent and solvent–solvent forces of interaction are unequal. These inequalities alter the effective concentration of each component so that it cannot be represented by a normal expression of concentration, such as the mole fraction term x that is used in Eqns 3.1 and 3.2. Consequently, deviations from Raoult's law are often exhibited by real solutions, and the previous equations are not obeyed in such cases. These equations can be modified, however, by substituting each concentration term (x) by a measure of the effective concentration; this is provided by the so-called *activity* (or thermodynamic activity), a. Thus, Eqn 3.2 is converted into Eqn 3.3:

$$p_1 = p_1^0 a_1 \qquad (3.3)$$

which is applicable to all systems whether they are ideal or non-ideal. It should be noted that if a solution exhibits ideal behaviour then a equals x, whereas a does not equal x if deviations from such behaviour are apparent. The ratio of activity/concentration is termed the *activity coefficient (f)* and it provides a measure of the deviation from ideality.

If the attractive forces between solute and solvent molecules are weaker than those exerted between the solute molecules themselves or the solvent molecules themselves, then the components will have little affinity for each other. The escaping tendency of the surface molecules in such a system is increased compared to that of an ideal solution. In other words, p_1, p_2 and P are greater than expected from Raoult's law, and the thermodynamic activities of the components are greater than their mole fractions, i.e. $a_1 > x_1$ and $3 > x_2$. This type of system is said to show a *positive deviation* from Raoult's law, and the extent of the deviation increases as the miscibility of the components decreases. For example, a mixture of alcohol and benzene shows a smaller deviation than the less miscible mixture of water + diethyl ether, whereas the virtually immiscible mixture of benzene + water exhibits a very large positive deviation.

Conversely, if the solute and the solvent have a strong mutual affinity that results in the formation of a complex or compound, then a negative deviation from Raoult's law occurs. Thus, p_1, p_2 and P are lower than expected and $a_1 < x_1$ and $3 < x_2$. Examples of systems that show this type of behaviour include chloroform + acetone, pyridine + acetic acid and water + nitric acid.

Although most systems are non-ideal and deviate either positively or negatively from Raoult's law, such deviations are small when a solution is dilute because the effects of a small amount of solute on interactions between solvent molecules are minimal. Thus, dilute solutions tend to exhibit ideal behaviour and the activities of their components approximate to their mole fractions, i.e. a_1 approximately equals x_1 and 3 approximately equals x_2. Conversely, large deviations may be observed when the concentration of a solution is high.

Knowledge of the consequences of such marked deviations is particularly important in relation to the distillation of liquid mixtures. For example, the complete separation of the components of a mixture by fractional distillation may not be achievable if large positive or negative deviations from Raoult's law give rise to the formation of so-called azeotropic mixtures with minimum and maximum boiling points, respectively

IONIZATION OF SOLUTES

Many solutes dissociate into ions if the dielectric constant of the solvent is high enough to cause sufficient separation of the attractive forces between the oppositely charged ions. Such solutes are termed *electrolytes*, and their ionization (or dissociation) has several consequences that are often important in pharmaceutical practice. Some of these are discussed below.

Hydrogen ion concentration and pH

The dissociation of water can be represented by Eqn 3.4:

$$H_2O \rightleftharpoons H^+ + OH^- \qquad (3.4)$$

It should be realized that this is a simplified representation because the hydrogen and hydroxyl ions do not exist in a free state but combine with undissociated water molecules to yield more complex ions, such as H_3O^+ and $H_7O_4^-$

In pure water the concentrations of H^+ and OH^- ions are equal, and at 25°C both have the values of 1×10^{-7} mol L^{-1}. As the Lowry–Brönsted theory of acids and bases defines an acid as a substance that donates a proton (or hydrogen ion), it follows that the addition of an acidic solute to water will result in a hydrogen ion concentration that exceeds this value. Conversely, the addition of a base, which is defined as a substance that accepts protons, will decrease the concentration of hydrogen ions. The hydrogen ion concentration range that can be obtained decreases from 1 mol L^{-1} for a strong acid to 1×10^{-14} mol L^{-1} for a strong base.

In order to avoid the frequent use of low values that arise from this range, the concept of pH has been introduced as a more convenient measure of hydrogen ion concentration. pH is defined as the negative logarithm of the hydrogen ion concentration $[H^+]$, as shown by Eqn 3.5:

$$pH = -\log_{10}[H^+] \qquad (3.5)$$

so that the pH of a neutral solution such as pure water is 7. This is because the concentration of H^+ ions (and thus OH^-) ions is 1×10^{-7} mol L^{-1}. The pH of acidic and alkaline solutions will be < 7 or > 7, respectively.

pH has several important implications in pharmaceutical practice. In addition to its effects on the solubilities of drugs that are weak acids or bases, pH may have a considerable effect on the stabilities of many drugs, be injurious to body tissues, and affect the ease of absorption of drugs from the gastrointestinal tract into the blood.

For example, many (indeed most) drugs are weak bases or their salts. These drugs dissolve more rapidly in the low pH of the acidic stomach. However, there will be little or no absorption of the

drug, as it will be too ionized (see Chapter 16). Absorption will normally have to wait until the more alkaline intestine, where the ionization of the dissolved base is reduced.

Dissociation (or ionization) constants and pK_a

Many drugs are either weak acids or weak bases. In solutions of these drugs equilibria exist between undissociated molecules and their ions. Thus, in a solution of a weakly acidic drug HA the equilibrium may be represented by Eqn 3.6:

$$HA \rightleftharpoons H^+ + A^- \qquad (3.6)$$

Similarly, the protonation of a weakly basic drug B can be represented by Eqn 3.7:

$$B + H^+ \rightleftharpoons BH^+ \qquad (3.7)$$

In solutions of most salts of strong acids or bases in water, such equilibria are shifted strongly to one side of the equation because these compounds are completely ionized.

The *ionization constant* (or *dissociation constant*) K_a of a weak acid can be obtained by applying the Law of Mass Action to Eqn 3.6 to yield:

$$K_a = \frac{[H^+][A^-]}{[HA]} \qquad (3.8)$$

Taking logarithms of both sides of Eqn 3.8 yields:

$$\log K_a = \log [H^+] + \log [A^-] - \log [HA]$$

The signs in this equation may be reversed to give:

$$-\log K_a = -\log [H^+] - \log [A^-] + \log [HA] \qquad (3.9)$$

The symbol pK_a, is used to represent the negative logarithm of the acid dissociation constant K_a in the same way that pH is used to represent the negative logarithm of the hydrogen ion concentration, and Eqn 3.9 may therefore be rewritten as:

$$pK_a = pH + \log [HA] - \log [A^-] \qquad (3.10)$$

or

$$pK_a = pH + \log \frac{[HA]}{[A^-]} \qquad (3.11)$$

A general equation may be written that is applicable to any acidic drug with one ionizable group, where c_u and c_i represent the concentrations of the unionized and ionized species, respectively. This is known as the *Henderson–Hasselbalch equation*, (Eqn 3.12):

$$pK_a = pH + \log \frac{c_u}{c_i}. \qquad (3.12)$$

Ionization constants are usually expressed in terms of pK_a for both acidic and basic drugs. From Eqn 3.7 it can be seen that the acid dissociation constant (K_a) of a protonated weak base is given by:

$$K_a = \frac{[H^+][B]}{[BH^+]} \quad (3.13)$$

Taking negative logarithms yields:

$$-\log K_a = -\log [H^+] - \log [B] + \log [BH^+] \quad (3.14)$$

or

$$pK_a = pH + \log \frac{[BH^+]}{[B]} \quad (3.15)$$

The Henderson–Hasselbalch equation for any weak base with one ionizable group may therefore be written as:

$$pK_a = pH + \log \frac{c_i}{c_u} \quad (3.16)$$

where c_i and c_u refer to the concentrations of the protonated and unionized species, respectively.

Various analytical techniques, e.g. spectrophotometric and potentiometric methods, may be used to determine ionization constants, but the temperature at which the determination is performed should be specified because the values of the constants vary with temperature.

There is a direct link for most polar ionic compounds between the degree of ionization and aqueous solubility, as is shown in Figure 3.1.

The degree of ionization of a drug in a solution can be calculated from the Henderson–Hasselbalch equations for weak acids and bases (Eqns 3.11 and 3.15, respectively) if the pK_a value of the drug and the pH of the solution are known. Such calculations are particularly useful in determining the degree of ionization of drugs in various parts of the gastrointestinal tract and in the plasma. The following examples are therefore related to this type of situation.

Calculation example

1. The pK_a value of aspirin, which is a weak acid, is about 3.5. If the pH of the gastric contents is 2.0, then from Eqn 3.12:

$$\log \frac{c_u}{c_i} = pK_a - pH = 3.5 - 2.0 = 1.5$$

so that the ratio of the concentration of unionized acetylsalicyclic acid to acetylsalicylate anion is given by:

$$c_u : c_i = \text{antilog } 1.5 = 31.62 : 1$$

2. The pH of plasma is 7.4, so that the ratio of unionized to ionized aspirin in this medium is given by:

$$\log \frac{c_u}{c_i} = pK_a - pH = 3.5 - 7.4 = -3.9$$

and

$$c_u : c_i = \text{antilog} - 3.9 = 1.259 \times 10^{-4} : 1$$

3. The pK_a of the weakly acidic drug sulphapyridine is about 8.0; if the pH of the intestinal contents is 5.0, then the ratio of unionized to ionized drug is given by:

$$\log \frac{c_u}{c_i} = pK_a - pH = 8.0 - 5.0 = 3.0$$

and

$$c_u : c_i = \text{antilog } 3.0 = 10^3 : 1$$

4. The pK_a of the basic drug amidopyrine is 5.0. In the stomach the ratio of ionized to unionized drug is calculated from Eqn 3.16 as follows:

$$\log \frac{c_i}{c_u} = pK_a - pH = 5.0 - 2.0 = 3.0$$

and

$$c_i : c_u = \text{antilog } 3.0 = 10^3 : 1$$

whereas in the intestine the ratio is given by:

$$\log \frac{c_i}{c_u} = 5.0 - 5.0 = 0$$

and

$$c_i : c_u = \text{antilog } 0 = 1 : 1$$

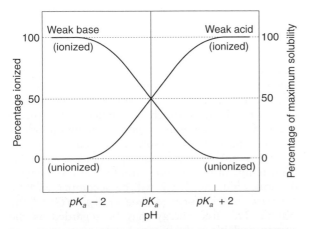

Fig. 3.1 Change in degree of ionization and relative solubility of weakly acidic and weakly basic drugs as a function of pH.

Buffer solutions and buffer capacity

Buffer solutions will maintain a constant pH even when small amounts of acid or alkali are added to the solution. Buffers usually contain mixtures of a weak acid and one of its salts, although mixtures of a weak base and one of its salts may be used. The latter suffer from the disadvantage that arises from the volatility of many bases.

The action of a buffer solution can be appreciated by considering a simple system such as a solution of acetic acid and sodium acetate in water. The acetic acid, being a weak acid, will be confined virtually to its undissociated form because its ionization will be suppressed by the presence of common acetate ions produced by complete dissociation of the sodium salt. The pH of this solution can be described by Eqn 3.17, which is a rearranged form of Eqn 3.12:

$$pH = pK_a + \log \frac{c_i}{c_u} \qquad (3.17)$$

It can be seen from Eqn 3.17 that the pH will remain constant as long as the logarithm of the ratio c_i/c_u does not change. When a small amount of acid is added to the solution it will convert some of the salt into acetic acid, but if the concentrations of both acetate ion and acetic acid are reasonably large then the effect of the change will be negligible and the pH will remain constant. Similarly, the addition of a small amount of base will convert some of the acetic acid into its salt form, but the pH will be virtually unaltered if the overall changes in concentrations of the two species are relatively small.

If large amounts of acid or base are added to a buffer then changes in the log c_i/c_u term become appreciable and the pH alters. The ability of a buffer to withstand the effects of acids and bases is an important property from a practical point of view. This ability is expressed in terms of *buffer capacity* (β). This can be defined as being equal to the amount of strong acid or strong base, expressed as moles of H^+ or OH^- ion, required to change the pH of 1 litre of the buffer by one pH unit. From the remarks above it should be clear that buffer capacity increases as the concentrations of the buffer components increase. In addition, the capacity is also affected by the ratio of the concentrations of weak acid and its salt, maximum capacity (β_{max}) being obtained when the ratio of acid to salt = 1. In such circumstances pH = pK_a of the acid and β_{max} = 0.576 (total buffer concentration).

The components of various buffer systems and the concentrations required to produce different pHs are listed in several reference books, such as the pharmacopoeias. When selecting a suitable buffer the pK_a value of the acid should be close to the required pH and the compatibility of its components with other ingredients in the system should be considered. The toxicity of buffer components must also be taken into account if the solution is to be used for medicinal purposes.

COLLIGATIVE PROPERTIES

When a non-volatile solute is dissolved in a solvent certain properties of the resultant solution are largely independent of the nature of the solute and are determined by the concentration of solute particles. These properties are known as *colligative properties*. In the case of a non-electrolyte the solute particles will be molecules, but if the solute is an electrolyte then its degree of dissociation will determine whether the particles will be ions only or a mixture of ions and undissociated molecules.

The most important colligative property from a pharmaceutical point of view is referred to as *osmotic pressure*. However, as all colligative properties are related to each other by virtue of their common dependency on the concentration of the solute molecules, the remaining colligative properties (which are lowering of vapour pressure of the solvent, elevation of its boiling point and depression of its freezing point) are of pharmaceutical interest. These other observations offer alternative means to osmotic pressure determinations as methods of comparing the colligative properties of different solutions.

Osmotic pressure

The osmotic pressure of a solution is the external pressure that must be applied to the solution in order to prevent it being diluted by the entry of solvent via a process known as *osmosis*. This refers to the spontaneous diffusion of solvent from a solution of low solute concentration (or a pure solvent) into a more concentrated one through a semipermeable membrane. Such a membrane separates the two solutions and is permeable only to solvent molecules.

Because the process occurs spontaneously at constant temperature and pressure, the laws of thermodynamics indicate that it will be accompanied by a decrease in the so-called *free energy (G)* of the system. This free energy may be regarded as the energy available in the system for the performance of useful work, and when an equilibrium position is attained then there is no difference between the states that are in equilibrium. The rate of increase in free energy of a solution caused by an increase in the number of moles of one component is termed the partial molar free energy $(\overline{G})$ or chemical potential (μ) of that component. For example, the chemical potential of the solvent in a binary solution is given by:

$$\left(\frac{\partial G}{\partial n_2} \right)_{T, P, n_1} = \overline{G}_2 = \mu_2 \qquad (3.18)$$

where the subscripts outside the bracket on the left-hand side indicate that temperature, pressure and amount of component 1 (the solute in this case) remain constant.

Because only solvent can pass across the semipermeable membrane, the driving force for osmosis arises from the inequality of the chemical potentials of the solvent on opposing sides of the membrane. Thus the direction of osmotic flow is from the dilute solution (or pure solvent), where the chemical potential of the solvent is highest because there are more moles of it, into the concentrated solution, where the number of moles and, consequently, the chemical potential of the solvent is reduced by the presence of more solute. The chemical potential of the solvent in the more concentrated solution can be increased by forcing its molecules closer together under the influence of an externally applied pressure. Osmosis can therefore be prevented by such means, hence the definition of osmotic pressure.

The relationship between osmotic pressure (π) and the concentration of a non-electrolyte is given for dilute solutions, which may be assumed to exhibit ideal behaviour, by the van't Hoff equation:

$$\pi V = n_2 R T \qquad (3.19)$$

where V is the volume of solution, n_2 is the number of moles of solute, T is the thermodynamic temperature and R is the gas constant. This equation, which is similar to the ideal gas equation, was derived empirically but it does correspond to a theoretically derived equation if approximations based on low solute concentrations are taken into account.

If the solute is an electrolyte, Eqn 3.19 must be modified to allow for the effect of ionic dissociation, because this will increase the number of particles in the solution. This modification is achieved by insertion of the van't Hoff correction factor (i) to give:

$$\pi V = i n_2 R T \qquad (3.20)$$

where $i = \dfrac{\text{observed colligative property}}{\begin{array}{c}\text{colligative property expected if}\\ \text{dissociation did not occur}\end{array}}$

Osmolality and osmolarity

The amount of osmotically active particles in a solution is sometimes expressed in terms of osmoles or milliosmoles (1 osmol = 1×10^3 mosmol). These may be either molecules or ions. The concentration of a solution may therefore be expressed in terms of its **osmolality** or its **osmolarity**, where osmolality is the number of osmoles per kilogram of water and osmolarity is the number of osmoles per litre of solution.

Iso-osmotic solutions

If two solutions are separated by a perfect semipermeable membrane, i.e. a membrane which is permeable only to solvent molecules, and no net movement of solvent occurs across the membrane, then the solutions are said to be **iso-osmotic** and will have equal osmotic pressures.

Isotonic solutions

Biological membranes do not always function as perfect semipermeable membranes and some solute molecules as well as water are able to pass through them. If two iso-osmotic solutions remain in osmotic equilibrium when separated by a biological membrane they may be described as being **isotonic** with respect to that particular membrane. Adjustment of isotonicity is particularly important for formulations intended for parenteral routes of administration.

DIFFUSION IN SOLUTION

By definition, the components of a solution form a single phase, which is homogeneous. This homogeneity arises from the process of diffusion, which occurs spontaneously and is consequently accompanied by a decrease in the free energy (G) of the system. **Diffusion** may be defined as the spontaneous transference of a component from a region in the system where it has a high chemical potential into one where its chemical potential is lower. Although such a gradient in chemical potential provides the driving force for diffusion, the laws that describe this phenomenon are usually expressed in terms of concentration gradients, for example Fick's first law, which is discussed in Chapter 2.

The most common explanation of the mechanism of diffusion in solution is based on the lattice theory of the structure of liquids.

Lattice theories postulate that liquids have crystalline or quasicrystalline structures. The concept of a crystal type of lattice is only intended to provide a convenient starting point and should not be interpreted as a suggestion that liquids possess rigid structures. The theories also postulate that a reasonable proportion of the volume occupied by the liquid is, at any moment, empty, i.e. there are 'holes' in the liquid lattice network, which constitute the so-called free volume of the liquid.

Diffusion can therefore be regarded as the process by which solute molecules move from hole to hole within a liquid lattice. In order to achieve such movement a solute molecule must acquire sufficient kinetic energy at the right time so that it can break away from any bonds that tend to anchor it in one hole and then jump into an adjacent hole. If the average distance of each jump is δ cm and the frequency with which the jumps occur is ϕ s^{-1}, then the **diffusion coefficient (D)** is given by:

$$D = \frac{\delta^2 \phi}{6} \text{ cm}^2 \text{ s}^{-1} \tag{3.21}$$

The diffusion coefficient is assumed to have a constant value for a particular system at a given temperature. This assumption is only strictly true at infinite dilution, and D may therefore exhibit some concentration dependency. In a given solvent the value of D decreases as the size of the diffusing solute molecule increases. In water, for example, D is of the order of 2×10^{-5} cm^2 s^{-1} for solutes with molecular weights of approximately 50 Da and it decreases to about 1×10^{-6} cm^2 s^{-1} when the molecular weight increases to a few thousand Da.

The value of δ for a given solute is unlikely to alter very much from one liquid to another. Differences in the diffusion coefficient of a substance in solution in various solvents arise mainly from changes in jump frequency (ϕ), which are determined in turn by the free volume or looseness of packing in the solvent.

When the size of the solute molecules is not appreciably larger than that of the solvent molecules then it has been shown that the diffusion coefficient of the former is related to its molecular weight (M) by the relationship:

$$DM^{1/2} = \text{constant} \tag{3.22}$$

When the solute is much greater in size than the solvent, diffusion arises largely from transport of solvent molecules in the opposite direction and the relationship becomes:

$$DM^{1/3} = \text{constant} \tag{3.23}$$

This latter agrees with the Stokes–Einstein equation (Eqn 3.24) for the diffusion of spherical particles that are larger than surrounding liquid molecules. Since the mass (m) of a spherical particle is proportional to the cube of its radius (r), i.e. $r \propto m^{1/3}$, it follows from Eqn 3.23 that $Dm^{1/3}$ and consequently D and r are constants for such a system. The Stokes–Einstein equation is usually written in the form:

$$D = \frac{kT}{6\pi r \eta} \tag{3.24}$$

where k is the Boltzmann constant, T is the thermodynamic temperature and η is the viscosity of the liquid. The appearance of a viscosity term in this type of equation is not unexpected because the reciprocal of viscosity, which is known as the **fluidity** of a liquid, is proportional to the free volume in a liquid. Thus, jump frequency (ϕ) and diffusion coefficient (D) will increase as the viscosity of a liquid decreases or as the number of holes in its structure increases.

The experimental determination of diffusion coefficients of solutes in liquid solvents is not easy because the effects of other factors that may influence the movement of solute in the system, e.g. temperature and density gradients, mechanical agitation and vibration, must be eliminated.

BIBLIOGRAPHY

Chang, R. (1981) *Physical Chemistry with Applications to Biological Systems*, 2nd edn. Macmillan.

Florence, A.T. and Attwood, D. (1998) *Physicochemical Principles of Pharmacy*, 3rd edn. MacMillan.

Martin A. (1993) *Physical Pharmacy*, 4th edn. Lea & Febiger.

4

Rheology

Chris Marriott

VISCOSITY, RHEOLOGY AND THE FLOW OF FLUIDS

The viscosity of a fluid may be described simply as its resistance to flow or movement. Thus water, which is easier to stir than syrup, is said to have the lower viscosity.

Historically the importance of rheology (a term invented by Bingham and formally adopted in 1929), which may be defined as the study of the flow and deformation properties of matter, in pharmacy was merely as a means of characterizing and classifying fluids and semisolids. For example, in the *British Pharmacopoeia* a viscosity standard has for many years been used to control substances such as liquid paraffin. However, the increased reliance on the dissolution testing of dosage forms and the use of polymers has given added importance to a knowledge of flow properties. Furthermore, advances in the methods of evaluation of the viscoelastic properties of semisolids and biological materials have produced useful correlations with bioavailability and function.

A proper understanding of the rheological properties of pharmaceutical materials is essential to the preparation, development, evaluation and performance of pharmaceutical dosage forms. This chapter describes rheological behaviour and techniques of measurement, and will form a basis for the applied studies described in later chapters.

NEWTONIAN FLUIDS

Viscosity coefficients for Newtonian fluids

Dynamic viscosity

The definition of viscosity was put on a quantitative basis by Newton, who was the first to realize that the

41

rate of flow (γ) was directly related to the applied stress (σ): the constant of proportionality is the coefficient of dynamic viscosity, (η), more usually referred to simply as the viscosity. Simple fluids which obey the relationship are referred to as Newtonian fluids and those which do not are known as non-Newtonian.

The phenomenon of viscosity is best understood by a consideration of a hypothetical cube of fluid made up of infinitely thin layers (laminae) which are able to slide over one another like a pack of playing cards (Fig. 4.1(a)).

When a tangential force is applied to the uppermost layer it is assumed that each subsequent layer will move at progressively decreasing velocity and that the bottom layer will be stationary (Fig. 4.1(b)). A velocity gradient will therefore exist, and this will be equal to the velocity of the upper layer in ms^{-1} divided by the height of the cube in metres. The resultant gradient, which is effectively the rate of flow but is usually referred to as the rate of shear, γ, will have units of reciprocal seconds (s^{-1}). The applied stress, known as the shear stress, σ, is derived by dividing the applied force by the area of the upper layer and will have units of N m^{-2}.

As Newton's law can be expressed as:

$$\sigma = \eta\gamma \qquad (4.1)$$

then

$$\eta = \frac{\sigma}{\gamma} \qquad (4.2)$$

and η will have units of N m^{-2} s. Thus by reference to Eqn 4.1 it can be seen that a Newtonian fluid of viscosity 1 N m^{-2} s would produce a velocity of 1 ms^{-1} for a cube of 1 m dimension with an applied force of 1 N. Because the name for the derived unit of force per unit area in the SI system is the pascal (Pa), then

Table 4.1 Viscosities of some fluids of pharmaceutical interest	
Fluid	Dynamic viscosity at 20°C (mPa s)
Chloroform	0.58
Water	1.002
Ethanol	1.20
Glyceryl trinitrate	36.0
Olive oil	84.0
Castor oil	986.0
Glycerol	1490

viscosity should be referred to in Pa s. It is common to use the submultiple mPa s, and the viscosity of water at 20°C is virtually 1 mPa s. (The latter is equivalent to 1 centipoise (cP), which is one hundredth of a Poise (1 dyn cm^{-2} s), the unit of viscosity in the now redundant cgs system of units. Although no longer official, its use is still relatively common.)

The values of the viscosity of water and some examples of other fluids of pharmaceutical interest are given in Table 4.1.

Kinematic viscosity

The dynamic viscosity is not the only coefficient that can be used to characterize a fluid. The kinematic viscosity (v) is also used and may be defined as the dynamic viscosity divided by the density of the fluid (ρ):

$$v = \frac{\eta}{\rho} \qquad (4.3)$$

and the SI units will be m^2 s^{-1} or, more usefully, mm^2 s^{-1}. (The cgs unit was the Stoke (10^{-4} m^2 s^{-1}), and the centistoke (cS) might still be found in the literature.)

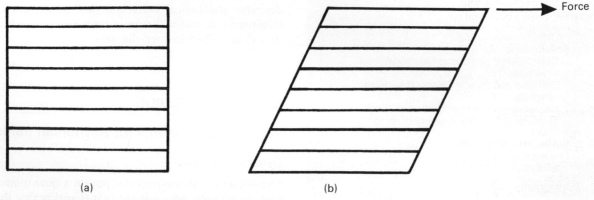

Force

(a)   (b)

Fig. 4.1 Representation of the effect of shearing a 'block' of fluid.

Relative and specific viscosities

The viscosity ratio or relative viscosity (η_r) of a solution is the ratio of the solution viscosity to the viscosity of the solvent (η_o):

$$\eta_r = \frac{\eta}{\eta_o} \qquad (4.4)$$

and the specific viscosity (η_{sp}) is given by

$$\eta_{sp} = \eta_r - 1 \qquad (4.5)$$

In these calculations the solvent can be of any nature, although in pharmaceutical products it is often water.

For a colloidal dispersion the equation derived by Einstein may be used:

$$\eta = \eta_o(1 + 2.5\phi) \qquad (4.6)$$

where ϕ is the volume fraction of the colloidal phase (the volume of the dispersed phase divided by the total volume of the dispersion). The Einstein equation may be rewritten as:

$$\frac{\eta}{\eta_o} = 1 + 2.5\ \phi \qquad (4.7)$$

when from Eqn 4.4 it can be seen that the left hand side of Eqn 4.7 is equal to the relative viscosity. It can also be rewritten as:

$$\frac{\eta}{\eta_o} - 1 = \frac{\eta - \eta_o}{\eta_o} = 2.5\ \phi \qquad (4.8)$$

when the left-hand side equals the specific viscosity. Equation 4.8 can be rearranged to produce:

$$\frac{\eta_{sp}}{\phi} = 2.5 \qquad (4.9)$$

and as the volume fraction will be directly related to concentration C, Eqn 4.9 can be rewritten as:

$$\frac{\eta_{sp}}{C} = k \qquad (4.10)$$

When the dispersed phase is a high molecular mass polymer then a colloidal solution will result and, provided moderate concentrations are used, then Eqn 4.10 can be expressed as a power series:

$$\frac{\eta_{sp}}{C} = k_1 + k_2 C + k_3 C^2 \qquad (4.11)$$

Intrinsic viscosity

If $\dfrac{\eta_{sp}}{C}$, the viscosity number or reduced viscosity is determined at a range of polymer concentrations and plotted as a function of concentration (Fig. 4.2), then a linear relationship should be obtained, and the intercept produced on extrapolation of the line to the ordinate will yield the constant k_1 which is referred to as the limiting viscosity number or the intrinsic viscosity, [η], when the units of concentration are in g dL^{-1}.

The limiting viscosity number may be used to determine the approximate molecular mass (M) of polymers using the Mark–Houwink equation:

$$[\eta] = KM^\alpha \qquad (4.12)$$

where K and α are constants that must be obtained at a given temperature for the specific polymer–solvent system. However, once these constants are known then viscosity determinations provide a quick and precise method of molecular mass determination of pharmaceutical polymers such as dextrans, which are used as plasma extenders. Also the values of the two constants provide an indication of the shape of the molecule in solution: spherical molecules yield values of $\alpha = 0$, whereas extended rods have values greater than 1.0. A randomly coiled molecule will yield an intermediate value (≈ 0.5).

The specific viscosity may be used in the following equation to determine the volume of a molecule in solution:

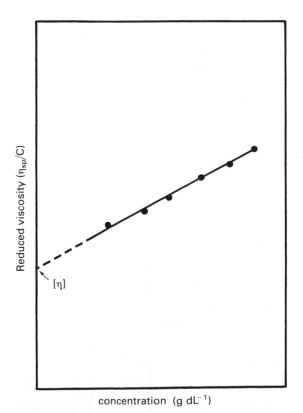

Fig. 4.2 Plot of concentration (g dL^{-1}) against reduced viscosity (η_{sp}/C), which by extrapolation gives the limiting viscosity number or intrinsic viscosity ([η]).

$$\eta_{sp} = 2.5C\,\frac{NV}{M} \qquad (4.13)$$

where C is concentration, N is Avogadro's number, V is the hydrodynamic volume of each molecule and M is the molecular mass. However, it does suffer from the obvious disadvantage that the assumption is made that all polymeric molecules form spheres in solution.

Huggins' constant

Finally, the constant k_2 in Eqn 4.11 is referred to as Huggins' constant and is equal to the slope of the plot shown in Figure 4.2. Its value gives an indication of the interaction between the polymer and the solvent, such that a positive slope is produced for a polymer that interacts weakly with the solvent, and the slope becomes less positive as the interaction increases. A change in the value of Huggins' constant can be used to evaluate the interaction of drug molecules with polymers.

Boundary layers

From Figure 4.1 it can be seen that the rate of flow of a fluid over an even surface will be dependent upon the distance from the surface. The velocity, which will be almost zero at the surface, increases with increasing distance from the surface until the bulk of the fluid is reached and the velocity becomes constant. The region over which differences in velocity are observed is referred to as the boundary layer. Its depth is dependent upon the viscosity of the fluid and the rate of flow in the bulk fluid: high viscosity and a low flow rate would result in a thick boundary layer, which will become thinner as either the viscosity falls or the flow rate is increased. The boundary layer, which arises because of the intermolecular forces between the liquid molecules and those of the surface resulting in reduction of movement of the

Fig. 4.3 Velocity distributions across a pipe.

layer adjacent to the wall to zero, represents an important barrier to heat and mass transfer. In the case of a capillary tube then the two boundary layers meet at the centre of the tube, such that the velocity distribution is parabolic (Fig. 4.3). With an increase in either the diameter of the tube or the fluid velocity, the proximity of the two boundary layers is reduced and the velocity profile becomes flattened at the centre (Fig. 4.3).

Laminar, transitional and turbulent flow

The conditions under which a fluid flows through a pipe, for example, can markedly affect the character of the flow. The type of flow that occurs can be best understood by reference to experiments conducted by Reynolds in 1883. The apparatus used (Fig. 4.4) consisted of a straight glass tube through which the fluid flowed under the influence of a force provided by a constant head of water. At the centre of the inlet of the tube a fine stream of dye was introduced. At low flow rates the dye formed a coherent thread which remained undisturbed in the centre of the

Fig. 4.4 Reynolds' apparatus.

tube and grew very little in thickness along the length. This type of flow is described as **streamlined** or **laminar**, and the liquid is considered to flow as a series of concentric cylinders in a manner analogous to an extending telescope.

If the speed of the fluid is increased a critical velocity is reached at which the thread begins to waver and then to break up, although no mixing occurs. This is known as **transitional flow**. When the velocity is increased to high values the dye instantaneously mixes with the fluid in the tube, as all order is lost and irregular motions are imposed on the overall movement of the fluid. Such flow is described as **turbulent**. In this type of flow the movement of molecules is totally haphazard, although the average movement will be in the direction of flow.

Reynolds' experiments indicated that the flow conditions were affected by four factors, namely the diameter of the pipe and the viscosity, density and velocity of the fluid. Furthermore, it was shown that these factors could be combined to give the following equation:

$$Re = \frac{\rho u d}{\eta} \qquad (4.14)$$

where ρ is the density, u is the velocity and η is the dynamic viscosity of the fluid; d is the diameter of the pipe. Re is known as Reynolds' number and, provided compatible units are used, it will be dimensionless.

Values of Reynolds' number have been determined that can be associated with a particular type of flow. If it is below 2000 then streamline flow will occur, but if it is above 4000 then flow will be turbulent. In between these two values the nature of the flow will depend upon the surface over which the fluid is flowing. For example, if the surface is smooth then streamline flow may not be disturbed and may exist at values of Reynolds' number above 2000. However, if the surface is rough or the channel tortuous then flow may well be turbulent at values below 4000, and even as low as 2000. Consequently, although it is tempting to state that values of Reynolds' number between 2000 and 4000 are indicative of transitional flow, such a statement would only be correct for a specific set of conditions. This also explains why it is difficult to demonstrate transitional flow practically. However, Reynolds' number is still an important parameter and can be used to predict the type of flow that will occur in a particular situation. The importance of knowing the type of flow lies in the fact that with streamline flow there is no component at right-angles to the direction of flow, so that fluid cannot move across the tube. This component is strong for turbulent flow

and interchange across the tube is rapid. Thus in the latter case, for example, mass will be rapidly transported, whereas in streamline flow the fluid layers will act as a barrier to such transfer, which can only occur by molecular diffusion.

Determination of the flow properties of simple fluids

A wide range of instruments exist that can be used to determine the flow properties of Newtonian fluids. However, only some of these are capable of providing data that can be used to calculate viscosities in fundamental units: the design of many instruments precludes the calculation of absolute viscosities, as they are capable of providing data only in terms of empirical units.

It is not possible to describe all of the types of instrument used to measure viscosity, and consequently this section is limited to simple instruments specified in the *European Pharmacopoeia* (Ph. Eur.) or the *British Pharmacopoeia* (BP).

Capillary viscometers

A capillary viscometer can be used to determine viscosity provided that the fluid is Newtonian and the flow is streamlined. The rate of flow of the fluid through the capillary is measured under the influence of gravity or an externally applied pressure.

Ostwald U-tube viscometer Such instruments are described in pharmacopoeias and are the subject of a specification of the International Standards Organization. A range of capillary bores are available and an appropriate one should be selected so that a flow time of approximately 200 s is obtained; the wider-bore viscometers are thus for use with fluids of higher viscosity. For fluids where there is a viscosity specification in the BP, the size of instrument that must be used in the determination of their viscosity is stated. The instrument is shown in Figure 4.5 and flow through the capillary occurs under the influence of gravity. The maximum shear rate, γ_m is given by:

$$\gamma_m = \frac{\rho g r_c}{2 \eta} \qquad (4.15)$$

where ρ is the density of the fluid, g the acceleration due to gravity, r_c the radius of the capillary and η the absolute viscosity. Consequently, for a fluid of viscosity 1 mPa s the maximum shear rate is approximately 2.10^3 s^{-1} if the capillary has a diameter of 0.64 mm, but it will be of the order of 10^2 s^{-1} for a fluid with a viscosity of 1490 mPa s if the capillary has a diameter of 2.74 mm.

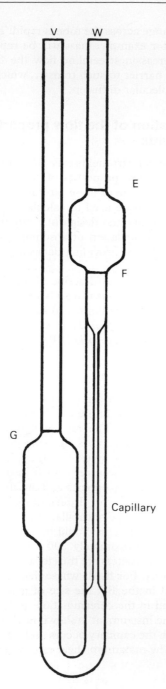

Fig. 4.5 A U-tube viscometer.

Fig. 4.6 A suspended-level viscometer.

The liquid is introduced into the viscometer up to mark G through arm V using a pipette long enough to prevent wetting the sides of the tube.

The viscometer is then clamped vertically in a constant-temperature water bath and allowed to reach the required temperature. The level of the liquid is adjusted and is then blown or sucked into tube W until the meniscus is just above mark E. The time for the meniscus to fall between marks E and F is recorded. Determinations should be repeated until three readings all within 0.5 s are obtained. Care should be taken not to introduce air bubbles and that the capillary does not become partially occluded with small particles.

Suspended-level viscometer This instrument is a modification of the U-tube viscometer which avoids the need to fill the instrument with a precise volume of fluid. Also, the fact that the pressure head in the U-tube is continually changing as the two menisci approach one another is avoided. This is also described in the BP and the Ph. Eur. and is shown in Figure 4.6.

A volume of liquid which will at least fill bulb C is introduced via tube V. The only upper limit on the volume used is that it should not block the ventilating tube Z. The viscometer is clamped vertically in a constant-temperature water bath and allowed to attain the required temperature. Tube Z is closed and fluid is drawn into bulb C by the application of suction through tube W until the meniscus is just above the mark E. Tube W is then closed and tube Z opened so that liquid can be drawn away from the bottom of the capillary. Tube W is then opened and the time the fluid takes to fall between marks E and F is recorded. If at any time during the determination the end of the ventilating tube Z becomes blocked by the liquid, the experiment must be repeated. The same criteria for reproducibility of timings described with the U-tube viscometer must be applied.

Because the volume of fluid introduced into the instrument can vary between the limits described above, this means that measurements can be made at a range of temperatures without the need to adjust the volume.

Calculation of viscosity from capillary viscometers

Poiseuille's law states that for a liquid flowing through a capillary tube

$$\eta = \frac{\pi r^4 t P}{8LV} \qquad (4.16)$$

where r is the radius of the capillary, t is the time of flow, P is the pressure difference across the ends of the tube, L is the length of the capillary and V is the volume of liquid. As the radius and length of the capillary as well as the volume flowing are constants for a given viscometer, then

$$\eta = KtP \qquad (4.17)$$

where K is equal to $\frac{\pi r^4}{8LV}$

The pressure difference, P, depends upon the density, ρ, of the liquid, the acceleration due to gravity, g, and the difference in heights of the two menisci in the two arms of the viscometer. Because the value of g and the level of the liquids are con-

stant, these can be included in a constant and Eqn 4.17 can be written for the viscosities of an unknown and a standard liquid:

$$\eta_1 = K't_1\rho_1 \qquad (4.18)$$
$$\eta_2 = K't_2\rho_2 \qquad (4.19)$$

Thus, when the flow times for two liquids are compared using the same viscometer, division of Eqn 4.18 by Eqn 4.19 gives:

$$\frac{\eta_1}{\eta_2} = \frac{K't_1\rho_1}{K't_2\rho_2} \qquad (4.20)$$

and reference to Eqn 4.4 shows that Eqn 4.20 will yield the viscosity ratio.

However, as Eqn 4.3 indicates that the kinematic viscosity is equal to the dynamic viscosity divided by the density, then Eqn 4.20 may be rewritten as:

$$\frac{\nu_1}{\nu_2} = \frac{t_1}{t_2} \qquad (4.21)$$

For a given viscometer a standard fluid such as water can be used for the purposes of calibration. Then, Eqn 4.21 may be rewritten as:

$$v = ct \qquad (4.22)$$

where c is the viscometer constant.

This is the equation that appears in the BP and explains the continued use of the kinematic viscosity as it means that liquids of known viscosity but of differing density from the test fluid can be used as the standard. A series of oils of given viscosity are available commercially and are recommended for the calibration of viscometers for which water cannot be used.

Falling-sphere viscometer

This viscometer is based upon Stokes' law (Chapter 6). When a body falls through a viscous medium it experiences a resistance or viscous drag which opposes the downward motion. Consequently, if a body falls through a liquid under the influence of gravity, an initial acceleration period is followed by motion at a uniform terminal velocity when the gravitational force is balanced by the viscous drag. Equation 4.23 will then apply to this terminal velocity when a sphere of density ρ_s and diameter d falls through a liquid of viscosity η and density ρ_1. The terminal velocity is u and g is the acceleration due to gravity:

$$3\pi\eta du = \frac{\pi}{6}d^3g(\rho_s - \rho_l) \qquad (4.23)$$

The viscous drag is given by the left-hand side of equation, whereas the right-hand side represents the force responsible for the downward motion of the sphere under the influence of gravity. Equation 4.23 may be used to calculate viscosity by rearranging it to give:

$$\eta = \frac{d^2 g\left(\rho_s - \rho_l\right)}{18u} \qquad (4.24)$$

Equation 4.3 gives the relationship between η and the kinematic viscosity, such that Eqn 4.24 may be rewritten as:

$$\nu = \frac{d^2 g\left(\rho_s - \rho_l\right)}{18u\rho_l} \qquad (4.25)$$

In the derivation of these equations it is assumed that the sphere is falling through a fluid of infinite dimensions. However, for practical purposes the fluid must be contained in a vessel of finite dimensions, and therefore it is necessary to include a correction factor to allow for the end and wall effects. The correction normally used is due to Faxen and may be given as:

$$F = 1 - 2.104\frac{d}{D} + 2.09\frac{d^3}{D^3} - 0.95\frac{d^5}{D^5} \qquad (4.26)$$

where D is the diameter of the measuring tube. The last term in Eqn 4.26 accounts for the end effect and may be ignored if the middle third of the depth is used for measuring the velocity of the sphere. In fact, the middle half of the tube can be used if D is at least 10 times d, and the second and third terms, which account for the wall effects, can be replaced by $2.1\frac{d}{D}$.

The apparatus used to determine u is shown in Figure 4.7. The liquid is placed in the fall tube which is clamped vertically in a constant-temperature bath. Sufficient time must be allowed for temperature equilibration to occur and for air bubbles to rise to the surface. A steel sphere which has been cleaned and brought to the temperature of the experiment is introduced into the fall tube through a narrow guide tube. The passage of the sphere is monitored by means of a telescope and the time it takes to fall between the etched marks A and B is recorded. It is usual to take the average of three readings, of which all are within 0.5%, as the fall time, t, to calculate the viscosity. If the same sphere and fall tube are used then Eqn 4.25 reduces to:

$$v = Kt\left(\frac{\rho_s}{\rho_l} - 1\right) \qquad (4.27)$$

where K is a constant that may be determined by the use of a liquid of known kinematic viscosity.

The BP specifies the use of a falling-sphere viscometer complying with British Standard 188: 1977 for the determination of the kinematic viscosity of a

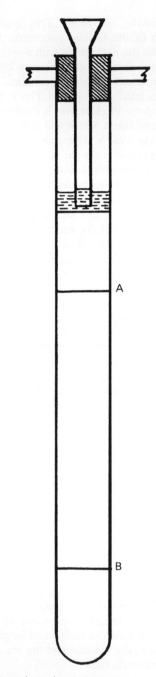

Fig. 4.7 A falling-sphere viscometer.

solution of pyroxylin in acetone and water. This type of viscometer is really only of use with Newtonian fluids, and a variation has involved measuring the time taken for a sphere to roll through the fluid contained in an inclined tube. This instrument can only be used after calibration with standard fluids, as fundamental derivation of viscosity is impossible.

NON-NEWTONIAN FLUIDS

The characteristics described in the previous sections apply only to fluids that obey Newton's law and which are consequently referred to as Newtonian. However, most pharmaceutical fluids do not follow this law because the viscosity of the fluid varies with the rate of shear. The reason for these deviations is that the fluids concerned are not simple fluids such as water and syrup, but are disperse or colloidal systems, including emulsions, suspensions and gels. These materials are known as non-Newtonian, and with the increasing use of sophisticated polymer-based delivery systems more examples of such behaviour are found in pharmacy.

Types of non-Newtonian behaviour

More than one type of deviation from Newton's law can be recognized, and it is the type of deviation that occurs which can be used to classify the particular material.

If a Newtonian fluid is subjected to an increasing rate of shear, γ, and the corresponding shear stress, σ, recorded then a plot of γ against σ will produce the linear relationship shown in Figure 4.8(a). Such a plot is usually referred to as a flow curve or rheogram. The slope of this plot will give the viscosity of the fluid and its reciprocal the fluidity. Equation 4.1 implies that this line will pass through the origin.

Plastic (or Bingham) flow

Figure 4.8(b) indicates an example of plastic or Bingham flow, when the rheogram does not pass through the origin but intersects with the shear stress axis at a point usually referred to as the yield value, σ_y. This implies that a plastic material does not flow until such a value of shear stress has been exceeded, and at lower stresses the substance behaves as a solid (elastic) material. Plastic materials are often referred to as Bingham bodies in honour of the worker who carried out many of the original studies with such materials. The equation he derived may be given as:

$$\sigma = \sigma_y + \eta_p \gamma \qquad (4.28)$$

where η_p is the plastic viscosity and σ_y the Bingham yield stress or value (Fig. 4.8(b)). The equation implies that the rheogram is a straight line intersecting the shear stress axis at the yield value σ_y. In practice, flow occurs at a lower shear stress than σ_y and the flow curve gradually approaches the extrapolation of the linear portion of the line shown in Figure 4.8(b). This extrapolation will also give the Bingham or apparent yield value; the slope is the plastic viscosity.

Plastic flow is exhibited by concentrated suspensions, particularly if the continuous phase is of high viscosity or if the particles are flocculated.

Pseudoplastic flow

The rheogram shown in Figure 4.8(c) arises at the origin and, as no yield value exists, the material will

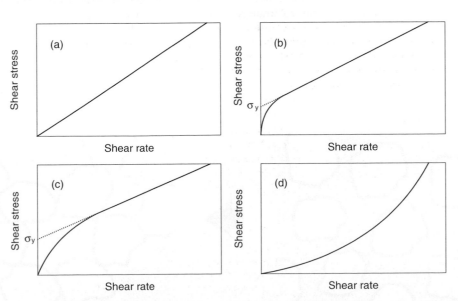

Fig. 4.8 Flow curves or rheograms representing the behaviour of various materials. (a) Newtonian, (b) plastic, (c) pseudoplastic and (d) dilatant.

flow as soon as a shear stress is applied; the slope of the curve gradually decreases with increasing rate of shear. The viscosity is derived from the slope and therefore decreases as the shear rate is increased. Materials exhibiting this behaviour are said to be pseudoplastic, and no single value of viscosity can be considered as characteristic. The viscosity can only be calculated from the slope of a tangent drawn to the curve at a specific point. Such viscosities are known as apparent viscosities and are only of any use if quoted in conjunction with the shear rate at which the determination was made. As it would need several apparent viscosities to characterize a pseudoplastic material, the most satisfactory representation is by means of the entire flow curve. However, it is frequently noted that at higher shear stresses the flow curve tends towards linearity, indicating that a minimum viscosity has been attained. When this is the case such a viscosity can be a useful means of classification.

There is no completely satisfactory quantitative explanation of pseudoplastic flow: probably the most widely used is the Power Law, which is given as:

$$\sigma^n = \eta' \gamma \qquad (4.29)$$

where η' is a viscosity coefficient and the exponent n an index of pseudoplasticity. When $n = 1$, then η' becomes the dynamic viscosity and Eqn 4.29 the same as Eqn 4.1, but as a material becomes more pseudoplastic then the value of n will fall. In order to obtain the values of the constants in Eqn 4.29, $\log \sigma$ must be plotted against $\log \gamma$, from which the slope will produce n and the intercept η'. The equation may only apply over a limited range (approximately one decade) of shear rates, and so it may not be applicable for all pharmaceutical materials and other models may have to be considered in order to fit the data. For example, the model known as Herschel–Bulkley, which can be given as:

$$\sigma = \sigma_y + K\gamma^n - 1 \qquad (4.30)$$

where K is a viscosity coefficient, is effectively a combination of Eqns 4.27 and 4.28 and can be of use for flow curves that are curvilinear and which intersect with the stress axis.

The materials that exhibit this type of flow include aqueous dispersions of natural and chemically modified hydrocolloids, such as tragacanth, methylcellulose and carmellose, and synthetic polymers such as polyvinylpyrrolidone and polyacrylic acid. The presence of long, high molecular weight molecules in solution results in entanglement together with the association of immobilized solvent. Under the influence of shear the molecules tend to become disentangled and align themselves in the direction of flow. They thus offer less resistance to flow and this, together with the release of some of the entrapped water, accounts for the lower viscosity. At any particular shear rate an equilibrium will be established between the shearing force and the re-entanglement brought about by Brownian motion.

Dilatant flow

The opposite type of flow to pseudoplasticity is depicted by the curve in Figure 4.8(d), in that the viscosity increases with increase in shear rate. As such materials increase in volume during shearing they are referred to as dilatant and exhibit shear thickening. An equation similar to that for pseudoplastic flow (Eqn 4.29) may be used to describe dilatant behaviour, but the value of the exponent n will be greater than 1 and will increase as dilatancy increases.

This type of behaviour is less common than plastic or pseudoplastic flow but may be exhibited by dispersions containing a high concentration ($\approx 50\%$) of small, deflocculated particles. Under conditions of

Fig. 4.9   Representation of the cause of dilatant behaviour

zero shear the particles are closely packed and the interparticulate voids are at a minimum (Fig. 4.9), which the vehicle is sufficient to fill. Consequently, at low shear rates such as those created during pouring this fluid can adequately lubricate the relative movement of the particles. As the shear rate is increased the particles become displaced from their even distribution and the clumps that are produced result in the creation of larger voids, into which the vehicle drains, so that the resistance to flow is increased and viscosity rises. The effect is progressive with increase in shear rate until eventually the material may appear paste-like as flow ceases. Fortunately, the effect is reversible and removal of the shear stress results in the re-establishment of the fluid nature.

Dilatancy can be a problem during the processing of dispersions and the granulation of tablet masses when high-speed blenders and mills are employed. If the material being processed becomes dilatant in nature then the resultant solidification could overload and damage the motor. Changing the batch or supplier of the material used could lead to processing problems, which can only be avoided by rheological evaluation of the dispersions prior to their introduction in the production process.

Time-dependent behaviour

In the description of the different types of non-Newtonian behaviour it was implied that although the viscosity of a fluid might vary with shear rate it was independent of the length of time that the shear rate was applied, and also that replicate determinations at the same shear rate would always produce the same viscosity. This must be considered as the ideal situation, as most non-Newtonian materials are colloidal in nature and, as such, the flowing elements, whether particles or macromolecules, may not adapt immediately to the new shearing conditions. Therefore, when such a material is subjected to a particular shear rate the shear stress, and consequently the viscosity, will decrease with time. Furthermore, once the shear stress has been removed, even if the structure which has been broken down is reversible, it may not return to its original structure (rheological ground state) instantly. The common feature of all these materials is that if they are subjected to a gradually increasing shear rate, followed immediately by a shear rate decreasing to zero, then the downcurve will be displaced with regard to the upcurve and the rheogram will exhibit a hysteresis loop (Fig. 4.10). In the case of plastic and pseudoplastic materials the downcurve will be displaced to the right of the upcurve

Fig. 4.10 Rheogram produced by a thixotropic pseudoplastic materials.

Fig. 4.11 Rheogram produced by a thixotropic dilatant material.

(Fig. 4.10), whereas for dilatant substances the reverse will be true (Fig. 4.11). The presence of the hysteresis loop indicates that a breakdown in structure has occurred, and the area within the loop may be used as an index of the degree of breakdown.

The term used to describe such behaviour is thixotropy, which means 'to change by touch', although strictly the term should only be applied to an isothermal sol–gel transformation. However, it has become common to describe as thixotropic any material that exhibits a reversible time-dependent decrease in apparent viscosity. Thixotropic systems are usually composed of asymmetric particles or macromolecules which are capable of interacting by numerous secondary bonds to produce a loose three-dimensional structure, so that the material is gel-like when unsheared. The energy imparted during shearing disrupts these bonds, so that the flowing elements become aligned and the viscosity falls, as a gel–sol transformation has occurred. When the shear stress is eventually removed the structure will tend to reform, although the process is not immediate and will increase with time as the molecules return to the original state under the influence of Brownian motion. Furthermore, the time taken for recovery, which can vary from minutes to days depending upon the system, will be directly related to the length of time the material was subjected to the shear stress, as this will affect the degree of breakdown.

In some cases the structure that has been destroyed is never recovered, no matter how long the system is left unsheared. Repeat determinations of the flow curve will then produce only the downcurve which was obtained in the experiment that resulted in the destruction. It is suggested that such behaviour be referred to as 'shear destruction' rather than thixotropy which, as will be appreciated from the above, is a misnomer in this case.

An example of such behaviour are the gels produced by high molecular weight polysaccharides which are stabilized by large numbers of secondary bonds. Such systems undergo extensive reorganization during shearing, such that the three-dimensional structure is reduced to a two-dimensional one: the gel-like nature of the original is then never recovered.

The occurrence of such complex behaviour creates problems in the quantitative classification because not only will the apparent viscosity change with shear rate, but there will also be two viscosities that can be calculated for any given shear rate (i.e. from the upcurve and the downcurve). It is usual to attempt to calculate one viscosity for the upcurve and another for the downcurve. This must of course assume that each of the curves achieves linearity over some of its length, otherwise a defined shear rate must be used; only the former situation is truly satisfactory. Each of the lines used to derive the viscosity may be extrapolated to the shear stress axis to give an associated yield value. However, only the one derived from the upcurve has any significance, as that derived from the downcurve will relate to the broken-down system. Consequently, the most useful index of thixotropy can be obtained by integration of the area contained within the loop. This will not of course take into account the shape of the up- and downcurves, and consequently two materials may produce loops of similar area but with completely different shapes representing totally different flow behaviours. In order to prevent confusion it is best to adopt a method whereby an estimate of area is accompanied by yield value(s). This is particularly important when complex upcurves exhibiting bulges are obtained, although it is now acknowledged that when these have been reported in the literature they might well have been a consequence of the design of the instrument, rather than providing information on three-dimensional structure. The evidence for this is based on the flow curves produced using more modern instruments, which do not exhibit the same, if any, bulges.

Determination of the flow properties of non-Newtonian fluids

With such a wide range of rheological behaviours it is extremely important to carry out measurements that will produce meaningful results. It is crucial therefore not to use a determination of viscosity at one shear rate (such as would be acceptable for a Newtonian fluid), as it could lead to completely erroneous comparative results. Figure 4.12 shows rheograms which are an example of the four different types of flow behaviour, all of which intersect at point A, which is equivalent to a shear rate of 100 s⁻¹. Therefore, if a measurement were made at this one shear rate, all four materials would be shown to have the same viscosity although they all possess different properties and behaviours. Single-point determinations are probably an extreme example but are used to emphasize the importance of properly designed experiments.

Rotational viscometers

These instruments rely on the viscous drag exerted on a body when it is rotated in the fluid to determine the viscosity of the fluid. The major advantage of such instruments is that wide ranges of shear rate can be achieved, and often a programme of shear rates can be produced automatically. Thus, the flow curve of a material may be obtained directly. A number of commercial instruments are available but each shares a common feature in that various measuring geometries can be used: often these have been concentric cylinder (or couette) and cone-

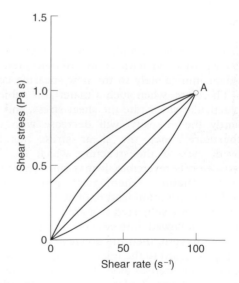

Fig. 4.12 Explanation of the effect of single-point viscosity determination and the resultant errors.

plate, although parallel-plate geometry is sometimes preferred.

Concentric cylinder In this geometry there are two coaxial cylinders of different diameters, the outer forming the cup containing the fluid in which the inner cylinder or bob is positioned centrally

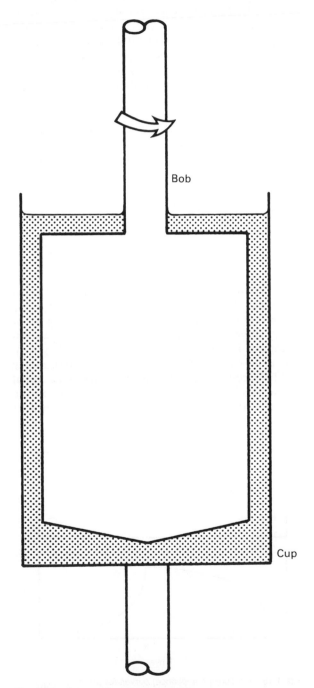

Fig. 4.13 Concentric cylinder geometry

(Fig. 4.13). In older types of instrument the outer cylinder is rotated and the viscous drag exerted by the fluid is transmitted to the inner cylinder as a torque, so that it rotates against a transducer such as a fine torsion wire. The stress on this inner cylinder is indicated by the angular deflection, θ, once equilibrium (i.e. steady flow) has been attained. The torque, T, can then be calculated from:

$$C\theta = T \qquad (4.31)$$

where C is the torsional constant of the wire. The viscosity is then given by:

$$\eta = \frac{\left(\dfrac{1}{r_1^2} - \dfrac{1}{r_2^2}\right) T}{4\pi h \omega} \qquad (4.32)$$

where r_1 and r_2 are the radii of the inner and outer cylinders, respectively, h is the height of the inner cylinder and ω is the angular velocity of the outer cylinder.

A rheometer of this type is described in the BP, although any instrument that has equivalent accuracy and precision may be used.

Cone–plate This geometry is composed of a flat circular plate with a wide-angle cone placed centrally above it (Fig. 4.14). The tip of the cone just touches the plate and the sample is loaded into the included gap. If the plate is rotated the cone will be caused to rotate against a torsion wire in the same way as the inner cylinder described above. Provided the angle is small (of the order of 1°) the viscosity will be given by:

$$\eta = \frac{3\omega T}{2\pi r^3 \alpha} \qquad (4.33)$$

where ω is the angular velocity of the plate, T is the torque, r is the radius of the cone and α is the angle between the cone and the plate.

Whether cone–plate or concentric cylinder geometry is used, instruments, particularly the

Fig. 4.14 Cone–plate geometry

more modern examples, have been modified to make measurements both easier and more accurate. The common modification is to make one part of the geometry, usually the plate or the outer cylinder, stationary and to rotate the other member at a constant speed. A torque sensor can then measure the developed shear stress. An alternative is to rotate the upper member under a constant stress when the developed shear rate is measured. Such controlled stress instruments consist of a specially designed induction motor which generates a torque that is independent of the degree or rate of rotation. Torque is not measured, as it is defined by the way the power is fed to the motor, which is connected to the measuring geometry through a rigid drive chain so that no motion is lost in the deflection of a torque sensor. It is then necessary only to detect the movement of the drive system and its associated measuring geometry by, for example, an optical encoder, in order to obtain the shear rate or strain. Both designs have been the subject of considerable sophistication, including the use of microcomputers for programming and data analysis. Also, having one part of the geometry stationary means that it can be circulated with water or other fluid at a temperature appropriate to the measurement.

Concentric cylinder viscometers are very useful for Newtonian and non-Newtonian fluids provided the latter are not too solid-like in nature. Wide ranges of shear rate can be achieved by varying the diameters of the cylinders. However, this geometry does suffer from disadvantages, the major one being that the shear rate across the gap is not constant, and this is especially the case when the gap is large. Also, the end effects can be significant, as Eqn 4.32 only takes into account the surfaces of the walls of the cylinders and not the ends. These end effects are usually accounted for by calibration of the instrument with a fluid of known viscosity. Frictional heating can be a problem at high shear rates, and so temperature control is essential with such instruments. Filling and cleaning are often difficult when the gap is small, but if it is large then the volume of sample required may be prohibitive.

Viscoelasticity

In the experiments described for rotational viscometers two observations are often made with pharmaceutical materials:

1. With cone-plate geometry the sample appears to 'roll up' and at high shear rates and is ejected from the gap.

2. With concentric cylinder geometry the sample will climb up the spindle of the rotating inner cylinder (Weissenberg effect).

The reason for both these phenomena is the same, in that the liquids are not exhibiting purely viscous behaviour but are viscoelastic. Such materials display solid and liquid properties simultaneously, and the factor that governs the actual behaviour is time. A whole spectrum of viscoelastic behaviour exists, from materials which are predominantly liquid to those that are predominantly solid. Under a constant stress all of these materials will dissipate some of the energy in viscous flow and store the remainder, which will be recovered when the stress is removed. The type of response can be seen in Figure 4.15(a), where a small, constant stress has been applied to a 2% gelatin gel and the resultant change in shape (strain) is measured. In the region A–B an initial elastic jump is observed, followed by a curved region B–C when the material is attempting to flow as a viscous fluid but is being retarded by its solid characteristics. At longer times equilibrium is established, such that for a system like this, which is ostensibly liquid, viscous flow will eventually predominate and the curve will become linear (C–D). If the concentration of gelatin in the gel had been increased to 30% then the resultant material would be more solid-like and no flow would be observed at longer times, and the curve would level out as shown in Figure 4.15(b). In the case of the liquid system, when the stress is removed only the stored energy will be recovered, and this is exhibited by an initial elastic recoil (D–E, Fig. 4.15(a)) equivalent to the region A–B and a retarded response E–F equivalent to B–C. There will be a displacement from the start-

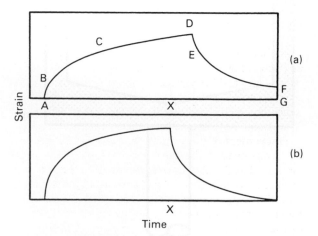

Fig. 4.15 Creep (or compliance) curves for (a) an uncrosslinked system and (b) a crosslinked system.

ing position (F–G) and this will be related to the amount of energy lost in viscous flow. For the higher-concentration gel all the energy will be recovered, so that only the regions D–E and E–F are observed.

This significance of time can be observed from the point X on the time axis. Although both systems are viscoelastic, and indeed are produced by different concentrations of the same biopolymer, in Figure 4.15(a) the sample is flowing like a high-viscosity fluid, whereas in Figure 4.15(b) it is behaving like a solid.

Creep testing

Both the experimental curves shown in Figure 4.15 are examples of a phenomenon known as creep. If the measured strain is divided by the stress – which, it should be remembered, is constant – then a compliance will be produced. The resultant curve, which will have the same shape as the original strain curve, then becomes known as a creep compliance curve and, as compliance is the reciprocal of elasticity, it will have the units $m^2 N^{-1}$ or Pa^{-1}. If the applied stress is below a certain limit (known as the linear viscoelastic limit) it will be directly related to the strain and the creep compliance curve will have the same shape and magnitude regardless of the stress used to obtain it. This curve therefore represents a fundamental property of the system, and derived parameters are characteristic and independent of the experimental method. For example, although it is common to use either cone-plate or concentric cylinders with viscoelastic pharmaceuticals, almost any measuring geometry can be used provided the shape of the sample can be defined.

It is common to analyse the creep compliance curve in terms of a mechanical model. An example of such a model is shown in Figure 4.16. This figure also indicates the regions on the curve shown in Figure 4.15(a) to which the components of the model relate. Thus, the instantaneous jump can be described by a perfectly elastic spring and the region of viscous flow by a piston fitted into a cylinder containing an ideal Newtonian fluid (this arrangement is referred to as a dashpot). In order to describe the behaviour in the intermediate region it is necessary to combine both these elements in parallel, such that the movement of the spring is retarded by the piston; this combination is known as a Voigt unit. It is implied that the elements of the model do not move until the preceding one has become fully extended, and although it is not feasible to associate the elements of the model with the molecular arrangement of the material it is possible to ascribe viscosities to the fluids in the cylinders and elasticities (or compliances) to the springs. Thus, a viscosity can be calcu-

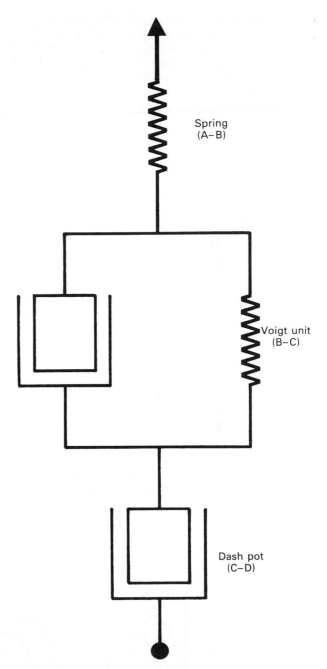

Fig. 4.16 Mechanical model representation of a creep compliance curve.

lated for the single dashpot (Fig. 4.16) from the reciprocal of the slope of the linear part of the creep compliance curve. This viscosity will be several orders of magnitude greater than that obtained by the conventional rotational techniques, and may be considered to be that of the rheological ground state

(η_0) as the creep test is non-destructive and should produce the same viscosity however many times it is repeated on the same sample. This is in direct contrast to continuous shear measurements, which destroy the structure being measured and with which it is seldom possible to obtain the same result on subsequent experiments on the same sample. The compliance (J_0) of the spring can be measured directly from the height of region A-B (Fig. 4.15(a)) and the reciprocal of this value will yield the elasticity, E_0. It is often the case that this value, together with η_0, provides an adequate characterization of the material. However, the remaining portion of the curve can be used to derive the viscosity and elasticity of the elements of the Voigt unit. The ratio of the viscosity to the elasticity is known as the retardation time, τ, and is a measure of the time taken for the unit to deform to $1/e$ of its total deformation. Consequently, more rigid materials will have longer retardation times and the more complex the material the greater number of Voigt units that are necessary to describe the creep curve.

It is also possible to use a mathematical expression to describe the creep compliance curve:

$$J(t) = J_o - \sum_{i=1}^{n} J_i \left(1 - e^{t/\tau_i}\right) + t/\eta_o \qquad (4.34)$$

where $J(t)$ is the compliance at time t, and J_i and τ_i are the compliance and retardation time, respectively, of the 'ith' Voigt unit. Both the model and the mathematical approach interpret the curve in terms of a line spectrum. It is also possible to produce a continuous spectrum in terms of the distribution of retardation times.

What is essentially the reverse of the creep compliance test is the stress relaxation test, where the sample is subjected to a predetermined strain and the stress required to maintain that strain is measured as a function of time. In this instance a spring and dashpot in series (Maxwell unit) can be used to describe the behaviour. Initially the spring will extend, and will then contract as the piston flows in the dashpot. Eventually the spring will be completely relaxed but the dashpot will be displaced, and in this case the ratio of viscosity to elasticity is referred to as the relaxation time.

Dynamic testing

Both creep and relaxation experiments are considered to be static tests. Viscoelastic materials can also be evaluated by means of dynamic experiments, whereby the sample is exposed to a forced sinusoidal oscillation and the transmitted stress measured. Once again, if the linear viscoelastic limit is not exceeded then the stress will also vary sinusoidally (Fig. 4.17). However, because of the nature of the material energy will be lost, so that the amplitude of the stress wave, will be less than that of the strain wave, it will also lag behind the strain wave. If the amplitude ratio and the phase lag can be measured, then the elasticity, referred to as the storage modulus, G', is given by:

$$G' = \left(\frac{\sigma}{\gamma}\right)\cos\delta \qquad (4.35)$$

where σ is the stress, γ is the strain and δ is the phase lag. A further modulus, G'', known as the loss modulus, is given by:

$$G'' = \left(\frac{\sigma}{\gamma}\right)\sin\delta \qquad (4.36)$$

This can be related to viscosity, η', by:

$$\eta' = \frac{G''}{\omega} \qquad (4.37)$$

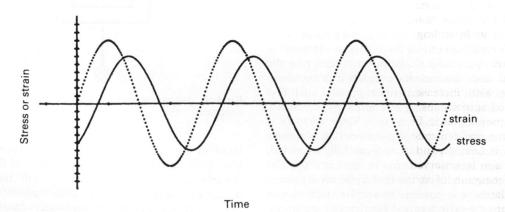

Fig. 4.17 Sine waves showing the stress wave lagging behind the strain wave by 60° during dynamic viscosity testing.

where ω is the frequency of oscillation in rad (s^{-1}). From Eqns 4.35 and 4.36 it can be seen that:

$$\frac{G''}{G'} = \tan\delta \qquad (4.38)$$

and tan δ is known as the loss tangent. Thus, a perfectly elastic material would produce a phase lag of 0°, whereas for a perfect fluid it would be 90°.

Finally, the concepts of liquid-like and solid-like behaviour can be explained by the dimensionless Deborah number (De), which finds expression as:

$$De = \frac{\tau}{T} \qquad (4.39)$$

where τ is a characteristic time of the material and T is a characteristic time of the deformation process. For a perfectly elastic material τ will be infinite, whereas for a Newtonian fluid it will be zero. High Deborah numbers can be produced either by high values of τ or as small values of T. The latter will occur in situations where high rates of strain are experienced, for example slapping water with the hand. Also, even solid materials would be predicted to flow if a high enough stress were applied for a sufficiently long time.

Suspensions

The rheological properties of suspensions are markedly affected by the degree of flocculation (see Chapter 6). The reason for this is that the amount of free continuous phase is reduced, as it becomes entrapped in the diffuse floccules. Consequently, the apparent viscosity of a flocculated suspension is normally higher than that of a suspension which is in all ways similar, with the exception that it is deflocculated. In addition, when a disperse system is highly flocculated then the possibility of interaction between floccules occurs and structured systems result. If the forces bonding floccules together are capable of withstanding weak stresses then a yield value will result, and below this value the suspension will behave like a solid. Once the yield value has been exceeded the amount of structural breakdown increases with increased shear stress. Therefore, flocculated suspensions will exhibit plastic or, more usually, pseudoplastic behaviour. Obviously, if the breakdown and reformation of the bonds between floccules is time dependent then thixotropic behaviour will also be observed.

The formation of structures does not occur in deflocculated suspensions and so their rheological behaviour is determined by that of the continuous phase together with the effect of distortion of the flow lines around the particles; in this situation the Einstein equation (Eqn 4.6) may apply. As the suspension becomes more concentrated and the particles come into contact, then dilatancy will occur.

Many pharmaceutical products, particularly those for children, are presented as suspensions and their rheological properties are important. In general these properties must be adjusted so that:

1. the product is easily administered (e.g. easily poured from a bottle or forced through a syringe needle);
2. sedimentation is either prevented or retarded; if it does occur, redispersion is easy;
3. the product has an elegant appearance.

Deflocculated particles in Newtonian vehicles

When such systems sediment a compact sediment or cake is produced which is difficult to redisperse. The rate of sedimentation can be reduced by increasing the viscosity of the continuous medium, which will remain Newtonian. However, there is a limit to which this viscosity can be increased because difficulty will be experienced, for example, in pouring the suspension from a bottle. Furthermore, if sedimentation does occur, then subsequent redispersion may be even more difficult.

Deflocculated particles in non-Newtonian vehicles

Only pseudoplastic or plastic dispersion media can be used in the formulation of suspensions and both will retard the sedimentation of small particles, as their apparent viscosities will be high under the small stresses associated with sedimentation. Also, as the medium will undergo structural breakdown under the higher stresses involved in shaking and pouring, both these processes are facilitated.

The hydrocolloids used as suspending agents, such as acacia, tragacanth, methylcellulose, gelatin and sodium carboxymethylcellulose, all impart non-Newtonian properties – normally pseudoplasticity – to the suspensions. Thixotropy can occur and this is particularly the case with the mineral clays, such as bentonite (which must only be used in suspensions for external use). The three-dimensional gel network traps the deflocculated particles at rest and their sedimentation is retarded and may be completely prevented. The gel network is destroyed during shaking so that administration is facilitated. It is desirable that the gel network is reformed quickly so that dispersion of the particles is maintained.

Flocculated particles in Newtonian vehicles

Such particles will still sediment, but because the aggregates are diffuse a large volume sediment is produced and, as such, is easier to disperse. These systems are seldom improved by an increase in the viscosity of the continuous phase as this will only influence the rate of sedimentation. The major problem is one of pharmaceutical inelegance, in that the sediment does not fill the whole of the fluid volume. Methods of improving such products are given in Chapters 6 and 23.

Flocculated particles in non-Newtonian vehicles

These systems combine the advantages of both methods. Furthermore, variations in the properties of the raw materials to be suspended are unlikely to influence the performance of a product made on production scale. Consequently, less difference will be observed between batches made by the same method and plant.

Emulsions

Because nearly all but the most dilute of medicinal emulsions exhibit non-Newtonian behaviour, their rheological characteristics have a marked effect on their usefulness. The fluid emulsions are usually pseudoplastic, and those approaching a semisolid nature behave plastically and exhibit marked yield values. The semisolid creams are usually viscoelastic. A considerable variety of pharmaceutical products can be formulated by altering the concentration of the disperse phase and the nature and concentration of the emulsifying agent. The latter can be used to confer viscoelastic properties on a topical cream merely by varying the ratio of surface-active agent to long-chain alcohol. These aspects are discussed further in Chapters 23 and 33.

THE EFFECT OF RHEOLOGICAL PROPERTIES ON BIOAVAILABILITY

The presence of the diffusion coefficient which is inversely related to viscosity in the constant k of the Noyes–Whitney equation (Chapter 2) means that the rate of dissolution of a drug particle will be decreased as the viscosity of the dissolution medium is increased. This will apply to both in vitro and in vivo situations, and usually the medium into which

the drug is dissolving will exhibit Newtonian behaviour. However, in the stomach the presence of the high molecular weight glycoproteins from mucus in acid solution will only be Newtonian up to a concentration of about 2%, beyond which it will exhibit non-Newtonian behaviour. In addition, the use of hydrocolloids will contribute to this effect and it has been shown that their inclusion in formulations can affect bioavailability. However, both increases and decreases in bioavailability have been reported, and it is not clear whether the effect is simply due to the modification of rheological properties or whether there has been an effect on gastrointestinal transit.

Attempts to predict this decrease in absorption have been made by the inclusion of natural or synthetic polymers in the dissolution medium used for in vitro studies. Some studies have shown that it is not the bulk viscosity of the dissolution medium that is of importance, but rather the 'effective viscosity'. Also, it is by no means certain that these polymers will behave in the same manner as the macromolecules that will be encountered in the gastrointestinal tract. Furthermore, it is impossible to carry out a dissolution test in an environment that relates to conditions in the region of the gut wall.

This viscosity effect will also operate at other drug delivery sites. For example, the absorption of drugs by the skin and from injection sites will be decreased by an increase in the viscosity of the vehicle. Indeed, in the case of injections the creation of a depot with a highly viscoelastic nature should result in prolonged delivery of the drug.

A proper understanding of rheological behaviour, both in the formulation and, if possible, at the absorption site, is essential in any evaluation of bioavailability.

BIBLIOGRAPHY

Barnes, H.A., Hutton, J.F. and Walters, K. (1989) *An Introduction to Rheology*, Elsevier Science, Amsterdam.

Barry, B.W. (1974) *Advances in Pharmaceutical Sciences*, (Eds H.S. Bean, A.W. Beckett and J.E. Carless), Vol 4, Chapter 1, Academic Press, London.

Ferry, J.D. (1980) *Viscoelastic Properties of Polymers*, John Wiley & Sons, New York.

Lapasin, R. and Pricl, S. (1999) *Rheology of Industrial Polysaccharides: Theory and Applications*, Aspen Publishers, Gaithersburg.

Ross-Murphy, S.B. (1994) In: *Physical Techniques for the Study of Food Biopolymers*, (Ed. S.B. Ross-Murphy), Chapter 7, Blackie Academic & Professional, Glasgow.

Schott, H. (1990) In: *Remington's Pharmaceutical Sciences*, 18th edn (Ed. R. Gennaro), Chapter 20, Mack Publishing Co., Easton, Pennsylvania.

5

Surface and interfacial phenomena

John Fell

The boundary between two phases is generally described as an interface. When one of the phases is a gas or a vapour, the term surface is frequently used. Matter at interfaces usually has different characteristics from that in the bulk of the media, and as a consequence the study of interfaces has developed into a separate branch of chemistry – surface chemistry. In pharmaceutical sciences interfacial phenomena play an important role in the processing of a wide variety of formulations. The subsequent behaviour of these formulations in vivo is often governed by an interfacial process.

Interfaces are categorized according to the phases they separate, as follows: liquid/liquid (L/L), liquid/vapour (L/V), solid/vapour (S/V) and solid/liquid (S/L). It is convenient to treat each interface separately.

SURFACE TENSION AND SURFACE FREE ENERGY

Consider the case of a single component liquid. The molecules in the liquid are subject to attractive forces from adjacent molecules. Figure 5.1 shows the attractive forces experienced by a molecule at the surface of the liquid. In the bulk of the liquid the molecules are subjected to equal attraction in all directions. At the surface, however, the net attractive force is towards the bulk of the liquid. This net

Fig. 5.1   Attractive forces at the surface and in the bulk of a material.

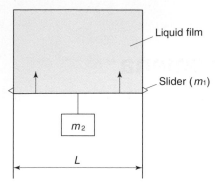

Liquid film

Slider (m_1)

m_2

L

Fig. 5.2 Liquid film attached to a freely moving slider.

inward attraction reduces the number of molecules in the surface and increases the intermolecular distance. It is this that gives the surface different characteristics from the bulk and gives rise to surface tension and surface free energy.

A useful approach to understanding these terms is to examine Figure 5.2. This shows parallel wires, joined at the top, on which there is a freely moving slider of length l and mass m_1. If a film of soap solution is formed between the upper wire and the slider, the film will rapidly contract owing to the surface tension forces (minimization of the free energy). The slider can be held in the original position by attaching a weight to it, (m_2), and this will give a measure of the surface tension. The same weight will hold the film in equilibrium even if it is expanded or contracted. This is because the surface is not stretched or contracted as such but remains the same, with molecules entering or leaving the bulk to compensate for the change in area.

The surface tension is therefore independent of the area of the film, but depends on the chemical nature of the interfaces and their length. In the example in Figure 5.2 there are two interfaces, on the front and the back of the film; the total length of the film/air interface is $2l$. The surface tension is the force acting parallel to the surface at right-angles to a line of 1 m length anywhere in the surface. Its units are typically mN m^{-1}. In the above example the surface tension (γ) is the force acting perpendicular to the surface, divided by the length of the surface, and is:

$$\gamma = \frac{(m_1 + m_2)g}{2l} = \frac{F}{2l} \qquad (5.1)$$

Where g is the acceleration due to gravity.

As explained earlier, if the film shown in Figure 5.2 is expanded no force is required. Work is done, however, because the area is increased. If the slider is moved a distance, x, the increase in total surface area

is $2lx$ as there are two surfaces, the front and back of the film. The work done is Fx. The surface free energy is defined as the work required to increase the surface area by 1 m^2. Typical units are mJ m^{-2}. The work done, per unit area, in expanding the film is

$$\frac{Fx}{2lx} = \frac{F}{2l} = \gamma \qquad (5.2)$$

The surface tension and the surface free energy are thus dimensionally equivalent (J = N m) and numerically equal.

The above concepts were derived from a consideration of a liquid/vapour system. Identical arguments can be used for liquid/liquid systems, the terminology being changed to interfacial free energy and interfacial tension. In principle the above argument also applies to solids, although it is easier to visualize the existence of the surface free energy of solids in terms of the unbalanced forces projecting from the interface, rather than the net inward attraction exerted on the molecules residing at the interface.

In this chapter, the symbol γ will be used to denote surface or interfacial tension. When it is necessary to distinguish between different surface or interfacial tensions, subscripts will be used. For example, $\gamma_{L/L}$ is the interfacial tension between two liquids and $\gamma_{L/V}$ is the surface tension between a liquid and its vapour. For more specific cases, γ_A will represent the surface tension of a liquid A and $\gamma_{A/B}$ the interfacial tension between liquids A and B.

Liquid/vapour systems

Curved surfaces

A pressure difference exists across curved surfaces to balance the influence of surface tension. A knowledge of this is important in some methods of the measurement of surface tension.

Consider a bubble of vapour in a liquid. In the absence of any external forces the bubble will be spherical in shape and will remain the same size because the surface tension forces are balanced by an internal excess pressure. This excess pressure is given by:

$$\Delta p = \frac{2\gamma}{r} \qquad (5.3)$$

where p is the excess pressure and r is the radius of the bubble. For non-spherical surfaces which can be described by two radii of curvature the equation becomes:

$$\Delta p = \gamma \left(\frac{1}{r_1} + \frac{1}{r_2} \right) \qquad (5.4)$$

This is known as the Laplace equation; γ is always positive. For p to be positive r must be positive, which means that the pressure is always greater on the concave side.

These equations (5.3 and 5.4) apply to any curved liquid interface, e.g. the system described above, a liquid film around a bubble in air, or the meniscus of a bulk liquid.

Influence of temperature

For the majority of liquids an increase in temperature leads to a decrease in surface tension. The exceptions are some molten metals. This decrease in surface tension with temperature is approximately linear. As the temperature approaches the critical temperature for a liquid (i.e. the temperature when the liquid structure is lost), the intermolecular cohesion forces approach zero and the surface tension becomes very small.

Liquid/liquid systems

The interfacial tension between two immiscible liquids arises as a result of imbalance of forces, in an identical manner to the surface tension between a liquid and its vapour. Interfacial tensions generally lie between the surface tensions of the two liquids under consideration. Table 5.1 lists the surface tensions of several liquids and their interfacial tensions against water.

Spreading

If a small quantity of an immiscible liquid is placed on a clean surface of a second liquid, it may spread to cover the surface with a film or remain as a drop or lens (Fig. 5.3). Which of the two applies depends

Fig. 5.3 Spreading of one liquid on another.

on the achievement of a state of minimum free energy. The ability of one liquid to spread over another can be assessed in terms of the spreading coefficient (S):

$$S = \gamma_A - (\gamma_B + \gamma_{A/B}) \qquad (5.5)$$

A positive or zero value of S is required for spreading to occur. An alternative approach is to examine spreading in terms of the work of cohesion and adhesion. The work of cohesion applies to a single liquid and is the work required to pull apart a column of liquid of unit cross-sectional area and create two liquid/air interfaces.

$$W_{A/A} = 2\gamma_A \qquad (5.6)$$

The work of adhesion is the work required to separate a unit cross-sectional area of a liquid/liquid interface to form two different liquid/air interfaces, and is given by the Dupre equation:

$$W_{A/B} = \gamma_A + \gamma_B - \gamma_{A/B} \qquad (5.7)$$

Hence, by substitution into Eqn 5.5:

$$S = W_{A/B} - W_{A/A} \qquad (5.8)$$

Therefore, spreading occurs when the liquid placed on, for example, a water surface adheres to the water more strongly than it coheres to itself.

In practice, when two immiscible liquids are placed in contact the bulk liquids will eventually become mutually saturated. This will change the values of the various surface and interfacial tensions. Hence, there is an initial spreading coefficient which is an immediate value, and a final spreading coefficient after mutual saturation has taken place. For benzene or hexanol on water the initial spreading coefficients are positive. When mutual saturation has occurred the values of the surface and interfacial tensions are reduced, so that the final spreading coefficients are negative. Hence benzene or hexanol spreads immediately on water and then the spreading stops, leaving a monomolecular layer of benzene or hexanol, with the remainder to the liquid in the form of flat lenses.

Measurement of surface and interfacial tension

There are several methods available for the measurement of surface and interfacial tension. Four will be

Table 5.1 The surface tensions of some common liquids and their interfacial tensions against water (mN m^{-1}), 20°C		
Liquid	Surface tension	Interfacial tension against water
Water	72	–
n-Octanol	27	8.5
Carbon tetrachloride	27	45
Chloroform	27	33
Olive oil	36	33
n-Hexane	18	51

described here. Further details and descriptions of other methods can be obtained by consulting the bibliography.

Wilhelmy plate methods

The apparatus consists of a thin mica, glass or platinum plate attached to a suitable balance (Fig. 5.4). When used as a detachment method, the plate is immersed in the liquid, and the liquid container is gradually lowered. The reading on the balance immediately prior to detachment is noted. The detachment force is equal to the surface tension multiplied by the perimeter of the surface detached:

$$W_L - W = 2(L + T)\gamma \qquad (5.9)$$

Where W_L is the reading on the balance prior to detachment, W is the weight of the plate in air and L and T are the length and the thickness of the plate, respectively. Immersion of the plate into the lower of two liquids in a container and subsequent detachment will give the interfacial tension.

Alternatively, the plate can be used in a static mode, where the change in force required to keep the plate at a constant depth is measured. This is useful for assessing changes in surface tension with time.

The method requires the contact angle that the liquid makes with the plate to be zero. This can be achieved by scrupulous cleaning and by roughening the surface of the plate. In addition, it must be ensured that the edge of the plate lies in a horizontal plane.

Ring method (du Nuoy tensiometer)

This method measures the force required to detach a platinum ring from a surface or an interface. Figure 5.5 shows the set-up for an interface. Again, the detachment force is equal to the surface tension multiplied by the perimeter of liquid detached, hence:

$$F = 2\pi(R_1 + R_2)\gamma \qquad (5.10)$$

Fig. 5.4 Wilhelmy plate method.

Fig. 5.5 Du Nuoy tensiometer being used to measure interfacial tension.

where F is the detachment force and R_1 and R_2 are the inner and outer radii of the ring. Again, a zero contact angle of the liquid on the ring must be assured or the equation will not hold. This can be achieved by careful cleaning and flaming of the platinum loop, or by the use of a silicone-treated ring for oils. The ring must also lie horizontally in the surface.

As the shape of the liquid supported by the ring during detachment is complex and hence the surface tension forces do not act vertically, the above simple equation is in error and correction factors must be applied for accurate determinations.

Drop weight and drop volume methods

If the volume or weight of a drop as it is detached from a tip of known radius is determined, the surface or interfacial tension can be calculated from:

$$\gamma = \frac{\phi mg}{2\pi r} = \frac{\phi V\rho g}{2\pi r} \qquad (5.11)$$

where m is the mass of the drop, V is the volume of the drop, ρ is the density of the liquid, r is the radius of the tip, g is the acceleration due to gravity and ϕ is a correction factor. A typical apparatus is shown in Figure 5.6. The method is easily adapted for both surface and interfacial tensions and is therefore popular. The correction factor is required as not all the drop leaves the tip on detachment. The correction factors are shown in Figure 5.7 and depend on the radius of the tip and the drop volume. It is important that the tip is completely wetted by the liquid, and that the drop does not 'climb' up the outside of the tube. The drop should also be formed slowly, especially in the stage immediately preceding detachment.

Capillary rise method

Although this method is used little in pharmaceutical research, it is considered to be the most accurate

Fig. 5.6 Drop volume or drop weight method.

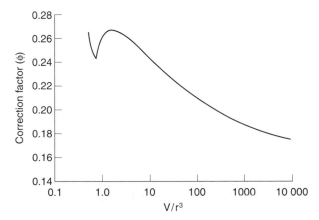

Fig. 5.7 Correction factors for the drop volume or drop weight method.

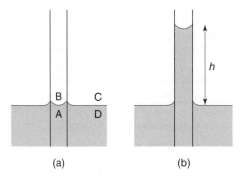

Fig. 5.8 Stages in the rise of a liquid up a capillary tube.

$$\Delta p = \frac{2\gamma \cos\theta}{r_t} \qquad (5.13)$$

which is the pressure difference between atmospheric and that immediately below the meniscus. Referring to Figure 5.8, the pressure at point B is atmospheric, whereas that at point A is less by an amount given by Eqn 5.4. At point C the pressure is atmospheric, as it also is at point D, as the liquid here is effectively flat, i.e. the radius of curvature of the meniscus is large. The pressure difference between D and A causes the liquid to rise in the capillary tube until the difference is balanced by the hydrostatic pressure of the column of liquid. At this equilibrium point:

$$\frac{2\gamma \cos\theta}{r_t} = h(\rho_L - \rho_V)g \qquad (5.14)$$

Where $\rho_L - \rho_V$ is the density difference between the liquid and its vapour, g is the acceleration due to gravity and h is the height of the liquid in the capillary tube.

As contact angles are difficult to reproduce, experiments are always run at $\theta = 0$, ($\cos\theta = 1$), achieved by careful cleaning. Hence the equation reduces to:

$$\gamma = \frac{r_t h(\rho_L - \rho_V)}{2}g \qquad (5.15)$$

The capillaries used must be circular in cross-section and of uniform bore. As with all methods of measuring surface and interfacial tension, cleanliness at all stages of the experiment is vital and adequate temperature control must be ensured.

Solid/vapour and solid/liquid systems

Liquid surfaces and interfaces are open to direct, simple experimental procedures for determining surface and interfacial tensions. Methods for determining similar parameters for solids are indirect and difficult. The system of most interest pharmaceutically is the behaviour of a liquid in contact with a solid.

way of measuring surface tension and has been used to establish values for many liquids. As the surface of the liquid is undisturbed during the measurement, time effects can be followed.

If a capillary tube is placed in a liquid, provided the angle of contact that the liquid makes with the capillary tube is less than 90°, the liquid will rise in the tube to a certain height. Figure 5.8 shows a diagrammatic representation of this.

If the tube is small in diameter the meniscus can be considered to be hemispherical, and the radius of curvature will be:

$$r_t = r_m\cos\theta \qquad (5.12)$$

where r_t is the radius of the capillary tube, r_m is the radius of curvature of the meniscus and θ is the contact angle. Hence, from the Laplace equation (Eqn 5.3) for this system:

Contact angle

If a drop of liquid is placed on a flat, smooth, horizontal solid surface it may spread completely, but is more likely to form a drop. This drop will exhibit a definite angle against the solid, known as the contact angle (Fig. 5.9). By equating the horizontal component of the various interfacial tensions, the following equation (Young's equation) is derived:

$$\gamma_{S/V} = \gamma_{S/L} + \gamma_{L/V}\cos\theta \qquad (5.16)$$

The work of adhesion between the solid and the liquid is given by the appropriate form of the Dupre equation (Eqn 5.7):

$$W_{S/L} = \gamma_{S/V} + \gamma_{L/V} - \gamma_{S/L} \qquad (5.17)$$

Combining this with Eqn 5.16 gives the following:

$$W_{S/L} = \gamma_{L/V}(1 + \cos\theta) \qquad (5.18)$$

This means that the work of adhesion between the solid and the liquid can be determined in terms of measurable quantities.

In a similar manner to liquids, a spreading coefficient (S) for a liquid on a solid may be defined as:

$$S = \gamma_{L/V}(\cos\theta - 1) \qquad (5.19)$$

which will give a measure of how well a liquid will spread on a solid. If a liquid is penetrating into a capillary, for example the pores in a powder bed or a tablet, the value of interest is the adhesion tension (AT), given by:

$$AT = \gamma_{L/V}\cos\theta \qquad (5.20)$$

As $\gamma_{L/V}$ is always positive, the spontaneity of these processes will be controlled by $\cos\theta$. For example, for penetration into capillaries under no extra applied pressure the adhesion tension must be positive, hence $\cos\theta$ must be positive, i.e. the contact angle, θ, must be less than 90°.

The determination of contact angles for materials that are available as flat smooth solid surfaces is relatively straightforward. A drop of liquid is placed on the surface and the angle it makes with the surface can be measured directly by magnifying the drop in some way. Unfortunately, most materials of pharmaceutical interest are powders, and direct measurement on individual particles is not usually possible. Direct measurement can be achieved by compressing the powder into a compact. The problem here is that the application of high pressure may change the characteristics of the particles and alter the contact angle. Figure 5.10 shows this has occurred with amylobarbitone, the measured contact angle changing as the pressure is increased. The h–ε method also uses a compact, but prepared at a lower pressure and saturated with the test liquid. A liquid drop is then formed on the surface of this saturated compact and the maximum height of this drop is related to the contact angle.

Another method that uses a compact is dynamic contact angle analysis. Here the powder is compressed into a thin rectangular plate and the method used is the same as the Wilhelmy plate method for measuring surface tension. The liquid forms a contact angle with the plate, as shown in Figure 5.11. The contact angle is given by:

$$\cos\theta = \frac{F}{\gamma\,2(L+T)} \qquad (5.21)$$

Fig. 5.10 Changes in the contact angle of amylobarbitone with the pressure used to form the compact (from Buckton et al. Powder Technology 1986; 46: 201–208, with permission from Elsevier Science).

Fig. 5.9 Contact angles of liquids on solids

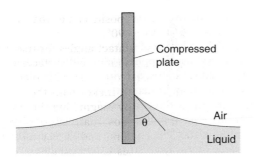

Fig. 5.11 Measurement of contact angles using dynamic contact angle analysis.

Table 5.2 The contact angles of some pharmaceutical solids against their saturated aqueous solutions	
Material	Contact angle (°)
Acetylsalicylic acid	74
Amylobarbitone	102
Diazepam	83
Lactose	30
Magnesium stearate	121
Paracetamol	59
Digoxin	49
Ampicillin	35
Indomethacin	90
Sulphanilamide	64

Compare this to the determination of surface tension by the Wilhelmy plate.

To measure the contact angle of a powder without compaction, the Washburn method can be used. Here, a powder bed is formed in a tube fitted with a sintered glass filter at the base. The base of the tube is immersed in liquid and the liquid will penetrate into the capillaries between the powder particles as shown earlier, in Figure 5.8. The rate of penetration is measured and, if the capillaries in the powder bed are regarded as being a bundle of capillary tubes, the rate of penetration is given by:

$$\frac{L^2}{t} = \gamma \frac{\cos\theta\; r}{2\;\eta} \qquad (5.22)$$

where L is the length penetrated in time t, r is the radius of the capillaries, η is the liquid viscosity and γ and θ are the surface tension and the contact angle of the liquid, respectively.

L^2/t is measured in the experiment, the liquid characteristics η and γ are known or can be easily measured; the problem is in determining r. This can be solved by measuring the rate of penetration, L^2/t, into the powder in an identical state of packing, using a liquid that has a zero contact angle against the powder. Substituting this into Eqn 5.22 gives a value for r which can then be used in the equation to determine the required value of θ.

Examples illustrating the range of contact angle values found for pharmaceutical powders are given in Table 5.2.

Pharmaceutical applications

Many pharmaceutical processes involve interactions at the interfaces described. The preparation of emulsions and suspensions, described in Chapters 6 and 23, involves interactions at the liquid/liquid and liquid/solid interfaces, respectively. Interactions between a liquid and a solid are particularly common. Granulation, prior to tabletting, involves the mixing of a powder with a liquid binder and the success of the process will, in part, depend on the spreading of the liquid over the solid. A rational approach to the selection of a granulating agent, based on the measurement of spreading coefficients and other surface properties, has been described by Rowe (1989). Similarly, film coating requires the spread of liquid over a tablet surface. The successful dissolution of a tablet or capsule necessitates penetration of the liquid into the pores of the dosage form. In all these examples the contact angle and the surface tension of the liquid are important. Surface-active agents are commonly employed in formulation as they reduce the contact angle and hence aid in the wetting of a solid by reducing $\gamma_{L/V}$, and also absorbing at the solid/liquid interface and reducing $\gamma_{S/V}$.

ADSORPTION

Liquid/vapour and liquid/liquid systems

Surface-active agents

Many compounds have structures that contain two separate regions, a hydrophilic (water-liking) region which confers on the compound a solubility in water, and a hydrophobic (water-hating) region which renders the material soluble in hydrocarbon solvents. Because of this dual structure, it is energetically favourable for these materials, when dissolved, to adsorb at interfaces, orientating themselves in such a manner that the regions are associated with the appropriate solvent or air. Such materials are termed surface-active agents (or surfactants). Details of their structures and properties are given in Chapters 6 and 23.

Pure liquid surfaces have a tendency to contract as a result of surface tension forces. The packing of the surface with surface-active molecules favours expansion of the surface. The surface-active molecules reduce the surface tension of the liquid by an amount equal to the expanding (or surface) pressure. Surfactants will lower surface tension to different degrees. An approximation, Traube's rule, states that for a particular homologous series of surfactants in dilute solution, the concentration necessary to produce an equal lowering of surface tension decreases by a factor of three for each additional CH_2 group. The formation of the adsorbed surface layer will not be instantaneous, but will be governed by the diffusion of the surfactant to the interface. The time taken to reach equilibrium will depend on factors such as molecular size, shape and the presence of impurities. For immiscible liquids, the reduction in interfacial tension may be such that emulsification takes place readily. Detailed aspects of this are dealt with in Chapter 6.

In certain cases a 'negative adsorption' may occur, i.e. the solute molecules migrate away from the surface. In these cases, examples of which are solutions of sugars and electrolytes, small increases in surface tension are observed.

Surface excess concentration

The extent of the distribution of a solute between an interface and the bulk phase is generally expressed in terms of a surface excess, n. This is the amount of a material present at the interface in excess of that which would have been there if the bulk phase extended to the interface without a change in composition.

The surface excess concentration, Γ, is n/A where A is the area of the interface.

The adsorption of material at any interface is given by the Gibbs adsorption equation. Its general form is:

$$d\gamma = -\Sigma \Gamma i du_i \qquad (5.23)$$

where d is the change in interfacial tension, Γ is the surface excess concentration of the ith component and u_i is the chemical potential of the ith component.

In the specific case of a solute partitioning between the surface and the bulk of a liquid, the equation becomes:

$$\Gamma = \frac{C}{RT}\frac{d\gamma_{L/V}}{dC} \qquad (5.24)$$

where C is the overall solute concentration, R is the gas constant, T is the absolute temperature and $d\gamma_{LV}/dC$ is the change of surface tension with concentration. The above is applicable to dilute solutions. For concentrated solutions, activities must be substituted for concentration. Equation 5.24 has been verified experimentally by direct measurement of surface concentrations after removal of the surface layer with a microtome blade. The equation enables calculation of the surface excess from surface tension data.

As the concentration of a surface-active agent in aqueous solution is increased, the surface layer will eventually become saturated. Figure 5.12 shows a typical plot of surface tension against concentration. When the surface layer is saturated, further increases in concentration can no longer change the surface tension and the surfactant molecules form micelles (small aggregates of molecules) as an alternative means of 'protecting' the hydrophobic regions. Details of these are given in Chapter 6.

The discontinuity of the plot in Figure 5.12 is called the critical micelle concentration. Immediately before this the surfactant molecules are closely packed at the surface, and this gives a method of determining the surface area occupied by each molecule, A, from:

$$A = \frac{1}{N_A \Gamma} \qquad (5.25)$$

Where N_A is the Avogadro constant and Γ is the surface excess concentration calculated from the slope of the plot $d\gamma_{LV}/d \log C$ immediately before the critical micelle concentration (remember that Γ is a concentration expressed in terms of surface area).

Because of their structures many drugs are surface active in nature, and this activity may play a part in their pharmacological effects. Examples are some

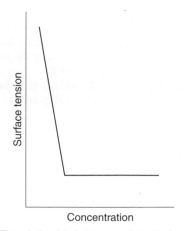

Fig. 5.12 The relationship between surface tension and concentration for a typical surfactant.

antihistamines, the phenothiazine tranquillizers and antidepressants.

Monomolecular films (monolayers)

Certain insoluble materials can, when dissolved in a suitable volatile solvent, be made to spread on the surface of water to form a film one molecule thick. This may be regarded as an extreme case of adsorption, as all the molecules are at the surface. Surface excess concentrations can be calculated directly from a knowledge of the amount of material and the surface area. The monolayer will reduce the surface tension of the water by an amount equal to the surface pressure. The surface pressure, which is the expanding pressure due to the monolayer opposing the contracting tension of the water, can be measured directly by enclosing the film between moveable barriers.

$$\pi = \gamma_o - \gamma_m \qquad (5.26)$$

where π is the surface pressure, γ_o is the surface tension of the 'clean' liquid and γ_m the surface tension of the liquid covered with a monolayer.

Monolayers exist in different physical states which are in some ways analogous to the three states of matter: solid, liquid and gas. Pharmaceutically, monolayers have been used to study polymers which are used for film coating and packaging, and as models for cell membranes.

Solid/vapour systems

Although adsorption in solid/liquid systems is of more interest pharmaceutically, the interpretation of results is often achieved using equations developed for solid/vapour systems. This system will therefore be described first.

If a gas or vapour is brought into contact with a solid, some of it will become attached to the surface. This reduces the imbalance of attractive forces and hence the surface free energy. Adsorption here must be distinguished from absorption, where penetration into the solid may take place. In some cases it may be impossible to distinguish between the two. Here the general term sorption is used. Adsorption may be by relatively weak non-specific forces (van der Waals forces), this being termed physical adsorption. Alternatively, the adsorption may be by stronger specific valence forces – chemisorption. Physical absorption is rapid and reversible, and multilayer adsorption is possible. Chemisorption is specific, may require an activation energy, and therefore be slow and not readily reversible. Only monomolecular chemisorbed layers are possible.

Adsorption studies using gases or vapour generally involve the determination of the amount of gas or vapour adsorbed, x, by a given mass, m, of the adsorbent at constant temperature. Determinations are carried out at different equilibrium pressures p, (the pressure attained after adsorption has taken place) to yield an adsorption isotherm. When vapours are used the results are generally expressed in terms of a relative vapour pressure p/p_o where p_o is the saturated vapour pressure. Prior to the studies the solid adsorbent must have any adsorbed material removed by placing it under vacuum or heating.

The isotherms obtained can generally be classified into five types, shown in Figure 5.13. Type I isotherms exhibit a rapid rise in adsorption up to a limiting value. They are referred to as Langmuir-type isotherms and are due to the adsorption being restricted to a monolayer. Hence adsorption of the chemisorption type will give this type of curve. Type II isotherms represent multilayer physical adsorption on non-porous materials. Types III and V occur when the adsorption in the first layer is weak, and are rare. Type IV is considered to be due to condensation of vapour in fine capillaries within a porous solid. There have been many attempts to develop equations to fit the experimentally observed isotherm. Among the most widely used expressions are the following.

Langmuir adsorption isotherm

The equation was derived by assuming that only monolayer coverage was possible, and so it is only

Fig. 5.13 Classification of isotherms for the adsorption of vapours by solids. Ordinates x/m, abscissae p/p_o.

applicable to type I isotherms. The equation is usefully written as:

$$p\frac{m}{x} = \frac{1}{b}p + \frac{1}{ab} \qquad (5.27)$$

where p, m and x are as defined previously and b and a are constants, b being the amount of gas required to produce a monolayer over the whole surface of the absorbent. Hence plotting pm/x against p should give a straight line with a slope $1/b$ and intercept $1/ab$.

Freundlich adsorption isotherm

This is given as:

$$\frac{x}{m} = kp^{1/n} \qquad (5.28)$$

where n and k are constants for a particular system. Plots of log x/m against log p should therefore give straight lines. The equation does not predict a limiting value as does the Langmuir equation.

Brunauer, Emmett and Teller (BET) equation

This equation takes into account multilayer adsorption and so describes type II isotherms. It is usually written in the form:

$$\frac{p}{V(p_0 - p)} = \frac{1}{V_m c} + \frac{c-1}{V_m c} x \frac{p}{p_0} \qquad (5.29)$$

Where p_0 is the saturation vapour pressure, V is the equilibrium volume of gas adsorbed per unit mass of adsorbent, V_m is the volume of gas required to cover unit mass of adsorbent with monolayer, and c is a constant. The equation reduces to the Langmuir equation if adsorption is restricted to monolayer formation.

One direct practical application of the adsorption of gases of pharmaceutical interest is the determination of the surface area of powders. If the isotherm is determined and the point of monolayer formation identified, a knowledge of the surface area of the adsorbing species will give a value for the surface area of the powder.

Solid/liquid systems

The adsorption of most interest is that of a solute, in solution, on to a solid. The equations most widely used to interpret the data are those of Langmuir and Freundlich. The pressure terms are replaced by concentration terms, hence the Langmuir equation becomes:

$$\frac{x}{m} = \frac{abC}{1+bC} \qquad (5.30)$$

where x is the amount of solute adsorbed by a weight, m, of adsorbent, C is the concentration of the solution at equilibrium, and b and a are constants.

Adsorption from solution

Several factors will affect the extent of adsorption from solution. These include the following.

Solute concentration An increase in the concentration of the solute will cause an increase in the amount of absorption that occurs at equilibrium until a limiting value is reached. It should be noted that for most cases of adsorption from solution, the relative amount of solute removed is greater in dilute solutions.

Temperature Adsorption is generally exothermic, and hence an increase in temperature leads to a decrease in adsorption.

pH The influence of pH is usually through a change in the ionization of the solute and the influence will depend on which species is more strongly adsorbed.

Surface area of adsorbent An increased surface area, achieved by a reduction in particle size or the use of a porous material, will increase the extent of adsorption.

Pharmaceutical applications of adsorption from solution

The phenomenon of adsorption from solution finds practical application of pharmaceutical interest in chromatographic techniques and in the removal of unwanted materials. In addition, adsorption may give rise to certain formulation problems.

The role of adsorption in chromatography is outside the scope of this book. Materials such as activated charcoal can be given in cases of orally taken poisons to adsorb the toxic materials. In addition, adsorbents may be used in haemodialysis to remove the products of dialysis from the dialysing solution, allowing the solution to be recycled. Adsorption may cause problems in formulation where drugs or other materials such as preservatives are adsorbed by containers, thereby reducing the effective concentration In addition, certain additives, such as the parabens, may be adsorbed on to the solid material present in a suspension, leading to a loss in antimicrobial activity (Allwood 1982). Glyceryl trinitrate is a volatile solid given in the form of tablets. The vapour may be sorbed by the container, leading to further volatilization and loss of potency. The adsorption of insulin on to intravenous administration sets has been reported, as has the sorption of phenylmercuric acetate, used as a preservative in eye drops, on to polyethylene containers (Aspinall et al 1980).

REFERENCES

Allwood, M.C. (1982) The adsorption of esters of *p*-hydroxybenzoic acid by magnesium trisilicate. *Int. J. Pharm.*, **11**, 101–107.
Aspinall, J.D., Duffy, T.D., Saunders, M.B. and Taylor, C.G. (1980) The effect of low density polyethylene containers on some hospital manufactured eye-drop formulations: sorption of phenyl mercuric acetate. *J. Clin. Hosp. Pharm.*, **5**, 21–30.
Rowe, R.C. (1989) Binder-substrate interactions in granulation: a theoretical approach based on surface free energy and polarity. *Int. J. Pharm.*, **52**, 149–154.

BIBLIOGRAPHY

Adamson, A.W. (1980) *Physical Chemistry of Surfaces*, 4th edn. John Wiley, New York.
Florence, A.T. and Attwood, D. (1998) *Physicochemical Principles of Pharmacy*, 3rd edn. Macmillan, London.
Shaw, D.J. (1992) *Introduction to Colloid and Surface Chemistry*, 4th edn. Butterworths, London.

6

Disperse systems

David Attwood

A disperse system consists essentially of one component, the ***disperse phase***, dispersed as particles or droplets throughout another component, the ***continuous phase***. By definition, dispersions in which the size of the dispersed particles is within the range 10^{-9} m (1 nm) to about 10^{-6} m (1 μm) are termed colloidal. However, the upper size limit is often extended to include emulsions and suspensions, which are very polydisperse systems in which the droplet size frequently exceeds 1 μm but which show many of the properties of colloidal systems. Some examples of colloidal systems of pharmaceutical interest are shown in Table 6.1. Many natural systems, such as suspensions of microorganisms, blood and isolated cells in culture, are also colloidal dispersions. In this chapter we will examine the properties of both coarse dispersions, such as emulsions, suspensions and aerosols, and fine dispersions, such as micellar systems, which fall within the defined size range of true colloidal dispersions.

Colloids can be broadly classified as those that are ***lyophobic*** (solvent-hating) and those that are ***lyophilic*** (solvent-liking). When the solvent is water the terms ***hydrophobic*** and ***hydrophilic*** are used. Surfactant molecules tend to associate in water into aggregates called micelles, and these constitute hydrophilic colloidal dispersions. Proteins and gums also form lyophilic colloidal systems because of a similar affinity between the dispersed particles and the continuous phase. On the other hand, dispersions of oil droplets in water or water droplets in oil are examples of lyophobic dispersions.

It is because of the subdivision of matter in colloidal systems that they have special properties. A common feature of these systems is a large surface-to-volume ratio of the dispersed particles. As a consequence there is a tendency for the particles to associate to reduce their surface area. Emulsion droplets, for example, eventually coalesce to form a macrophase, thereby attaining a minimum surface area and hence an equilibrium state. In this chapter we will examine how the stability of colloidal dispersions can be understood by a consideration of the forces acting between the dispersed particles. Approaches to the formulation of emulsions, suspensions and aerosols will be described and the instability of these coarse dispersions will be discussed using a theory of colloid stability. The association of surface-active agents into micelles and the applications of these colloidal dispersions in the solubilization of poorly water-soluble drugs will also be considered.

Table 6.1	Types of disperse systems		
Dispersed phase	Dispersion medium	Name	Examples
Liquid	Gas	Liquid aerosol	Fogs, mists, aerosols
Solid	Gas	Solid aerosol	Smoke, powder aerosols
Gas	Liquid	Foam	Foam on surfactant solutions
Liquid	Liquid	Emulsion	Milk, pharmaceutical emulsions
Solid	Liquid	Sol, suspension	Silver iodide sol, aluminium hydroxide suspension
Gas	Solid	Solid foam	Expanded polystyrene
Liquid	Solid	Solid emulsion	Liquids dispersed in soft paraffin, opals, pearls
Solid	Solid	Solid suspension	Pigmented plastics, colloidal gold in glass, ruby glass

COLLOIDS

Preparation and purification of colloidal systems

Lyophilic colloids

The affinity of lyophilic colloids for the dispersion medium leads to the spontaneous formation of colloidal dispersions. For example, acacia, tragacanth, methylcellulose and certain other cellulose derivatives readily disperse in water. This simple method of dispersion is a general one for the formation of lyophilic colloids.

Lyophobic colloids

The preparative methods for lyophobic colloids may be divided into those methods that involve the breakdown of larger particles into particles of colloidal dimensions (dispersion methods) and those in which the colloidal particles are formed by the aggregation of smaller particles such as molecules (condensation methods).

Dispersion methods The breakdown of coarse material may be effected by the use of a colloid mill or ultrasonics.

Colloid mills These cause the dispersion of coarse material by shearing in a narrow gap between a static cone (the stator) and a rapidly rotating cone (the rotor).

Ultrasonic treatment The passage of ultrasonic waves through a dispersion medium produces alternating regions of cavitation and compression in the medium. The cavities collapse with great force and cause the breakdown of coarse particles dispersed in the liquid.

With both these methods the particles will tend to reunite unless a stabilizing agent such as a surface-active agent is added.

Condensation methods These involve the rapid production of supersaturated solutions of the colloidal material under conditions in which it is deposited in the dispersion medium as colloidal particles and not as a precipitate. The supersaturation is often obtained by means of a chemical reaction that results in the formation of the colloidal material. For example, colloidal silver iodide may be obtained by reacting together dilute solutions of silver nitrate and potassium iodide; colloidal sulphur is produced from sodium thiosulphate and hydrochloric acid solutions; and ferric chloride boiled with an excess of water produces colloidal hydrated ferric oxide.

A change of solvent may also cause the production of colloidal particles by condensation methods. If a saturated solution of sulphur in acetone is poured slowly into hot water the acetone vaporizes, leaving a colloidal dispersion of sulphur. A similar dispersion may be obtained when a solution of a resin, such as benzoin in alcohol, is poured into water.

Dialysis

Colloidal particles are not retained by conventional filter papers but are too large to diffuse through the pores of membranes such as those made from regenerated cellulose products, e.g. collodion (cellulose nitrate evaporated from a solution in alcohol and ether) and cellophane. The smaller particles in solution are able to pass through these membranes. Use is made of this difference in diffusibility to separate micromolecular impurities from colloidal dispersions. The process is known as dialysis. The process of dialysis may be hastened by stirring, so as to maintain a high concentration gradient of diffusible molecules across the membrane and by renewing the outer liquid from time to time.

Ultrafiltration By applying pressure (or suction) the solvent and small particles may be forced across a membrane but the larger colloidal particles are retained. This process is referred to as ultrafiltration.

It is possible to prepare membrane filters with a known pore size, and the use of these allows the particle size of a colloid to be determined. However, particle size and pore size cannot be properly correlated because the membrane permeability is affected by factors such as electrical repulsion, when both the membrane and the particle carry the same charge, and particle adsorption, which can lead to blocking of the pores.

Electrodialysis An electric potential may be used to increase the rate of movement of ionic impurities through a dialysing membrane and so provide a more rapid means of purification. The concentration of charged colloidal particles at one side and at the base of the membrane is termed electrodecantation.

Pharmaceutical applications of dialysis Dialysis is the basis of a method – haemodialysis – whereby small molecular weight impurities from the body are removed by passage through a membrane. Other applications involving dialysis include the use of membranes for filtration, and as models for the diffusion of drugs through natural membranes.

Properties of colloids

Size and shape of colloidal particles

Size distribution Within the size range of colloidal dimensions specified above there is often a wide distribution of sizes of the dispersed colloidal particles. The molecular weight or particle size is therefore an average value, the magnitude of which is dependent on the experimental technique used in its measurement. When determined by the measurement of colligative properties such as osmotic pressure a number average value, M_n, is obtained, which in a mixture containing $n_1, n_2, n_3, \ldots$ moles of particle of mass $M_1, M_2, M_3 \ldots$, respectively, is defined by:

$$M_n = \frac{n_1 M_1 + n_2 M_2 + n_3 M_3 + \ldots}{n_1 + n_2 + n_3 + \ldots} = \frac{\Sigma n_i M_i}{\Sigma n_i} \quad (6.1)$$

In the light-scattering method for the measurement of particle size, larger particles produce greater scattering and the weight rather than the number of particles is important, giving a weight average value, M_w, defined by:

$$M_w = \frac{m_1 M_1 + m_2 M_2 + m_3 M_3 + \ldots}{m_1 + m_2 + m_3 + \ldots} = \frac{\Sigma n_i M_i^2}{\Sigma n_i M_i} \quad (6.2)$$

In Eqn 6.2 m_1, m_2, and m_3 ... are the masses of each species, and m_i is obtained by multiplying the mass of each species by the number of particles of that species, that is, $m_i = n_i M_i$. A consequence is that $M_w > M_n$, and only when the system is monodisperse will the two averages be identical. The ratio M_w/M_n expresses the degree of polydispersity of the system.

Shape Many colloidal systems, including emulsions, liquid aerosols and most dilute micellar solutions, contain spherical particles. Small deviations from sphericity are often treated using ellipsoidal models. Ellipsoids of revolution are characterized by their axial ratio, which is the ratio of the half-axis a to the radius of revolution b (Fig. 6.1). Where this ratio is greater than unity, the ellipsoid is said to be a prolate (rugby ball-shaped) ellipsoid, and when less than unity an oblate (discus-shaped).

High molecular weight polymers and naturally occurring macromolecules often form random coils in aqueous solution. Clay suspensions are examples of systems containing plate-like particles.

Kinetic properties

This section considers several properties of colloidal systems that relate to the motion of particles with respect to the dispersion medium. Thermal motion manifests itself in the form of Brownian motion, diffusion and osmosis. Gravity (or a centrifugal field) leads to sedimentation. Viscous flow is the result of an externally applied force. Measurement of these properties enables molecular weight or particle size to be determined.

Brownian motion Colloidal particles are subject to random collisions with the molecules of the dispersion medium, with the result that each particle pursues an irregular and complicated zigzag path. If the particles (up to about 2 μm diameter) are observed under a microscope or the light scattered by colloidal particles is viewed using an ultramicroscope, an erratic motion is seen. This movement is referred to as Brownian motion, after Robert Brown who first reported his observation of this phenomenon with pollen grains suspended in water in 1827.

Diffusion As a result of Brownian motion colloidal particles spontaneously diffuse from a region of higher concentration to one of lower concentration. The rate of diffusion is expressed by Fick's first law:

$$\frac{dm}{dt} = -DA\frac{dC}{dx} \quad (6.3)$$

where dm is the mass of substance diffusing in time dt across an area A under the influence of a concentration gradient dC/dx (the minus sign denotes that diffusion takes place in the direction of decreasing concentration). D is the diffusion coefficient and has the dimensions of area per unit time. The diffusion coefficient of a dispersed material is related to the frictional coefficient, f, of the particles by Einstein's law of diffusion:

$$Df = k_B T \quad (6.4)$$

where k_B is the Boltzmann constant and T is temperature.

Therefore, as the frictional coefficient is given by the Stokes equation:

$$f = 6\pi\eta a \quad (6.5)$$

where η is the viscosity of the medium and a the radius of the particle, (assuming sphericity), then

$$D = kT/6\pi\eta a = RT/6\pi\eta a N_A \quad (6.6)$$

where N_A is the Avogadro number and R is the universal gas constant. The diffusion coefficient may be obtained by an experiment measuring the change in concentration, via refractive index gradients, when the solvent is carefully layered over the solution to form a sharp boundary and diffusion is allowed to proceed. A more commonly used method is that of dynamic light scattering, which is based on the frequency shift of laser light as it is scattered by a moving particle – the so-called Doppler shift. The diffusion coefficient can be used to obtain the molecular weight of an approximately spherical particle, such as egg albumin and haemoglobin, by using Eqn 6.6 in the form

$$D = \frac{RT}{6\pi\eta N_A}\sqrt[3]{\frac{4\pi N_A}{3M\bar{v}}} \quad (6.7)$$

where M is the molecular weight and $\bar{v}$ the partial specific volume of the colloidal material.

Sedimentation Consider a spherical particle of radius a and density σ falling in a liquid of density ρ and viscosity η. The velocity v of sedimentation is given by Stokes' law:

$$v = 2a^2g(\sigma - \rho)/9\eta \quad (6.8)$$

where g is acceleration due to gravity.

If the particles are subjected only to the force of gravity, then as a result of Brownian motion, the

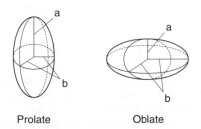

Prolate · Oblate

Fig. 6.1 Model representation of ellipsoids of revolution.

lower size limit of particles obeying Eqn 6.8 is about 0.5 μm. A stronger force than gravity is therefore needed for colloidal particles to sediment, and use is made of a high-speed centrifuge, usually termed an ultracentrifuge, which can produce a force of about $10^6 g$. In a centrifuge, g is replaced by $\omega^2 x$, where ω is the angular velocity and x the distance of the particle from the centre of rotation, and Eqn 6.8 becomes:

$$v = \frac{2a^2 g(\sigma - \rho)\, \omega^2 x}{9\eta} \qquad (6.9)$$

The ultracentrifuge is used in two distinct ways in investigating colloidal material. In the **sedimentation velocity** method a high centrifugal field is applied – up to about $4 \times 10^5 g$ – and the movement of the particles, monitored by changes in concentration, is measured at specified time intervals. In the **sedimentation equilibrium** method the colloidal material is subjected to a much lower centrifugal field until sedimentation and diffusion tendencies balance one another, and an equilibrium distribution of particles throughout the sample is attained.

Sedimentation velocity The velocity dx/dt of a particle in a unit centrifugal force can be expressed in terms of the Svedberg coefficient s:

$$s = (dx/dt)/\omega^2 x \qquad (6.10)$$

Under the influence of the centrifugal force particles pass from position x_1 at time t_1 to position x_2 at time t_2: the differences in concentration with time can be measured using changes in refractive index and the application of the schlieren optical arrangement, whereby photographs can be taken showing these concentrations as peaks. Integration of Eqn 6.10 using the above limits gives:

$$s = \frac{\ln x_2 / x_1}{\omega^2 (t_2 - t_1)} \qquad (6.11)$$

By suitable manipulation of Eqns 6.9, 6.10 and 6.11 an expression giving molecular weight M can be obtained:

$$M = \frac{RTs}{D(1 - \bar{v}\rho)} = \frac{RT \ln x_2 / x_1}{D(1 - \bar{v}\rho)(t_2 - t_1)\omega^2} \qquad (6.12)$$

where $\bar{v}$ is the specific volume of the particle.

Sedimentation equilibrium Equilibrium is established when sedimentation and diffusional forces balance. Sedimentation and diffusion equations are combined in the analysis, giving:

$$M = \frac{2RT \ln C_2 / C_1}{\omega^2 (1 - \bar{v}\rho)(x_2^2 - x_1^2)} \qquad (6.13)$$

where C_1 and C_2 are the sedimentation equilibrium concentrations at distances x_1 and x_2 from the axis of rotation. A disadvantage of the sedimentation equilibrium method is the length of time required to attain equilibrium, often as long as several days. A modification of the method in which measurements are made in the early stages of the approach to equilibrium significantly reduces the overall measurement time.

Osmotic pressure The determination of molecular weights of dissolved substances from colligative properties such as the depression of freezing point or the elevation of boiling point is a standard procedure. However, of the available methods only osmotic pressure has a practical value in the study of colloidal particles because of the magnitude of the changes in the properties. For example, the depression of freezing point of a 1% w/v solution of a macromolecule of molecular weight 70 kDa is only 0.0026 K, far too small to be measured with sufficient accuracy by conventional methods and also very sensitive to the presence of low molecular weight impurities. In contrast, the osmotic pressure of this solution at 20°C would be 350 N m^{-2}, or about 35 mmH$_2$O. Not only does the osmotic pressure provide an effect that is measurable, but also the effect of any low molecular weight material that can pass through the membrane is virtually eliminated.

However, the usefulness of osmotic pressure measurement is limited to a molecular weight range of about 10^4–10^6; below 10^4 the membrane may be permeable to the molecules under consideration and above 10^6 the osmotic pressure will be too small to permit accurate measurement.

If a solution and a solvent are separated by a semipermeable membrane the tendency to equalize chemical potentials (and hence concentrations) on either side of the membrane results in a net diffusion of solvent across the membrane. The pressure necessary to balance this osmotic flow is termed the osmotic pressure.

For a colloidal solution the osmotic pressure π can be described by

$$\pi/C = RT/M + BC \qquad (6.14)$$

where C is the concentration of the solution, M the molecular weight of the solute and B a constant depending on the degree of interaction between the solvent and solute molecules.

Thus a plot of π/C versus C is linear, with the value of the intercept as $C \to 0$ giving RT/M, enabling the molecular weight of the colloid to be calculated. The molecular weight obtained from osmotic pressure measurements is a number average value.

A potential source of error in the determination of molecular weight from osmotic pressure measurements arises from the **Donnan membrane effect**. The diffusion of small ions through a membrane will be affected by the presence of a charged macromolecule that is unable to penetrate the membrane because of its size. At equilibrium the distribution of the diffusible ions is unequal, being greater on the side of the membrane containing the non-diffusible ions. Consequently, unless precautions are taken to correct for this effect or to eliminate it, the results of osmotic pressure measurements on charged colloidal particles such as proteins will be invalid.

Viscosity Viscosity is an expression of the resistance to flow of a system under an applied stress. An equation of flow applicable to colloidal dispersions of spherical particles was developed by Einstein:

$$\eta = \eta_0 (1 + 2.5\ \phi) \qquad (6.15)$$

where η_0 is the viscosity of the dispersion medium and η the viscosity of the dispersion when the volume fraction of colloidal particles present is ϕ.

A number of viscosity coefficients may be defined with respect to Eqn 6.15. These include **relative viscosity**:

$$\eta_{rel} = \eta/\eta_0 = 1 + 2.5\ \phi \qquad (6.16)$$

and **specific viscosity**:

$$\eta_{sp} = \eta/\eta_0 - 1 = (\eta - \eta_0)/\eta_0 = 2.5\ \phi$$

or

$$\eta_{sp}/\phi = 2.5 \qquad (6.17)$$

Because volume fraction is directly related to concentration, Eqn 6.17 may be written as:

$$\eta_{sp}/C = K \qquad (6.18)$$

where C is the concentration expressed as grams of colloidal particles per 100 ml of total dispersion. If η is determined for a number of concentrations of macromolecular material in solution and η_{sp}/C is plotted versus C, then the intercept obtained on extrapolation of the linear plot to infinite dilution is known as the **intrinsic viscosity** $[\eta]$.

This constant may be used to calculate the molecular weight of the macromolecular material by making use of the Mark–Houwink equation:

$$[\eta] = KM^\alpha \qquad (6.19)$$

where K and α are constants characteristic of the particular polymer–solvent system. These constants are obtained initially by determining $[\eta]$ for a polymer fraction whose molecular weight has been determined by another method, such as sedimentation, osmotic pressure or light scattering. The molecular weight of the unknown polymer fraction may

then be calculated. This method is suitable for use with polymers such as the dextrans used as blood plasma substitutes.

Optical properties

Light scattering When a beam of light is passed through a colloidal sol some of the light may be absorbed (when light of certain wavelengths is selectively absorbed a colour is produced), some is scattered and the remainder is transmitted undisturbed through the sample. Because of the scattered light the sol appears turbid: this is known as the Tyndall effect. The turbidity of a sol is given by the expression:

$$I = I_0\ \exp^{-\tau l} \qquad (6.20)$$

where I_0 is the intensity of the incident beam, I that of the transmitted light beam, l the length of the sample and τ the turbidity.

Light scattering measurements are of great value for estimating particle size, shape and interactions, particularly of dissolved macromolecular materials, as the turbidity depends on the size (molecular weight) of the colloidal material involved. Measurements are simple in principle but experimentally difficult because of the need to keep the sample free from dust, the particles of which would scatter light strongly and introduce large errors.

As most colloids show very low turbidities, instead of measuring the transmitted light (which may differ only marginally from the incident beam), it is more convenient and accurate to measure the scattered light, at an angle (usually 90°) relative to the incident beam. The turbidity can then be calculated from the intensity of the scattered light, provided the dimensions of the particle are small compared to the wavelength of the incident light, by the expression:

$$\tau = \frac{16\pi}{3}\ R_{90} \qquad (6.21)$$

R_{90} is given by $I_\theta r^2/I_0$ known as the Rayleigh ratio after Lord Rayleigh, who laid the foundations of the light-scattering theory in 1871. I_θ is the intensity of the scattered light and I_0 that of the incident light; r is the distance from the scattering particle to the point of observation. The light-scattering theory was modified for use in the determination of the molecular weight of colloidal particles by Debye in 1947, who derived the following relationship between turbidity and molecular weight:

$$HC/\tau = 1/M + 2BC \qquad (6.22)$$

where C is the concentration of the solute and B an interaction constant allowing for non-ideality. H is an optical constant for a particular system, depending on the refractive index change with concentration and the wavelength of light used. A plot of HC/τ against concentration results in a straight line of slope $2B$. The intercept on the HC/τ axis is $1/M$, allowing the molecular weight to be calculated. The molecular weight derived by the light-scattering technique is a weight average value.

Light-scattering measurements are particularly suitable for finding the size of the micelles of surface-active agents and for the study of proteins and natural and synthetic polymers.

For spherical particles the upper limit of the Debye equation is a diameter of approximately 1/20th of the wavelength λ of the incident light, that is, about 20–25 nm. The light-scattering theory becomes more complex when one or more dimensions exceeds $\lambda/20$, because the particles can no longer be considered as point sources of scattered light. By measuring the light scattering from such particles as a function of both the scattering angle θ and the concentration C, and extrapolating the data to zero angle and zero concentration, it is possible to obtain information not only on the molecular weight but also on the particle shape.

Because the intensity of the scattered light is inversely proportional to the wavelength of the light used, blue light ($\lambda \approx 450$ nm) is scattered much more than red light ($\lambda \approx 650$ nm). With incident white light a scattering material will therefore tend to be blue when viewed at right-angles to the incident beam, which is why the sky appears to be blue, the scattering arising from dust particles in the atmosphere.

Ultramicroscopy Colloidal particles are too small to be seen with an optical microscope. Light scattering is made use of in the ultramicroscope first developed by Zsigmondy, in which a cell containing the colloid is viewed against a dark background at right-angles to an intense beam of incident light. The particles, which exhibit Brownian motion, appear as spots of light against the dark background. The ultramicroscope is used in the technique of microelectrophoresis for measuring particle charge.

Electron microscopy The electron microscope, capable of giving actual pictures of the particles, is used to observe the size, shape and structure of colloidal particles. The success of the electron microscope is due to its high resolving power, defined in terms of d, the smallest distance by which two objects can be separated yet remain distinguishable. The smaller the wavelength of the radiation used the smaller is d and the greater the resolving power. An optical microscope, using visible light as its radiation source, gives a d of about 0.2 μm. The radiation source of the electron microscope is a beam of high-energy electrons having wavelengths in the region of 0.01 nm, d is thus about 0.5 nm. The electron beams are focused using electromagnets and the whole system is under a high vacuum of about 10^{-3}–10^{-5} Pa to give the electrons a free path. With wavelengths of the order indicated the image cannot be viewed directly, so use is made of a fluorescent screen.

One big disadvantage of the electron microscope for viewing colloidal particles is that normally only dried samples can be examined. Consequently it usually gives no information on solvation or configuration in solution, and moreover, the particles may be affected by sample preparation. A recent development that overcomes these problems is environmental scanning electron microscopy (ESSEM), which allows the observation of material in the wet state.

Electrical properties

Electrical properties of interfaces Most surfaces acquire a surface electric charge when brought into contact with an aqueous medium, the principal charging mechanisms being as follows.

Ion dissolution Ionic substances can acquire a surface charge by virtue of unequal dissolution of the oppositely charged ions of which they are composed. For example, the particles of silver iodide in a solution with excess [I⁻] will carry a negative charge, but the charge will be positive if excess [Ag⁺] is present. Because the concentrations of Ag^+ and I^- determine the electric potential at the particle surface, they are termed potential determining ions. In a similar way H^+ and OH^- are potential determining ions for metal oxides and hydroxides such as magnesium and aluminium hydroxides.

Ionization Here the charge is controlled by the ionization of surface groupings; examples include the model system of polystyrene latex, which frequently has carboxylic acid groupings at the surface which ionize to give negatively charged particles. In a similar way acidic drugs such as ibuprofen and nalidixic acid also acquire a negative charge.

Amino acids and proteins acquire their charge mainly through the ionization of carboxyl and amino groups to give $-COO^-$ and NH_3^+ ions. The ionization of these groups and hence the net molecular charge depends on the pH of the system. At a pH below the pK_a of the COO⁻ group the protein will be positively charged because of the protonation of this group, $-COO^- \rightarrow COOH$, and the ionization of the amino group $-NH_2 \rightarrow -NH_3^+$, which has a much higher pK_a; whereas at higher pH, where the amino group is no longer ionized, the net charge on the molecule is now negative because of the ionization of the carboxyl group. At a certain definite pH, specific for each individual protein, the total number of positive charges will equal the total number of negative charges and the net charge will be zero. This pH is termed the isoelectric point of the protein and the protein exists as its zwitterion. This may be represented as follows:

R—NH$_2$—COO$^-$ Alkaline solution

$\downarrow\uparrow$

R—NH$_3^+$—COO$^-$ Isoelectric point (zwitterion)

$\downarrow\uparrow$

R—NH$_3^+$—COOH   Acidic solution

A protein is least soluble (the colloidal sol is least stable) at its isoelectric point and is readily desolvated by very water-soluble salts such as ammonium sulphate. Thus insulin may be precipitated from aqueous alcohol at pH 5.2.

Erythrocytes and bacteria usually acquire their charge by ionization of surface chemical groups such as sialic acid.

Ion adsorption   A net surface charge can be acquired by the unequal adsorption of oppositely charged ions. Surfaces in water are more often negatively charged than positively charged, because cations are generally more hydrated than anions. Consequently, the former have the greater tendency to reside in the bulk aqueous medium, whereas the smaller, less hydrated and more polarizing anions have a greater tendency to reside at the particle surface; Surface-active agents are strongly adsorbed and have a pronounced influence on the surface charge, imparting either a positive or negative charge depending on their ionic character.

The electrical double layer   Consider a solid charged surface in contact with an aqueous solution containing positive and negative ions. The surface charge influences the distribution of ions in the aqueous medium; ions of opposite charge to that of the surface, termed counter-ions, are attracted towards the surface; ions of like charge, termed co-ions, are repelled away from the surface. However, the distribution of the ions will also be affected by thermal agitation, which will tend to redisperse the ions in solution. The result is the formation of an electrical double layer, made up of the charged surface and a neutralizing excess of counter-ions over co-ions (the system must be electrically neutral) distributed in a diffuse manner in the aqueous medium.

The theory of the electric double layer deals with this distribution of ions and hence with the magnitude of the electric potentials that occur in the locality of the charged surface. For a fuller explanation of what is a rather complicated mathematical approach the reader is referred to a textbook of colloid science (e.g. Shaw 1992). A somewhat simplified picture of what pertains from the theories of Gouy, Chapman and Stern follows.

The double layer is divided into two parts (Fig. 6.2(a)), the inner, which may include adsorbed ions, and the diffuse part where ions are distributed as influenced by electrical forces and random thermal motion. The two parts of the double layer are separated by a plane, the Stern plane, at about a hydrated ion radius from the surface: thus counter-ions may be held at the surface by electrostatic attraction, and the centre of these hydrated ions forms the Stern plane.

The potential changes linearly from ψ_0 (the surface potential) to ψ_δ, (the Stern potential) in the Stern layer and decays exponentially from ψ_δ to zero in the diffuse double layer (Fig. 6.2(b)). A plane of shear is also indicated in Figure 6.2 (a) and (b). In addition to ions in the Stern layer a certain amount of solvent will be bound to the ions and the charged surface. This solvating layer is held to the surface and the edge of the layer, termed the surface or plane of shear, represents the boundary of relative movement between the solid (and attached material) and the liquid. The potential at the plane of shear is termed the zeta, ζ, or electrokinetic, potential and its magnitude may be measured using microelectrophoresis or any other of the electrokinetic phenomena. The thickness of the solvating layer is ill-defined and the zeta potential therefore represents a potential at an unknown distance from the particle surface; its value, however, is usually taken as being slightly less than that of the Stern potential.

In the discussion above it was stated that the Stern plane existed at a hydrated ion radius from the particle surface; the hydrated ions are electrostatically attracted to the particle surface. It is possible for ions/molecules to be more strongly adsorbed at the surface – termed specific adsorption – than by simple electrostatic attraction. In fact, the specifically adsorbed ion/molecule may be uncharged, as in the case with non-ionic surface-active agents. Surface-active ions specifically adsorb by the hydrophobic effect and can have a significant effect on the Stern potential, causing ψ_0 and ψ_δ to have opposite signs as in Figure 6.3(a), or for ψ_δ to have the same sign as ψ_0 but be greater in magnitude, as in Figure 6.3(b).

Figure 6.2(b) shows an exponential decay of the potential to zero with distance from the Stern plane. The distance over which this occurs is $1/\kappa$, referred

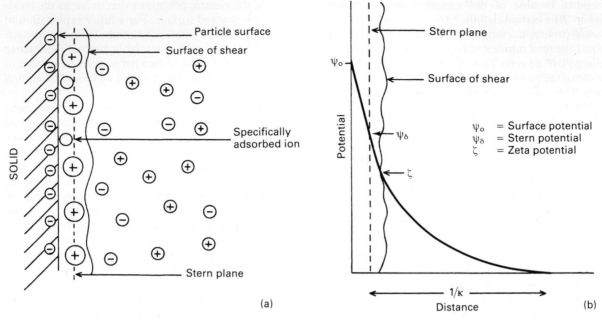

Fig. 6.2 The electric double layer. (a) Schematic representation; (b) changes in potential with distance from particle surface.

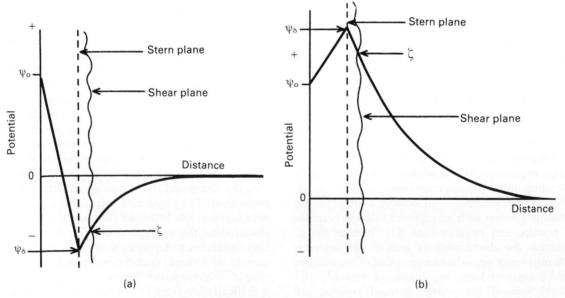

Fig. 6.3 Changes in potential with distance from solid surface. (a) Reversal of charge sign of Stern potential Ψ_δ, due to adsorption of surface-active or polyvalent counter ion. (b) Increase in magnitude of Stern potential Ψ_δ, due to adsorption of surface-active co-ions.

to as the Debye–Huckel length parameter, or the thickness of the electrical double layer. The parameter κ is dependent on the electrolyte concentration of the aqueous medium. Increasing the electrolyte concentration increases the value of κ and consequently decreases the value of $1/\kappa$, that is, it compresses the

double layer. As ψ_δ stays constant this means that the zeta potential will be lowered.

As indicated earlier, the effect of specifically adsorbed ions may be to lower the Stern potential and hence the zeta potential without compressing the double layer. Thus the zeta potential may be reduced by additives to the aqueous system in either (or both) of two different ways.

Electrokinetic phenomena This is the general description applied to the phenomena that arise when attempts are made to shear off the mobile part of the electrical double layer from a charged surface. There are four such phenomena: electrophoresis, sedimentation potential, streaming potential and electro-osmosis, all of which may be used to measure the zeta potential, but electrophoresis is the easiest to use and has the greatest pharmaceutical application.

Electrophoresis The movement of a charged particle (plus attached ions) relative to a stationary liquid under the influence of an applied electric field is termed electrophoresis. When the movement of the particles is observed with a microscope, or the movement of light spots scattered by particles too small to be observed with the microscope is observed using an ultramicroscope, this constitutes microelectrophoresis.

A microscope equipped with an eyepiece graticule is used and the speed of movement of the particle under the influence of a known electric field is measured. This is the electrophoretic velocity, v, and the electrophoretic mobility, u, is given by:

$$u = v/E \qquad (6.23)$$

where v is measured in m s^{-1}, and E, the applied field strength, in V m^{-1}, so that u has the dimensions of m^2 s^{-1} V^{-1}. Typically a stable lyophobic colloidal particle may have an electrophoretic mobility of 4×10^{-8} m^2 s^{-1} V^{-1}. The equation used to convert the electrophoretic mobility, u, into the zeta potential depends on the value of κa (κ is the Debye–Huckel reciprocal length parameter described previously and a the particle radius). For values of κa >100 (as is the case for particles of radius 1 μm dispersed in 10^{-3} mol dm^{-3} sodium chloride solution) the Smoluchowski equation can be used:

$$u = \epsilon\zeta/\eta \qquad (6.24)$$

where ϵ is the permittivity and η the viscosity of the liquid used. For particles in water at 25°C, $\zeta = 12.85 \times 10^{-5} u$ volts, so that for the mobility given above a zeta potential of 0.0514 V or 51.4 mV is obtained. For values of $\kappa a < 100$ a more complex relationship which is a function of κa and the zeta potential is used.

The technique of microelectrophoresis finds application in the measurement of zeta potentials, of model systems (such as polystyrene latex dispersions) to test colloid stability theory, of coarse dispersions (e.g. suspensions and emulsions) to assess their stability, and in the identification of charge groups and other surface characteristics of water-insoluble drugs and cells such as blood and bacteria.

Other electrokinetic phenomena The other electrokinetic phenomena are as follows: **sedimentation potential**, the reverse of electrophoresis, is the electric field created when particles sediment; **streaming potential**, the electric field created when liquid is made to flow along a stationary charged surface, e.g. a glass tube or a packed powder bed; and **electro-osmosis**, the opposite of streaming potential, the movement of liquid relative to a stationary charged surface, e.g. a glass tube, by an applied electric field.

Physical stability of colloidal systems

In colloidal dispersions frequent encounters between the particles occur as a result of Brownian movement. Whether these collisions result in permanent contact of the particles (coagulation), which leads eventually to the destruction of the colloidal system as the large aggregates formed sediment out, or temporary contact (flocculation), or whether the particles rebound and remain freely dispersed (a stable colloidal system), depends on the forces of interaction between the particles.

These forces can be divided into three groups: electrical forces of repulsion, forces of attraction, and forces arising from solvation. An understanding of the first two explains the stability of lyophobic systems, and all three must be considered in a discussion of the stability of lyophilic dispersions. Before considering the interaction of these forces it is necessary to define the terms **aggregation, coagulation** and **flocculation**, as used in colloid science.

Aggregation is a general term signifying the collection of particles into groups. Coagulation signifies that the particles are closely aggregated and difficult to redisperse – a primary minimum phenomenon of the DLVO theory of colloid stability (see next section). In flocculation the aggregates have an open structure in which the particles remain a small distance apart from one another. This may be a secondary minimum phenomenon (see the DLVO theory) or a consequence of bridging by a polymer or polyelectrolyte, as explained later in this chapter.

As a preliminary to discussion on the stability of colloidal dispersions a comparison of the general properties of lyophobic and lyophilic sols is given in Table 6.2.

Stability of lyophobic systems

DLVO theory In considering the interaction between two colloidal particles Derjaguin and Landau and, independently, Verwey and Overbeek, in the 1940s produced a quantitative approach to the stability of hydrophobic sols. In what has come to be known as the **DLVO theory of colloid stability**

Table 6.2   Comparison of properties of lyophobic and lyophilic sols

Property	Lyophobic	Lyophilic
Effect of electrolytes	Very sensitive to added electrolyte, leading to aggregation in an irreversible manner. Depends on: (a) type and valency of counter ion of electrolyte, e.g. with a negatively charged sol, $La^{3+} > Ba^{2+} > Na^+$ (b) Concentration of electrolyte. At a particular concentration sol passes from disperse to aggregated state. For the electrolyte types in (a) the concentrations are about 10^{-4}, 10^{-3}, 10^{-1} mol dm^{-3} respectively. These generalizations, (a) and (b), form what is known as the Schulze–Hardy rule	Dispersions are stable generally in the presence of electrolytes. May be salted out by high concentrations of very soluble electrolytes. Effect is due to desolvation of the lyophilic molecules and depends on the tendency of the electrolyte ions to become hydrated. Proteins more sensitive to electrolytes at their isoelectric points. Lyophilic colloids when salted out may appear as amorphous droplets known as a coacervate
Stability	Controlled by charge on particles	Controlled by charge and solvation of particles
Formation of dispersion	Dispersions usually of metals, inorganic crystals etc., with a high interfacial surface-free energy due to large increase in surface area on formation. A positive ΔG of formation, dispersion will never form spontaneously and is thermodynamically unstable. Particles of sol remain dispersed due to electrical repulsion	Generally proteins, macromolecules etc., which disperse spontaneously in a solvent. Interfacial free energy is low. There is a large increase in entropy when rigidly held chains of a polymer in the dry state unfold in solution. The free energy of formation is negative, a stable thermodynamic system
Viscosity	Sols of low viscosity, particles unsolvated and usually symmetrical	Usually high at sufficiently high concentration of disperse phase a gel may be formed. Particles solvated and usually asymmetric

they assumed that the only interactions involved are electrical repulsion, V_R, and van der Waals attraction, V_A, and that these parameters are additive. Therefore, the total potential energy of interaction V_T (expressed schematically in the curve shown in Fig. 6.4) is given by:

$$V_T = V_A + V_R \qquad (6.25)$$

Repulsive forces between particles Repulsion between particles arises because of the osmotic effect produced by the increase in the number of charged species on overlap of the diffuse parts of the electrical double layer. No simple equations can be given for repulsive interactions; however, it can be shown that the repulsive energy that exists between two spheres of equal but small surface potential is given by:

$$V_R = 2\pi \varepsilon a \omega_0^2 \exp[-\kappa H] \qquad (6.26)$$

where ε is the permittivity of the polar liquid, a the radius of the spherical particle of surface potential ψ_0, κ is the Debye–Huckel reciprocal length parameter and H the distance between particles. An estimation of the surface potential can be obtained from zeta potential measurements. As can be seen, the repulsion energy is an exponential function of the distance between the particles and has a range of the order of the thickness of the double layer.

Attractive forces between particles The energy of attraction, V_A, arises from van der Waals universal forces of attraction, the so-called dispersion forces, the major contribution to which are the electromagnetic attractions described by London in 1930. For an assembly of molecules dispersion forces are additive, summation leading to long-range attraction between colloidal particles. As a result of the work of de Boer and Hamaker in 1936 it can be shown that the attractive interaction between spheres of the same radius, a, can be approximated to:

$$V_A = -Aa/12\,H \qquad (6.27)$$

where A is the Hamaker constant for the particular material derived from London dispersion forces. Equation 6.27 shows that the energy of attraction varies as the inverse of the distance between particles.

Total potential energy of interaction Consideration of the curve of total potential energy of interaction V_T versus distance between particles, H (Fig. 6.4), shows that attraction predominates at small distances, hence the very deep primary minimum. The attraction at large interparticle distances that produces the secondary minimum arises because the fall-off in repulsive energy with distance is more rapid than that of attractive energy. At intermediate distances double-layer repulsion may predominate,

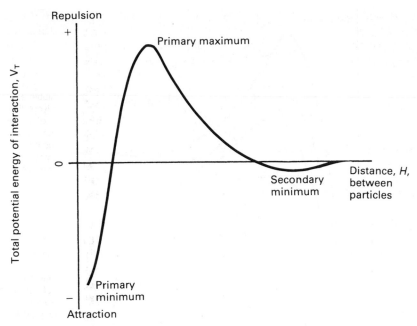

Fig. 6.4 Schematic curve of total potential energy of interaction, V_T, versus distance of separation, H, for two particles. $V_T = V_R + V_A$.

giving a primary maximum in the curve. If this maximum is large compared to the thermal energy $k_B T$ of the particles the colloidal system should be stable, i.e. the particles should stay dispersed. Otherwise, the interacting particles will reach the energy depth of the primary minimum and irreversible aggregation, i.e. coagulation, occurs. If the secondary minimum is smaller than $k_B T$ the particles will not aggregate but will always repel one another, but if it is significantly larger than $k_B T$ a loose assemblage of particles will form which can be easily redispersed by shaking, i.e. flocculation occurs.

The depth of the secondary minimum depends on particle size, and particles may need to be of radius 1 μm or greater before the attractive force is sufficiently great for flocculation to occur.

The height of the primary maximum energy barrier to coagulation depends upon the magnitude of V_R, which is dependent on ω_o and hence the zeta potential. In addition, it depends on electrolyte concentration via κ, the Debye–Huckel reciprocal length parameter. The addition of electrolyte compresses the double layer and reduces the zeta potential: this has the effect of lowering the primary maximum and deepening the secondary minimum (Fig. 6.5). This latter means that there will be an increased tendency for particles to flocculate in the secondary minimum and is the principle of the **controlled flocculation** approach to pharmaceutical suspension formulation described later. The primary maximum may also be lowered (and the secondary minimum deepened) by adding substances, such as ionic surface-active agents, which are specifically adsorbed within the Stern layer. Here ω_δ is reduced and hence the zeta potential; the double layer is usually not compressed.

Stability of lyophilic systems Solutions of macromolecules, lyophilic colloidal sols, are stabilized by a combination of electrical double-layer interaction and solvation, and both of these factors must be sufficiently weakened before attraction predominates and the colloidal particles coagulate. For example, gelatin has a sufficiently strong affinity for water to be soluble even at its isoelectric pH, where there is no double-layer interaction.

Hydrophilic colloids are unaffected by the small amounts of added electrolyte that cause hydrophobic sols to coagulate; however, when the concentration of electrolyte is high, particularly with an electrolyte whose ions become strongly hydrated, the colloidal material loses its water of solvation to these ions and coagulates, i.e. a 'salting-out' effect occurs.

Variation in the degree of solvation of different hydrophilic colloids affects the concentration of soluble electrolyte required to produce their coagulation and precipitation. The components of a mixture of hydrophilic colloids can therefore be separated by a process of fractional precipitation, which involves the 'salting out' of the various components at different concentrations of electrolyte. This technique is used in the purification of antitoxins.

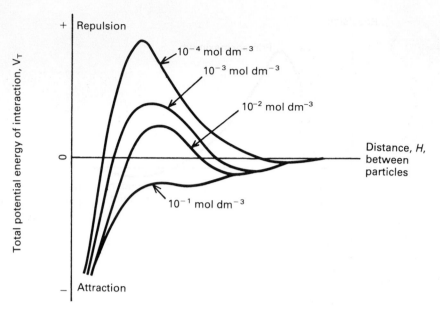

Fig. 6.5 Schematic curves of total potential energy of interaction, V_T, versus distance of separation, H, showing the effect of adding electrolyte at constant surface potential.

Lyophilic colloids can be considered to become lyophobic by the addition ·of solvents such as acetone and alcohol. The particles become desolvated and are then very sensitive to precipitation by added electrolyte.

Coacervation and microencapsulation Coacervation is the separation of a colloid-rich layer from a lyophilic sol on the addition of another substance. This layer, which is present in the form of an amorphous liquid, constitutes the coacervate. Simple coacervation may be brought about by a 'salting-out' effect on the addition of electrolyte or of a non-solvent. Complex coacervation occurs when two oppositely charged lyophilic colloids are mixed, e.g. gelatin and acacia. Gelatin at a pH below its isoelectric point is positively charged, acacia above about pH 3 is negatively charged; a combination of solutions at about pH 4 results in coacervation. Any large ions of opposite charge, for example cationic surface-active agents (positively charged) and dyes used for colouring aqueous mixtures (negatively charged), may react in a similar way.

If the coacervate is formed in a stirred suspension of an insoluble solid the macromolecular material will surround the solid particles. The coated particles can be separated and dried, and this technique forms the basis of one method of microencapsulation. A number of drugs, including aspirin, have been coated in this manner. The coating protects the drug from chemical attack, and microcapsules may be given orally to prolong the action of the medicament.

Effect of addition of macromolecular material to lyophobic colloidal sols When added in small amounts many polyelectrolyte and polymer molecules (lyophilic colloids) can adsorb simultaneously on to two particles and are long enough to bridge across the energy barrier between the particles. This can even occur with neutral polymers when the lyophobic particles have a high zeta potential (and would thus be considered a stable sol). The result is a structured floc (Fig. 6.6(a)).

With polyelectrolytes, where the particles and the polyelectrolyte have the same sign, flocculation can often occur when divalent and trivalent ions are added to the system (Fig. 6.6(b)). These complete the 'bridge' and only very low concentrations of these ions are needed. Use is made of this property of small quantities of polyelectrolytes and polymers in water purification, to remove colloidal material resulting from sewage.

On the other hand, if larger amounts of polymer are added, sufficient to cover the surface of the particles, then a lyophobic sol may be stabilized to coagulation by added electrolyte – the so-called steric stabilization or protective colloid effect.

Steric stabilization (protective colloid action) It has long been known that non-ionic polymeric materials such as gums, non-ionic surface-active agents and methylcellulose adsorbed at the particle surface can stabilize a lyophobic sol to coagulation even in the absence of a significant zeta potential. The approach

Fig. 6.6 Diagram of flocs formed by (a) polymer bridging and (b) polyelectrolyte bridging in the presence of divalent ions of opposite charge.

of two particles with adsorbed polymer layers results in a steric interaction when the layers overlap, leading to repulsion. In general, the particles do not approach each other closer than about twice the thickness of the adsorbed layer, and hence passage into the primary minimum is inhibited. An additional term has thus to be included in the potential energy of interaction for what is called steric stabilization, V_S:

$$V_T = V_A + V_R + V_S \qquad (6.28)$$

The effect of V_S on the potential energy against distance between particles curve is seen in Figure 6.7, showing that repulsion is generally seen at all shorter distances provided that the adsorbed polymeric material does not move from the particle surface.

Steric repulsion can be explained by reference to the free energy changes that take place when two polymer-covered particles interact. Free energy ΔG, enthalpy ΔH and entropy ΔS changes are related according to:

$$\Delta G = \Delta H - T\Delta S \qquad (6.29)$$

The second law of thermodynamics implies that a positive value of ΔG is necessary for dispersion stability, a negative value indicating that the particles have aggregated.

A positive value of ΔG can arise in a number of ways, for example when ΔH and ΔS are both negative and $T\Delta S > \Delta H$. Here the effect of the entropy change opposes aggregation and outweighs the enthalpy term; this is termed **entropic stabilization**. Interpenetration and compression of the polymer chains decreases the entropy as these chains become more ordered. Such a process is not spontaneous: work must be expended to interpenetrate and compress any polymer chains existing between the colloidal particles, and this work is a reflection of the repulsive potential energy. The enthalpy of mixing of these polymer chains will also be negative. Stabilization by these effects occurs in non-aqueous dispersions.

Again, a positive ΔG occurs if both ΔH and ΔS are positive and $T\Delta S > \Delta H$. Here enthalpy aids stabilization, entropy aids aggregation. Consequently, this effect is termed **enthalpic stabilization** and is common with aqueous dispersions, particularly where the stabilizing polymer has polyoxyethylene chains. Such chains are hydrated in aqueous solution due to H-bonding between water molecules and the 'ether oxygens' of the ethylene oxide groups. The water molecules have thus become more structured and lost degrees of freedom. When interpenetration and compression of ethylene oxide chains occurs there is an increased probability of contact between ethylene oxide groups, resulting in some of the bound water molecules being released (Fig. 6.8). The released water molecules have greater degrees of freedom than those in the bound state. For this to occur they must be supplied with energy, obtained from heat absorption, i.e. there is a positive enthalpy change. Although there is a decrease in entropy in the interaction zone, as with entropic stabilization, this is overridden by the increase in the configurational entropy of the released water molecules.

Fig. 6.7 Schematic curves of the total potential energy of interaction versus distance for two particles, showing the effect of the steric stabilization term V_S (a) in the absence of electrostatic repulsion, the solid line representing $V_T = V_A + V_S$; (b) in the presence of electrostatic repulsion, the solid line representing $V_T = V_R + V_A + V_S$.

Fig. 6.8 Enthalpic stabilization. (a) Particles with stabilizing polyoxyethylene chains and H-bonded water molecules. (b) Stabilizing chains overlap, water molecules released $\rightarrow +\ \Delta H$.

GELS

The majority of gels are formed by aggregation of colloidal sol particles, the solid or semisolid system so formed being interpenetrated by a liquid. The particles link together to form an interlaced network, thereby imparting rigidity to the structure; the continuous phase is held within the meshes. Often only a small percentage of disperse phase is required to impart rigidity, for example 1% of agar in water produces a firm gel. A gel rich in liquid may be called a jelly; if the liquid is removed and only the gel framework remains this is termed a xerogel. Sheet gelatin, acacia tears and tragacanth flakes are all xerogels.

Types of gel

Gelation of lyophobic sols Gels may be flocculated lyophobic sols where the gel can be looked upon as a continuous floccule (Fig. 6.9(a)). Examples are aluminium hydroxide and magnesium hydroxide gels.

Clays such as bentonite, aluminium magnesium silicate (Veegum) and to some extent kaolin form gels by flocculation in a special manner. They are hydrated aluminium (aluminium/magnesium) silicates whose crystal structure is such that they exist as flat plates; the flat part or 'face' of the particle carries a negative charge due to O^- atoms and the edge of the plate carries a positive charge due to Al^{3+}/Mg^{2+} atoms. As a result of electrostatic attraction between the face and the edge of different particles a gel structure is built up, forming what is usually known as a 'card house floc' (Fig. 6.9(b)).

The forces holding the particles together in this type of gel are relatively weak – van der Waals forces in the secondary minimum flocculation of aluminium hydroxide, electrostatic attraction in the case of the clays – and because of this these gels show the phenomenon of **thixotropy**, a non-chemical isothermal gel–sol–gel transformation. If a thixotropic gel is sheared (for example by simple shaking) these weak bonds are broken and a lyophobic sol is formed. On standing the particles collide, flocculation occurs and the gel is reformed. Flocculation in gels is the reason for their anomalous rheological properties (Chapter 4). This phenomenon of thixotropy is made use of in the formulation of pharmaceutical suspensions, e.g. bentonite in calamine lotion, and in the paint industry.

Gelation of lyophilic sols Gels formed by lyophilic sols can be divided into two groups depending on the nature of the bonds between the chains of the network. Gels of **type I** are irreversible systems with a three-dimensional network formed by covalent bonds between the macromolecules. Typical examples are the swollen networks that have been formed by the polymerization of monomers of water-soluble polymers in the presence of a crosslinking agent. For example, poly (2-hydroxyethylmethacrylate), [poly (HEMA)], crosslinked with ethylene glycol dimethacrylate, [EGDMA], forms a three-dimensional structure, see below, that swells in water but cannot dissolve because the crosslinks are stable. Such polymers have been used in the fabrication of expanding implants that imbide body fluids and swell to a predetermined volume. Implanted in the dehydrated state these polymers swell to fill a body cavity or give form to surrounding tissues. They also find use in the fabrication of implants for the prolonged release of drugs, such as antibiotics, into the immediate environment of the implant.

Type II gels are held together by much weaker intermolecular bonds such as hydrogen bonds. These gels are heat reversible, a transition from the sol to gel occurring on either heating or cooling. Poly (vinyl

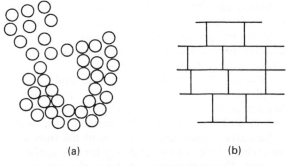

(a)   (b)

Fig. 6.9 Gel structure. (a) Flocculated lyophobic sol, e.g. aluminium hydroxide. (b) 'Card house' floc of clays, e.g. bentonite.

Poly (HEMA):poly (2-hydroxyethyl methacrylate) cross-linked with ethylene glycol dimethacrylate (EGDMA)

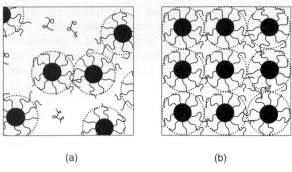

(a) (b)

Fig. 6.10 Poly(oxyethylene)-poly(oxypropylene)-poly(oxyethylene) block copolymers. (a) Micelle formation. (b) Formation of a cubic gel phase by packing of micelles.

alcohol) solutions, for example, gel on cooling below a certain temperature referred to as the gel point. Because of their gelling properties poly (vinyl alcohol)s are used as jellies for the application of drugs to the skin. On application the gel dries rapidly, leaving a plastic film with the drug in intimate contact with the skin. Concentrated aqueous solutions of high molecular weight poly(oxyethylene)-poly(oxypropylene)-poly(oxyethylene) block copolymers, commercially available as Pluronic™ or Synperonic™ surfactants, form gels on heating. These compounds are amphiphilic, and many form micelles with a hydrophobic core comprising the poly(oxypropylene) blocks surrounded by a shell of the hydrophilic poly(oxyethylene) chains. Unusually, water is a poorer solvent for these compounds at higher temperatures and consequently warming a solution with a concentration above the critical micelle concentration leads to the formation of more micelles. If the solution is sufficiently concentrated gelation may occur as the micelles pack so closely as to prevent their movement (Fig. 6.10). Gelation is a reversible process, the gels returning to the sol state on cooling.

SURFACE ACTIVE AGENTS

Certain compounds, because of their chemical structure, have a tendency to accumulate at the boundary between two phases. Such compounds are termed amphiphiles, surface-active agents, or surfactants. The adsorption at the various interfaces between solids, liquids and gases results in changes in the nature of the interface which are of considerable importance in pharmacy. Thus, the lowering of the interfacial tension between oil and water phases facilitates emulsion formation, the adsorption of surfactants on insoluble particles enable these particles to be dispersed in the form of a suspension, their

adsorption on solid surfaces enables these surfaces to be more readily wetted, and the incorporation of insoluble compounds within micelles of the surfactant can lead to the production of clear solutions.

Surface-active compounds are characterized by having two distinct regions in their chemical structure, termed hydrophilic (water-liking) and hydrophobic (water-hating). The existence of two such regions in a molecule is referred to as amphipathy and the molecules are consequently often referred to as amphipathic molecules. The hydrophobic portions are usually saturated or unsaturated hydrocarbon chains or, less commonly, heterocyclic or aromatic ring systems. The hydrophilic regions can be anionic, cationic or non-ionic. Surfactants are generally classified according to the nature of the hydrophilic group. Typical examples are given in Table 6.3.

A wide variety of drugs have also been reported to be surface active, this being a consequence of their amphipathic nature. The hydrophobic portions of the drug molecules are usually more complex than those of typical surface-active agents, being composed of aromatic or heterocyclic ring systems. Examples include the tranquillizers, such as chlorpromazine, which are based on the large tricyclic phenothiazine ring system; the antidepressant drugs such as imipramine, which also possess tricyclic ring systems; and the antihistamines such as diphenhydramine, which are based on a diphenylmethane group. Further examples of surface-active drugs are given in Attwood and Florence (1983).

Surface activity

The dual structure of amphipathic molecules is the unique feature that is responsible for the surface activity of these compounds. It is a consequence of their adsorption at the solution–air interface – the means by which the hydrophobic region of the molecule 'escapes' from the hostile aqueous environment by protruding into the vapour phase above. Similarly, adsorption at the interface between non-aqueous solutions occurs in such a way that the hydrophobic group is in the solution in the non-aqueous phase, leaving the hydrophilic group in contact with the aqueous solution.

The molecules at the surface of a liquid are not completely surrounded by other like molecules as they are in the bulk of the liquid. As a result there is a net inward force of attraction exerted on a molecule at the surface from the molecules in the bulk solution, which results in a tendency for the surface to contract. The contraction of the surface is spontaneous, that is, it is accompanied by a decrease in free

Table 6.3 Classification of surface-active agents

	Hydrophobic	Hydrophilic
Anionic		
Sodium dodecanoate	$CH_3(CH_2)_{10}$	COO^-Na^+
Sodium dodecyl (lauryl) sulphate	$CH_3(CH_2)_{11}$	$OSO_3^-Na^+$
Sodium dioctyl sulphosuccinate	$CH_3(CH_2)_7.OOC.CHSO_3^-Na^+$	
	$CH_3(CH_2)_7.OOC.CH_2$	
Cationic		
Hexadecyl trimethyl ammonium bromide (Cetrimide)	$CH_3(CH_2)_{15}$	$N^+-CH_3Br^-$ (with CH_3 above and CH_3 below)
Dodecyl pyridinium iodide	$CH_3(CH_2)_{11}$	pyridinium ring N^+H I^-
Non-ionic		
Hexaoxyethylene monohexadecyl ether	$CH_3(CH_2)_{15}$	$(OCH_2CH_2)_6OH$
Polyoxyethylene sorbitan mono-oleate (polysorbate 80)	$C_{17}H_{33}$	$COOCH_2 \cdot CH_2(CH_2CH_2O)_nOCH_2$
		$HO(CH_2CH_2O)_nCH$ O
		$HO(OCH_2CH_2)_n$ $(CH_2CH_2O)_nOH$
		$HO(OCH_2CH_2)_n$ $(CH_2CH_2O)_nOH$
		$(CH_3CH_2O)_nOH$
Sorbitan mono-oleate	$C_{17}H_{33}$	$COOCH_2CH$ O, OH, HO, OH
Ampholytic N-dodecyl alanine	$CH_3(CH_2)_{11}$	$\overset{+}{N}H_2.CH_2.CH_2.COO^-$
Lecithin	$C_{17}H_{35}$	$COO.CH_2$
	$C_{17}H_{35}$	$COO.CH$
		$CH_2-O-\overset{O^-}{\underset{O}{P}}-O(CH_2)_2.\overset{+}{N}(CH_3)_3$

energy. The contracted surface thus represents a minimum free energy state, and any attempt to expand the surface must involve an increase in the free energy. The surface tension is a measure of the contracting power of the surface. Surface-active molecules in aqueous solution orientate themselves at the surface in such a way as to remove the hydrophobic group from the aqueous phase and hence achieve a minimum free energy state. As a result, some of the water molecules at the surface are replaced by non-polar groups. The attractive forces between these groups and the water molecules, or between the groups themselves, are less than those existing between water molecules. The contracting power of the surface is thus reduced and so, therefore, is the surface tension.

A similar imbalance of attractive forces exists at the interface between two immiscible liquids. The value of the interfacial tension is generally between those of the surface tensions of the two liquids involved, except where there is interaction between them. Intrusion of surface-active molecules at the interface between two immiscible liquids leads to a reduction of interfacial tension, in some cases to such a low level that spontaneous emulsification of the two liquids occurs.

Micelle formation

The surface tension of a surfactant solution decreases progressively with increase of concentration as more surfactant molecules enter the surface or interfacial layer. However, at a certain concentration this layer becomes saturated and an alternative means of shielding the hydrophobic group of the surfactant from the aqueous environment occurs through the formation of aggregates (usually spherical) of colloidal dimensions, called *micelles*. The hydrophobic chains form the core of the micelle and are shielded from the aqueous environment by the surrounding shell composed of the hydrophilic groups that serve to maintain solubility in water.

The concentration at which micelles first form in solution is termed the *critical micelle concentration* or CMC. This onset of micelle formation can be detected by a variety of experimental techniques. A change of slope occurs when physical properties such as surface tension, conductivity, osmotic pressure, solubility and light-scattering intensity are plotted as a function of concentration (Fig. 6.11), and such techniques can be used to measure the CMC. The CMC decreases with an increase in the length of the hydrophobic chain. With non-ionic surfactants, which are typically composed of a hydrocarbon chain and an oxyethylene chain (see Table 6.3), an increase in the hydrophilic oxyethylene chain length causes an increase in the CMC. The addition of electrolytes to ionic surfactants decreases the CMC and increases the micellar size. The effect is simply explained in terms of a reduc-

tion in the magnitude of the forces of repulsion between the charged head groups in the micelle, allowing the micelles to grow and also reducing the work required for their formation.

The primary reason for micelle formation is the attainment of a state of minimum free energy. The free energy change, ΔG, of a system is dependent on changes in both entropy, S, and enthalpy, H, which are related by the expression $\Delta G = \Delta H - T\Delta S$. For a micellar system at normal temperatures the entropy term is by far the most important in determining the free energy changes ($T\Delta S$ constitutes approximately 90–95% of the ΔG value). The explanation most generally accepted for the entropy change is concerned with the structure of water. Water possesses a relatively high degree of structure owing to hydrogen bonding between adjacent molecules. If an ionic or strongly polar solute is added to water it will disrupt this structure, but the solute molecules can form hydrogen bonds with the water molecules that more than compensate for the disruption or distortion of the bonds existing in pure water. Ionic and polar materials thus tend to be easily soluble in water. No such compensation occurs with non-polar groups and their solution in water is accordingly resisted, the water molecules forming extra structured clusters around the non-polar region. This increase in structure of the water molecules around the hydrophobic groups leads to a large negative entropy change. To counteract this and achieve a state of minimum free energy, the hydrophobic groups tend to withdraw from the aqueous phase either by orientating themselves at the interface with the hydrocarbon chain away from the aqueous phase or by self-association into micelles. This tendency for hydrophobic materials to be removed from water as a result of the strong attraction of water molecules for each other and not for the hydrophobic solute, has been termed *hydrophobic bonding*. However, because there is in fact no actual bonding between the hydrophobic groups the phenomenon is best described as the hydrophobic effect. When the non-polar groups approach each other until they are in contact, there will be a decrease in the total number of water molecules in contact with the non-polar groups. The formation of the hydrophobic bond in this way is thus equivalent to the partial removal of hydrocarbon from an aqueous environment and a consequent loss of the ice-like structuring that always surrounds the hydrophobic molecules. The increase in entropy and decrease in free energy that accompany the loss of structuring make the formation of the hydrophobic bond an energetically favourable process. An alternative explanation of the free energy decrease empha-

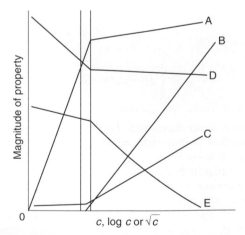

Fig. 6.11 Solution properties of an ionic surfactant as a function of concentration, *c*. (A) Osmotic pressure (against *c*); (B) solubility of a water-insoluble solubilizate (against *c*); (C) intensity of light scattered by the solution (against *c*); (D) surface tension (against log *c*); (E) molar conductivity (against √*c*).

sizes the increase in internal freedom of the hydrocarbon chains that occurs when these chains are transferred from the aqueous environment, where their motion is restrained by the hydrogen-bonded water molecules, to the interior of the micelle. It has been suggested that the increased mobility of the hydrocarbon chains, and of course their mutual attraction, constitutes the principal hydrophobic factor in micellization.

It should be emphasized that micelles are in dynamic equilibrium with monomer molecules in solution, continuously breaking down and reforming. It is this factor that distinguishes micelles from other colloidal particles and the reason why they are called *association colloids*. The concentration of surfactant monomers in equilibrium with the micelles stays approximately constant at the CMC value when the solution concentration is increased above the CMC, i.e. the added surfactant all goes to form micelles.

A typical micelle is a spherical or near-spherical structure composed of some 50–100 surfactant molecules. The radius of the micelle will be slightly less than that of the extended hydrocarbon chain (approximately 2.5 nm), with the interior core having the properties of a liquid hydrocarbon. For ionic micelles, about 70–80% of the counter-ions will be attracted close to the micelle, thereby reducing the overall charge. The compact layer around the core of an ionic micelle, which contains the head groups and the bound counter-ions, is called the *Stern layer* (Fig. 6.12a). The outer surface of the Stern layer is the shear surface of the micelle. The core and the Stern layer together constitute what is termed the 'kinetic micelle'. Surrounding the Stern layer is a diffuse layer called the *Gouy–Chapman electrical double layer* that contains the remaining counterions required to neutralize the charge on the kinetic micelle. The thickness of the double layer is dependent on the ionic strength of the solution and is greatly compressed in the presence of electrolyte. Non-ionic micelles have a hydrophobic core surrounded by a shell of oxyethylene chains which is often termed the *palisade layer* (Fig. 6.12b). As well as the water molecules that are hydrogen bonded to the oxyethylene chains, this layer is also capable of mechanically entrapping a considerable number of water molecules. Micelles of non-ionic surfactants tend, as a consequence, to be highly hydrated. The outer surface of the palisade layer forms the shear surface; that is, the hydrating molecules form part of the kinetic micelle.

Solubilization

As mentioned previously, the interior core of a micelle can be considered as having the properties of a liquid hydrocarbon and is thus capable of dissolving materials that are soluble in such liquids. This process, whereby water-insoluble or partly soluble substances are brought into aqueous solution by incorporation into micelles, is termed solubilization. The site of solubilization within the micelle is closely related to the chemical nature of the solubilizate. It is generally accepted that non-polar solubilizates (aliphatic hydrocarbons, for example) are dissolved in the hydrocarbon core (Fig. 6.13a). Water-insoluble compounds containing polar groups are orientated with the polar group at the surface of the ionic micelle among the micellar charged head groups, and the hydrophobic group buried inside the hydrocarbon core of the micelle (Fig. 6.13b). Slightly polar solubilizates without a distinct amphiphilic structure partition between the micelle surface and the core (Fig. 6.13c). Solubilization in non-ionic polyoxyethylated surfactants can also occur in the polyoxyethylene shell (palisade layer) that surrounds

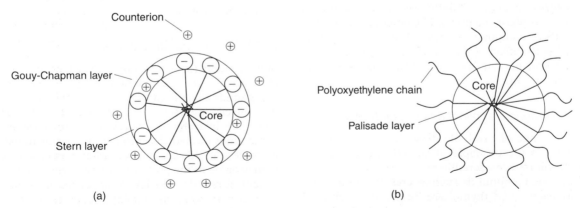

(a)

(b)

Fig. 6.12 Schematic representation of micelles of (a) ionic and (b) non-ionic surfactants.

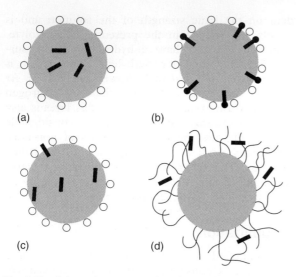

Fig. 6.13 Schematic representation of sites of solubilization in ionic and non-ionic micelles. (a) Non-polar solubilizate; (b) amphipathic solubilzate; (c) slightly polar solubilizate; (d) polar solubilizate in polyoxyethylene shell of a non-ionic micelle.

the core (Fig. 6.13d); thus *p*-hydroxy benzoic acid is entirely within this region, hydrogen-bonded to the ethylene oxide groups, whereas esters such as the parabens are located at the shell core junction.

The maximum amount of solubilizate that can be incorporated into a given system at a fixed concentration is termed the ***maximum additive concentration*** (MAC). The simplest method of determining the MAC is to prepare a series of vials containing surfactant solution of known concentration. Increasing concentrations of solubilizate are added and the vials are then sealed and agitated until equilibrium conditions are established. The maximum concentration of solubilizate forming a clear solution can be determined by visual inspection, or from extinction or turbidity measurements on the solutions. Solubility data are expressed as a solubility versus concentration curve, or as phase diagrams. The latter are preferable, as a three-component phase diagram completely describes the effect of varying all three components of the system, namely the solubilizate, the solubilizer and the solvent.

Pharmaceutical applications of solubilization

A wide range of insoluble drugs have been formulated using the principle of solubilization, some of which will be considered here.

Phenolic compounds such as cresol, chlorocresol, chloroxylenol and thymol are frequently solubilized with soap to form clear solutions which are widely used for disinfection. Solution of Chloroxylenol BP, for example, contains 5% v/v chloroxylenol with terpineol in an alcoholic soap solution.

Non-ionic surfactants can be used to solubilize iodine; such iodine–surfactant systems (referred to as iodophors) are more stable than iodine–iodide systems. They are preferable in instrument sterilization as corrosion problems are reduced. Loss of iodine by sublimation from iodophor solutions is significantly less than from simple iodine solutions such as iodine solution NF. There is also evidence of an ability of the iodophor solution to penetrate hair follicles of the skin, thereby enhancing its activity.

The low solubility of steroids in water presents a problem in their formulation for ophthalmic use. Because such formulations are required to be optically clear it is not possible to use oily solutions or suspensions, and there are many examples of the use of non-ionic surfactants as a means of producing clear solutions which are stable to sterilization. In most formulations solubilization has been effected using polysorbates or polyoxyethylene sorbitan esters of fatty acids.

The polysorbate non-ionics have also been employed in the preparation of aqueous injections of the water-insoluble vitamins A, D, E and K.

Although solubilization is an excellent means of producing an aqueous solution of a water-insoluble drug, it should be realized that it may well have effects on the drug's activity and absorption characteristics. As a generalization it may be said that low concentrations of surface-active agents increase absorption, possibly owing to enhanced contact of the drug with the absorbing membrane, whereas concentrations above the CMC either produce no additional effect or cause decreased absorption. In the latter case the drug may be held within the micelles, so that the concentration available for absorption is reduced. For a survey of this topic the review by Attwood and Florence (1983) should be consulted.

Solubilization and drug stability

Solubilization has been shown to have a modifying effect on the rate of hydrolysis of drugs. Non-polar compounds solubilized deep in the hydrocarbon core of a micelle are likely to be better protected against attack by hydrolysing species than are more polar compounds located closer to the micellar surface. For example, the alkaline hydrolysis of benzocaine and homatropine in the presence of several non-ionic surfactants is retarded, the less polar benzocaine showing a greater increase in stability compared to homatropine because of its deeper penetration into the micelle. An important factor in considering the breakdown of a drug located close to the micellar surface is the ionic nature of the surface-active agent. For base-catalysed hydrolysis anionic micelles should give an enhanced protection owing to repulsion of the attacking OH$^-$ group. For cationic micelles there should be the converse effect. Although this pattern has been found, enhanced protection by cationic micelles also occurs, suggesting that in these cases the positively charged polar head groups hold the OH$^-$ groups and thus block their penetration into the micelle.

Protection from oxidative degradation has also been found with solubilized systems.

As indicated earlier, drugs may be surface active. Such drugs form micelles and this self-association has been found in some cases to increase the drug's stability. Thus micellar solutions of penicillin G have been reported to be 2.5 times as stable as monomeric solutions under conditions of constant pH and ionic strength.

Detergency

Detergency is a complex process whereby surfactants are used for the removal of foreign matter from solid surfaces, be it the removal of dirt from clothes or the cleansing of body surfaces. The process includes many of the actions characteristic of specific surfactants. Thus the surfactant must have good wetting characteristics, so that the detergent can come into intimate contact with the surface to be cleaned. The detergent must have the ability to remove the dirt into the bulk of the liquid; the dirt/water and solid/water interfacial tensions are lowered, and thus the work of adhesion between the dirt and solid is reduced, so that the dirt particle may be easily detached. Once removed, the surfactant can be adsorbed at the particle surface, creating charge and hydration barriers that prevent deposition. If the dirt is oily it may be emulsified or solubilized.

COARSE DISPERSE SYSTEMS

Suspensions

A pharmaceutical suspension is a coarse dispersion in which insoluble particles, generally greater than 1 μm in diameter, are dispersed in a liquid medium, usually aqueous.

An aqueous suspension is a useful formulation system for administering an insoluble or poorly soluble drug. The large surface area of dispersed drug ensures a high availability for dissolution and hence absorption. Aqueous suspensions may also be used for parenteral and ophthalmic use, and provide a suitable form for the applications of dermatological materials to the skin. Suspensions are similarly used in veterinary practice, and a closely allied field is that of pest control. Pesticides are frequently presented as suspensions for use as fungicides, insecticides, ascaricides and herbicides.

An acceptable suspension possesses certain desirable qualities, among which are the following: the suspended material should not settle too rapidly; the particles that do settle to the bottom of the container must not form a hard mass but should be readily dispersed into a uniform mixture when the container is shaken; and the suspension must not be too viscous to pour freely from the bottle or to flow through a syringe needle.

The physical stability of a pharmaceutical suspension may be defined as the condition in which the particles do not aggregate and in which they remain uniformly distributed throughout the dispersion. As this ideal situation is seldom realized it is appropriate to add that if the particles do settle they should be easily resuspended by a moderate amount of agitation.

The major difference between a pharmaceutical suspension and a colloidal dispersion is one of size of the dispersed particles, with the relatively large particles of a suspension liable to sedimentation owing to gravitational forces. Apart from this, suspensions show most of the properties of colloidal systems. The reader is referred to Chapter 23 for a detailed account of the formulation of suspensions.

Controlled flocculation

A suspension in which all the particles remain discrete would, in terms of the DLVO theory, be considered to be stable. However, with pharmaceutical suspensions, in which the solid particles are very much coarser, such a system would sediment because of the size of the particles. The electrical repulsive forces between the particles allow them to slip past one another to form a close-packed arrangement at the bottom of the container, with the small particles filling the voids between the larger ones. The supernatant liquid may remain cloudy after sedimentation owing to the presence of colloidal particles that remain dispersed. Those particles lowermost in the sediment are gradually pressed together by the weight of the ones above. The repulsive barrier is thus overcome, allowing the particles to pack closely together. Physical bonding, leading to 'cake' or 'clay' formation, may then occur owing to the formation of bridges between the particles resulting from crystal growth and hydration effects, forces greater than agitation usually being required to disperse the sediment. Coagulation in the primary minimum, resulting from a reduction in the zeta potential to a point where attractive forces predominate, thus produces coarse compact masses with a 'curdled' appearance, which may not be readily dispersed.

On the other hand, particles flocculated in the secondary minimum form a loosely bonded structure, called a **flocculate** or **floc**. A suspension consisting of particles in this state is said to be flocculated. Although sedimentation of flocculated suspensions is fairly rapid, a loosely packed, high-volume sediment is obtained in which the flocs retain their structure and the particles are easily resuspended. The supernatant liquid is clear because the colloidal particles are trapped within the flocs and sediment with them. Secondary minimum flocculation is therefore a desirable state for a pharmaceutical suspension.

Particles greater than 1 μm radius should, unless highly charged, show a sufficiently deep secondary minimum for flocculation to occur because the attractive force between particles, V_A, depends on particle size. Other factors contributing to secondary minimum flocculation are shape (asymmetric particles, especially those that are elongated, being more satisfactory than spherical ones) and concentration. The rate of flocculation depends on the number of particles present, so that the greater the number of particles the more collisions there will be and the more flocculation is likely to occur. However, it may be necessary, as with highly charged particles, to control the depth of the secondary minimum to induce a satisfactory flocculation state. This can be achieved by the addition of electrolytes or ionic surface-active agents that reduce the zeta potential and hence V_R, resulting in the displacement of the whole of the DLVO plot to give a satisfactory secondary minimum, as indicated in Figure 6.5. The production of a satisfactory secondary minimum leading to floc formation in this manner is termed **controlled flocculation**.

A convenient parameter for assessing a suspension is the sedimentation volume ratio, F, which is defined as the ratio of the final settled volume V_u to the original volume V_o.

$$F = V_u/V_o \qquad (6.30)$$

The ratio F gives a measure of the aggregated–deflocculated state of a suspension and may usefully be plotted, together with the measured zeta potential, against concentration of additive, enabling an assessment of the state of the dispersion to be made

in terms of the DLVO theory. The appearance of the supernatant liquid should be noted and the redispersibility of the suspension evaluated.

It should be pointed out that in using the controlled flocculation approach to suspension formulation it is important to work at a constant, or narrow, pH range because the magnitude of the charge on the drug particle can vary greatly with pH.

Other additives, such as flavouring agents, may also affect particle charge.

Steric stabilization of suspensions

As described earlier, colloidal particles may be stabilized against coagulation in the absence of a charge on the particles by the use of non-ionic polymeric material – the concept of steric stabilization or protective colloid action. This concept may be applied to pharmaceutical suspensions where naturally occurring gums such as tragacanth, and synthetic materials such as non-ionic surfactants and cellulose polymers, may be used to produce satisfactory suspensions. These materials may increase the viscosity of the aqueous vehicle and thus slow the rate of sedimentation of the particles, but they will also form adsorbed layers around the particles so that the approach of their surfaces and aggregation to the coagulated state is hindered.

Repulsive forces arise as the adsorbed layers interpenetrate and, as explained above, these have an enthalpic component owing to the release of water of solvation from the polymer chains, and an entropic component due to movement restriction. As a result the particles will not usually approach one another closer than twice the thickness of the adsorbed layer.

However, as indicated above in the discussion on controlled flocculation, from a pharmaceutical point of view an easily dispersed aggregated system is desirable. To produce this state a balance between attractive and repulsive forces is required. This is not achieved by all polymeric materials, and the equivalent of deflocculated and caked systems may be produced. The balance of forces appears to depend on both the thickness and the concentration of the polymer in the adsorbed layer. These parameters determine the Hamaker constant and hence the attractive force, which must be large enough to cause aggregation of the particles comparable to flocculation. The steric repulsive force, which depends on the concentration and degree of solvation of the polymer chains, must be of sufficient magnitude to prevent close approach of the uncoated particles, but low enough so that the attractive force is dominant, leading to aggregation at about twice the adsorbed layer thickness. It has been found, for example, that adsorbed layers of certain polyoxyethylene–polyoxypropylene block copolymers will product satisfactory flocculated systems, whereas many nonyl phenyl ethoxylates will not. With both types of surfactant the molecular moieties producing steric repulsion are hydrated ethylene oxide chains, but the concentration of these in the adsorbed layers varies, giving the results indicated above.

Wetting problems

One of the problems encountered in dispersing solid materials in water is that the powder may not be readily wetted (see Chapter 5). This may be due to entrapped air or to the fact that the solid surface is hydrophobic. The wettability of a powder may be described in terms of the contact angle, θ, that the powder makes with surface of the liquid. This is described by:

$$\gamma_{S/V} = \gamma_{S/L} + \gamma_{L/V} \cos \theta$$

or

$$\cos \theta = \frac{\gamma_{S/V} - \gamma_{S/L}}{\gamma_{L/V}} \qquad (6.31)$$

where $\gamma_{S/V}$, $\gamma_{S/L}$ and $\gamma_{L/V}$ are the respective interfacial tensions.

For a liquid to wet a powder completely there should be a decrease in the surface free energy as a result of the immersion process. Once the particle is submerged in the liquid, the process of spreading wetting becomes important. In most cases where water is involved the reduction of contact angle may only be achieved by reducing the magnitude of $\gamma_{L/V}$ and $\gamma_{S/L}$ by the use of a wetting agent. The wetting agents are surfactants that not only reduce $\gamma_{L/V}$ but also adsorb on to the surface of the powder, thereby reducing $\gamma_{S/V}$. Both of these effects reduce the contact angle and improve the dispersibility of the powder.

Problems may arise because of the build-up of an adherent layer of suspension particles on the walls of the container just above the liquid line that occurs as the walls are repeatedly wetted by the suspension. This layer subsequently dries to form a hard, thick crust. Surfactants reduce this adsorption by coating both the glass and particle surfaces such that they repel each other.

Rheological properties of suspensions

Flocculated suspensions tend to exhibit plastic or pseudoplastic flow, depending on concentration, whereas concentrated deflocculated dispersions tend to be dilatant. This means that the apparent viscosity of flocculated suspensions is relatively high when the applied shearing stress is low, but it decreases as the applied stress increases and the attractive forces producing the flocculation are overcome. Conversely, the apparent viscosity of a concentrated deflocculated suspension is low at low shearing stress, but increases as the applied stress increases. This effect is due to the electrical repulsion that occurs when the charged particles are forced close together (see the DLVO plot of potential energy of interaction between particles; Fig. 6.4), causing the particles to rebound and creating voids into which the liquid flows, leaving other parts of the dispersion dry. In addition to the rheological problems associated with particle charge, the sedimentation behaviour is also of course influenced by the rheological properties of the liquid continuous phase.

Emulsions

An emulsion is a system consisting of two immiscible liquid phases, one of which is dispersed throughout the other in the form of fine droplets. A third component, the emulsifying agent, is necessary to stabilize the emulsion.

The phase that is present as fine droplets is called the disperse phase and the phase in which the droplets are suspended is the continuous phase. Most emulsions will have droplets with diameters of 0.1–100 μm and are inherently unstable systems; smaller globules exhibit colloidal behaviour and the stability of a hydrophobic colloidal dispersion.

Pharmaceutical emulsions usually consist of water and an oil. Two main types can exist: oil-in-water (o/w) and water-in-oil (w/o), depending upon whether the continuous phase is aqueous or oily. More complicated emulsion systems may exist: for example, an oil droplet enclosing a water droplet may be suspended in water to form a water-in-oil-in-water emulsion (w/o/w). Such systems or their o/w/o counterparts are termed ***multiple emulsions*** and are of interest as delayed-action drug delivery systems. Traditionally, emulsions have been used to render oily substances such as castor oil and liquid paraffin in a more palatable form. It is possible to formulate together oil-soluble and water-soluble medicaments in emulsions, and drugs may be more easily absorbed owing to the finely divided condition of emulsified substances.

A large number of bases used for topical preparations are emulsions, water miscible being o/w type and greasy bases w/o. The administration of oils and fats by intravenous infusion, as part of a total parenteral nutrition programme, has been made possible by the use of suitable non-toxic emulsifying agents such as lecithin. Here, the control of particle size of the emulsion droplets is of paramount importance in the prevention of embolus formation.

Microemulsions Unlike the coarse emulsions described above, microemulsions are homogeneous, transparent systems that are thermodynamically stable. Moreover, they form spontaneously when the components are mixed in the appropriate ratios. They can be dispersions of oil in water or water in oil, but the droplet size is very much smaller – 5–140 nm – than in coarse emulsions. They are essentially swollen micellar systems, but obviously the distinction between a micelle containing solubilized oil and an oil droplet surrounded by an interfacial layer largely composed of surfactant, is difficult to assess.

An essential requirement for their formation and stability is the attainment of a very low interfacial tension. It is generally not possible to achieve the required lowering of interfacial tension with a single surfactant, and it is necessary to include a second amphiphile, usually a medium chain length alcohol, in the formulation. The second amphiphile is referred to as the **cosurfactant**.

Although microemulsions have many advantages over coarse emulsions, particularly their transparency and stability, they require much larger amounts of surfactant for their formulation, which restricts the choice of acceptable components.

Theory of emulsion stabilization

Interfacial films When two immiscible liquids, e.g. liquid paraffin and water, are shaken together a temporary emulsion will be formed. The subdivision of one of the phases into small globules results in a large increase in surface area and hence the interfacial free energy of the system. The system is thus thermodynamically unstable, which results first in the dispersed phase being in the form of spherical droplets (the shape of minimum surface area for a given volume), and secondly in coalescence of these droplets, causing phase separation, the state of minimum surface free energy.

The adsorption of a surface-active agent at the globule interface will lower the o/w interfacial tension, the process of emulsification will be made easier and the stability may be enhanced. However, if a surface-active agent such as sodium dodecyl sulphate is used, the emulsion, after standing for a short while, will still separate out into its constituent phases. On the other hand, substances such as acacia, which are only slightly surface active,

produce stable emulsions. Acacia forms a strong viscous interfacial film around the globules, and it is thought that the characteristics of the interfacial film are most important in considering the stability of emulsions.

Pioneering work on emulsion stability by Schulman and Cockbain in 1940 showed that a mixture of an oil-soluble alcohol such as cholesterol and a surface-active agent such as sodium cetyl (hexadecyl) sulphate was able to form a stable complex condensed film at the oil/water interface. This film was of high viscosity, sufficiently flexible to permit distortion of the droplets, resisted rupture, and gave an interfacial tension lower than that produced by either component alone. The emulsion produced was stable, the charge arising from the sodium cetyl sulphate contributing to the stability, as described for lyophobic colloidal dispersions. For complex formation at the interface the correct 'shape' of molecule is necessary, thus Schulman and Cockbain found that sodium cetyl sulphate stabilized an emulsion of liquid paraffin when elaidyl alcohol (the *trans* isomer) was the oil-soluble component, but not when the *cis* isomer, oleyl alcohol, was used.

In practice, the oil-soluble and water-soluble components are dissolved in the appropriate phases and when the two phases are mixed the complex is formed at the interface. Alternatively, an emulsifying wax may be used consisting of a blend of the two components. The wax is dispersed in the oil phase and the aqueous phase is added at the same temperature. Examples of such mixtures are given in Table 6.4.

This principle is also applied with the non-ionic emulsifying agents. For example, mixtures of sorbitan mono-oleate and polyoxyethylene sorbitan esters (e.g. polysorbate 80) have good emulsifying properties. Non-ionic surfactants are widely used in the production of stable emulsions and have the advantages over ionic surfactants of being less toxic and

Table 6.4 Emulsifying waxes		
Product	Oil-soluble component	Water-soluble component
Emulsifying wax (anionic)	Cetostearyl alcohol	Sodium lauryl (dodecyl) sulphate
Cetrimide emulsifying wax (cationic)	Cetostearyl alcohol	Cetrimide (hexadecyl trimethyl ammonium bromide)
Cetomacrogol emulsifying wax (non-ionic)	Cetostearyl alcohol	Cetomacrogol (polyoxyethylene monohexadecyl ether)

less sensitive to electrolytes and pH variation. These emulsifying agents are not charged and there is no electrical repulsive force contributing to stability. It is likely, however, that these substances, and the cetomacrogol emulsifying wax included in Table 6.4, sterically stabilize the emulsions, as discussed above.

Hydrophilic colloids as emulsion stabilizers A number of hydrophilic colloids are used as emulsifying agents in pharmacy. These include proteins (gelatin, casein) and polysaccharides (acacia, cellulose derivatives and alginates). These materials, which generally exhibit little surface activity, adsorb at the oil/water interface and form multilayers. Such multilayers have viscoelastic properties, resist rupture and presumably form mechanical barriers to coalescence. However, some of these substance have chemical groups that ionize, e.g. acacia consists of salts of arabic acid, and proteins contain both amino and carboxylic acid groupings, thus providing electrostatic repulsion as an additional barrier to coalescence. Most cellulose derivatives are not charged. There is evidence, however, from studies on solid suspensions, that these substances sterically stabilize and it would appear probable that there will be a similar effect with emulsions.

Solid particles in emulsion stabilization Emulsions may be stabilized by finely divided solid particles if they are preferentially wetted by one phase and possess sufficient adhesion for one another so that they form a film around the dispersed droplets.

Solid particles will remain at the interface as long as a stable contact angle, θ, is formed by the liquid/liquid interface and the solid surface. The particles must also be of sufficiently low mass for gravitational forces not to affect the equilibrium. If the solid is preferentially wetted by one of the phases, then more particles can be accommodated at the interface if the interface is convex towards that phase. In other words, the liquid whose contact angle (measured through the liquid) is less than 90° will form the continuous phase (Fig. 6.14). Aluminium and

magnesium hydroxides and clays such as bentonite are preferentially wetted by water and thus stabilize o/w emulsions, e.g. liquid paraffin and magnesium hydroxide emulsion. Carbon black and talc are more readily wetted by oils and stabilize w/o emulsions.

Emulsion type

When an oil, water and an emulsifying agent are shaken together, what decides whether an o/w or w/o emulsion will be produced? A number of simultaneous processes have to be considered, for example droplet formation, aggregation and coalescence of droplets, and interfacial film formation. When oil and water are shaken together both phases initially form droplets. The phase that persists in droplet form for longer should become the disperse phase, and it should be surrounded by the continuous phase formed from the more rapidly coalescing droplets. The phase volumes and interfacial tensions will determine the relative number of droplets produced and hence the probability of collision, i.e. the greater the number of droplets the higher the chance of collision, so that the phase present in greater amount should finally become the continuous phase. However, emulsions containing well over 50% of disperse phase are common.

A more important consideration is the interfacial film produced by the adsorption of emulsifier at the o/w interface. Such films significantly alter the rates of coalescence by acting as physical and chemical barriers to coalescence. As indicated in the previous section, the barrier at the surface of an oil droplet may arise because of electrically charged groups producing repulsion between approaching droplets, or because of the steric repulsion, enthalpic in origin, from hydrated polymer chains. The greater the number of charged molecules present, or the greater the number of hydrated polymer chains at the interface, the greater will be the tendency to reduce oil droplet coalescence. On the other hand, the interfacial barrier for approaching water droplets arises primarily because of the non-polar or hydrocarbon portion of the interfacial film. The longer the hydrocarbon chain length and the greater the number of molecules present per unit area of film, the greater the tendency for water droplets to be prevented from coalescing. Thus it may be said generally that it is the dominance of the polar or non-polar characteristics of the emulsifying agent that plays a major contribution to the type of emulsion produced.

It would appear, then, that the type of emulsion formed, depending as it does on the polar/non-polar characteristics of the emulsifying agent, is a function

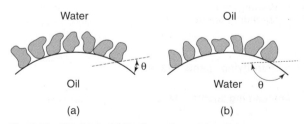

Fig. 6.14 Emulsion stabilization using solid particles. (a) Preferential wetting of solid by water, leading to an o/w emulsion; (b) preferential wetting of solid by oil, leading to a w/o emulsion.

of the relative solubility of the emulsifying agent, the phase in which it is more soluble being the continuous phase. This is a statement of what is termed the Bancroft rule, an empirical observation made in 1913.

The foregoing helps to explain why charged surface-active agents such as sodium and potassium oleates, which are highly ionized and possess strong polar groups, favour o/w emulsions, whereas calcium and magnesium soaps, which are little dissociated, tend to produce w/o emulsions. Similarly, non-ionic sorbitan esters favour w/o emulsions, whereas o/w emulsions are produced by the more hydrophilic polyoxyethylene sorbitan esters.

Because of the stabilizing mechanism involved, polar groups are far better barriers to coalescence than their non-polar counterparts. It is thus possible to see why o/w emulsions can be made with greater than 50% disperse phase, and w/o emulsions are limited in this respect and invert (change type) if the amount of water present is significant.

Hydrophile–lipophile balance The fact that a more hydrophilic interfacial barrier favours o/w emulsions whereas a more non-polar barrier favours w/o emulsions is made use of in the hydrophile–lipophile balance (HLB) system for assessing surfactants and emulsifying agents, which was introduced by Griffin in 1949. Here an HLB number is assigned to an emulsifying agent which is characteristic of its relative polarity. Although originally conceived for non-ionic emulsifying agents with polyoxyethylene hydrophilic groups, it has since been applied with varying success to other surfactant groups, both ionic and non-ionic.

By means of this number system an HLB range of optimum efficiency for each class of surfactant is established, as seen in Figure 6.15. This approach is empirical but it does allow comparison between different chemical types of emulsifying agent.

There are several formulae for calculating HLB values of non-ionic surfactants. We can estimate values for polysorbates (Tweens) and sorbitan esters (Spans) from:

$$HLB = (E + P)/5 \qquad (6.32)$$

where E is the percentage by weight of oxyethylene chains and P is the percentage by weight of polyhydric alcohol groups (glycerol or sorbitol) in the molecule. If the surfactant contains only polyoxyethylene as the hydrophilic group then we can use a simpler form of the equation:

$$HLB = E/5 \qquad (6.33)$$

Alternatively, we can calculate HLB values directly from the chemical formula using empirically determined group numbers. The formula is then:

$$HLB = 7 + \Sigma(\text{hydrophilic group numbers}) - \Sigma(\text{lipophilic group numbers}) \qquad (6.34)$$

Fig. 6.15 HLB scale showing classification of surfactant function.

Table 6.5 Group contributions to HLB values

Group	Contribution	Group	Contribution
SO$_4$Na	+38.7	COOK	+21.1
COONa	+19.1	SO$_3$Na	+11.0
N (tertiary amine)	+9.4	Ester (sorbitan ring)	+6.8
Ester (free)	+2.4	COOH	+2.1
OH (free)	+1.9	-O-(ether)	+1.3
OH (sorbitan)	+0.5	CH, CH$_2$ etc (alkyl)	-0.475
CF$_2$, CF$_3$	-0.870		
OCH$_2$CH$_2$	+0.33	OCH(CH$_3$)CH$_2$	-0.15

Group numbers of some commonly occurring groups are given in Table 6.5. Finally, the HLB of polyhydric alcohol fatty acid esters such as glyceryl monostearate may be obtained from the saponification value, S, of the ester, and the acid number, A, of the fatty acid using:

$$HLB = 20\,[1 - S/A] \qquad (6.35)$$

In addition, it has been suggested that certain emulsifying agents of a given HLB value appear to work best with a particular oil phase, and this has given rise to the concept of a *required HLB value* for any oil or combination of oils. However, this does not necessarily mean that every surfactant having the required HLB value will produce a good emulsion, as specific surfactants may interact with the oil, with another component of the emulsion, or even with each other.

For reasons mentioned earlier, mixtures of surface-active agents give more stable emulsions than when used singly. The HLB of a mixture of surfactants, consisting of fraction x of A and $(1 - x)$ of B, is assumed to be an algebraic mean of the two HLB numbers:

$$HLB_{mixt} = x\,HLB_A + (1 - x)\,HLB_B \qquad (6.36)$$

It has been found that at the optimum HLB for a particular emulsion the mean particle size of the emulsion is at a minimum, and this factor contributes to the stability of the emulsion system. The use of HLB values in the formulation of emulsions is discussed in Chapter 23.

Phase viscosity The emulsification process and the type of emulsion formed are influenced to some extent by the viscosity of the two phases. Viscosity can be expected to affect interfacial film formation because the migration of molecules of emulsifying agent to the oil/water interface is diffusion con-

trolled. Droplet movement prior to coalescence is also affected by the viscosity of the medium in which the droplets are dispersed.

Stability of emulsions

A stable emulsion may be defined as a system in which the globules retain their initial character and remain uniformly distributed throughout the continuous phase. The function of the emulsifying agent is to form an interfacial film around the dispersed droplets; the physical nature of this barrier controls whether or not the droplets will coalesce as they approach one another. If the film is electrically charged then repulsive forces will contribute to stability.

Separation of an emulsion into its constituent phases is termed **cracking** or **breaking**. It follows that any agent that will destroy the interfacial film will crack the emulsion. Some of the factors that cause an emulsion to crack are:

- the addition of a chemical that is incompatible with the emulsifying agent, thus destroying its emulsifying ability. Examples include surface-active agents of opposite ionic charge, e.g. the addition of cetrimide (cationic) to an emulsion stabilized with sodium oleate (anionic); the addition of large ions of opposite charge, e.g. neomycin sulphate (cationic) to aqueous cream (anionic); and the addition of electrolytes such as calcium and magnesium salts to emulsion stabilized with anionic surface-active agents;
- bacterial growth: protein materials and non-ionic surface-active agents are excellent media for bacterial growth;
- temperature change: protein emulsifying agents may be denatured and the solubility characteristics of non-ionic emulsifying agents change with a rise in temperature, heating above 70°C destroys most emulsions. Freezing will also crack an emulsion; this may be due to the ice formed disrupting the interfacial film around the droplets.

Other ways in which an emulsion may show instability are as follows.

Flocculation Even though a satisfactory interfacial film is present around the oil droplets, secondary minimum flocculation, as described earlier in this chapter under the discussion on the DLVO theory of colloid stability, is likely to occur with most pharmaceutical emulsions. The globules do not coalesce and may be redispersed by shaking. However, because of the closeness of approach of droplets in the floccule, if any weaknesses in the interfacial films occur then coalescence may follow. Flocculation should not be confused with creaming (see below). The former is due to the interaction of attractive and repulsive forces and the latter to density differences in the two phases; both may occur.

Phase inversion As indicated under the section on emulsion type, phase volume ratio is a contributory factor to the type of emulsion formed. Although it was stated there that stable emulsions containing more than 50% of disperse phase are common, attempts to incorporate excessive amounts of disperse phase may cause cracking of the emulsion or phase inversion (conversion of an o/w emulsion to w/o, or vice versa). It can be shown that uniform spheres arranged in the closest packing will occupy 74.02% of the total volume irrespective of their size. Thus Ostwald suggested that an emulsion which resembles such an arrangement of spheres would have a maximum disperse phase concentration of the same order. Although it is possible to obtain more concentrated emulsions than this, because of the non-uniformity of size of the globules and the possibility of deformation of shape of the globules, there is a tendency for emulsions containing more than about 70% disperse phase to crack or invert.

Further, any additive that alters the hydrophile–lipophile balance of an emulsifying agent may alter the emulsion type, thus the addition of a magnesium salt to an emulsion stabilized with sodium oleate will cause the emulsion to crack or invert.

The addition of an electrolyte to anionic and cationic surfactants may suppress their ionization owing to the common ion effect, and so a w/o emulsion may result even though normally an o/w emulsion would be produced. For example, White Liniment BP is formed from turpentine oil, ammonium oleate, ammonium chloride and water. With ammonium oleate as the emulsifying agent an o/w emulsion would be expected, but the suppression of ionization of the ammonium oleate by the ammonium chloride (the common ion effect) and a relatively large volume of turpentine oil produce a w/o emulsion.

Emulsions stabilized with non-ionic emulsifying agents such as the polysorbates may invert on heating. This is caused by the breaking of the H-bonds responsible for the hydrophilic characteristics of the polysorbate; its HLB value is thus altered and the emulsion inverts.

Creaming Many emulsions cream on standing. The disperse phase, according to its density relative to that of the continuous phase, rises to the top or sinks to the bottom of the emulsion, forming a layer of more concentrated emulsion. A common example

is milk, an o/w emulsion, with cream rising to the top of the emulsion.

As mentioned earlier, flocculation may occur as well as creaming, but not necessarily so. Droplets of the creamed layer do not coalesce, as may be found by gentle shaking which redistributes the droplets throughout the continuous phase. Although not so serious an instability factor as cracking, creaming is undesirable from a pharmaceutical point of view because a creamed emulsion is inelegant in appearance, provides the possibility of inaccurate dosage, and increases the likelihood of coalescence as the globules are close together in the cream.

Those factors that influence the rate of creaming are similar to those involved in the sedimentation rate of suspension particles and are indicated by Stokes' law, as follows:

$$v = \frac{2a^2 g(\sigma - \rho)}{9\eta} \qquad (6.37)$$

where v is the velocity of creaming, a the globule radius, σ and ρ the densities of disperse phase and dispersion medium, respectively, and η the viscosity of the dispersion medium. A consideration of this equation shows that the rate of creaming will be decreased by:

1. a reduction in the globule size
2. a decrease in the density difference between the two phases
3. an increase in the viscosity of the continuous phase.

A decrease of creaming rate may therefore be achieved by homogenizing the emulsion to reduce the globule size and increasing the viscosity of the continuous phase η by the use of thickening agents such as tragacanth or methyl cellulose. It is seldom possible to adjust the densities of the two phases satisfactorily.

Assessment of emulsion stability Approximate assessments of the relative stabilities of a series of emulsions may be obtained from estimations of the degree of separation of the disperse phase as a distinct layer, or from the degree of creaming. Whereas separation of the emulsion into two layers, i.e. cracking, indicates gross instability, a stable emulsion may cream, creaming being due simply to density differences and easily reversed by shaking. Some coalescence may, however, take place owing to the close proximity of the globules in the cream, similar problems occur with flocculation.

However, instability in an emulsion results from any process that causes a progressive increase in particle size and a broadening of the particle size distribution, so that eventually the dispersed particles become so large that they separate out as free liquid. Accordingly, a more precise method for assessing emulsion stability is to follow the globule size distribution with time. An emulsion approaching the unstable state is characterized by the appearance of large globules as a result of the coalescence of others.

Foams

A foam is a coarse dispersion of a gas in a liquid which is present as thin films or lamellae of colloidal dimensions between the gas bubbles.

Foams find application in pharmacy as aqueous and non-aqueous spray preparations for topical, rectal and vaginal medications and for burn dressings. Equally important, however, is the destruction of foams and the use of antifoaming agents. These are important in manufacturing processes, preventing foam in liquid preparations, for example. In addition, foam inhibitors such as the silicones are used in the treatment of flatulence, for the elimination of gas, air or foam from the gastrointestinal tract prior to radiography, and for the relief of abdominal distension and dyspepsia.

Because of their high interfacial area (and surface free energy) all foams are unstable in the thermodynamic sense. Their stability depends on two major factors, the tendency for the liquid films to drain and become thinner, and their tendency to rupture due to random disturbances such as vibration, heat and diffusion of gas from small bubbles to large bubbles. Gas diffuses from the small bubbles to the large because the pressure in the former is greater. This is a phenomenon of curved interfaces, the pressure difference Δp being a function of the interfacial tension, γ, and the radius, r, of the droplet according to $\Delta p = 2\gamma/r$.

Pure liquids do not foam. Transient or unstable foams are obtained with solutes such as short-chain acids and alcohols which are mildly surface active. However, persistent foams are formed by solutions of surfactants. The film in such foams consists of two monolayers of adsorbed surface-active molecules separated by an aqueous core. The surfactants stabilize the film by means of electrical double-layer repulsion or steric stabilization, as described for colloidal dispersions.

Foams are often troublesome, and knowledge of the action of substances that cause their destruction is useful. There are two types of antifoaming agent:

1. **Foam breakers**, such as ether and *n*-octanol. These substances are highly surface active and are thought to act by lowering the surface tension over small regions of the liquid film. These regions are rapidly pulled out by surrounding regions of higher tension, small areas of film are therefore thinned out and left without the properties to resist rupture.
2. **Foam inhibitors**, such as polyamides and silicones. It is thought that these are adsorbed at the air/water interface in preference to the foaming agent, but they do not have the requisite ability to form a stable foam. They have a low interfacial tension in the pure state and may be effective by virtue of rapid adsorption.

Aerosols

Aerosols are colloidal dispersions of liquids or solids in gases. In general, mists and fogs possess liquid disperse phases whereas smoke is a dispersion of solid particles in gases. However, no sharp distinction can be made between the two kinds because liquid is often associated with the solid particles. A mist consists of fine droplets of liquid that may or may not contain dissolved or suspended material. If the concentration of droplets becomes high it may be called a *fog*.

Although all the disperse systems mentioned above are less stable than colloids that have a liquid as dispersion medium, they have many properties in common with the latter and can be investigated in the same way. Particle size is usually within the colloidal range, but if it is larger than 1 μm the life of an aerosol is short because the particles settle out too quickly.

Preparation of aerosols In common with other colloidal dispersions, aerosols may be prepared by either dispersion or condensation methods. The latter involve the initial production of supersaturated vapour of the material that is to be dispersed. This may be achieved by supercooling the vapour. The supersaturation eventually leads to the formation of nuclei, which grow into particles of colloidal dimensions. The preparation of aerosols by dispersion methods is of greater interest in pharmacy and may be achieved by the use of pressurized containers with, for example, liquefied gases such as propellants. If a solution or suspension of active ingredients is contained in the liquid propellant, or in a mixture of this liquid and an additional solvent, then when the valve on the container is opened the vapour pressure of the propellant forces the mixture out of the container. The large expansion of the propellant at room temperature and atmospheric pressure produces a dispersion of the active ingredients in air. Although the particles in such dispersions are often larger than those in colloidal systems, these dispersions are still generally referred to as aerosols.

Application of aerosols in pharmacy The use of aerosols as a dosage form is particularly important in the administration of drugs via the respiratory system. In addition to local effects, systemic effects may be obtained if the drug is absorbed into the bloodstream from the lungs. Topical preparations are also well suited for presentation as aerosols. Therapeutic aerosols are discussed in more detail in Chapter 31.

BIBLIOGRAPHY

Attwood, D. and Florence, A.T. (1983) *Surfactant Systems, their Chemistry, Pharmacy and Biology.* Chapman & Hall, London.

Florence, A.T. and Attwood, D. (1998) *Physicochemical Principles of Pharmacy*, 3rd Edn. Palgrave, London.

Rosen, M.J. (1989) *Surfactants and Interfacial Phenomena*, 2nd Edn. John Wiley and Sons, New York.

Shaw, D.J. (1992) *Colloid and Surface Chemistry*, 4th Edn. Butterworth-Heinemann, Oxford.

7

Kinetics and product stability

John Pugh

KINETICS

Introduction

Kinetics is the study of the rate at which processes occur. The changes may be chemical (decomposition of a drug, radiochemical decay) or physical (transfer across a boundary, such as the intestinal lining or skin). Kinetic studies are useful in providing information that:

1. gives an insight into the mechanisms of the changes involved, and
2. allows a prediction of the degree of change that will occur after a given time has elapsed.

In general, the theories and laws of chemical kinetics are well founded and provide a sound basis for the application of such studies to pharmaceutical problems that involve chemical reactions, e.g. the decomposition of medical compounds. This chapter is concerned with chemical reactions: it is not the intention to discuss in detail the chemistry of instability and methods of prolonging the effective life of a medicine, the preformulation consideration of which is discussed briefly in Chapter 8.

Homogeneous and heterogeneous reactions

Homogeneous reactions occur in a single phase, i.e. true solutions or gases, and proceed uniformly throughout the whole of the system. **Heterogeneous reactions** involve more than one phase and are often confined to the phase boundary, their rates being dependent on the supply of fresh reactants to that boundary. Examples are decomposition of drugs in suspensions and enzyme-catalysed reactions.

Molecularity

Molecularity is the number of molecules involved in forming the product. This follows from the balanced (stoichiometric) equation describing the reaction. For example, $N_2O_5 \rightarrow 2NO_2 + \frac{1}{2}O_2$ is a slow unimolecular reaction and $\frac{1}{2}O_2 + \frac{1}{2}O_2 \rightarrow O_2$ is a fast bimolecular reaction.

Order

This is the number of concentration terms that determine the rate. In an unimolecular process a molecule will react if it has sufficiently high-energy. The number of high-energy molecules depends on how many molecules are present, i.e. their concentration in solution (or pressure in a gas). In a bimolecular process two molecules must collide to react, and the likelihood of collision depends on the concentrations of each species. The law of mass action states that the rate depends on the product of concentrations of the reactants.

Thus in the first step of the example reaction,

$$N_2O_5 = 2NO_2 + \frac{1}{2}O_2$$

the rate of reaction $= k_1 [N_2O_5]$, i.e. there is only one concentration term and the reaction is known as *first order*.

In the second step,

$$\frac{1}{2}O_2 + \frac{1}{2}O_2$$

the rate of reaction $= k_2 [\frac{1}{2}O_2] [\frac{1}{2}O_2] = k_2 [\frac{1}{2}O_2]^2$, where k_1 and k_2 are the reaction rate constants. Thus there are two concentration terms and the reaction is known as *second order*.

Each of these is discussed in more detail below.

First order

The rate is determined by one concentration term. These are by far the most important processes in pharmaceutical science. Many drug decompositions on storage and the passage of drugs from one body compartment to another, e.g. lumen of the intestine into blood, follow first-order kinetics. The rate of reaction is most simply defined as the concentration change divided by the corresponding time change:

$$\frac{dc}{dt} = -kc \tag{7.1}$$

The negative sign is used because concentration falls as time increases. This makes the rate constant, k, positive.

The differential equation above describes infinitely small changes. For real changes these small changes are summed (integrated), usually from the start of the process (time = 0, concentration = c_0) to the concentration, c, remaining at any other time, t.

$$\int_{c}^{c_0} \frac{dc}{c} = -k \int_{t}^{o} dt$$

$$[\ln c]_{c}^{c_0} = -k[t]_{t}^{o}$$

$$\ln c_o - \ln c = -k\{(0) - (t)\}$$

$$\ln c = \ln c_o - kt \tag{7.2}$$

$$(y) \qquad a \quad +b(x)$$

Thus a plot of $\ln c$ against t is a straight line with intercept c_0 and gradient $-k$.

The units of k are given by rearranging Eqn 7.1:

$$\frac{dc}{c\,dt} = k$$

i.e. the rate constant has the dimensions of time^{-1} and typical units of s^{-1}.

Note that because k contains no concentration term it is not necessary to convert experimental data to concentration values in order to estimate it. Any convenient property of the system that is directly proportional to concentration can be used, such as UV absorbance, conductivity, pressure or radioactivity. For example, absorbance (A) is related to concentration, c, by Beer's law, i.e. $c = \alpha A$, where α is a proportionality constant.

Substitution into Eqn 7.2 gives: $\ln \alpha A = \ln \alpha A_o - kt$ hence $\ln A = \ln A_o - kt$. Thus, although the intercept of the graph will alter, the gradient remains the same.

Example 7.1

Consider the following. A tritiated cardiac stimulant is administered by i.v. injection. Blood samples have the following radioactivity counts per second (cps):

t (min)	0	30	60	90	120	150
cps	59.7	24.3	9.87	4.01	1.63	0.67
ln (cps)	4.09	3.19	2.29	1.39	0.49	−0.41

From Figure 7.1 the rate constant for absorption from the blood is 0.03 min^{-1}.

Pseudo first order

Consider the hydrolysis of ethyl acetate:

$$CH_3COOEt + H_2O \rightarrow CH_3COOH + EtOH$$

Fig. 7.1 First order.

Strictly the reaction is second order and the rate of reaction is expressed as:

$$\text{Rate} = k\,[CH_3COOEt]\,[H_2O]$$

However, in a dilute aqueous solution of ethyl acetate, $[H_2O]$ is very large compared to $[CH_3COOEt]$ and hardly alters during the course of the reaction. $[H_2O]$ can be taken as a constant and incorporated into the second-order rate constant, k':

$$\text{Rate} = k'\,[CH_3COOEt]$$

where $k' = k[H_2O]$.

Thus the reaction is, in effect, first order with a rate constant k'. This applies to many drug decompositions by hydrolysis in aqueous solution.

Second order

Rate depends on the product of two concentration terms. In the simplest case they refer to the same species. For example:

$$2HI \rightarrow H_2 + I_2$$

Here the reaction is not simply a matter of an HI molecule falling apart, but relies on the collision of two HI molecules. The rate of reaction from the law of mass action is given by:

$$\text{Rate} = k[HI]\,[HI] = k[HI]^2$$

$$\frac{dc}{dt} = -kc^2 \tag{7.3}$$

$$\int_{c}^{c_o} \frac{c^{-2}}{dc} = -k \int_{t}^{o} dt$$

$$\left[-c^{-1}\right]_{c}^{c_o} = -k\left[t\right]_{t}^{o}$$

$$\frac{1}{c} = \frac{1}{c_o} + kt$$

$$(y)\quad a\ +b(x)$$

Thus the gradient of a plot of $1/c$ against t gives the rate constant, k.

Units of k from Eqn 7.3 are:

$$\frac{dc}{c^2 dt} = -k$$

i.e. conc^{-1} time^{-1} and typical units are L mol^{-1} s^{-1} or similar.

Example 7.2

Consider the following decomposition data:

t (days)	0	30	60	90	120	150
c (mmol L^{-1})	100	2.17	1.10	0.74	0.56	0.44

From Figure 7.2 the rate constant is 0.015 L mmol^{-1} day^{-1}.

If the reaction is between two different species, A and B, it is unlikely that their starting concentrations will be equal. Let their initial concentrations be a_o and b_o (where $a_o > b_o$), falling to a and b at time t. As equal numbers of molecules of A and B are lost in the decomposition, the rate can be defined as da/dt (or db/dt). Thus:

$$\frac{da}{dt} = -kab \tag{7.4}$$

Integration by partial fractions gives:

$$\ln(a/b) = \ln(a_o/b_o) + k(a_o - b_o)t$$
$$(y)\quad = \quad a \quad + \quad b(x)$$

Thus a plot of $\ln(a/b)$ against t is a straight line with gradient $k(a_o - b_o)$.

Fig. 7.2 Second order.

Zero order

In a zero-order reaction the rate of reaction (decomposition, dissolution, drug release) is independent of the concentration of the reactants, i.e. the rate is constant. A constant rate of drug release from a dosage form is highly desirable. Zero-order kinetics often apply to processes occurring at phase boundaries, where the concentration at the surface remains constant either because reaction sites are saturated (enzyme kinetics, drug receptor interaction) or are constantly replenished by diffusion of fresh material from within the bulk of one phase. This diffusion criterion applies to the hydrolysis of drugs in suspensions or delivery from controlled-release dosage forms such as transdermal patches.

$$\frac{dc}{dt} = -k \qquad (7.5)$$

$$\int_c^{c_o} c \ dc = k \int_t^o dt$$
$$[c]_c^{c_o} = -k[t]_t^o$$
$$c_o - c = -k\{(0) - (t)\}$$
$$c = c_o - kt \qquad (7.6)$$
$$(y)a + b(x)$$

Thus, a plot of c against t is a straight line with gradient k. Units of k from Eqn 7.5 are conc time^{-1}, with typical units of mole L^{-1} s^{-1} or similar.

Example 7.3

The concentration of steroid remaining in a transdermal patch is as follows:

Time (h)	0	30	60	90	120	150
Amount (μg)	20	16.4	12.8	9.2	5.6	2

Note: strictly speaking, 'amount' is not the same as 'concentration'. In this case concentration is μg patch^{-1}.

Fig. 7.3 Zero order.

From Figure 7.3 the rate constant is 0.12 μg h^{-1}(patch^{-1}).

Half-life ($t_{\frac{1}{2}}$)

This is the time taken for the concentration (of, say, a drug in solution) to reduce by a half. Rearrangement of the integrated equations for t (Eqns 7.2, 7.4 and 7.6) gives:

	Zero order	First order	Second order
$t =$	$(c - c_o)/k$	$\ln(c_o/c)/k$	$(1/c - 1/c_o)/k$

and substituting $c = c_o/2$ at $t_{\frac{1}{2}}$

$t_{\frac{1}{2}}$ $\quad c_o/2k$	$0.693/k$	$1/c_ok$

Note that for first-order reactions the half life, $t_{\frac{1}{2}}$, is independent of concentration.

Table 7.1 summarizes the parameters for zero-order, first-order and second-order processes.

Determination of order and rate constant from experimental data

This can achieved in two ways:

1. Substituting the data into the integrated equations and observing which plot is a straight line;

Table 7.1   Summary of parameters

	Zero order	First order	Second order ($a = b$)
Linear equation	$c = c_o - kt$	$\ln c = \ln c_o - kt$	$1/c = 1/c_o + kt$
Intercept	c_o	$\ln c_o$	$1/c_o$
Gradient	$-k$	$-k$	k
Units of k	conc time^{-1}	time^{-1}	conc^{-1} time^{-1}
e.g.	mole L^{-1} s^{-1}	s^{-1}	L mole^{-1} s^{-1}
Half-life($t_{\frac{1}{2}}$)	$c_o/2k$	$0.693/k$	$1/c_ok$

2. Finding $t_{\frac{1}{2}}$ values at different stages of the reaction and noting whether and how they vary with 'starting' concentration.

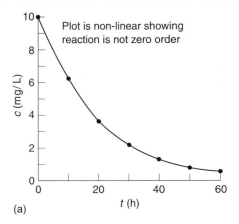

Plot is non-linear showing reaction is not zero order

(a)

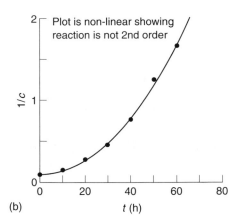

Plot is non-linear showing reaction is not 2nd order

(b)

Linear relationship shows 1st order process
Gradient $(-k) = -0.048$ h^{-1}
1st order rate constant $(k) = 0.048$ h^{-1}

(c)

Fig. 7.4 (a) Plot of concentration against time. (b) Plot of 1/concentration against time: (c) Plot of ln (concentration) against time.

Example 7.4

The following data apply to the decomposition of a drug:

t (h)	0	10	20	30	40	50	60
c (mg L^{-1})	10	6.2	3.6	2.2	1.3	0.8	0.6
$\ln c$	2.30	1.83	1.28	0.79	0.26	−0.22	−0.51
$1/c$	0.10	0.161	0.278	0.455	0.769	1.250	1.667

Data plotting method

The data are plotted in Figure 7.4. The plot of c against t (Fig. 7.4(a)) is obviously not linear and so the reaction is not zero order. A plot of $1/c$ against time (Fig. 7.4(b)) is not linear, so the reaction is not second order.

The plot of $\ln c$ against t (Fig. 7.4(c)) is linear and so the reaction is first order. From the graph, the gradient (i.e. $-k$) is -0.048 h^{-1} and the first-order rate constant is 0.048 h^{-1}.

Half-life method

This involves the selection of a set of convenient 'initial' concentrations and then determining the times taken to fall to half these values.

Example 7.5

The 'c_0' values are obtained by interpolation of the concentration versus time plot of the data in Example 7.4.

'c_0'	10	8	6	4	2
t at 'c_0'	0	5	11	18	32
t at 'c_0'/2	12	18	24	32	45
$t_{\frac{1}{2}}$	12	13	13	14	13

Within experimental error $t_{\frac{1}{2}}$ seems independent of 'c_0', suggesting that the reaction is first order. To confirm this it is necessary to check whether $t_{\frac{1}{2}}$ values correspond to zero- or to second-order kinetics.

If the reaction were zero order, then $c_0/2t_{\frac{1}{2}}$ would be a constant value (k). Similarly, for a second-order reaction $k = 1/c_0 t_{\frac{1}{2}}$ would be constant. Calculating these gives:

'c_0'	10	8	6	4	2
'c_0'/$2t_{\frac{1}{2}}$	0.42	0.31	0.23	0.14	0.08
$1/$'c_0'$t_{\frac{1}{2}}$	0.008	0.009	0.013	0.018	0.038

Thus neither set of values is constant, confirming that the reaction is neither zero or second order.

The first-order rate constant is found from the mean $t_{\frac{1}{2}}$ value of 13 h, i.e. $k = 0.693/t_{\frac{1}{2}} = 0.053$ h^{-1}.

Complex reactions

The theories so far have assumed that a single reaction pathway is involved and that the product does not affect the kinetics. Neither of these assumptions may be true and the overall order, being the result of several reactions, may not be zero, first or second order but have a fractional value.

There are three basic types of complex behaviour:

Parallel (side) reactions

Here reactants A form a mixture of products:

$$B \xleftarrow{k_1} A \xrightarrow{k_2} C$$

Usually only one of the products is desirable, the others being byproducts.

$$\text{(Yield of B/Yield of C)} = k_1/k_2$$

Series (consecutive) reactions

$$A \xrightarrow{k_1} B \xrightarrow{k_2} C$$

If $k_2 \ll k_1$ then a build-up of B occurs. The second step is then the rate-determining step of the reaction, and the overall order is approximately that of the rate-determining step. Thus the reaction:

$$2N_2O_5 \rightarrow 4NO_2 + O_2$$

is comprised of two consecutive reactions:

$N_2O_5 \rightarrow 2NO_2 + \frac{1}{2}O_2$ (slow – first order)
$\frac{1}{2}O_2 + \frac{1}{2}O_2 \rightarrow O_2$ (fast – second order)

and the overall reaction is first order, defined by the slower first step.

Reversible reactions

Here the product reforms the reactants:

$$A \underset{k_{-1}}{\overset{k_1}{\Longleftrightarrow}} B + C$$

Here there are two reactions occurring simultaneously: first-order decomposition of A, rate constant k_1, and second-order formation of A from B and C. The rate constant is often written as k_{-1}. This can cause confusion. The negative sign merely implies that it

refers to the reverse of a reaction numbered 1 (A → B + C): it does *not* mean that if k_1 is 0.5 h^{-1} then the rate constant for the reverse reaction is –0.5 h^{-1}.

Michaelis–Menten equation

These three basic reaction types can be combined in different ways. One important combination describes processes that occur at interfaces. These appear repeatedly in the life sciences, e.g. enzyme–substrate, transmitter–receptor, drug–receptor binding. The kinetics are described by the Michaelis–Menten equation, which assumes that the enzyme E and the substrate S form an unstable complex ES, which can either reform S or form a new product, P:

$$E + S \underset{k_2}{\overset{k_1}{\Longleftrightarrow}} ES \xrightarrow{k_3} P + E$$

The overall reaction rate is the rate at which P is formed. This is first order depending on $[ES]$. (The square brackets mean concentration of ES), thus $dP/dt = k_3[ES]$ (note no negative sign because P increases as t increases).

Unfortunately, we normally have no way of measuring $[ES]$. However, the rate at which $[ES]$ changes is the rate at which it forms from E and S, $(k_1[E][S])$, minus the rates at which it decomposes to reform E and S, $(k_2[ES])$, or to form P, $(k_3[ES])$. Thus:

$$\frac{d[ES]}{dt} = k_1[E][S] - k_2[ES] - k_3[ES]$$

$$\frac{d[ES]}{dt} = k_1[E][S] - (k_2 + k_3)[ES].$$

In practice $[ES]$ is small as the complex decomposes rapidly. Changes in $[ES]$ soon become negligible compared to other concentration changes in the system. Then $[ES]$ is almost a constant, $d[ES]/dt = 0$, and the system is said to be at a **steady state**.

Thus at the steady state:

$$\frac{d[ES]}{dt} = 0 = k_1[E][S] - (k_2 + k_3)[ES].$$

and rearrangement gives:

$$[ES] = \frac{k_1[E][S]}{(k_2 + k_3)}$$

Writing $(k_2 + k_3)/k_1$ as K gives:

or

$$[ES] = \frac{[E][S]}{K}$$

$$[ES] = \frac{[E]}{K/[S]} \qquad (7.7)$$

To proceed we need to know $[ES]$, i.e. the concentration of the unstable intermediate. In practice we only know the total concentration of enzyme that we put into the mixture, $[E_o]$. As this now exists in free and complexed forms, then

$$[E_o] = [E] + [ES]$$

Substituting $[E] = [E_o] - [ES]$ into Eqn 7.7 and then writing $J = K/[S]$ gives:

$$[ES] = \frac{[E_o] - [ES]}{K/[S]} = \frac{[E_o]}{J} - \frac{[ES]}{J}$$

$$[ES] + \frac{[ES]}{J} = \frac{[E_o]}{J}$$

$$[ES]\left(1 + \frac{1}{J}\right) = \frac{[E_o]}{J}$$

$$[ES]\left(\frac{J+1}{J}\right) = \frac{[E_o]}{J}$$

$$[ES] = \frac{[E_o]}{(J+1)} = \frac{[E_o]}{\left((K/[S])+1\right)}$$

The overall rate of reaction, V, is given by the Michaelis–Menten equation:

$$V = \frac{dP}{dt} = k_3 [ES]$$

$$V = \frac{k_3 [E_o]}{\dfrac{K}{[S]} + 1} \qquad (7.8)$$

Thus the rate, V, is not constant but declines from its initial value, V_o, as $[S]$ falls, i.e. as the substrate is used up. V_o is found from the initial gradient of the plot of $[P]$ against t (Fig. 7.5).

If these V_o values are found for a range of substrate concentrations, $[S]$, keeping the same enzyme concentration $[E_o]$, the familiar plateau curve results (Fig. 7.6).

The plateau shape arises from the mathematical properties of the Michaelis–Menten equation.

(a) At low $[S]$ values $\dfrac{K}{[S]}$ is large, so that

$$\left(\frac{K}{[S]} + 1\right) \approx \frac{K}{[S]}$$

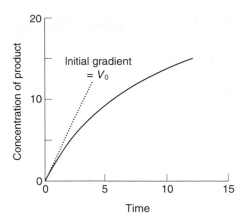

Fig. 7.5 Estimation of initial velocity of enzyme-catalysed reaction.

Fig. 7.6 Michaelis–Menten plot for enzyme-catalysed reaction.

Substitution into Eqn 7.8 gives:

$$V_o = \frac{k_3 [E_o]}{K}[S] \qquad (7.9)$$

i.e. the reaction is first order with respect to $[S]$ and the plot has gradient $= \dfrac{k_3 [E_o]}{K}$

(b) At high $[S]$ values $\dfrac{K}{[S]}$ is small and $\left(\dfrac{K}{[S]} + 1\right) \approx 1$

Substitution into Eqn 7.8 gives:

$$V_o = k_3 [E_o] \qquad (7.10)$$

k_3 and $[E_o]$ are constants and so this process is zero order. $k_3 [E_o]$ is the maximum rate, V_{max}, for a given enzyme concentration.

Viewed simply, the enzyme reactive sites are saturated by substrate molecules.

This plateau curve is very common and often signifies a process occurring at a saturatable interphase, a heterogeneous process.

Fig. 7.7 Lineweaver–Burke plot of data in Figure 7.6.

Equation 7.8 is often inverted to give a linear relationship between $1/V_0$ and $1/[S]$:

$$\frac{1}{V_0} = \frac{1}{k_3 E_0} + \frac{K}{k_3 E_0}\left(\frac{1}{[S]}\right)$$

$$\frac{1}{V_0} = \frac{1}{V_{max}} + \frac{K}{V_{max}}\left(\frac{1}{[S]}\right) \quad (7.11)$$

V_{max}, K and k_3 are found from the gradient and intercept of this Lineweaver–Burke plot (Fig. 7.7). Workers in the field of enzyme inhibition or drug–receptor interaction often estimate K from the intercept on the abscissa (x-axis) of the plot. This is the value of $1/[S]$ where $1/V_0 = 0$. Substitution into Eqn 7.11 gives:

$$1/[S] = -1/K.$$

Thus from Figure 7.7, $V_{max} = 15.1$ mmol L^{-1} s^{-1} and $K = 5.7$. The way in which these parameters are altered by inhibitors enables us to say whether the inhibition is reversible or irreversible and competitive or non-competitive (see York 1992 for further details).

Effect of temperature on reaction rate

Generally, increasing temperature increases the rate of reaction, and an often-quoted rough guide is that a 10°C rise doubles the rate constant. Better descriptions are given by the Arrhenius theory and the more rigorous transition state theory (see, for example, Martin 1993).

Arrhenius theory

This can be developed from simple basic ideas and leads to an equation that is formally identical with the transition state theory.

Consider the simple bimolecular reaction:

$$2HI \rightarrow H_2 + I_2$$

The original proposition was that if two molecules collided they would react. The collision number, Z, can be calculated from the kinetic theory of gases, and it was found that the number of molecules reacting per second, μ, was much smaller than Z. The theory was modified to propose that the colliding molecules must have sufficient energy to form an unstable intermediate, which breaks down to form the product.

The fraction of molecules with at least this activation energy, E, was calculated by Boltzmann as $e^{-E/RT}$, so that $\mu = Ze^{-E/RT}$.

This equation adequately describes simple reactions such as the decomposition of HI, but for even slightly more complex reactions, such as:

$$N(CH_3)_3 + CH_3I = N(CH_3)_4I$$

μ is thousands of times smaller than $Ze^{-E/RT}$.

This is because the nitrogen atom is shielded by a mass of C and H atoms, so that only very few collisions occur between the nitrogen and the carbon of the approaching CH_3I. Thus an orientation factor, P, often with a very small value, must also be included:

$$\mu = PZe^{-E/RT}.$$

The rate constant k is proportional to μ. So, writing k as $\alpha\mu$ gives:

$$k = \alpha PZe^{-E/RT}$$

Over a small temperature range the change in Z with T is negligible compared to that in the $e^{-E/RT}$ term, so that αPZ is a constant, A. A is called the 'frequency factor', as it is related to the frequency of correctly aligned collisions.

$$k = Ae^{-E/RT} \quad (7.12)$$

This is the Arrhenius equation, and may also be written as:

$$\ln k = \ln A - \frac{E}{R}\left(\frac{1}{T}\right)$$
$$(y) \qquad a \qquad +b(x) \quad (7.13)$$

or, in $\log_{10}$ form:

$$\log k = \log A - \frac{E}{2.303R}\left(\frac{1}{T}\right)$$

so that a plot of $\ln k$ (or $\log k$) against $(1/T)$ is a straight line, enabling the calculation of E and A from the gradient and intercept (remember that T must be in K, not °C). The same equation holds for zero- and first-order reactions. Here the molecule will react if it has energy $\geq E$. The collision and orientation factors are inapplicable and A is now the proportionality constant α, although it is still termed the frequency factor.

ACCELERATED STABILITY TESTING

All medicinal products decompose with time. Paradoxically, when this decomposition is being assessed the skilled formulator becomes a victim of his own expertise, as a good formulation will take a long time to decompose. Instabilities in modern formulations are often detectable only after considerable storage periods under normal conditions. To assess the stability of a formulated product it is usual to expose it to 'high stress', i.e. conditions of temperature, humidity and light intensity that are known from experience to be likely causes of breakdown. High stress conditions enhance the deterioration of the product and therefore reduce the time required for testing. This enables more data to be gathered in a shorter time, which in turn will allow unsatisfactory formulations to be eliminated early in a study and will also reduce the time for a successful product to reach the market. It must be emphasized that extrapolations to 'normal' storage conditions must be made with care, and that the formulator must be sure that such extrapolations are valid. It is advisable therefore to run concurrently a batch under expected normal conditions to confirm later that these assumptions are valid.

The objectives of such accelerated tests may be defined as:

1. The rapid detection of deterioration in different initial formulations of the same product. This is of use in selecting the best formulation from a series of possible choices;
2. The prediction of shelf-life, which is the time a product will remain satisfactory when stored under expected or directed storage conditions;
3. The provision of a rapid means of quality control, which ensures that no unexpected change has occurred in the stored product.

Good formulations will invariably break down more slowly than poor ones. Even though no absolute conclusions can be drawn about their predicted stability under normal storage from data obtained under stress conditions, such tests allow formulations to be optimized relatively quickly.

When the perceived optimal formulation is decided, attempts can be made to predict its likely stability at proposed storage conditions. These may be at 25°C for ambient room temperature (or 30°C for use in hot climates), or 0–4°C for a refrigerator. The amount of decomposition that is acceptable in fixing an expiry date depends on the particular drug. This will be small if the therapeutic index (ratio of toxic dose/effective dose) is low, e.g. digoxin, or if the decomposition products are toxic. It might be decided to fix the shelf-life as being the time taken for 10% of the drug to decompose at 25°C.

Stability testing protocols

Accelerated stability testing requires the careful design of protocols which must define clearly the following:

1. The temperature and humidity for storage
2. Storage time before sampling
3. The number of batches to be sampled
4. The number of replicates within each batch
5. A suitable light challenge
6. Details of assay.

Although all pharmaceutical products have to satisfy government regulatory authorities, surprisingly there are no nationally or internationally standardized storage conditions. Storage conditions during stability testing vary from company to company and even within a single company. Often different types of products are given different challenges. Two alternative stability protocol strategies are discussed below.

Factorial analysis

Factorial analysis is a simple approach for gauging the likely effect of additional factors for which no simple descriptive relationship such as the Arrhenius equation exists. For example, it may reasonably be suspected that light and humidity cause the degradation of a freeze-dried antibiotic powder. The powder is therefore stored under low and high stresses in sealed vessels over water or desiccant on windowsills and in cupboards. After a suitable time the amount of decomposition is measured and typical results are:

$hl = 8\%$; $Hl = 39\%$; $hL = 16\%$; $HL = 47\%$.
(where, for example, hL = low humidity, high light intensity).

Average decomposition at high humidity,
$H = (39 + 47)/2 = 42\%$

Average decomposition at low humidity, $h = 12\%$

Thus the scaled effect of humidity is $(42 - 12) = 30\%$.
Similarly, the effect of light is 8%.

Thus although both light and humidity cause decomposition, humidity poses the greater threat to stability.

A structured approach

A typical protocol is shown in Table 7.2. At least two, possibly three, batches are stored as indicated and subsequently tested in duplicate. Products are usually stored in their final container. If at this stage the final pack has not been confirmed, a range of packs and pack materials must be tested. For example, tablets may be stored in glass bottles, HDPE containers, aluminium foil and PVC or PVC/PVDC blisters (see Chapter 36). Some batches

Table 7.2 A typical storage and testing protocol for accelerated stability assessment of pharmaceutical products

Time of sampling	Storage temperature (°C) and humidity (%RH)						
	4	RT	30	37	37/75%	50	75
6 weeks	S	S		T	T		T	T
3 months	S	S	T	T	T		T	T
6 months	S	S	T	T	T		T	
12 months	S	S	T	T				
18 months	S	S	T	T				
2 years	S	S	T	T				
3 years	S	S	T					
4 years	S	S	T					
5 years	T	T	T					

Notes

Apart from one, or rarely two, high humidity challenges, the remaining storage temperatures are at ambient humidities.

RT: (room temperature) – often an uncontrolled cabinet in which the temperature can be between 15 and 25°C.

S: the 4°C and 25°C samples are often retained as spares in the event of any problems with the analysis of any of the other samples.

T: testing is performed on these samples. To give an example – in the case of tablets these tests may consist of:
   assay for active ingredient(s) by HPLC;
   assay for degradation product(s) by TLC;
   an assessment of appearance;
   tablet weight;
   tablet thickness;
   friability;
   crushing strength;
   moisture content;
   disintegration;
   dissolution.

of liquid products may be stored in an inverted position to check for interaction between the ingredients and the liner of the cap.

It is important that stability studies are performed at all stages of product development. Stability testing during preformulation is discussed in Chapter 8 of this book and by Monkhouse (1984). Stability programmes for formulation studies have been discussed by Dukes (1984) and during clinical trials and scale-up by Lantz (1984). Stability programmes for marketed batches are described by Kaminski (1984) and Thompson (1984). The products may also be exposed to an additional light challenge. This may be in the form of a standard fluorescent-tube light cabinet or more simply, a south facing window.

Prediction of shelf-life from accelerated stability testing data

The mathematical prediction of shelf-life is based on the application of the Arrhenius equation, Eqn 7.12, which indicates the effect of temperature on the rate constant, k, of a chemical reaction. Figure 7.8 shows that a graph of ln k versus the reciprocal of thermodynamic temperature, $1/T$, is a straight line. If the slope of this line is determined from the results of accelerated tests at high temperatures it is possible to determine the value of the rate constant at other temperatures (e.g. normal room temperature) by extrapolation. Substitution of this value of k into the appropriate order of reaction (i.e. the rate equation that applies to the reaction involved in the particular decomposition) allows the amount of decomposition after a given time to be calculated. As pointed out, this approach involves a knowledge of the order of the reaction involved, and preliminary experiments are therefore necessary to determine this order.

Several difficulties and limitations are involved in this aspect of accelerated stability testing. First, as in all accelerated tests, there is the possibility that the application of high stresses may cause reactions that would not take place under the lower stresses associated with normal storage conditions. Secondly, the uncertainty surrounding the term 'normal storage conditions' introduces a difficulty when attempting to forecast the shelf-life of a product. Unless the storage conditions are defined precisely on the container, allowance should be made for variations in the conditions likely to be encountered under normal storage. Attempts to allow for such a contingency often involve accepting the shortest shelf-life for the range of conditions likely to be encountered. The climate of the country in which a product is to be marketed is particularly important in defining this range.

Decompositions in formulated products often proceed via a complex reaction series and may involve simultaneous, consecutive or chain reactions, because the formulated products themselves are complex systems. In addition, the order of a reaction may change after a certain time. Predictions of the extent of decomposition at future times are then impracticable, and prolonged tests under normal storage conditions must be carried out.

In spite of these difficulties the application of accelerated testing to pharmaceutical products is often useful, and predicted shelf-lives are sufficiently accurate. Statistical methods of designing such tests have therefore been reported which allow the selection of the number of replicates, sampling times and other factors involved in the tests to be made on a logical basis to attain the required degree of accuracy without wasting time on unnecessary experimentation.

Common high stresses or challenges

Temperature challenge

An increase in temperature causes an increase in the rate of chemical reactions. The products are therefore stored at temperatures higher than room temperature. The nature of the product often determines the range covered in the accelerated test. Samples are removed at various time intervals and the extent of decomposition is determined by analysis. Sensitive analytical methods should be used in all stability tests of this nature, as small changes may be detected after very short storage periods.

The effects caused by high temperatures should not be confused with those that arise from the effect of low humidity. Such confusion is possible because the relative humidity inside a high-temperature storage cabinet will be lower than that in the room. This low humidity causes loss of moisture, which may lead to apparent increases in the concentration of ingredients. If these concentration changes are not allowed for in subsequent analyses decomposition may be unsuspected.

The most useful feature of the Arrhenius equation in pharmacy is that it allows the prediction of reaction rates at proposed storage temperatures from data at high temperatures. Preparations are stored at high temperatures, thus saving time in developmental formulation studies. However, extrapolation of results is always a risky business, even from a purely statistical standpoint, when it is assumed that the plot remains linear over the extrapolated range. Added to this is the (small) variation in A with temperature and the possibility of change in reaction mechanism with temperature, i.e. variation in E.

Example 7.6

From the following data, estimate the rate constant at 25°C:

Temp (°C)	k (day^{-1})	T (K)	$1/T$	ln k
70	0.0196	343	2.92×10^{-3}	−3.93
60	0.0082	333	3.00×10^{-3}	−4.80
50	0.0028	323	3.10×10^{-3}	−5.88
40	0.0011	313	3.20×10^{-3}	−6.81
25		298	3.36×10^{-3}	

A plot of ln k against $1/T$ is a good straight line (Fig. 7.8).

Reading ln k from the graph at $1/T = 3.36 \times 10^{-3}$ (corresponding to 25°C) is −8.5, giving $k_{25} = 2.03 \times 10^{-4}$ day^{-1}.

Regression analysis (see, for example, Bolton 1984) gives the equation for the best straight line as:

ln k = 26.4 − 10408 $1/T$; correlation coefficient, r, of 0.999. Hence $k_{25} = 1.98 \times 10^{-4}$ day^{-1}.

The 95% confidence interval is $(1.35–2.95) \times 10^{-4}$ day^{-1}, showing that even good-quality experimental data yield disappointingly imprecise results on extrapolation.

The decomposition is first order and so obeys the equation

$$\ln c = \ln c_o - kt.$$

At the shelf-life, $t_{10\%}$, $c = 0.9c_o$, thus

$$t_{10\%} = \frac{\ln(c_o / 0.9c_o)}{k} = \frac{\ln 1.11}{1.98 \times 10^{-4}}$$

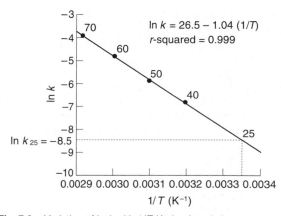

Fig. 7.8 Variation of ln k with $1/T$ (Arrhenius plot).

Thus, $t_{10\%}$ = 527 days (95% confidence interval = 354–773 days).

A scheme for continually increasing the storage temperature is sometimes employed. Curvature of the final plot indicates a change in reaction mechanism, and data collected at low temperatures are used in the assessment, thereby reducing extrapolation errors.

The Arrhenius equation involves only one rate constant and therefore applies to a simple (single step) decomposition mechanism. It cannot be used for complex reactions (consecutive, parallel etc.) or heterogeneous processes involving phase boundaries. Here additional factors, such as rate of dissolution, diffusion from within a matrix, and melting, are important determinants of decomposition. All sorts of confounding factors may invalidate the procedure. For example, the higher temperatures may reduce the moisture content of the product, thus slowing hydrolysis, gelatin may soften or melt, tablet coatings may split; the effects of temperature on photochemical and microbiological destruction are unpredictable.

Humidity challenge

Storage of the product in atmospheres of high humidity will accelerate decompositions that result from hydrolysis. Marked acceleration will be obtained if the 'naked' product (i.e. not enclosed in a container) is subjected to these tests, which usually indicate the minimum humidity tolerated by the product without undue decomposition, and are therefore useful in determining the degree of protection that should be afforded by a container.

Light challenge

A source of artificial light is used to accelerate the effects of sunlight or sky light. The source should emit a similar distribution of radiant energy to that in sunlight because photochemical reactions involve the absorption of light of definite wavelengths. Daylight fluorescent lamps provide a satisfactory source, and banks of such lamps may be used to accelerate the effects of light. However, although these lamps do not have a marked heating effect the use of glass plates to reduce such an effect is recommended, otherwise it is difficult to separate the accelerated decomposition caused by light from that caused by increased temperatures.

Concluding comments

Even if the Arrhenius equation can be applied successfully to predict the effect of temperature, and the effect of other factors, such as the influence of light and humidity can now be predicted with some certainty, other factors beyond the control of the formulator must be foreseen. The end user may store bottles lying down, so that reaction with materials in the cap may occur; if the preparation is to be used as bulk stock, e.g. 2 L of a cough mixture, it may well be left half-filled with air after opening for a prolonged period and oxidation may occur; stock containers of tablets will be continually opened and resealed, admitting moisture from the atmosphere.

It must be remembered that although accelerated storage testing is a useful tool for formulation studies, the results can only be a guide and may not apply to actual usage. It is essential that final formulations in their final packaging be stored under conditions that will be encountered in practice, to provide acceptable data for the licensing authorities.

REFERENCES

Bolton, S. (1984) *Pharmaceutical Statistics.* Marcel Dekker, New York, pp. 198–200
Dukes, G.R. (1984) Stability programs for formulation studies. *Drug Dev. Ind. Pharm.*, **10**(8&9), 1413–1424.
Kaminski, E.E. (1984) Stability program for marketed batches. *Drug Dev. Ind. Pharm.*, **10**(8&9), 1433–1448.
Lanz, R.J. (1984) Stability aspects of clinical supplies and scale-up studies. *Drug Dev. Ind. Pharm.*, **10**(8&9), 1425–1432.
Martin, A. (1993) *Physical Pharmacy*, 4th edn. Lea and Febiger, Philadelphia, pp. 297–298
Monkhouse, D.C. (1984) Stability aspects of preformulation and formulation of solid pharmaceutical. *Drug Dev. Ind. Pharm.*, **10**(8&9), 1373–1412.
Thompson, K. (1984) Stability programs for marketed batches. *Drug Dev. Ind. Pharm.*, **10**(8&9), 1449–1462.
York, J.L. (1992) Enzymes: classification, kinetics and control. Chapter 4 in *Textbook of Biochemistry*, 3rd edn. (ed.) T.M. Devlin. Wiley, New York, pp. 157–162.

Pharmaceutical preformulation: the physicochemical properties of drug substances

James Wells

CHAPTER CONTENTS

THE CONCEPT OF PREFORMULATION

Almost all new drugs are marketed as tablets, capsules or both (Table 8.1). Although only a few are marketed as an injection (25% of those marketed as tablets) the intravenous route is always required during early toxicity, metabolic, bioavailability and clinical studies to provide a precise drug and dose deposition. Other dosage forms may be required (Table 8.1) but these are drug specific and depend to a large extent on the successful development of tablets, capsules and injections.

Prior to the development of these three major dosage forms, it is essential that certain *fundamental* physical and chemical properties of the drug molecule and other *derived* properties of the drug powder are determined. This information dictates many of the subsequent events and approaches in formulation development. This first learning phase is known as *preformulation*.

A recommended list of the information required in preformulation is shown in Table 8.2. This is assembled, recognizing the relative importance and probable existence of only limited quantities of new bulk drug (mg rather than g). Investigators must be pragmatic and generate data of immediate relevance, especially if the likely dosage forms are known.

Two fundamental properties are mandatory for a new compound:

1. Intrinsic solubility (C_o),
2. Dissociation constant (pK_a).

Table 8.1 Frequency distribution of dosage form types manufactured in the UK

Dosage form	Frequency (%)
Tablets	46
Liquid oral	16
Capsules	15
Injections	13
Suppositories and pessaries	3
Topicals	3
Eye preparations	2
Aerosols (inhalation)	1
Others	1

Independent of this pharmaceutical profiling (Table 8.2), analysts will generate data (Table 8.3) to confirm structure and purity, and this should be used to complement and confirm pharmaceutical data. Their greater training and knowledge in analysis will assist in the identification of suitable stability-indicating assays by high-performance liquid chromatography (HPLC).

SPECTROSCOPY

The first step in preformulation is to establish a simple analytical method. Most drugs absorb light in the ultraviolet wavelengths (190–390 nm) as they are

Table 8.2 Preformulation drug characterization

Test	Method/function/characterization
Spectroscopy	Simple UV assay
Solubility	Phase solubility, purity
aqueous	Intrinsic solubility, pH effects
pK_a	Solubility control, salt formation
salts	Solubility, hygroscopicity, stability
solvents	Vehicles, extraction
partition coeff K^o_w	Lipophilicity, structure activity
dissolution	Biopharmacy
Melting point	DSC – polymorphism, hydrates, solvates
Assay development	UV, TLC, HPLC
Stability (in solution and solid state)	Thermal, hydrolysis, oxidation, photolysis, metal ions, pH.
Microscopy	Morphology, particle size
Powder flow	Tablet and capsule formulation
bulk density	
angle of repose	
Compression properties	Tablet and capsule formation
Excipient compatibility	Excipient choice

Table 8.3	Analytical preformulation
Attribute	Test
Identity	Nuclear magnetic resonance (NMR) Infra red spectroscopy (IR) Ultraviolet spectroscopy (UV) Thin-layer chromatography (TLC) Differential scanning calorimetry (DSC) Optical rotation, where applicable
Purity	Moisture (water and solvents) Inorganic elements Heavy metals Organic impurities Differential scanning calorimetry (DSC)
Assay	Titration Ultraviolet spectroscopy (UV) High-performance liquid chromatography (HPLC)
Quality	Appearance Odour Solution colour pH of slurry (saturated solution) Melting point

generally aromatic and contain double bonds. The acidic or basic nature of the molecule can be predicted from functional groups (Perrin et al 1981). Using the UV spectrum of the drug, it is possible to choose an analytical wavelength (often λ_{max}) suitable to quantify the amount of drug in a particular solution. Excitation of the molecule in solution causes a loss in light energy, and the net change from the intensity of the incident light (I_o) and the transmitted light (I) can be measured. The amount of light absorbed by a solution of drug is proportional to the concentration (C) and the path length of the solution (l) through which the light has passed. Equation 8.1 is the Beer–Lambert law, where e is the molar extinction coefficient.

$$\text{Absorbance } (A) = \log_{10} (I_o/I) = eCl \qquad (8.1)$$

In pharmacy it is usual to use the **specific absorption coefficient** $E_{1\,cm}^{1\%}$ (E_1^1), where the pathlength is 1 cm and the solution concentration is 1% w/v (10 mg mL^{-1}), as doses of drugs and concentrations are generally in unit weights rather than molarity ($E_1^1 = 10e/MW$).

SOLUBILITY

Aqueous solubility

The availability of a drug is always limited and the preformulation scientist may only have 50 mg. As the

compound is new the quality is invariably poor, so that a large number of impurities may be present and often the first crystals come down as a metastable polymorph. Accordingly, as a minimum, the solubility and pK_a must be determined. Solubility dictates the ease with which formulations for oral gavage and intravenous injection studies in animals are obtained. The pK_a allows the informed use of pH to maintain solubility and to choose salts required to achieve good bioavailability from the solid state (Chapter 9) and improve stability (Chapter 7) and powder properties (Chapter 13 and 14).

Kaplan (1972) suggested that unless a compound has an aqueous solubility in excess of 1% (10 mg mL^{-1}) over the pH range 1–7 at 37°C, potential bioabsorption problems may occur. If the intrinsic dissolution rate was greater than 1 mg cm^{-2} min^{-1} then absorption was unimpeded. Dissolution rates less than 0.1 mg cm^{-2} min^{-1} were likely to give dissolution rate-limited absorption. This tenfold difference in dissolution rate translates to a lower limit for solubility of 1 mg mL^{-1}. Under sink conditions, dissolution rate and solubilities are proportional.

A solubility of less than 1 mg mL^{-1} indicates the need for a salt, particularly if the drug will be formulated as a tablet or capsule. In the range 1–10 mg mL^{-1} serious consideration should be given to salt formation. When the solubility of the drug cannot be manipulated in this way (neutral molecules, glycosides, steroids, alcohols, or where the pK_a is less than 3 for a base or greater than 10 for an acid) then liquid filling in soft or hard gelatin capsules may be necessary.

Intrinsic solubility (C_o)

An increase in solubility in acid compared to aqueous solubility suggests a weak base, and an increase in alkali a weak acid. In both cases a dissociation constant (pK_a) can be measured and salts should form. An increase in acidic and alkaline solubility suggests either amphoteric or zwitterion behaviour. In this case there will be two pK_as, one acidic and one basic. No change in solubility suggests a non-ionizable neutral molecule with no measurable pK_a, and solubility manipulation will require either solvents or complexation.

When the purity of the drug sample can be assured, the solubility value obtained in acid for a weak acid or alkali for a weak base can be assumed to be the intrinsic solubility (C_o), ie. the fundemental solubility when completely unionized. The solubility should ideally be measured at two temperatures:

1. 4°C to ensure physical stability and extend short-term storage and chemical stability until more definitive data are available. The maximum density of water occurs at 4°C. This leads to a minimum aqueous solubility.
2. 37°C to support biopharmaceutical evaluation.

However, as absolute purity is often in doubt it is more accurate to determine this crucial solubility by the use of a phase-solubility diagram (Fig. 8.1). The data are obtained from a series of experiments in which the ratio of the amount of drug to the amount of dissolving solvent is varied.

Any deviation from the horizontal is indicative of impurities, which a higher drug loading and its inherent impurities either promotes or suppresses solubility. In cases where the observed result changes with the amount of solvent, the line is extrapolated to zero phase ratio, where solubility will be independent of solvent level and the true intrinsic solubility of the drug. The United States Pharmacopoeia uses this method to estimate the purity of mecamylamine hydrochloride.

pK$_a$ from solubility data

Seventy-five per cent of all drugs are weak bases; 20% are weak acids and only 5% are non-ionic, amphoteric or alcohols. It is therefore appropriate to consider the Henderson–Hasselbalch equations for weak bases and acids.

For weak bases: $$pH = pK_a + \log_{10}([B]/[BH^+])\ (8.2)$$

and for weak acids: $$pH = pK_a + \log_{10}([A^-]/[HA])\ (8.3)$$

Equations 8.2 and 8.3 can be used:

1. to determine pK$_a$ by following changes in solubility
2. to predict solubility at any pH, provided that the intrinsic solubility (C_o) and pK$_a$ are known
3. to facilitate the selection of suitable salt-forming compounds and predict the solubility and pH properties of the salts.

Albert and Serjeant (1984) give a detailed account of how to obtain precise pK$_a$ values by potentiometry, spectroscopy and conductivity.

Salts

A major improvement in solubility can be achieved by forming a salt. Acceptable pharmaceutical salt counter-ions are shown in Table 8.4. As an example, the consequence of changing chlordiazepoxide to various salt forms is shown in Table 8.5.

In some cases, salts prepared from strong acids or bases are freely soluble but very hygroscopic. This does lead to instability in tablet or capsule formulations, as some drug will dissolve in its own adsorbed films of moisture. It is often better to use a weaker acid or base to form the salt, provided any solubility requirements are met. A less soluble salt will gener-

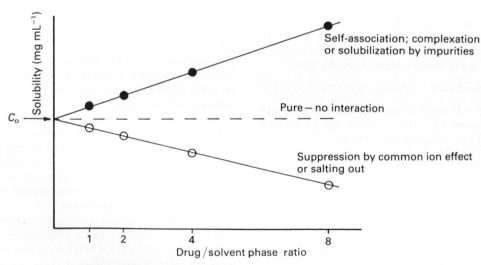

Fig. 8.1 Effect of drug: solvent ratio on solubility when the drug is impure. Assuming the compound is a base and the estimate of its solubility in 0.1 M NaOH was 1 mg mL^{-1}, four solutions of 3 mL should be set up containing 3, 6, 12 and 24 mg of drug. These give the phase ratios shown here. 3 mL is the smallest volume that can be manipulated for either centrifugation or filtration and dilution of UV analysis. The vials should be agitated continuously overnight and then the concentration in solution determined.

Table 8.4 Potential pharmaceutical salts

Basic drugs			Acidic drugs		
Anion	pK_a	% Usage	Cation	pK_a	% Usage
Hydrochloride	−6.10	43.0	Potassium	16.00	10.8
Sulphate	−3.00, +1.96	7.5	Sodium	14.77	62.0
Mesylate	−1.20	2.0	Lithium	13.82	1.6
Maleate	1.92, 6.23	3.0	Calcium	12.90	10.5
Phosphate	2.15, 7.20, 12.38	3.2	Magnesium	11.42	1.3
Salicylate	3.00	0.9	Diethanolamine	9.65	1.0
Tartrate	3.00	3.5	Zinc	8.96	3.0
Lactate	3.10	0.8	Choline	8.90	0.3
Citrate	3.13, 4.76, 6.40	3.0	Aluminium	5.00	0.7
Succinate	4.21, 5.64	0.4			
Acetate	4.76	1.3			
Others		31.4	Others		8.8

Table 8.5 Theoretical solubility and pH of salts of chlordiazepoxide

Salt	pK_a	Salt pH	Solubility (mg mL^{-1})
Base	4.80	8.30	2.0
Hydrochloride	−6.10	2.53	<165[a]
Maleate	1.92	3.36	57.1
Tartrate	3.00	3.90	17.9
Benzoate	4.20	4.50	6.0
Acetate [b]	4.76	4.78	4.1

[a] Maximum solubility of chlordiazepoxide hydrochloride, achieved at pH 2.89, is governed by crystal lattice energy and common ions.
[b] Chlordiazepoxide acetate may not form; pK_a of acetate too high and too close to that of drug ion.

ally be less hygroscopic and form less acidic or basic solutions (Table 8.5). Injections should ideally lie in the pH range 3–9 to prevent vessel or tissue damage and pain at the injection site. Oral syrups should not be too acidic, to enhance palatability. Packaging may also be susceptible: undue alkalinity will attack glass, and hydrochloride salts should not be used in aerosol cans as a propellant–acid reaction will corrode the canister.

From Table 8.5, not only does the intrinsic pH of the base solution fall significantly if salt forms are produced but, as a consequence, the solubility increases exponentially (Eqns 8.2 and 8.3). This has important implications in vivo. A weak base with an intrinsic solubility greater than 1 mg mL^{-1} will be freely soluble in the gastrointestinal tract, especially in the stomach. However, it is usually better to formulate with a salt, as it will control the pH of the diffusion layer (the saturated solution immediately adjacent to the dissolving surface, known as the pH microenviroment). For example, although chlordiazepoxide base (C_s = 2 mg mL^{-1} at pH_{sat} 8.3) meets the requirements for in vivo 'solubility' (Kaplan, 1972); commercial capsules contain chlordiazepoxide hydrochloride (C_s = 165 mg mL^{-1} at pH_{sat} 2.53).

A weak base will have a high dissolution rate in the stomach, but as it moves down the gastrointestinal tract the pH rises and dissolution rate falls. Conversely, a weak acid has minimal dissolution in the stomach but becomes more soluble and dissolution rate increases down the gut. Paradoxically, as dissolution rate increases so absorption falls because the drug is ionized.

The dissolution rate of a particular salt is usually much greater than that of the parent drug. Sodium and potassium salts of weak acids dissolve much more rapidly than do the parent acids, and some comparative data are shown in Table 8.6. On the basis of bulk pH these salts would be expected to have lower dissolution rates in the stomach. However, the pH of the diffusion layer (found by measuring the pH of a saturated bulk solution) is higher than that of gastric fluid (which is approximately 1.5) because of its buffering action. The pH is the saturated unbuffered aqueous solution (calculated pH in Table 8.6) and the dissolution rate is governed by this pH and not the bulk medium pH.

In the intestine the salt does not depress the pH, unlike the acid which is neutralized, and the diffusion layer pH is again raised to promote dissolution. Providing that the acid forming the salt is strong, the pH of the solution adjacent to the dissolving surface will be that of the salt, whereas for the dissolving free base it will be the pH of the bulk dissolving medium. With weak bases, their salts dissolve rapidly in the stomach but there is no absorption, as the drug is ionized and absorption is delayed until the intestine. Any undissolved drug, as salt, rapidly dissolves, as the higher diffusion layer pH compensates for the higher bulk pH, which would be extremely unfavourable to the free base. Data for chlordiazepoxide are shown in Table 8.5. The maleate salt has a predicted solubility of 57 mg mL^{-1} but, more importantly, reduces the pH by 5 units. By controlling diffusion layer pH the dissolution rate can increase manyfold, independently of its position in the gastrointestinal tract. This is particularly important in the development of controlled-release products.

Different salts of a drug rarely change pharmacology, but only physical properties. This statement has been qualified to acknowledge that salts do affect the intensity of response. However, the salt form does change the physiochemical properties of the drug. Changes in dissolution rate and solubility affect the rate and extent of absorption (bioavailability), and changes on hygroscopicity and stability influence formulation.

Consequently each new drug candidate has to be examined to choose the most suitable salt, because each potential salt will behave differently and require separate preformulation screening. The regulatory authorities also treat each salt as a different chemical entity, particularly in the context of toxicity testing.

Solvents

It is generally necessary to formulate an injection even if there is no intention to market. The first-choice solvent is obviously water. However, although the drug may be freely soluble, it may be unstable in aqueous solution. Chlordiazepoxide HCl is such an example. Accordingly, water-miscible solvents are used:

1. in formulations to improve solubility or stability
2. in analysis to facilitate extraction and separation (e.g. chromatography).

Oils are used in emulsions, topicals (creams and ointments), intramuscular injections and liquid-fill oral preparations (soft and hard gelatin capsules) when aqueous pH and solvent solubility and stability are unattainable Table 8.7 shows a range of solvents to fulfil these needs.

Aqueous methanol is widely used in HPLC and is the standard solvent in sample extraction during analysis and stability testing. It is often made acidic or alkaline to increase solvent power and ensure consistent ionic conditions for UV analysis. Other pharmaceutical solvents are available but are generally only required in special cases. The most acceptable non-aqueous solvents pharmaceutically are glycerol, propylene glycol and ethanol. Generally for a lipophilic drug (i.e. a partition coefficient ($\log P > 1$), solubility doubles through this series.

Where bulk is limited and the aqueous solubility is inadequate, it is better to measure the solubility in

Table 8.6 Dissolution rates of weak acids and their sodium salts				
Drug	pK_a	pH (at C_s)	Dissolution rate (mg cm^{-2} min^{-1}) × 10^2	
			Dissolution media	
			0.1 M HCl (pH 1.5)	Phosphate (pH 6.8)
Salicylic acid	3.0	2.40	1.7	27
Sodium salicylate		8.78	1870	2500
Benzoic acid	4.2	2.88	2.1	14
Sodium benzoate		9.35	980	1770
Sulphathiazole	7.3	4.97	<0.1	0.5
Sodium sulphathiazole		10.75	550	810

Table 8.7 Recommended solvents for preformulation screening

Solvent	Dielectric constant (ϵ)	Solubility parameter (δ)	Application
Water	80	24.4	All
Methanol	32	14.7	Extraction, separation
0.1 M HCl (pH 1.1)			Dissolution (gastric), basic extraction
0.1 M NaOH (pH 13.1)			Acidic extraction
Buffer (pH 6–7)			Dissolution (intestinal)
Ethanol	24	12.7	Formulation
Propylene glycol	32	12.6	
Glycerol	43	16.5	
PEG 300 or 400	35		

aqueous solvent mixtures rather than in a pure organic solvent. Whereas solubilities at other levels and their mixtures can be predicted, the solubility in pure solvent is often inconsistent because of cosolvent effects. Furthermore, formulations rarely use pure non-aqueous solvent, particularly injections. For example, ethanol should only be used up to 10% in an injection to prevent haemolysis and pain at the injection site, and include isotonic salts.

Partition coefficient (K_w^o)

Partition coefficient (the solvent:water quotient of drug distribution) has a number of applications which are relevant to preformulation:

1. Solubility: both aqueous and in mixed solvents
2. Drug absorption in vivo: applied to a homologous series for structure activity relationships (SAR)
3. Partition chromatography: choice of column (HPLC) or plate (TLC) and choice of mobile phase (eluant).

Solvent solubility

The relative polarities of solvents can be scaled using dielectric constant (ε), solubility parameter (δ), interfacial (γ) and hydrophilic–lipophilic balance (HLB). The best solvent in any given application is one whose polarity matches that of the solute; an ideal, fully compatible solution exists when $\delta_{solvent} = \delta_{solute}$. This can be ascertained by determining solubility maxima, using a substituent contribution approach or the dielectric requirement of the system.

The most useful scale of polarity for a solute is K_w^o (oil:water partition coefficient), as the other

approaches do not allow easy estimates for the behaviour of crystalline solids. For a wide range of drugs it is possible to relate solvent solubility and the partition coefficient ($\log K_w^o = \log P$). Yalkowsky and Roseman (1981) derived the following expression for 48 drugs in propylene glycol:

$$\log C_s = \log C_w + \int (0.89 \log P + 0.03) \qquad (8.4)$$

Equation 8.4 can be applied more generally by introducing a factor ϕ to account for the relative solvent power of pharmaceutical solvents (see Table 8.8 for examples).

For a wide range of solvents Eqn 8.4 now becomes:

$$\log C_s = \log C_o + \int (\log \phi + 0.89 \log P + 0.03) \qquad (8.5)$$

Methodology and structure activity prediction

Choice of non-aqueous solvent (oil)   The oil:water partition (K_w^o) is a measure of the relative lipophilicity (oil-loving) nature of a compound, usually in the unionized state (HA or B), between an aqueous phase and an immiscible lipophilic solvent or oil.

Table 8.8 Solvent power (ϕ) of some pharmaceutical solvents

Solvent	Relative solvent power (ϕ)
Glycerol	0.5
Propylene glycol	1
PEG 300 or 400	1
Ethanol	2
DNA, DMF	4

Many partition solvents have been used. The largest database has been generated using n-octanol. The solubility parameter of octanol ($\delta = 10.24$) lies midway in the range for drugs (8–12), although some non-polar ($\delta < 7$) and polar drugs ($\delta > 13$) are encountered. This allows measurable results between equal volumes of oil and aqueous phases.

In the ***shake flask method*** the drug, dissolved in one of the phases, is shaken with the other partitioning solvent for 30 minutes, allowed to stand for 5 minutes, and then the majority of the lower aqueous phase (density of octanol = 0.8258 g mL^{-1}) is run off and centrifuged for 60 minutes at 2000 rpm. The aqueous phase is assayed before (ΣC) and after partitioning (C_w) [the aqueous concentration] to give $K_w^o = (\Sigma C - C_w)/(C_w)$.

If the transfer of solute to the oil phase is small, ΔC_w is small, and any analytical error increases error in the estimate of K_w^o. Indeed, to encourage greater aqueous loss ($> \Delta C_w$) a considerably more polar solvent, n-butanol, has been used. Where the partition coefficient is high, it is usual to reduce the ratio of the oil phase from 1:1 to 1:4 or 1:9 in order to increase the aqueous concentration (C_w) to a measurable level.

For a 1:9 oil:water ratio $K_w^o = (10\ \Sigma C - C_w)/C_w$.

The partition of a polar solute between an inert non-polar hydrocarbon e.g. hexane, and water is quite different from that of hydrogen bonding solvents such as octanol. The behaviour of the weak acid phenol ($pK_a = 10$) and weak base nicotine ($pK_a = 3.1$) is worthy of note. For phenol, $K_w^{octanol} = 29.5$, whereas $K_w^{hexane} = 0.11$. The acidic solvent chloroform suppresses partition ($K_w^o = 2.239$), whereas ethyl acetate and diethyl ether are more polar. The basic behaviour of the solvents give higher K_w^o values. With solvents capable of both hydrogen donation and acceptance (octanol, nitrobenzene and oleyl alcohol), K_w^o is intermediate. For nicotine the behaviour is reversed, and the hydrogen donor (acidic) solvent chloroform partitions most strongly $K_w^o = 77.63$), even though the neutral solvent nitrobenzene, which is marginally more lipophilic (log $P = 1.87$ against 1.96 for chloroform), gives similar values for both phenol and nicotine. Clearly both solute and solvent characteristics are important.

In general, polar solvents are advocated to correlate biological activity with physicochemical properties. Solvents less polar than octanol, measured by water solvency, have been termed hyperdiscriminating, whereas more polar solvents such as butanols and pentanols, are hypodiscriminating. This concept refers to the discriminating power of a partitioning solvent within a homologous series. With n-butanol

the values of log P tend to be close, whereas with heptane and other inert hydrocarbons the differences in solute lipophilicities are exaggerated. n-Octanol generally gives a range consistent with other physicochemical properties when compared to drug absorption in the GI tract. Hyperdiscriminating solvents reflect more closely the transport across the blood–brain barrier, whereas hypodiscriminating solvents give values consistent with buccal absorption (Fig. 8.2). In rationalizing the effects of different partitioning solvents, a good correlation was found to exist between the solvent water content at saturation and solvent lipophilicity.

Certainly it is imperative to standardize on methodology, especially for the solvent. Where solubility constraints allow, this should be n-octanol, especially as the existing data bank is extensive.

Structure–activity relationships Since the pioneering work of Meyer and Overton numerous studies on correlating molecular structure and biological activity have been reported. These structure–activity relationships (SAR) can rationalize drug activity and, particularly in modern medicinal chemistry, facilitate a scientific approach to the design of more effective, elegant structural analogues.

The application of SAR depends on a sound knowledge of the physicochemical properties of each new drug candidate in a therapeutic class, and preformulation is an essential information source.

It is assumed in SAR that:

$$\log K_w^o = a \times \log k_w^{octanol} + b \qquad (8.6)$$

This relationship holds for all polar and semipolar solvents, but with non-polar solvents (hexane to isooctane) correlations are poor, and this seems to be related to water content. Given the importance of water, it is imperative that the octanol is saturated with the aqueous phase and the aqueous phase with octanol prior to any determination, otherwise the partitioning behaviour of the drug will be confounded by the mutual partitioning of the two solvents.

Although the aqueous phase is often water, it is better to measure log P under controlled pH. All drugs capable of ionization and with a measurable pK_a will have intrinsic buffer capacity that affects the aqueous pH. Depending on the degree of dissociation, this will lead to an apparent K_w^o rather than the true (absolute) value, when the drug is unionized.

Because the ionized species will have greater aqueous solubility and lower lipophilicity to HA or BOH, the measured K_w^o (apparent) will be inevitably lower. Accordingly, K_w^o (true) should be measured at >2 pH units away from the pK_a (pK_a − 2 (acid); pK_a + 2 (base)) and the aqueous phase should contain a

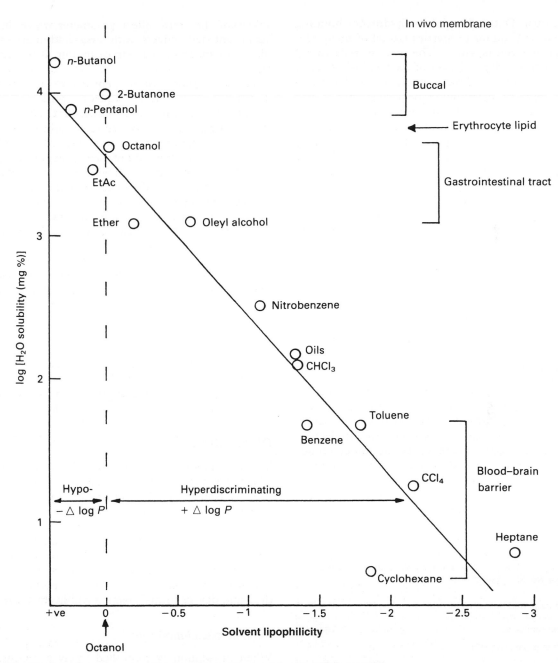

Fig. 8.2 Discriminating power of partitioning solvents as a function of their water capacity

suitable buffer. Given the importance of log P (log K_w^o) in SAR, comparative data generated in a therapeutic class (R_nX, where X is the therapeutic nucleus and n is a number of substituents R) should also be determined at physiological pH 7.4.

Quantitative SAR (QSAR) is based on the premise that drug absorption is a multipartitioning process (repeated adsorption and desorption) across cellular membranes and dependent on the lipophilicity of the drug, and the rate of penetration is proportional to the drug partition coefficient in vitro. Clearly the ionic condition in vivo will affect any correlation and, accordingly, for dissociating drugs the in vitro conditions should be similar. The widespread use of octanol in these studies and the existence of many excellent correlations in vivo is probably not fortuitous. Octanol exhibits hydrogen bonding acceptor and donor properties typical of many biological macromolecules. The partial polarity of octanol allows the inclusion of water, which is also a feature of biological lipid membranes and leads to a more complex partitioning behaviour than a less polar, essentially anhydrous solvent.

The effect of salt formation on the measured log P is shown in Table 8.9. Generally the log P differs between 3 and 4 (K_w^o from 1000 to 10 000). The lipophilicity falls by three to four orders of magnitude, which accounts for the significant increase in solubility of the salt. The physicochemical model for biological activity assumes that activity of a compound is related to the following factors associated with molecular structure:

• Electronic (charge)
• Steric (spatial size)
• Hydrophobic effects (partitioning).

Account must also be taken of structural and theoretical aspects, so that:

Biological activity = f [(electronic) + (steric) +
(hydrophobic) + structural/theoretical) (8.7)

The electronic parameter in Eqn. 8.7 is quantified by the sigma (σ) substituent constant of Hammett and reflects chemical reactivity in a homologous series. The substituent constant (σ) is positive for electron withdrawal (acids), whereas electron donor groups (bases) give a negative value. It can be used to predict pK_a (Perrin et al 1981).

Steric effects occur when there is a direct interaction between the substituent and the parent nucleus, and is related to substituent bulk. High positive values of the steric effect parameter, E_s, indicate significant steric effects, with intra- and intermolecular hindrance to a reaction or finding at the active site.

The hydrophobic component is measured by the distribution between an aqueous phase and an immiscible lipid phase and parallels drug adsorption and distribution in vivo. A relationship between partition coefficients has been demonstrated within a series by quantifying differences using an additive substituent constant (π). The constant is related almost completely to the effect of a particular substituent and much less to the parent compound, and this allows the prediction of the partition coefficient, log P, of a new derivative with reasonable accuracy. In addition, π can be related to biological effect as it is an additive component of the partition coefficient, and this has led to the wider application of SAR, with other modifications, notably taking into account of aromatic electron density and steric effects, to give *quantitative* SAR (i.e. QSAR).

Although all these substituents are useful, log P remains the most useful physical parameter and undoubtedly the most reliable data and correlations still come from experimentally derived partition values for the analogues in a series.

Dissolution

The dissolution rate of a drug is only important where it is the rate-limiting step in the absorption process. Kaplan (1972) suggested that provided the solubility of a drug exceeded 10 mg mL^{-1} at pH <7, no bioavailability- or dissolution-related problems were to be expected. Below 1 mg mL^{-1} such problems were quite possible, and salt formation could improve absorption and solubility by controlling the pH of the microenvironment independently of the drug and dosage forms' position within the GI tract.

Intrinsic dissolution rate

When dissolution is controlled solely by diffusion (transport control), the rate of diffusion is directly proportional to the saturated concentration of the drug in solution (i.e. solubility). Under these conditions the rate constant K_1 is defined by:

$$K_1 = 0.62 \, D^{2/3} \, \nu^{1/6} \, \omega^{1/2} \qquad (8.8)$$

where ν is the kinematic viscosity and ω is the angular velocity of a rotating disc of drug. By maintaining the dissolution fluid viscosity and rotational speed of the sample constant, the dissolution rate

Table 8.9 The effect of salt formation on the log P of some weakly basic drugs

Free base and hydrochloride salt	log P	Δlog P
Chlorpromazine	5.35	3.84
Chlorpromazine HCl	1.51	
Promazine	4.49	3.58
Promazine HCl	0.91	
Trifluopromazine	5.19	4.28
Trifluopromazine HCl	1.78	
Trifluoperazine	5.01	3.34
Trifluoperazine HCl	1.69	
Diphenylhydramine	3.30	3.42
Diphenylhydramine HCl	−0.12	

(dc/dt) from a constant surface area (A) will be constant and related solely to solubility. Under sink conditions ($C_s >>> C$) gives:

$$dc/dt = \frac{A}{V}K_1C_s \qquad (8.9)$$

Intrinsic dissolution rate (IDR) is given by:

$$IDR = K_1C_s \text{ (mg cm}^2 \text{ min}^{-1}) \qquad (8.10)$$

This constant rate differs from the dissolution from conventional dosage forms, which is known as total dissolution (mg mL^{-1}), where the exposed surface area (A) is uncontrolled as disintegration, deaggregation and dissolution proceed. Accordingly, the IDR is independent of formulation effects and measures the intrinsic properties of the drug and salts as a function of dissolution media, e.g. pH, ionic strength and counter-ions.

Measurement of intrinsic dissolution rate A compressed disc of material can be made by slow compression of 500 mg of drug in a 13 mm IR disc punch and die set to a high compaction pressure greater than 500 MPa (to ensure zero porosity) and a long dwell time (to improve compaction). The metal surfaces in contact should be prelubricated with, for example, stearic acid (5% w/v in chloroform). The compressed disc is fixed to the holder of the rotating basket apparatus using a low-melting paraffin wax and successively dipped so that the top and sides of the disc are coated. The lower circular face should be cleared of residual wax using a scalpel and carefully scraped to remove any stearic acid transferred from the punch face.

The coated disc is rotated at 100 rpm, 20 mm from the bottom of a 1 L flat-bottomed dissolution flask containing 1 L of fluid at 37°C. The amount of drug release is then monitored, usually by UV spectrometry, with time. The slope of the line divided by the exposed surface area gives the IDR (mg cm^2 min^{-1}).

Each candidate should be measured in 0.05 M HCl (gastric) and phosphate buffer pH 7 (intestinal), and distilled water especially if sink conditions are not possible for a weak base at pH 7 or a weak acid in 0.05 M HCl. Sink conditions maintain the bulk concentration (C) at a low level otherwise the rate of dissolution is progressively reduced and the plot of concentration against time becomes nonlinear. It is recommended that C should not exceed $0.1C_S$.

By comparing the IDR of a salt in water with that obtained in acid and alkali, or the free base with its salts in the same medium, a measure of the salt's ability to control its immediate microenvironment will emerge.

The equation derived from the Henderson–Hasselbalch equation:

$$IDR = k' [C_o(1 + \text{antilog } [pK_a - pH])] \quad (8.11)$$

shows that the rate of dissolution of a drug candidate is clearly a function of its intrinsic solution (C_o), its dissociation constant (pK_a), and the pH of either the bulk dissolution medium or the microenvironment created by the dissolving salt. Using the measured rate of the free base at known bulk pH, expected rates in other media, using the experimental salts, can be calculated and compared with experimental values.

The importance of improvements in the IDR due to microenvironmental pH control lies in the improvement in vivo of a salt over the parent drug. Where no increase is found there is likely to be no advantage in using that particular salt. Improvements are obviously more likely if the salt former is strong. For a weak base, the hydrochloride ($pK_a = -6.10$) offers the best advantage, but in some instances this may prove disappointing because of Cl$^-$ ions. Thus the measurement of IDR can be useful diagnostically.

Common ion effect

An often overlooked interaction is the common ion effect. A common ion often significantly reduces the solubility of a slightly soluble electrolyte. The 'salting out' results from the removal of water molecules as solvent owing to the competing hydration of other ions. The reverse process, 'salting in', arises with larger anions, e.g. benzoate, salicylate, which open the water structure. These hydrotropes increase the solubility of poorly water-soluble compounds such as diazepam.

Hydrochloride salts often exhibit suboptimal solubility in gastric juice owing to the abundance of Cl$^-$ ions (Table 8.10). Counter-ions other than Cl$^-$, such

Table 8.10 Examples of weakly basic drugs which have decreased solubility in acidic and Cl$^-$ solutions

Chlortetracycline

Demethylchlortetracycline

Methacycline

Demeclocyline

Phenazopyridine

Cyproheptadine

Bromhexine

Triamterine

as nitrate, sulphate and phosphate, have also been implicated. They are usually inorganic, because of their small size.

To identify a common ion interaction the IDR of the hydrochloride (or inorganic) salt should be compared between:

- water and water containing 1.2% w/v NaCl, and
- 0.05 M HCl and 0.9% w/v NaCl in 0.05 M HCl.

Both saline media contain 0.2M Cl⁻, which is typically encountered in fluids in vivo.

A common ion effect with Cl⁻ will result in a significantly reduced IDR in the presence of sodium chloride. Other salt forms are then indicated, e.g. tosylate, mesylate etc., but the parent molecule will still remain sensitive to Cl⁻ and solubilities will be suppressed in the presence of saline, although not to the same extent as Cl⁻ is not involved in the dissolving microenvironment. Any improvement with the new salt can be assessed by again measuring the IDR with and without saline. As some compounds are sensitive to other counter-ions, e.g. nitrate, sulphate and phosphate can be demonstrated by including the appropriate sodium salt in the dissolution medium. Phase solubility studies have indicated that basic amine drugs are more soluble in organic acids than inorganic. Where a hydrochloride salt exhibits suboptimal solubility then the next logical choice is probably a salt of toluene sulphonic acid (tosylate: $pK_a = -1.34$). Mesylate, napsylate, besylate and maleate salts offer progressively more weaker acidic alternatives.

With low-solubility amine drugs, the salts of poly-hydroxy acids, e.g. lactate, often give the greatest aqueous solubility because of their accessible hydroxy groupings.

MELTING POINT

Techniques

The melting point of a drug can be measured using three techniques:

1. Capillary melting
2. Hot stage microscopy
3. Differential scanning calorimetry or thermal analysis.

Capillary melting

Capillary melting (the observation of melting in a capillary tube in a heated metal block) gives infor-

mation about the melting range but it is difficult to assign an accurate melting point.

Hot stage microscopy

This is the visual observation of melting under a microscope equipped with a heated and lagged sample stage. The heating rate is controllable and up to three transitions can be registered. It is more precise as the phase transitions (first melt, 50% melt and completion) can be registered on a recorder as the melting proceeds, and because of the high magnification the values are more accurate.

Differential scanning calorimetry and thermal analysis

Neither of the previous methods is as versatile as either differential thermal analysis (DTA) or differential scanning calorimetry (DSC). An additional advantage is that the sample size required is only 2–5 mg.

DTA measures the temperature difference between the sample and a reference as a function of temperature or time when heating at a constant rate. DSC is similar to DTA, except that the instrument measures the amount of energy required to keep the sample at the same temperature as the reference, i.e. it measures the enthalpy of transition.

When no physical or chemical change occurs within the sample then there is neither a temperature change nor input energy to maintain an isotherm. However, when phase changes occur then latent heat suppresses a temperature change and the isothermal energy required registers as an electrical signal generated by thermocouples. Crystalline transitions, fusion, evaporation and sublimation are obvious changes in state which can be quantified (Fig. 8.3).

The major concern in preformulation is polymorphism, and the measurement of melting point and other phase changes is the primary diagnostic tool. Confirmation by IR spectroscopy and X-ray diffraction is usually required.

Polymorphism

A polymorph is a solid material with at least two different molecular arrangements that give distinct crystal species. These differences disappear in the liquid or the vapour state. Of concern are their relative stabilities and solubility. The highest-melting species is generally stable; other polymorphs are metastable and convert to the stable form. There are also potentially large differences in their physical

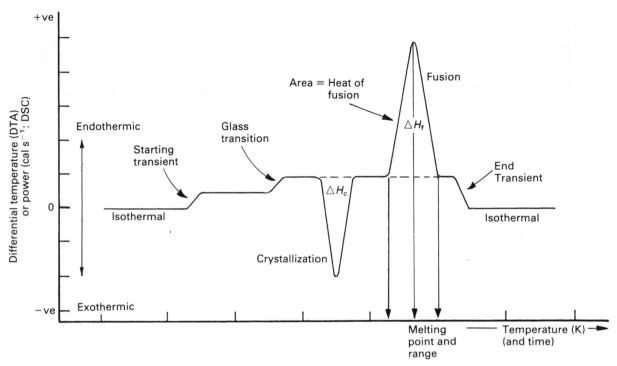

Fig. 8.3 Schematic differential scanning calorimeter thermogram.

properties so that they behave as distinct chemical entities. Solubility (particularly important in suspensions and biopharmaceutically), melting point, density, crystal shape, optical and electrical properties and vapour pressure are often very different for each polymorph.

Polymorphism is remarkably common, particularly within certain structural groups: 63% of barbiturates, 67% of steroids and 40% of sulphonamides exhibit polymorphism.

The steroid progesterone has five polymorphs, whereas the sulphonamide sulphabenzamide has four polymorphs and three solvates. The importance of polymorphism is illustrated by the biopharmaceutical data for fluprednisolone (Fig. 8.4).

It is convention to number the polymorphs in order of stability at room temperature, starting with form I using Roman numerals. Form I usually has the highest melting point and the lowest solubility; in suspension formulation it is essential to use the least soluble polymorph because of Ostwald ripening.

Accordingly, in preformulation the following should be considered.

- How many polymorphs exist?
- How stable are the metastable forms?
- Is there an amorphous glass?
- Can the metastable forms be stabilized?

- What is the solubility of each form?
- Will a more soluble form survive processing and storage?

Pseudopolymorphism (solvates)

Prior to this, the presence of solvates or false polymorphs, sometimes (incorrectly and confusingly) called pseudopolymorphs, should be identified, as most polymorphs can be obtained by changing the recrystallizing solvent. Typical solvents inducing polymorphic change are water, methanol, ethanol, acetone, chloroform, *n*-propanol, isopropanol alcohol, *n*-butanol, *n*-pentanol, toluene and benzene. Trace levels of solvent are usual in early batches of new drug candidates (residues from the final crystallization). These can become molecular additions to the crystal and change habit. These hydrates (water) and solvates (e.g. methanolate, ethanolate) have been confused with true polymorphism and have led to the term pseudopolymorphism.

The distinction between these false forms and true polymorphs can be ascertained by observing the melting behaviour of the compound dispersed in silicone oil using hot-stage microscopy.

Pseudopolymorphs will evolve a gas (steam or solvent vapour), causing the oil to bubble. True

125

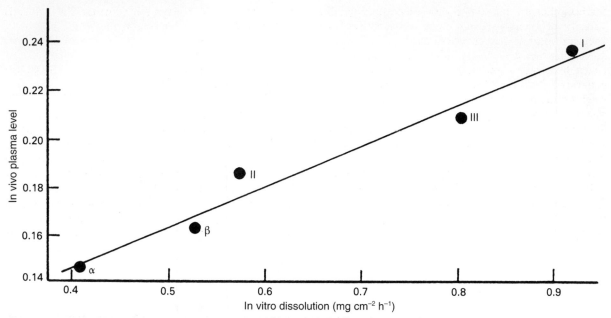

Fig. 8.4 The relationship between in vitro and in vivo release from fluprednisolone implants.

polymorphs merely melt, forming a second globular phase. The temperature at which the solvent volatilizes will be close to the boiling point of the solvent.

True polymorphism

After the study of pseudopolymorphism (see also Chapter 9 for further discussion on polymorphism), the evaluation of true polymorphism can proceed unconfounded. Most polymorphs are obtained by solvent manipulation. Others can be produced without the presence of solvent by thermal techniques, notably sublimation and recrystallization from the melt. Supercooling of the melt is particularly useful in discovering unstable modifications.

The initial difficulty is to measure the melting point of the metastable form, and here heating rate is critical. Too-rapid heating will obscure the endotherm, whereas too slow a heating rate may allow transition or encourage decomposition. Often, therefore, comparison at two rates, e.g. 2 and 20°C min^{-1}, is necessary.

The difference in melting point (ΔT_m) between polymorphs is a measure of the metastable polymorph stability. Where $\Delta T_m < 1$°C then neither is significantly more stable and either may be obtained upon conventional crystallization. If ΔT_m is 25–50°C then the lower melting species will be difficult to crystallize and will rapidly revert. The closer the two melting points ($\Delta T_m \rightarrow 1$–25°C) then the unstable form(s) can be obtained easily before a solid–solid

transformation occurs. This can be suppressed by using small samples, as individual crystals of even highly unstable forms can be melted.

If it appears that polymorphism is occurring or likely, then a cooperative study with the bulk chemists should determine the most stable form (chemical and physical). Differences in solubility and melting point must also be assessed and then a decision made to determine which form to progress through to the next stage of formulation. Small differences in stability but higher solubility of a relatively metastable form may lead to a preferential choice of a polymorph other than form I, but this is unlikely and is not encouraged by regulatory authorities.

Crystal purity

Thermal analysis has been widely used as a method of purity determination and the USP includes an appendix describing the methods. This is particularly pertinent at the preformulation stage, because early samples of a new drug are inevitably 'dirty' while improvements in synthetic route are made. Thermal analysis is rapid and will discriminate 0.002 mole% of impurity.

Solubility

The most important reason to determine melting point during preformulation is crystalline solubility.

Such studies are particularly important because the scarcity of available drug powder often precludes accurate solubility determinations.

Melting point and solubility are related via the latent heat of fusion, which is the amount of heat generated during melting or fusion. A crystal with weak bonds has a low melting point and low heat of fusion. Conversely, a strong crystal lattice leads to a high melting point and a high heat of fusion. Because solubility also requires the disruption of crystal structure to allow molecular dispersion in the solvent, it is also influenced by intermolecular forces.

Polymorphs differ in melting point and solubility. The existence of different crystal arrangements for the same compound inevitably leads to differences in crystal lattice energy, as intermolecular distances will be different in the alternative forms. This effect is shown in Figure 8.5 for riboflavine.

ASSAY DEVELOPMENT

The assumption that the drug is stable may not be valid as drugs are notoriously unstable, particularly as hydrolysis is often the predominant cause. In order to follow drug stability, in both solution and solid phase, it is mandatory to have suitable stability-indicating assays. In some cases UV spectroscopy can be used, but in general chromatography is required to separate the drug from its degradation products and any excipients. Thin-layer

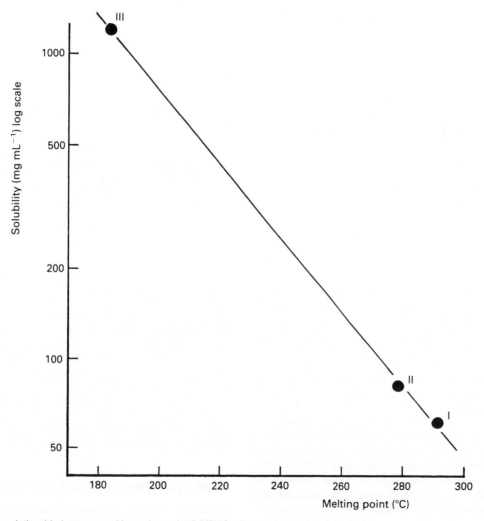

Fig. 8.5   The relationship between melting point and solubility for three polymorphs of riboflavine.

chromatography (TLC) is widely used in a semi-quantitative mode to estimate impurity levels, to establish the number of impurities, and to collect samples from the plate for subsequent HPLC (high-performance (pressure) liquid chromatography. HPLC is now acknowledged as the most versatile and powerful technique in pharmaceutical analysis and is the method of choice in preformulation stability assessment.

UV spectroscopy

The principles of UV spectroscopy were enumerated earlier and will serve to quantify many of the subsequent physical constants and solubilities above. TLC, and particularly HPLC, has largely superseded UV spectroscopy as a basic analytical tool in stability assessment. However, certain UV techniques are worthy of discussion:

- Solubility
- Molecular weight
- pK_a
- Assay (potency)
- Mixtures:
  - resolving compound products
  - stability: hydrolysis, oxidation (coloured products).

Molecular weight

To a first approximation the molar extinction coefficient (e) of a chromophore (absorbing molecular group) is unaffected by distant substituent groups in a molecule. Therefore, if e of the chromophore is known from another related compound in the series, the molecular weight of the new derivative can be calculated from the absorbance of a solution of known concentration, as mol. wt. = 10 e/E.

pK_a

pK_a measurement by spectroscopy is indicated when solubility is too low, or when the pK_a is particularly low (<2) or high (>11) for determination by potentiometry. The method depends on determining the ratio of molecular species (neutral molecular at pH < pK_a − 2 (acid), pH > pK_a + 2 (base)) to the ionized species in a series of seven buffers (pH = ±1 of pK_a). An analytical wavelength (λ) is chosen where the greatest difference in absorbance exists between the molecular species and the pure ionized moiety at two pH units from the pK_a.

Thin-layer chromatography

All chromatographic procedures emanate from the Russian botanist Tswett (1906), who separated plant pigments by pipetting solutions on to the top of packed glass tubes. Tswett's work led to the development of column chromatography and, under pressure, to HPLC. Other workers used paper as a support, and before the advent of HPLC paper chromatography was used for simplicity and speed. TLC arose from a need to satisfactorily separate lipids, which paper techniques could not achieve, but it was soon realized that the technique was also considerably more flexible. Paper chromatography is limited by the cellulose support, whereas the thin layer of material on a glass plate can be prepared from a slurry of a wide variety of different chemical types, e.g. silica gel, celite, alumina, cellulose (analogous to paper chromatography) and chemically modified celluloses; and more recently with the advent of reversed-phase chromatography, C_2, C_8 and C_{18} silanized and diphenyl silica.

Modern TLC was established by Stahl (1956) and separations were found to be considerably shorter than on paper, spots were more compact, resolution better, and submicrogram samples could be separated and recovered if necessary (by scraping away the spot using a fine spatula), re-extracted and injected on to HPLC.

TLC is now generally regarded as a reliable and sensitive qualitative technique for the separation of complex mixtures in stability samples. In a typical analysis, extracted samples are spotted 20 mm from the bottom of a square glass plate, 200 × 200 mm, coated with a dry slurry of silica (250 μm thick) and placed in a closed tank containing a 10 mm layer of eluting solvent, which has produced a saturated vapour phase. The sample is developed (separated) by the capillary movement of the solvent up the plate and is therefore similar to HPLC. It is a thin flat column (stationary phase) with solvent (mobile phase) pumped by capillary flux, and much of the theory (Snyder 1968) is the same. Consequently, TLC and HPLC are complementary. TLC will quantify the number of components (as they can be seen) and estimate their concentration by reference to standards run concurrently, whereas HPLC can quantify their level, confident that all have been separated. The developing solvent for TLC (particularly HPTLC (high-performance TLC) and reverse phase) is also a useful guide to identify the mobile phase for HPLC.

High-performance liquid chromatography

High-performance (pressure) liquid chromatography (HPLC) is essentially column chromatography performed by eluting under pressure. By pumping the eluting solvent (mobile phase) under a pressure of up to 40 MPa (6000 psi) and a flow rate of up to 3 mL min^{-1}, the column can be much smaller and use much smaller particle size packing material (stationary phase). This results in shorter retention times (solute time on column), high sensitivity (typically 1 ng), the need for only a small sample volume (0–50 μL) and yet high selectivity (separation power) for the resolution of complex mixtures.

HPLC methods can be divided into two distinct modes.

Normal-phase HPLC

Normal phase HPLC is performed by eluting a silica-packed column, which is hydrophilic, with a non-polar mobile phase. The mobile phase is usually hexane, to which is added one or more of the following, in increasing order of polarity: chloroform ($CHCl_3$), tetrahydrofuran (THF), acetonitrile (ACN), isopropyl alcohol (IPA) or methanol (MeOH). Separation is achieved by partition with differential adsorption and desorption of both the solute and solvents during passage down the column. Polar solutes are retained, but more lipophilic molecules are not. By increasing the polarity of the mobile phase (e.g. by adding MeOH or IPA), polar solutes are eluted more quickly, whereas non-polar solutes are better retained and their order of retention is changed. Decreasing solvent polarity increases polar solute retention and facilitates the elution of lipophilic molecules.

In general, normal-phase HPLC is used for moderately polar solutes (freely soluble in methanol). Non-polar hydrocarbon-soluble solutes are difficult to retain and very polar and water-soluble solutes are difficult to elute sufficiently.

Reverse-phase HPLC

When the solute is eluted by a polar (largely aqueous) mobile phase over a hydrophobic stationary phase, the chromatography is known as reverse phase. Solute behaviour is the reverse of that described for normal phase HPLC, which uses a hydrophilic silica stationary phase. Separation between the stationary phase and the mobile phase is solvophobic, analogous to partitioning.

Hydrophobicity of the stationary phase is achieved by bonding a coating on to the silica support. The most common bonded phases are alkyl silanes of C_{18} (octodecysiolane, ODS), C_8 (octysilane, OS), and C_1 (trimethysilane). The predominantly aqueous mobile phase usually contains methanol, ACN and/or THF to modify solvent polarity by matching the lipophilicity of the solutes in order to facilitate good chromatography. Ionization control can be achieved in the range pH 2–8. The inclusion of 1–2% acetic acid or diethylamine is used to suppress the ionization of weak acids and bases respectively (***ion-suppression chromatography*** is used to increase lipophilicity and improve the retention of polar solutes).

In general polar solutes have short retention times on reverse phase, whereas non-polar compounds are retained. Increasing the mobile phase polarity (by increasing the water concentration) shortens retention for polar solutes while retaining fewer polar compounds. Decreasing solvent polarity (by decreasing water concentration) helps retain polar compounds, but more lipophilic solutes are eluted more rapidly. Non-aqueous reverse phase (NARP HPLC, where THF or methylene chloride replaces water in the mobile phase) is used to separate lipophilic solutes.

The great flexibility of choice in mobile phase (by using solvents ranging from water to hexane), the increasing number of available stationary phases (particularly bonded phases) and the inherent sensitivity of HPLC produces a powerful analytical technique. It is the method of choice in preformulation stability studies.

DRUG AND PRODUCT STABILITY

Wherever possible, commercial pharmaceutical products should have a shelf-life of 3 years. The potency should not fall below 95% under the recommended storage conditions and the product should still look and perform as it did when first manufactured.

By investigating the intrinsic stability of the drug it is possible to advise on formulation approaches and indicate types of excipient, specific protective additives and packaging which are likely to improve the integrity of the drug and product. Typical stress conditions are shown in Table 8.11.

Drug degradation occurs by four main processes:

- Hydrolysis
- Oxidation
- Photolysis
- Trace metal catalysis.

Hydrolysis and oxidation are the most common pathways, and in general light (*c*) and metal ions catalyse a subsequent oxidative process.

Table 8.11 Stress conditions used in preformulation stability assessment

Test	Conditions
Solid	
Heat (°C)	4, 20, 30, 40, 40/75% RH, 50 and 75
Moisture uptake	30, 45, 60, 75 and 90% RH at RT[a,b]
Physical stress	Ball milling
Aqueous solution	
pH	1, 3, 5, 7, 9 and 11 at RT and 37°C. Reflux in 1 M HCl and 1 M NaOH
Light[c]	UV (254 and 366 nm) and visible (south-facing window) at RT
Oxidation[c]	Sparging with oxygen at RT; UV may accelerate breakdown

[a] RT is ambient room temperature. Can vary between 15 and 25°C.
[b] Saturated solutions of $MgBr_2$, KNO_2, NaBr, NaCl and KNO_3 respectively.
[c] At pH of maximum stability in simple aqueous solution.

Temperature

Thermal effects are superimposed on all four chemical processes. Typically a 10°C increase in temperature can produce a 2–5-fold increase in decay. Often the increase in reaction rate with temperature follows an Arrhenius-type relationship: a plot of the log of the rate of reaction against the reciprocal of absolute temperature yields a straight line. The reaction rate can then be calculated at any temperature and allows a prediction of shelf-life at room temperature by extrapolation. This assumption forms the basis of accelerated stability tests. However, the mechanism or pathway of the chemical breakdown often changes with temperature. This will be indicated by a discontinuity or 'knee joint' in the Arrhenius plot. This is not easily detected and would inevitably lead to erroneous conclusions, based on elevated temperature data, to predict shelf-lives at room temperature or under refrigeration. Reactions often change at about 50°C, and this is a sensible ceiling.

Order of reaction

The time course of degradation depends on the number of reactants, whose concentration influences the rate. It is often more convenient to express reaction rates in terms of time. The most common is the *half-life*, the time at which the concentration has halved ($t_{1/2}$ or t_{50}). The shelf-life of a product can be likewise expressed as t_{95} (i.e. the time for 5% loss) etc.

In the absence of a definitive value for the activation energy (E_a), which can be obtained from the slope of the Arrhenius plot, it is prudent to assume a low value (e.g. 10 kcal mol^{-1}), as this will lead to higher reaction rates and any prediction of shelf-life will be conservative. Values for a wide range of drug degradation reactions are 10–100 kcal mol^{-1}, but are usually in the range 15–60 kcal mol^{-1} with a mean of 19.8. Most occur by first-order kinetics (logarithmic) but some are zero order, e.g. aspirin in aqueous suspension, and a few are second order, e.g. chlorbutol hydrolysis.

Hydrolysis

The most likely cause of drug instability is hydrolysis. Water plays a dominant role and in many cases it is implicated passively as a solvent vector between two reacting species in solution. The solution is often saturated, so that studies in dilute solution can be completely misleading (see Solid-state stability, later in this chapter).

Hydrolytic reactions involve nucleophilic attack of labile bonds, e.g. lactam > ester > amide > imide, by water on the drug in solution, and are first order. When this attack is by a solvent other than water it is known as *solvolysis*.

A number of conditions catalyse the breakdown:

- The presence of OH$^-$
- The presence of H_3O^+
- The presence of divalent metal ions
- Ionic hydrolysis (protolysis) is quicker than molecular
- Heat
- Light
- Solution polarity and ionic strength
- High drug concentrations.

The influence of pH

The degradation of most drugs is catalysed by extremes of pH, i.e. high [H_3O^+] and [OH$^-$], and many drugs are most stable between pH 4 and 8.

Where maximum stability dictates wider values, it is important for injections that there is low buffer capacity to prevent unnecessary challenge to the homeostatic pH (7.4) of blood.

Weakly acidic and basic drugs are most soluble when ionized, and it is then that instability is most likely as they are charged. This leads to a problem, as many potent drugs are extremely poorly soluble and pH ionization is the most obvious method to obtain a solution. In some cases, therefore, the inclusion of a water-miscible solvent in the formulation will increase stability by:

1. Suppressing ionization
2. Reducing the extreme of pH required to achieve solubility
3. Reducing water activity by reducing the polarity of the solvent, e.g. 20% propylene glycol in chlordiazepoxide HCl injection.

Reactions in aqueous solution are usually catalysed by pH, and this is monitored by measuring degradation rates (usually pseudo first order) against pH, keeping temperature, ionic strength and solvent concentration constant. Suitable buffers include acetate, citrate, lactate, phosphate and ascorbate (an intrinsic antioxidant).

Solvolysis

Where the reacting solvent is not water, then breakdown is termed solvolysis. Furthermore, the definition can be extended to include any change in solvent polarity (usually measured as dielectric constant) as a result of increased ionic strength. Phenobarbitone is considerably more stable in preparations containing water-miscible solvents, whereas aspirin, which undergoes extensive hydrolysis, is degraded further by aqueous solvents. Both effects are directly related to the dielectric constant (polarity) of the solvent. In general, if a compound produces degradation products which are more polar then the addition of a less polar solvent will stabilize the formulation. If the degradation products are less polar, then the vehicle should be more polar to improve stability. With the hydrolysis of neutral non-polar drugs, e.g. steroids, the transition state will be non-polar with no net charge. In this case solvents will not affect the rate of decomposition and can be used with impunity to increase solubility.

Oxidation

Oxidation is controlled by the environment, i.e. light, trace metals, oxygen and oxidizing agents. Reduction is a complimentary reaction (redox) and there is a mutual exchange of electrons. Oxidation is a loss of electrons and an oxidizing agent must be able to take electrons. In organic chemistry, oxidation is synonymous with dehydrogenation (the loss of hydrogen) and this is the mode of action of polyhydroxphenol antioxidants, e.g. hydroquinone. However, most antioxidants function by providing electrons or labile H^+, which will be accepted by any free radical to terminate the chain reaction. A prerequisite for effective antioxidant activity in any particular preparation is that the antioxidant is more readily oxidized than the drug.

Chelating agents

Chelating agents are complexes, unlike simple ligands, e.g. ferrocyanide ($Fe(CN_6^{4-})$), which form complex salts by a single bond provided by a lone electron pair. Chelating agents are capable of forming more than one bond. For example, ethylene diamine is bidentate (two links), tripyridyl is tridentate (three) and ethylene diamine tetra-acetic acid (EDTA) is hexadentate (six), which makes it particularly effective as a pharmaceutical chelating agent.

Photolysis

Oxidation, and to some extent hydrolysis, is often catalysed by light. The energy associated with this radiation increases as wavelength decreases, so that the energy of UV visible is greater than that of IR and is independent of temperature (Table 8.12).

When molecules are exposed to electromagnetic radiation they absorb light (photons) at characteristic wavelengths which causes an increase in energy, which can:

• cause decomposition
• be retained or transferred
• be converted to heat
• result in light emission at a new wavelength (fluorescence, phosphorescence).

Table 8.12 Relationship between wavelength and associated energy of various forms of light		
Type of radiation	Wavelength (nm)	Energy (kcal mol^{-1})
UV	50–400	287–72
Visible	400–750	72–36
IR	750–10 000	36–1

Natural sunlight lies in the wavelength range 290–780 nm, of which only the higher energy (UV) range (290–320 nm) causes photodegradation of drugs, and sunburn. Fluorescent lighting tubes emit visible light and potentially deleterious UV radiation in the range 320–380 nm, whereas conventional tungsten filament light bulbs are safe, emitting radiations > 390 nm.

Thus photolysis is prevented by suitable packaging: low actinic amber glass bottles, cardboard outers and aluminium foil overwraps and blisters. Clear flint glass absorbs around 80% in the 290–320 nm range, whereas amber glass absorbs more than 95%. Plastic containers, by comparison, absorb only 50%.

Solid-state stability

Many of the processes of composition apply generally, particularly when the drug is in solution. However, certain important distinctions arise with the stability of drugs in the solid state, e.g. in tablets and capsules. There is limited information in the pharmaceutical literature, owing largely to the complexities of formulated systems and the difficulties in obtaining quantitative data. This paucity of data must not be interpreted to mean that this area is unimportant, especially given the popularity of tablets and capsules.

In all solid dose formulations there will be some free moisture (contributed by excipients as well as the drug), and certainly in tablets a significant percentage, typically 2% w/w, is required to facilitate good compression. This free water acts as a vector for chemical reactions between drug and excipients, and the adsorbed moisture films are saturated with drug compared to the dilute solutions encountered in injectables. The ionic equilibria are quite different and comparison is meaningless. They should not be extrapolated glibly to the solid state.

Hygroscopicity

A substance that absorbs sufficient moisture from the atmosphere to dissolve itself is deliquescent. A substance that loses water to form a lower hydrate or becomes anhydrous is termed efflorescent. These are extreme cases, and most pharmaceutical compounds are usually either impassive to the water available in the surrounding atmosphere or lose or gain water from the atmosphere, depending on the relative humidity (RH). Materials unaffected by RH are termed non-hygroscopic, whereas those in dynamic equilibrium with water in the atmosphere are hygro-

scopic. Ambient RH (0% poles and desert, 55% temperate and 87% tropics) can vary widely and continually depending on the weather and air temperature, and these cyclic changes lead to constant variations in the moisture content of unprotected bulk drug and excipients. The constant sinusoidal change in day and night temperatures is the major influence. For this reason pharmaceutical air conditioning is usually set below 50% RH, and very hygroscopic products, e.g. effervescents, which are particularly moisture sensitive, are stored and made below 40% RH. Tablets and capsules must be hydrophilic to facilitate wetting and the process of deaggregation and drug dissolution. As a paradox they must have limited hygroscopicity to ensure good chemical and physical stability under all reasonable climatic conditions. Good packaging will accommodate moisture challenge, e.g. glass bottles, foil blisters and dessicant. However, preformulation studies on the drug and potential excipient combinations should provide the basis for more robust formulations and a wider, more flexible and cheaper choice of pack, while still reducing significantly any hydrolytic instability due to absorbed free moisture. Pharmaceutical bulk, i.e. drug salts, should be chosen as being non-hygroscopic. As a working limit this should be <0.5% H_2O at <95% RH.

Stability assessment

The testing protocols used in preformulation to ascertain the stability of formulated products must be performed in solution and in the solid state since the same drug (salt) will be used in both an injection and a capsule, for example. These protocols are discussed briefly in Chapter 7, and a suggested scheme for preformulation samples has been shown in Table 8.11.

MICROSCOPY

The microscope has two major applications in pharmaceutical preformulation:

1. Basic crystallography, to determine crystal morphology (structure and habit), polymorphism and solvates
2. Particle size analysis.

Most pharmaceutical powders have crystals in the range 0.5–300 μm. However, the distributions are often smaller, typically 0.5–50 μm, to ensure good blend homogeneity and rapid dissolution. These are the major reasons for particle size control.

A lamp-illuminated mono-objective microscope fitted with polarizing filters above and below the stage is more than adequate. For most preformulation work a 10 × eyepiece and a 10 × objective are ideal, although occasionally, with micronized powders and when following solid–solid and liquid–liquid transitions in polymorphism, 10 × 20 may be required.

Crystal morphology

Crystals are characterized by repetition of atoms or molecules in a regular three-dimensional structure, which is absent in glasses and some polymers. There are six crystal systems (cubic, tetragonal, orthorhombic, monoclinic, triclinic and hexagonal) which have different internal structures and spatial arrangements. Although not changing their internal structure, which occurs with polymorphism, crystals can adopt different external structures. This is known as crystal habit, of which five types are recognized:

- Tabular: moderate expansion of two parallel faces
- Platy: plates
- Prismatic: columns
- Acicular: needle-like
- Bladed: flat acicular.

These occur in all six crystal systems.

Conditions during crystallization will contribute to changes in crystal habit and may be encountered in early batches of a new drug substance until the synthetic route has been optimized. Crystal habit can be modified by:

1. Excessive supersaturation, which tends to transform a prism or isodiametric (granular) crystals to a needle shape.
2. Cooling rate and agitation, which changes habit as it changes the degree of supersaturation. Naphthalene gives thin plates (platy) if rapidly recrystallized in cold ethanol or methanol, whereas slow evaporation yields prisms.
3. The crystallizing solvent affects habit by preferential absorption on to certain faces, inhibiting their growth. Resorcinol produces needles from benzene and squat prisms from butyl acetate.
4. The addition of cosolvents or other solutes and ions which change habit by poisoning crystal growth in one or more directions. Sodium chloride is usually cubic, but urea produces an octahedral habit.

Particle size analysis

Small particles are particularly important in low-dose high-potency drug candidates, as large particle populations are necessary to ensure adequate blend homogeneity (coefficient of variation <1–2%), and for any drug whose aqueous solubility is poor (<1 mg mL^{-1}), as dissolution rate is directly proportional to surface area (inversely proportional to particle size).

There are numerous methods of particle sizing. Sieving is usually unsuitable during preformulation owing to the lack of bulk material. The simplest (but unfortunately the most tedious) method for small quantities is the microscope. The Coulter Counter (a conductivity method based on electrolyte displacement as the sample is drawn through a small hole) and laser light scattering are widely used for routine bulk analysis and research.

POWDER FLOW PROPERTIES

Of primary importance when handling a drug powder is flow. When limited amounts of drug are available this can be evaluated by measurements of bulk density and angle of repose. These are extremely useful derived parameters to assess the impact of changes in drug powder properties as new batches become available. Changes in particle size and shape are generally very apparent; an increase in crystal size or a more uniform shape will lead to a smaller angle of repose and a smaller Carr's index.

Bulk density

A simple test has been developed to evaluate the flowability of a powder by comparing the poured (fluff) density (ρ_{Bmin}) and tapped density (ρ_{Bmax}) of a powder and the rate at which it packed down. A useful empirical guide is given by Carr's compressibility index ('Compressibility' is a misnomer, as compression is not involved):

$$\text{Carr's index (\%)} = \frac{\text{Tapped} - \text{Poured density}}{\text{Tapped density}} \times 100 \tag{8.12}$$

This is a simple index that can be determined on small quantities of powder and may be interpreted as in Table 8.13.

A similar index has been defined by Hausner (1967):

$$\text{Hausner ratio} = \frac{\text{Tapped density} \left(\rho_{Bmax} \right)}{\text{Poured density} \left(\rho_{Bmin} \right)} \times 100 \tag{8.13}$$

Table 8.13 Carr's index as an indication of powder flow	
Carr's index (%)	Type of flow
5–15	Excellent
12–16	Good
18–21	Fair to passable[a]
23–35	Poor[a]
33–38	Very poor
>40	Extremely poor

[a] May be improved by glidant, e.g. 0.2% Aerosil.

Table 8.14 Angle of repose as an indication of powder flow properties	
Angle of repose (degrees)	Type of flow
<20	Excellent
20–30	Good
30–34	Passable[a]
>40	Very poor

[a] May be improved by a glidant, e.g. 0.2% Aerosil.

Values less than 1.25 indicate good flow (= 20% Carr), whereas greater than 1.25 indicates poor flow (= 33% Carr). Between 1.25 and 1.5, added glidant normally improves flow.

Carr's index is a one-point determination and does not always reflect the ease or speed with which the powder consolidates. Indeed, some materials have a high index (suggesting poor flow) but may consolidate rapidly. Rapid consolidation is essential for uniform filling on tablet machines, when the powder flows at ρ_{Bmin} into the die and consolidates, approaching ρ_{Bmax}, at compression. An empirical linear relationship exists between the change in bulk density and the log number of taps in a jolting volumeter. Non-linearity occurs up to two taps and after 30 taps when the bed consolidates more slowly. The slope is a measure of the speed of consolidation and is useful for assessing powders or blends with similar Carr's indices and the benefit of glidants.

Angle of repose

A static heap of powder, with only gravity acting upon it, will tend to form a conical mound. One limitation exists: the angle to the horizontal cannot exceed a certain value, and this is known as the angle of repose (θ). If any particle temporarily lies outside this limiting angle, it will slide down the adjacent surface under the influence of gravity until the gravitational pull is balanced by the friction caused by interparticulate forces. Accordingly, there is an empirical relationship between θ and the ability of the powder to flow. However, the exact value for angle of repose does depend on the method of measurement. The angles of repose given in Table 8.14 may be used as a guide to flow.

A simple relationship between angle of repose, Carr's index and the expected powder flow is shown in Figure 8.6. When only small quantities of powder are available, an alternative is to determine the 'angle of spatula' by picking up a quantity of powder on a

spatula and estimating the angle of the triangular section of the powder heap viewed from the end of the spatula. This is obviously crude but is useful during preformulation, when only small quantities of drug are available.

COMPRESSION PROPERTIES

The compression properties of most drug powders are extremely poor and necessitate the addition of compression aids. When the dose is less than 50 mg, tablets can usually be prepared by direct compression with the addition of modern direct compression bases. At higher doses the preferred method would be wet massing.

Nonetheless, information on the compression properties of the pure drug is extremely useful. Although it is true that the tableted material should be plastic, i.e. capable of permanent deformation, it should also exhibit a degree of brittleness (fragmentation). Thus if the drug dose is high and it behaves plastically, the chosen excipients should fragment, e.g. lactose, calcium phosphate. If the drug is brittle or elastic, the excipients should be plastic, i.e. microcrystalline cellulose, or plastic binders should be used in wet massing. Obviously, as the dose is reduced this becomes less important as the diluent vehicle dominates compressibility.

The compression properties (elasticity, plasticity, fragmentation and punch filming propensity) for small quantities of a new drug candidate can be established by the sequence outlined in Table 8.15. An interpretation of the results follows.

Plastic material

When materials are ductile they deform by changing shape (plastic flow). As there is no fracture, no new surfaces are generated during compression and a

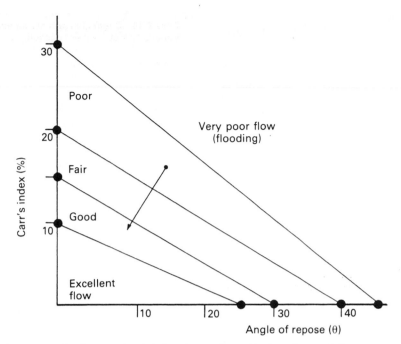

Fig. 8.6   Relationship between angle of repose, Carr's index of a powder and its flow characteristics.

Table 8.15   Scheme for the evaluation of drug compression properties

	500 mg drug + 1% magnesium stearate		
Sample code	A	B	C
Blend in a tumbler mixer for	5 min	5 min	30 min
Compress 13 mm diam. compacts in a IR hydraulic press at	75 MPa	75 MPa	75 MPa
for a dwell time of	2 s	30 s	2 s
Store tablets in a sealed container at room temperature to allow equilibration	24 h	24 h	24 h
Perform crushing strength on tablets and record load	*A* N	*B* N	*C* N

more intimate mix of magnesium stearate (as in sample C, Table 8.15) leads to poorer bonding. Because these materials bond after viscoelastic deformation, and because this is time dependent, increasing the dwell time at compression (*B*) will increase bonding strength. Thus, a material exhibiting crushing strengths in order *B* > *A* > *C* would probably have plastic tendencies.

Fragmentation

If a material is predominantly fragmenting, neither lubricant mixing time (*C*) nor dwell time (*B*) should affect tablet strength. Thus materials which show crushing strengths which are independent of the method of manufacture outlined in Table 8.15 are likely to exhibit fragmenting properties during compression, with a high friability.

Elastic material

Some materials, e.g. paracetamol, are elastic and there is very little permanent change (either plastic flow or fragmentation) caused by compression: the material rebounds (recovers elastically) when the compression load is released. If bonding is weak the compact will self-destruct and the top will detach (capping), or the whole cylinder cracks into horizontal layers (lamination). An elastic body will give as follows:

135

A will cap or laminate.

B will probably maintain integrity but will be very weak.

C will cap or laminate.

Elastic materials require a particularly plastic tableting matrix or wet massing to induce plasticity.

Punch filming (sticking)

Finally, the surface of the top and bottom punches should be examined for drug adhesion. The punches can be dipped into a suitable extraction solvent, e.g. MeOH, and the drug level determined. This will probably be higher for *A* and *B* (Table 8.15), as magnesium stearate is an effective antiadherent and 30 minutes' mixing (*C*) should produce a monolayer and suppress adhesion more effectively.

Sticky materials can be improved by a change in salt form; by using high excipient ratios; by using abrasive inorganic excipients; by wet massing; and/or by the addition of up to 2% magnesium stearate.

EXCIPIENT COMPATIBILITY

The successful formulation of a stable and effective solid dosage form depends on the careful selection of the excipients that are added to facilitate administration, promote the consistent release and bioavailability of the drug and protect it from degradation.

Thermal analysis can be used to investigate and predict any physicochemical interactions between components in a formulation and can therefore be applied to the selection of suitable chemically compatible excipients. Primary excipients recommended for initial screening for tablet and capsule formulations are shown in Table 8.16.

Method

The preformulation screening of drug–excipient interactions requires 5 mg of drug, in a 50% mixture with the excipient, to maximize the likelihood of observing an interaction. Mixtures should be examined under nitrogen to eliminate oxidative and pyrolytic effects at a standard heating rate (2, 5 or 10°C min^{-1}) on the DSC apparatus, over a temperature range which will encompass any thermal changes due to both the drug and excipient.

The melting range and any other transitions of the drug will be known from earlier investigations into purity, polymorphism and solvates. For all

Table 8.16 Suggested primary candidates as excipients for tablet and capsule formulations

Excipient	Function[a]
Lactose monohydrate	F
Dicalcium phosphate dihydate	F
Dicalcium phosphate anhydrous	F
Microcrystalline cellulose	F
Maize starch	D
Modified starch	D
Polyvinylpyrrolidone	B
Sodium starch glycollate	D
Sodium croscarmellose	D
Magnesium stearate	L
Stearic acid	L
Colloidal silica	G

[a] B, binder; D, disintegrant; F filler/diluent; G, glidant: L, lubricant.

potential excipients (Table 8.16) it is sensible to retain representative thermograms in a reference file for comparison.

Interpretation

A scheme for interpreting DSC data from individual components and their mixtures is shown in Figure 8.7. Basically, the thermal properties of a physical mixture are the sum of the individual components, and this thermogram can be compared with those of the drug and the excipient alone. An interaction on DSC will show as changes in melting point, peak shape and area and/or the appearance of a transition. However, there is invariably some change in transition temperature and peak shape and area by virtue of mixing two components, and this is not due to any detrimental interaction. In general, provided that no new thermal events occur, no interaction can be assigned. Chemical interactions are indicated by the appearance of new peaks, or where there is gross broadening or elongation of an exo- or endothermic change. Second-order transitions produce changes in the baseline. Such observations may be indicative of the production of eutectic or solid solution-type melts. The excipient is then probably chemically reactive and incompatible with the drug, and should be avoided. Where an interaction is suspected but the thermal changes are small, the incompatibility should be confirmed by TLC.

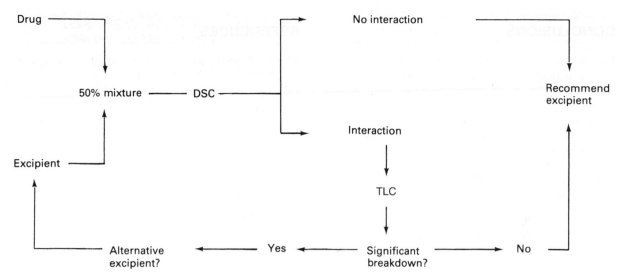

Fig. 8.7 Scheme to identify chemically compatible excipients using DSC with confirmatory TLC.

The advantages of DSC over more traditional, routine compatibility screens, typically TLC, is that no long-term storage of the mixture is required prior to evaluation, nor is any inappropriate thermal stress (other than the DSC itself, which had drug and excipient controls) required to accelerate the interactions. This, in itself, may be misleading if the mode of breakdown changes with temperature and elevated temperatures fail to reflect the degradation path occurring under normal (room temperature) storage.

Where confirmation is required by TLC, samples (50:50 mixtures of drug and excipient) should be sealed in small neutral glass test tubes and stored for either 7 days at 50°C or 14 days at 37°C.

It is important to view the results of such incompatibility testing with caution. For example, magnesium stearate is notoriously incompatible with a wide range of compounds when tested, yet because it is only used at low levels – typically 0.5–1% – such apparent incompatibility rarely produces a problem in practice in long-term storage and use.

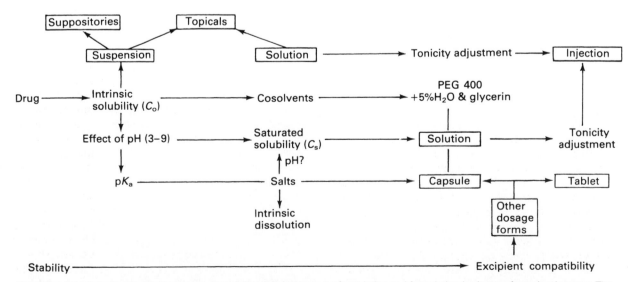

Fig. 8.8 A generic development pathway: the relationship between preformulation and formulation in dosage form development. The formulation stages are shown in boxes and the preformulation stages are unboxed.

CONCLUSIONS

Preformulation studies have a significant part to play in anticipating formulation problems and identifying logical paths in both liquid and solid dosage form technology (Fig. 8.8). The need for adequate drug solubility cannot be overemphasized. The availability of good solubility data should allow the selection of the most appropriate salt for development. Stability studies in solution will indicate the feasibility of parenteral or other liquid dosage forms, and can identify methods of stabilization. In parallel, solid-state stability by DSC, TLC and HPLC, and in the presence of tablet and capsule excipients, will indicate the most acceptable vehicles for solid dosage forms.

By comparing the physicochemical properties of each drug candidate within a therapeutic group (using C_s, pK_a, melting point, K_w^o) the preformulation scientist can assist the synthetic chemist to identify the optimum molecule, provide the biologist with suitable vehicles to elicit pharmacological response, and advise the bulk chemist about the selection and production of the best salt with appropriate particle size and morphology for subsequent processing.

REFERENCES

Albert, A.A. and Serjeant, E.P. (1984) *Ionization Constants of Acids and Bases*. Wiley, New York.
Kaplan, S.A. (1972) *Drug Metab. Rev*, **1**, 15–32.
Meyer, H. (1899) *Arch. Exp. Pathol. Pharmacol.*, **42**, 109
Perrin, D.D. Dempsey, B. and Serjeant, E.P. (1981) *pK_a Predictions for Organic Acids and Bases*. Chapman & Hall, London.
Yalkowski, S.H. and Roseman, T.J. (1981) *Techniques of Solubilization of Drugs*, ed. S.H. Yalkowski, Marcel Dekker, New York, Chapter 3.

BIBLIOGRAPHY

Albert, A.A. and Serjeant, E.P. (1984) *Ionization Constants of Acids and Bases*, Wiley, New York
Davies, S.S. and Higuchi, T. (1970) *J. Pharm Sci.*, **59**, 1376.
Hamilton, R.J. and Sewell, P.A. (1977) *Introduction to High Performance Liquidity Chromatography*. Chapman & Hall, London.
Jones, T.M. (1981) *Int. J. Pharm. Tech. Prod. Mfr.*, **2**, 17.
Kennon, L. (1964) *J. Pharm. Sci.* **53**, 815–818.
Pryde, A. and Gilbert M.T. (1979) *Applications of High Performance Liquid Chromatography*. Chapman & Hall, London.
Smith, A. (1982) *Anal. Proc.*, **19**, 559.
Yalkowski, S.H., Amidon, G.L., Zografi, G. and Flynn, G.L. (1975) *J. Pharm Sci.*, **64**, 48.
Yalkowski, S.H. and Roseman, T.J. (1981) *Techniques of Solubilization of Drugs*, Chapter 3, ed. S.H. Yalkowski, Marcel Dekker, New York.

PARTICLE SCIENCE AND POWDER TECHNOLOGY

PARTICLE SCIENCE AND POWDER TECHNOLOGY

9

Solid-state properties

Graham Buckton

THE SOLID STATE

The three states of matter are solid, liquid and gas (or vapour).

In a sealed container vapours will diffuse to occupy the total space, liquids will flow to fill part of the container completely, but solids will retain their original shape unless a compressive force is applied to them. From this simple consideration it becomes clear that solids are unique because their physical form (the packing of the molecules and the size and shape of the particles) can have an influence on the way the material will behave. At normal room temperature and pressure the majority of drugs and excipients exist as solids, and so the study of solid-state properties is of enormous pharmaceutical importance.

Solid particles are made up of molecules that are held in close proximity to each other by intermolecular forces. The strength of interaction between two molecules is due to the individual atoms within the molecular structure. For example, hydrogen bonds occur as a result of an electrostatic attraction involving one hydrogen atom and one electronegative atom, such as oxygen. For molecules that cannot hydrogen bond, attraction is due to van der Waal's forces. The term van der Waal's forces is generally taken to include dipole–dipole (Keesom), dipole-induced dipole (Debye) and induced dipole–induced dipole (London) forces. Here a dipole is where the molecule has a small imbalance of charge from one end to the other, making it behave like a small bar magnet. When the molecules pack together to form a solid, these dipoles align and give attraction between the positive pole of one and the negative pole on the next. Induced dipoles are where the free molecule does not have an imbalance of charge, but an imbalance is caused by bringing a second molecule into close proximity with the first.

CRYSTALLIZATION

Materials in the solid state can be crystalline or amorphous (or a combination of both). Crystalline materials are those in which the molecules are packed in a defined order, and this same order repeats over and over again throughout the particle. In Figure 9.1(a) an ordered packing of a molecule is shown, here the shape of the molecule is represented by a 'hockey-stick' style image, illustrating a planar structure with a functional group pointing up at the end. (This is not a real molecule: it has been drawn to provide an easy representation of a possible crystal packing arrangement.) A characteristic property of a crystal is that it has a melting point. This is the temperature at which the crystal lattice breaks down, owing to the molecules having gained sufficient energy from the heating process to overcome the attractive forces that hold the crystal together. It follows that crystals with weak forces holding the molecules together (such as paraffins, which only have van der Waals interactions) have low melting points, whereas crystals with strong lattices (i.e. those held together with strong attractive forces, such as extensive hydrogen bonding) have high melting points.

Crystals are produced by inducing a change from the liquid to the solid state. There are two options: one is to cool a molten sample to below its melting point. Pharmaceutical examples of crystallizing through cooling include the formation of suppositories, creams and semisolid matrix oral dosage forms. The other method of crystallization is to have a solution of the material and to change the system so that the solid is formed. At a given temperature and pressure, any solute (where the solute is the material that has been dissolved and the liquid is the solvent) has a certain maximum amount that can be dissolved in any liquid (called a saturated solution). If crystals are to be formed from a solution, it is necessary to have more solute present than can be dissolved at that temperature; this will eventually result in the formation of a solid in equilibrium with a saturated solution. In order to make a solid precipitate out of solution one can either:

- remove the liquid by evaporation (this is the way sea salt is prepared)
- cool the solution, as most materials become less soluble as the temperature is decreased
- add another liquid which will mix with the solution, but in which the solute has a low solubility. This second liquid is often called an antisolvent.

Many drugs are crystallized by adding water as an antisolvent to a solution of the drug in an organic liquid. For example, if a drug is almost insoluble in water but freely soluble in ethanol, the drug could be crystallized by adding water to a near-saturated solution of the drug in ethanol.

The processes by which a crystal forms are called **nucleation** and **growth**. Nucleation is the formation of a small mass on to which a crystal can grow. Growth is the addition of more solute molecules to the nucleation site. In order to achieve nucleation and growth, it is necessary to have a supersaturated solution, i.e. one where the amount of solute dissolved in the liquid is greater than the true solubility. Supersaturated solutions are not thermodynamically stable; in these circumstances the system will adjust in order to move back to the true solubility, and to do this the excess solute will precipitate. However, in some circumstances the process of nucleation can be slow. Most students will at some stage have a supersaturated solution which has not crystallized; then, simply by scratching the side of the beaker with a glass rod, crystallization can be induced. The scratching action produces a small amount of rough surface or glass spicule that acts as a nucleation site and causes the supersaturated solute to precipitate rapidly.

POLYMORPHISM

If the crystallization conditions are changed in any way, it is possible that the molecules may start to

Polymorphism of molecule ⎯⎯⎯⎯⎯

(a)

(b)

Fig. 9.1 Representation of two polymorphic forms of a crystal consisting of a molecule represented by a 'hockey-stick' shape.

form crystals with a different packing pattern from that which occurred when the original conditions were used. The change in conditions could be a different solvent, or a change in the stirring, or different impurities being present. Figure 9.1(b) shows an alternative packing arrangement from that which occurred for the same molecule in Figure 9.1(a). As both the packing arrangements in Figure 9.1 are repeating ordered systems, they are both crystals; these would be called polymorphic forms.

By looking at the packing arrangements in Figure 9.1 it can be seen that the molecules in (a) are more spaced out than those in (b), which means that the two crystal forms would have different densities (i.e. the same mass of material would be housed in different volumes). It looks as though it would be easier to physically pull a molecule off structure (a) than off (b), as the molecules in (b) are more interwoven into the structure. If this were the case then (a) would have a lower melting point than (b) and might dissolve more easily. Also, if an attempt were made to mill the two crystals, it appears that (a) would break easily, as there are natural break lines (either vertically or horizontally), whereas (b) does not seem to have an obvious weak line to allow easy breakage. This could mean that the milling and compaction (tabletting) properties of the two forms will differ. In summary, a change in the packing arrangement of the same molecule, giving two different crystal forms, could result in significant changes in the properties of the solid.

Many organic molecules, including drugs and excipients, exhibit polymorphism. Usually this is of a form known as monotropic, which means that only one polymorphic form is stable and any other polymorph that is formed will eventually convert to the stable form. However, some materials exhibit enantropic polymorphism, which means that under different conditions (temperature and pressure) the material can reversibly transform between alternative stable forms; however, this type of behaviour is less common and will not be considered further. Considering the more usual monotropic polymorphism, the true stable form has the highest melting point and all other forms are described as metastable. This means that the other forms exist for a period of time and thus appear stable, but given a chance they will convert to the true stable form. Different metastable forms can exist for very short times or for many months before they convert to the stable form, depending upon the conditions under which they are stored.

In general there will be a correlation between the melting point of the different polymorphs and the rate of dissolution, because the one with the lowest melting point will most easily give up molecules to dissolve, whereas the most stable form (highest melting point) will not give up molecules to the solvent.

High melting point = strong lattice = hard to remove a molecule = low dissolution rate (and vice versa).

It is relatively easy to understand that changes in polymorphic form can cause changes in the rate at which a drug will dissolve. However, it is less easy to understand why this can lead to a change in the apparent solubility. None the less, it is true that when a metastable polymorphic form is dissolved it can give a greater amount of material in solution than the saturated solubility. In other words, metastable forms can dissolve to give supersaturated solutions. These supersaturated solutions will eventually return to the equilibrium solubility, owing to the stable crystal form precipitating from solution, but this process may not be instantaneous. In fact, the supersaturated solution can often exist long enough to cause an increase in bioavailability of a poorly soluble drug. Figure 9.2 shows the solubility of two different polymorphs of sulphamethoxydiazine. It can be seen that Form III has a higher solubility than Form II, and that this lasts throughout

Fig. 9.2 The solubility time relationship for sulphamethoxydiazine. ○, solubility of polymorphic Form III, which rises to the drug's equilibrium solubility and plateaus. ●, solubility of polymorphic Form II, which dissolves to twice the extent of Form III and then shows a gradual decline with time, as the stable form crystallizes from solution. △, the effect of adding crystals of Form III to the solution of Form II at the peak of solubility. It can be seen that the amount dissolved falls rapidly from the supersaturated level to the true equilibrium solubility because the added crystals of Form II act as nucleation sites. (Reproduced from Ebian et al 1973, with permission.)

the 90-minute experiment. However, if crystals of Form II are added to the solution of Form III, then the solubility reverts rapidly to that of Form II because the excess solute in the supersaturated solution will have seed crystals of Form II on which to precipitate.

Polymorphism and bioavailability

Many drugs are hydrophobic and have very limited solubility in water. Owing to the limited aqueous solubility of such drugs the rate at which they dissolve (slow dissolution rate) can result in only a small percentage of the administered drug actually being available to the patient (low bioavailability). A classic example of the importance of polymorphism on bioavailability is that of chloramphenicol palmitate suspensions. In Figure 9.3 the blood serum level is plotted as a function of time after dosing. It can be seen that the stable α-polymorph produces low serum levels, whereas the metastable β-polymorph yields much higher serum levels when the same dose is administered.

For drugs that are freely soluble in water the bioavailability is not likely to be limited by the dissolution, so it would be surprising for polymorphism to influence bioavailability in this way. However, for drugs with low aqueous solubility the polymorphic form must be well controlled to ensure that the bioavailability is the same each time the product is made, and throughout the shelf-life of the product. It would be risky to deliberately make a product using anything other than the stable form of a drug, as other polymorphic forms could convert to the stable form during the shelf-life of the product, which could result in a reduction in bioavailability and hence the therapeutic effect of the product.

In conclusion, the stable polymorphic form will have the slowest dissolution rate, and so there may be occasions when it would be desirable to speed the dissolution by using a metastable form. However, the risk associated with using the metastable form is that it will convert back to the stable form during the product's life, and give a consequent change in properties. As polymorphism can have such serious consequences for the bioavailability of drugs with low aqueous solubility, it is essential that manufacturers check for the existence of polymorphism and ensure that they use the same appropriate polymorphic form every time they make a product.

As mentioned above, many properties other than rate of solution can change when a material is in a different polymorphic form. For example, paracetamol is a high-dose drug with poor compression properties, which can make it difficult to form into tablets. Consequently, researchers have tried to use different polymorphic forms of paracetamol to find one that is more compressible.

HYDRATES AND SOLVATES

It is possible for materials to crystallize and in so doing to trap molecules of the solvent within the lattice. If the solvent used is water, the material will be described as a hydrate. This entrapment is often in an exact molar ratio with the crystallizing material: for example, a monohydrate will have one molecule of water for each molecule of the crystallizing material. It is possible to have many different levels of hydrate: for example, some drugs can exist as a monohydrate, a dihydrate and a trihydrate (respectively one, two and three molecules of water to each molecule of drug). Morris (1999) notes that about 11% (over 16000 compounds) of all structures recorded on the Cambridge Structural Database exist as hydrates. Of the classes of hydrate materials that were similar to drugs, about 50% were monohydrates (one water molecule for each one of host), over 20% were dihydrates (two water molecules to one of host), 8% were trihydrates (three water molecules to one host) and 8% were hemihydrates (one water molecule to two of host); other hydrate levels (up to 10 water to one host) became progressively less common.

Fig. 9.3 Comparison of mean blood serum levels after the administration of chloramphenicol palmitate suspensions using varying ratios of the stable (α) and the metastable (β) polymorphs. M, 100% α polymorph; N, 25:75 β:α; O, 50:50 β:α; P, 75:25 β:α; L, 100% β polymorph. (Reproduced from Aguiar et al 1976, with permission.)

If solvents other than water are present in a crystal lattice the material is called a solvate. For example, if ethanol is present it would be an ethanolate. In general it is undesirable to use solvates for pharmaceuticals as the presence of retained organic vapours would be regarded as an unnecessary impurity in the product. If the organic vapour were toxic in any way it would obviously be inappropriate for pharmaceuticals. For this reason discussion will be limited to hydrates.

Hydrates often have very different properties from the anhydrous form, in the same way as two different polymorphs have different properties from each other. For this reason the difference between hydrates and anhydrous forms is described as pseudopolymorphism. With polymorphism the stable form has the highest melting point and the slowest dissolution rate (see above); however, with hydrates it is possible for the hydrate form to have either a faster or a slower dissolution rate than the anhydrous form. The most usual situation is for the anhydrous form to have a faster dissolution rate than the hydrate; an example of this is shown in Figure 9.4 for theophylline. In this situation, water could hydrogen bond between two drug molecules and tie the lattice together; this would give a much stronger, more stable lattice and hence a slower dissolution rate. It can be seen from Figure 9.4 that the anhydrous theophylline rises to a high concentration in solution and then falls again until the amount dissolved is the same as that recorded for the hydrate. The reason for this is that the hydrate has reached true equilibrium solubility, whereas the anhydrous form had initially formed a supersaturated solution (as has been described for metastable polymorphic forms above).

Although anhydrous forms are usually more rapidly soluble than the hydrate, there are examples of the opposite being true. In such circumstances one could think of water as a wedge pushing two molecules apart and preventing the optimum interaction between the molecules in the lattice. Here water would be weakening the lattice and would result in a more rapid dissolution rate. An example of the hydrate form speeding up dissolution is shown in Figure 9.5 for erythromycin.

THE AMORPHOUS STATE

When a material is in the solid state but the molecules are not packed in a repeating long-range ordered fashion, it is said to be amorphous. Amorphous solids have very different properties from the crystal form of the same material. For example, crystals have a melting point (the break-up of the crystal lattice), whereas the amorphous form does not (as it does not have a crystal lattice to break).

Polymeric materials (or other large molecular weight species) have molecules that are so large and flexible that it is not possible for them to align perfectly to form crystals. For these materials it will be usual to have ordered regions within the structure

Fig. 9.4 The dissolution of theophylline monohydrate rising to an equilibrium solubility, compared with that for theophylline anhydrous which forms a supersaturated solution with a peak over twice that of the dissolving hydrate, before crystallizing to form the true equilibrium solubility. (Reproduced from Shefter and Higuchi 1963, with permission.)

Fig. 9.5 The dissolution behaviour for erythromycin as anhydrate, monohydrate and dihydrate, showing a progressively faster dissolution rate as the level of hydrate is increased. (Reproduced from Allen et al 1978, with permission.)

surrounded by disorder, so they are described as semicrystalline. For materials such as these it will not be possible to produce a completely crystalline sample; however, the degree of crystallinity can vary depending upon processing conditions. This can affect the properties of the material and hence how they function in pharmaceutical products.

For low molecular weight materials the amorphous form may be produced if the solidification process was too fast for the molecules to have a chance to align in the correct way to form a crystal (this could happen when a solution is spray-dried). Alternatively, a crystal may be formed but then broken, for example if the crystal were exposed to energy, such as milling. A simple analogy that can be used here is that a crystal is like a brick wall, which has ordered long-range packing. If the wall is hit hard, perhaps during demolition, the bricks will separate (Figure 9.6). Unlike the brick wall, however, a disrupted crystal will be unstable and will revert back to the crystal form. This conversion may be rapid or very slow and, as with polymorphism, its pharmaceutical significance will depend on how long the partially amorphous form survives.

Amorphous forms have a characteristic temperature at which there is a major change in properties. This is called the glass transition temperature (T_g). If the sample is stored below the T_g the amorphous form will be brittle and is described as the glassy state. If the sample is above its T_g it becomes rubbery. The T_g, although not well understood, is a point where the molecules in the glass exhibit a major change in mobility. The lack of mobility when the sample is glassy allows the amorphous form to exist for longer, whereas when T_g is below the storage temperature the increased molecular mobility allows rapid conversion to the crystalline form.

The glass transition temperature of an amorphous material can be lowered by adding a small molecule, called a plasticizer, that fits between the glassy molecules, giving them greater mobility. Water is a good plasticizer for many materials, and so the glass transition temperature will usually reduce in the presence of water vapour. Most amorphous materials are able to absorb large quantities of water vapour. Absorption is a process whereby one molecule passes into the bulk of another material and should not be confused with adsorption, which is when something concentrates at the surface of another material. Figure 9.6 shows the way in which water can access amorphous regions. Figure 9.7 shows the amount of water that is adsorbed to a crystalline material (Figure 9.7(a)), compared to that absorbed into an amorphous form of the same material (Figure 9.7(b)). It can be seen that the amount absorbed is many times greater than that adsorbed. This large difference in water content at any selected relative humidity is important in many materials. For example, it is possible that certain drugs can degrade by hydrolysis when amorphous, but remain stable when crystalline. The extent of hydrolysis of an antibiotic which had been processed to yield different levels of crystalline:amorphous forms is shown in Table 9.1; the extent of degradation is greater when the amorphous content is increased.

In Figure 9.7 it can be seen that the amorphous form absorbs a very large amount of water until 50% RH, after which there is a weight loss, the reason for which is that the sample has crystallized. Crystallization occurs because the absorbed water has plasticized the sample to such an extent that the T_g has dropped below room temperature and allowed sufficient molecular mobility that the molecules are able to align and crystallize. The water is lost during this process, as absorption can only occur in the amorphous form and so cannot endure

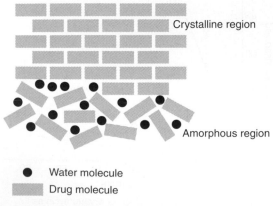

Water molecule

Drug molecule

Fig. 9.6 The disruption of a crystal (represented as a brick wall), giving the possibility for water vapour absorption in the amorphous region

Table 9.1 The chemical stability of cephalothin sodium related to the amorphous content of the sample. Data derived from Pikal et al 1978

Sample	% amorphous	% stable drug after storage at 31%RH 50°C
Crystalline	0	100
Freeze dried	12	100
Freeze dried	46	85
Spray dried	53	44

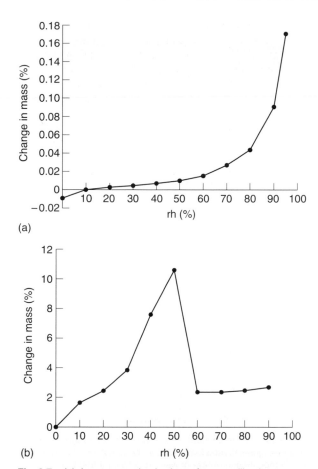

Fig. 9.7 (a) A water sorption isotherm for crystalline lactose monohydrate. The quantity of water adsorbed to the crystal surface is small. (b) Water sorption isotherm for amorphous lactose, showing a rise to about 11% water content due to absorption, followed by water loss as the sample crystallizes and the absorbed water is expelled.

not necessarily make all materials partially amorphous, the chance of seeing disruption to the crystalline lattice will increase with the amount of energy used in the milling.

The fact that processing can make crystalline materials partially amorphous means that it is possible for very complex materials to form that contain different metastable states. For example, in Figure 9.3 the plasma levels of two polymorphs of chloramphenicol palmitate were shown, however if the β-polymorph were milled it is possible that it might also become partially amorphous, which could make the plasma level even higher than when the crystalline form were used. However, milling the β-polymorph could also provide the necessary energy to convert it to the stable α-polymorph, which would reduce the effective plasma level. Equally, milling could disrupt the α-polymorph, giving a partially amorphous form that might have a higher bioavailability than the crystal. In other words, the effect of processing on the physical form can be very complicated, and often unpredictable. It is possible to produce a physical form that is partially amorphous and partially crystalline. The crystalline component could then be

Fig. 9.8 The amorphous content induced in crystalline lactose as a consequence of milling in an air-jet mill at different air pressures. (Redrawn from Briggner et al 1994, with permission.)

into the crystalline state. However, some water is retained in this example (Fig. 9.7(a) and (b)), because lactose is able to form a monohydrate. The amount of water required to form a monohydrate with lactose is 5% w/w (calculated from the molecular weight of lactose and water), which is much less than the 11% that was present in the amorphous form (Figure 9.7(b)).

In Figure 9.8 the amorphous content of lactose is seen to increase in proportion to the length of time it was left in an air-jet mill (micronizer). In Figure 9.9 it can be seen that a drug substance became partially amorphous when treated in a simple ball mill, and extensively amorphous when micronized. Although the example in Figure 9.9 is an extreme behaviour it is not unusual for highly processed materials to become partially amorphous. Although milling does

Fig. 9.9 The amorphous content of a model drug substance following milling in a ball mill and a micronizer. (Redrawn from Ahmed et al 1996, with permission.)

stable or metastable. Inevitably, with time (for low molecular weight species) the sample will revert to contain only the stable crystalline form, with no amorphous content and none of the metastable polymorph(s), but as this does not necessarily happen instantly the physical form and its complexity are of great importance.

CRYSTAL HABIT

All of the above discussion relates to the internal packing of molecules. It has been shown that they may have no long-range order (amorphous), or have different repeating packing arrangements (polymorphic crystals), or have solvent included (solvates and hydrates). Each of these changes in internal packing of a solid will give rise to changes in properties. However, it is also possible to change the external shape of a crystal. The external shape is called the crystal habit and this is a consequence of the rate at which different faces grow. Changes in internal packing usually (but not always) give an easily distinguishable change in habit. However, for the same crystal packing it is possible to change the external appearance by changing the crystallization conditions.

With any crystalline material, the largest face is always the slowest growing. The reason for this is shown in Figure 9.10, where it can be seen that if drug is deposited on two faces of the hexagonal crystal habit, then the first consequence is that the face where drug is deposited actually becomes a smaller part of the crystal, whereas the other faces become larger. Eventually, the fastest growing faces will no longer exist (Figure 9.10). The growth on different faces will depend on the relative affinities of the solute for the solvent and the growing faces of the crystal. Every molecule is made up of different functional groups, some being relatively polar (such as carboxylic acid groups) whereas others are nonpolar (such as a methyl group). Depending on the packing geometry of the molecules into the lattice, some crystal faces may have more exposed polar groups and others may be relatively non-polar. If the crystal were growing from an aqueous solution, drug would deposit on the faces that make the crystal more polar (i.e. the non-polar faces would grow, making the more polar faces dominate). If, however, the same crystal form were growing from a non-polar solvent, then the opposite would be true.

Obviously the external shape can alter the properties of drugs and excipients. For example, the disso-

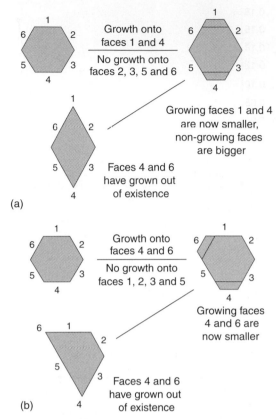

Fig. 9.10 (a) Demonstration of how growth on to faces 1 and 4 of a hexagonal crystal form result in the formation of a diamond. (b) Demonstration of how growth on to faces 4 and 6 of a hexagonal crystal result in the formation of a trapezium.

lution rate of a drug can change if the surface area to volume ratio is altered. An extreme difference would be between a long needle and a sphere (Figure 9.11). A sphere of 20 μm radius has approximately the same volume (mass) as a needle of $335 \times 10 \times 10$ μm, but the surface area of the needle is 2.7 times greater than that of the sphere. As dissolution rate is directly proportional to surface area, the needle would dissolve much faster than the sphere. Crystals do not grow to make spheres, although through milling they can develop rounded geometries; the closest to a sphere would be a cube, which would still have under half the surface area of the needle shown in Figure 9.11.

As well as changes in dissolution rate, different crystal habits can cause changes in powder flow (which is important as, for example, the die of a tabletting machine is filled by volume and requires good powder flow to guarantee content uniformity of the product) and sedimentation and caking of suspensions.

Sphere:
radius 20 μm
volume 33,515 μm³
surface area 5,027 μm²

Cube:
length, width and
thickness 32.2 μm
volume 33,386 μm³
surface area 6,221 μm²

Needle:
length 335 μm, width
and thickness 10 μm
volume 33,500 μm³
surface area 13,600 μm²

Fig. 9.11 The relative surface areas of a sphere, a cube and a needle that each have similar volumes of material.

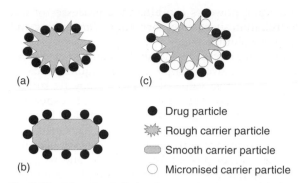

(a)   (c)

(b)

● Drug particle
✳ Rough carrier particle
▱ Smooth carrier particle
○ Micronised carrier particle

Fig. 9.12 A hypothesis that surface roughness may relate to dry release from carrier particles in dry powder inhalers. (a) Micronized drug trapped in the rough regions of the carrier particle, giving low inhaled dose. (b) Micronized drug can be readily removed from a smooth carrier particle. (c) Micronized drug may be removed readily (hence a high inhaled dose) if the carrier is first treated with micronized carrier particles in order to fill the rough voids.

It is technically possible to engineer changes in crystal habit by deliberately manipulating the rate of growth of different faces of the crystal. This is done by intentionally adding a small amount of impurity to the solution. The impurity must interact preferentially with one face of the growing crystal, and in so doing it will stop growth on that face, causing the remaining face(s) to grow more rapidly. The impurity would either be a very similar molecule to that of the crystallizing material, so that part of the molecule is included in the lattice but the remainder blocks further layers from attaching, or it may be a surfactant that adsorbs to one growing face.

SURFACE NATURE OF PARTICLES

Dry powder inhalers

Dry powder inhalers (see Chapter 31) often have a micronized drug, which must be small enough to be inhaled, mixed with a larger carrier particle which is often lactose. The carrier particle is there to make the powder suitable for handling and dosing, as micronized particles have poor flow properties. The shape and surface properties of the drug and/or carrier particles can be critical in controlling the dose of drug that is delivered. It may be necessary to adjust the surface roughness of carrier particles. In Figure 9.12(a) there is a cartoon of a rough carrier particle: this would hold the micronized drug too strongly, essentially trapped within the rough regions of the carrier, and so the inhaled dose would be very low. In Figure 9.12(b) a smooth particle of the same carrier is seen: here the drug will be easily displaced from the carrier during inhalation, but it may not stay mixed with the carrier during filling of the inhaler and dosing. In Figure 9.12(c) a rough carrier particle has been mixed first with micronized carrier and then with micronized drug. Using this approach

the drug is free to detach, as the micronized carrier is trapped in all the crevices on the carrier surface. The hypothesis relating to the use of fine carrier particles to enhance the delivery of micronized drug from large carrier particles is not proved beyond doubt. It remains possible that interactions between the fine carrier and fine drug may be the reason for the enhanced delivery.

For products such as these it is becoming increasingly important first to measure the surface nature of samples and then to control the form in order to achieve the desired delivery of drug. The surface shape of the carrier is an important consideration for the design of this type of product. A further concern is the surface energy, as this can influence the way in which the drug and the carrier are attached to each other.

Surface energy

Molecules at the surface of a material have a net inward force exerted on them from the molecules in the bulk: this is the basis of surface energy. Surface energy is important, as every interaction (except the mixing of two gases) starts with an initial contact between two surfaces. If this surface interaction is favoured then the process will probably proceed, whereas if it is not favoured then it will be limited. A good example of the role of surface energy is the wetting of a powder by a liquid, where the powder cannot dissolve until the liquid makes good contact with it. A practical example is instant coffee, where some brands are hard to wet and dissolve whereas others dissolve easily. Changes in the wetting of powders can affect the processes of wet granulation, suspension formation, film coating and drug dissolution.

The measurement and understanding of surface energy is relatively simple for pure liquids, because there is a single value of surface energy (= surface tension). However, for solids, and especially powders, the situation is far more complex. Even on the same crystal form it would be expected that every crystal face, edge and defect could experience different forces pulling from the bulk, and so could have a different surface energy. From the discussion above, it would be reasonable to assume that different physical forms of the same drug could have quite different surface energies. Thus for the same drug it is possible that changes in habit and/or polymorphic form and/or the presence of a solvate or hydrate would change the surface energy. For amorphous forms the molecules at the surface have greater freedom to move and reorientate than do molecules in crystal surfaces, and so the amorphous form could have changes in surface energy with time (and with physical state in relation to T_g).

The conventional way of determining the surface energy of a solid is to place a drop of liquid on to the solid surface and measure the contact angle. This is defined as the angle between the solid surface and the tangent drawn at the three-phase interface, measured through the liquid. Examples of contact angles are shown in Chapter 5. Perfect wetting of a solid by a liquid will result in a contact angle of 0°. Contact angles are the result of a balance of three interfacial forces γ_{LV} being the liquid surface tension, γ_{LS} between the liquid and the solid, and γ_{SV} between the solid and the vapour. The relative magnitude of these forces will determine whether the drop of liquid spreads on the solid or not, and consequently, by use of the contact angle (θ) it is possible to calculate the solid surface energy if the surface tension of the liquid is known:

$$\gamma_{SV} = \gamma_{SL} + \gamma_{LV} \cos \theta$$

This is known as Young's equation.

For smooth solid surfaces contact angles are an ideal way of assessing surface energy; however, powders present a problem as it is not possible to place a drop of liquid on their surface. Consequently, a compromise will always be required when measuring a contact angle for powdered systems. An example of such a compromise would be to make a compact of the powder so as to produce a smooth flat surface; the disadvantage of this is that the process of compaction may well change the surface energy of the powder.

A preferred option by which to assess the surface energy of powders would be vapour sorption.

Vapour sorption

When a powder is exposed to a vapour or gas, the interaction will take one of the following forms:

1. Adsorption of the vapour to the powder surface (adsorption is described in Chapter 5)
2. Absorption into the bulk
3. Deliquescence
4. Hydrate/solvate formation.

Absorption into the bulk can occur if the sample is amorphous, whereas the interaction will be limited to adsorption if the powder is crystalline. The extent and energetics of interaction between vapours and powder surfaces allows the surface energy to be calculated. The other processes listed are deliquescence, which is where the powder dissolves in the vapour, and hydrate formation, which is discussed above.

It is therefore possible to use adsorption and/or absorption behaviour to determine powder surface energy. There are three basic approaches to this: gravimetric, calorimetric and chromatographic. Each of these techniques has found application in studies of batch-to-batch variability of materials. An example of a critical case could be that a certain drug shows extensive variability in respirable dose from a dry powder inhaler. Assuming that the size distribution was acceptable in all cases, it would be necessary to understand why some batches yielded unacceptable doses. These vapour sorption techniques could then be used to assess the surface energy and define values that would be acceptable in order to obtain good drug dosing, and equally to define batches of drug that will give unacceptable products.

Gravimetric methods use sensitive microbalances as a means of determining the extent of vapour sorption to a powder surface. The calorimetric approaches measure the enthalpy change associated with vapour–powder interaction, which gives clear information on the nature of the powder surface. Using the principles of gas chromatography it is possible to pack the powder for which the surface energy is required into a column, and then to inject different vapours into the column with a carrier gas. Obviously the time taken for the vapour to come out of the other end of the column is a measure of how favourable was the interaction between the powder and the vapour. It is then possible to calculate the surface energy of the powder from the retention time of different vapours in the column. Gas chromatography is normally used with a column of known properties with unknown vapours; however, in this experiment the unknown is the solid column and the materials with known properties are the injected vapours. For this reason this technique is called inverse phase gas chromatography.

REFERENCES

Aguiar, A.J., Krc, J.Jr., Kinkel, A.W. and Sanyn, J.C. (1967) *J. Pharm. Sci.*, **56**, 847–853.

Ahmed, H., Buckton, G. and Rawlins, D.A. (1996) *Int. J. Pharm.*, **130**, 195–201.

Allen, P.V., Rahn, P.D., Sarapu, A.C. and Vanderwielen, A.J. (1978) *J. Pharm. Sci.*, **67**, 1087–1093.

Briggner, L.-E., Buckton, G., Bystrom, K. and Darcy, P. (1994) *Int. J. Pharm.*, **105**, 125–135.

Ebian, A.R., Moustafa, M.A., Khalil, S.A. and Motawi, M.M. (1973) *J. Pharm. Pharmacol*, **25**, 13–20.

Morris, K.R. (1999) Structural aspects of hydrates and solvates. In Brittain, H.G. (ed.) *Polymorphism in Pharmaceutical Solids*. Marcel Dekker, New York, pp. 125–181.

Pikal, M.J., Lukes, A.L., Lang, J.E. and Gaines, K. (1978) *J. Pharm. Sci.*, **67**, 767–773.

Shefter, E. and Higuchi, T. (1963) *J. Pharm. Sci.*, **52**, 781–791.

BIBLIOGRAPHY

Brittain, H.G. (ed.) (1999) *Polymorphism in Pharmaceutical Solids*. Marcel Dekker, New York.

Buckton, G. (1995) *Interfacial Phenomena in Drug Delivery and Targeting*. Harwood Academic Press, Amsterdam.

Florence, A.T. and Attwood, D. (1998) *Physicochemical Principles of Pharmacy*, 3rd edn. Macmillan, London.

Mersmann, A. (ed.) (1994) *Crystallization Technology Handbook*. Marcel Dekker, New York.

10
Particle-size analysis

John Staniforth

PARTICLE SIZE AND THE LIFETIME OF A DRUG

The dimensions of particulate solids are important in achieving optimum production of efficacious medicines. Figure 10.1 shows an outline of the lifetime of a drug; during stages 1 and 2, when a drug is synthesized and formulated, the particle size of drug and other powders is determined and influences the subsequent physical performance of the medicine and the pharmacological performance of the drug.

Particle size influences the production of formulated medicines (stage 3, Fig. 10.1) as solid dosage forms. Both tablets and capsules are produced using equipment that controls the mass of drug and other particles by volumetric filling. Therefore, any interference with the uniformity of fill volumes may alter the mass of drug incorporated into the tablet or capsule and hence reduce the content uniformity of the medicine. Powders with different particle sizes have different flow and packing properties, which alter the volumes of powder during each encapsulation or tablet compression event. In order to avoid such problems the particle sizes of drug and other powder may be defined during formulation so that problems during production are avoided.

Following administration of the medicine (stage 4, Fig. 10.1), the dosage form should release the drug into solution at the optimum rate. This depends on several factors, one of which will be the particle size of drug as predicted from the following theoretical considerations. Noyes and Whitney first showed that the rate of solution of a solid was related to the law of diffusion, and proposed that the following equations could be used to predict the rate of solution of a wide variety of solutes.

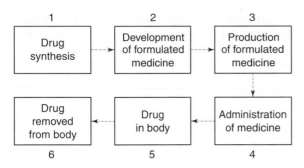

Fig. 10.1 Schematic representation of the lifetime of a drug.

$$\frac{dx}{dt} = c(C_s - C) \qquad (10.1)$$

$$c = \frac{1}{t} \log_e \frac{C_s}{C_s - C} \qquad (10.2)$$

where C is the concentration of solute in solution at time, t, C_s is the solubility of solute and c is a constant which can be determined from a knowledge of solute solubility. The constant c was more precisely defined by Danckwerts, who showed that the mean rate of solution per unit area under turbulent conditions was given by:

$$\frac{dx}{dt} = D\sigma(C_s - C) \qquad (10.3)$$

where D is a diffusion coefficient and σ is the rate of production of fresh surface. $D\sigma$ can be interpreted as a liquid film mass transfer coefficient, which will tend to vary inversely with particle size as a reduction in size generally increases the specific surface area of particles. Thus particles having small dimensions will tend to increase the rate of solution. For example, the drug griseofulvin has a low solubility by oral administration but is rapidly distributed following absorption; the solubility of griseofulvin can be greatly enhanced by particle size reduction, so that blood levels equivalent to, or better than, those obtained with crystalline griseofulvin can be produced using a microcrystalline form of the drug. A reduction of particle size to improve rate of solution and hence bioavailability is not always beneficial. For example, small particle-size nitrofurantoin has an increased rate of solution which produces toxic side-effects because of its more rapid absorption.

It is clear from the lifetime of a drug outlined above that a knowledge and control of particle size is of importance both for the production of medicines containing particulate solids and in the efficacy of the medicine following administration.

PARTICLE SIZE

Dimensions

When determining the size of a relatively large solid it would be unusual to measure fewer than three dimensions, but if the same solid was broken up and the fragments milled, the resulting fine particles would be irregular with different numbers of faces and it would be difficult or impractical to determine more than a single dimension. For this reason a solid particle is often considered to approximate to a sphere which can then be characterized by determining its diameter. Because measurement is then based on a hypothetical sphere, which represents only an approximation to the true shape of the particle, the dimension is referred to as the ***equivalent diameter*** of the particle.

Equivalent diameters

It is possible to generate more than one sphere which is equivalent to a given irregular particle shape. Figure 10.2 shows the two-dimensional projection of a particle with two different diameters constructed about it.

The projected area diameter is based on a circle of equivalent area to that of the projected image of a solid particle; the projected perimeter diameter is based on a circle having the same perimeter as the particle. Unless the particles are unsymmetrical in three dimensions then these two diameters will be independent of particle orientation. This is not true for Feret's and Martin's diameters (Fig. 10.3), the values of which are dependent on both the orientation and the shape of the particles. These are statistical diameters which are averaged over many different orientations to produce a mean value for each particle diameter. Feret's diameter is determined from the mean distance between two parallel

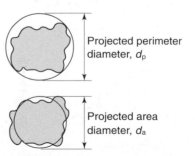

Fig. 10.2 Different equivalent diameters constructed around the same particle.

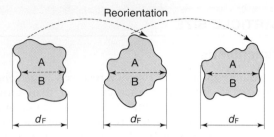

Fig. 10.3 Influence of particle orientation on statistical diameters. The change in Feret's diameter is shown by the distances, d_F; Martins diameter d_M corresponds to the dotted lines in the midpart of each image.

tangents to the projected particle perimeter. Martin's diameter is the mean chord length of the projected particle perimeter, which can be considered as the boundary separating equal particle areas (A and B in Fig. 10.3).

It is also possible to determine particle size based on spheres of, for example, equivalent volume, sedimentation volume, mass or sieve mass of a given particle. In general, the method used to determine particle size dictates the type of equivalent diameter that is measured, although interconversion may be carried out and this is sometimes done automatically as part of the size analysis.

Particle size distribution

A particle population which consists of spheres or equivalent spheres with uniform dimensions is monosized and its characteristics can be described by a single diameter or equivalent diameter.

However, it is unusual for particles to be completely monosized: most powders contain particles with a large number of different equivalent diameters. In order to be able to define a size distribution or compare the characteristics of two or more powders consisting of particles with many different diameters, the size distribution can be broken down

into different size ranges, which can be presented in the form of a histogram plotted from data such as that in Table 10.1. Such a histogram presents an interpretation of the particle size distribution and enables the percentage of particles having a given equivalent diameter to be determined. A histogram representation allows different particle size distributions to be compared; for example, the size distribution shown in Fig. 10.4(b) contains a larger proportion of fine particles than the powder in Fig. 10.4(a) in which the particles are ***normally distributed***. The peak frequency value, known as the ***mode***, separates the ***normal curve*** into two identical halves, because the size distribution is fully symmetrical.

Not all particle populations are characterized by symmetrical normal size distributions and the frequency distributions of such populations exhibit skewness (Fig. 10.4(b)). A frequency curve with an elongated tail towards higher size ranges is ***positively skewed*** (Fig. 10.4(b)); the reverse case exhibits ***negative skewness***. These skewed distributions can sometimes be normalized by replotting the equivalent particle diameters using a logarithmic scale, and are thus usually referred to as log normal distributions.

In some size distributions more than one mode occurs: Figure 10.4(c) shows bimodal frequency distribution for a powder which has been subjected to milling. Some of the coarser particles from the unmilled population remain unbroken and produce a mode towards the highest particle size, whereas the fractured particles have a new mode which appears lower down the size range.

An alternative to the histogram representation of a particle size distribution is obtained by sequentially adding the percent frequency values as shown in Table 10.2 to produce a cumulative percent frequency distribution. If the addition sequence begins with the coarsest particles, the values obtained will be cumulative percent frequency undersize; the

Fig. 10.4 Frequency distribution curves corresponding to (a) a normal distribution, (b) a positively skewed distribution and (c) a bimodal distribution.

reverse case produces a cumulative percent oversize. Figure 10.5 shows two cumulative percent frequency distributions. Once again it is possible to compare two or more particle populations using the cumulation distribution representation. For example, the size distribution in Fig. 10.5(a) shows that this powder has a larger range or spread of equivalent diameters than the powder represented in Figure 10.5(b). The particle diameter corresponds to the point that separates the cumulative frequency curve into two equal halves, above and below which 50% of the particles lie (point *a* in Fig. 10.5(a)). Just as the median divides a symmetrical cumulative size distribution curve into two equal halves, so the lower and upper quartile points at 25% and 75% divide the upper and lower ranges of a symmetrical curve into equal parts (points *b* and *c*, respectively, in Fig. 10.5(a)).

Statistics to summarize data

Although it is possible to describe particle size distributions qualitatively it is always more satisfactory to compare particle size data quantitatively. This is made possible by summarizing the distributions using statistical methods.

In order to quantify the degree of skewness of a particle population, the interquartile coefficient of skewness (IQCS) can be determined as follows:

$$IQCS = \frac{(c-a)-(a-b)}{(c-a)+(a-b)} \qquad (10.4)$$

where *a* is the median diameter and *b* and *c* are the lower and upper quartile points (Fig. 10.5).

The IQCS can take any value between −1 and +1. If the IQCS is zero then the size distribution is practically symmetrical between the quartile points. To ensure unambiguity in interpreting values for IQCS a large number of size intervals are required.

Fig. 10.5 Cumulative frequency distribution curves. Point *a* corresponds to the median diameter; *b* is the lower quartile point and *c* is the upper quartile point.

To quantify the degree of symmetry of a particle size distribution a property known as **kurtosis** can be determined. The symmetry of a distribution is based on a comparison of the height or thickness of the tails and the 'sharpness' of the peaks with those of a normal distribution. 'Thick'-tailed 'sharp' peaked curves are described as **leptokurtic**, whereas 'thin'-tailed 'blunt' peaked curves are **platykurtic** and the normal distribution is **mesokurtic**.

The coefficient of kurtosis, *k* (Eqn. 10.5), has a value of 0 for a normal curve, a negative value for curves showing platykurtosis and positive values for leptokurtic size distributions:

$$k = \frac{n\Sigma(x-\bar{x})^4}{(\Sigma(x-\bar{x})^2)^2} - 3 \qquad (10.5)$$

where *x* is any particle diameter, $\bar{x}$ is mean particle diameter and *n* is number of particles.

Again, a large number of data points are required to provide an accurate analysis.

The mean of the particle population referred to above in Eqn 10.5, together with the median (Fig. 10.5) and the mode (Fig. 10.4) are all measures

Table 10.1 Frequency distribution data

Equivalent particle diameter (µm)	Number of particles in each diameter range (frequency)	Per cent particles in each diameter range (per cent frequency)
20	100	4.5
40	200	9.1
60	400	18.2
80	800	36.4
100	400	18.2
120	200	9.1
140	100	4.5

Table 10.2 Cumulative frequency distribution data

Equivalent particle diameter (µm)	Per cent frequency (from Table 10.1)	Cumulative per cent frequency Undersize	Oversize
20	4.5	4.5	100
40	9.1	13.6	95.5
60	18.2	31.8	86.4
80	36.4	68.2	68.2
100	18.2	86.4	31.8
120	9.1	95.5	13.6
140	4.5	100	4.5

of central tendency and provide a single value near the middle of the size distribution, which represents a central particle diameter. Whereas the mode and median diameters can be obtained for an incomplete particle size distribution, the mean diameter can only be determined when the size distribution is complete and the upper and lower size limits are known. It is also possible to define and determine the mean in several ways and, for log-normal distributions, a series of relationships known as Hatch–Choate equations link the different mean diameters of a size distribution (Table 10.3).

In a log-normal distribution the frequency, f, of the occurrence of any given particle of equivalent diameter d is given by:

$$f = \frac{\Sigma\, n}{2\pi\, \ln\sigma_g} \cdot \exp\left[-\frac{(\ln d - \ln M)^2}{2\ln^2\sigma_g}\right] \quad (10.6)$$

where M is the geometric mean diameter and σ_g is the geometric standard deviation.

Influence of particle shape

The techniques discussed above for representing particle size distribution are all based on the assumption that particles could be adequately represented by an equivalent circle or sphere. In some cases particles deviate markedly from circularity and sphericity, and the use of a single equivalent diameter measurement may be inappropriate. For example, a powder consisting of monosized fibrous particles would appear to have a wider size distribution according to statistical diameter measurements. However, the use of an equivalent diameter based on projected area would also be

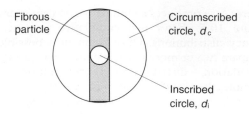

Fig. 10.6 A simple shape factor is shown which can be used to quantify circularity. The ratio of two different diameters (d_i/d_c) is unity for a circle and falls for acicular particles.

misleading. Under such circumstances it may be desirable to return to the concept of characterizing a particle using more than one dimension. Thus, the breadth of the fibre could be obtained using a projected circle inscribed within the fibre (d_i) and the fibre length could be measured using a projected circle circumscribed around the fibre d_c (Fig. 10.6).

The ratio of inscribed circle to circumscribed circle diameters can also be used as a simple shape factor to provide information about the circularity of a particle. The ratio d_i/d_c will be 1 for a circle and diminish as the particle becomes more acicular.

Such comparisons of equivalent diameters determined by different methods offer considerable scope for both particle size and particle shape analysis. For example, measurement of particle size to obtain a projected area diameter, a, and an equivalent volume diameter, v, provides information concerning the surface:volume (a/v) ratio or bulkiness of a group of particles, which can also be useful in interpreting particle size data.

Table 10.3   Hatch–Choate relationships
$\ln d_n = \ln M + 0.5 \ln^2 \sigma_g$
$\ln d_s = \ln M + \ln^2 \sigma_g$
$\ln d_v = \ln M + 1.5 \ln^2 \sigma_g$
$\ln d_{sv} = \ln M + 2.5 \ln^2 \sigma_g k^1$
$\ln M = \ln d_g + 2.5 \ln^2 \sigma_g k^1$
$\ln d_n = \ln d_g - 2.5 \ln^2 \sigma_w$
$\ln d_s = \ln d_g - 2.0 \ln^2 \sigma_w$
$\ln d_v = \ln d_g - 1.5 \ln^2 \sigma_w$
$\ln d_{sv} = \ln d_g - 0.5 \ln^2 \sigma_w$
Key: M, geometric mean diameter by number (see Eqn 10.6); d_n, number mean diameter; d_s, surface mean diameter; d_v volume diameter; d_{sv}, surface volume or surface weighted diameter; d_g, geometric mean diameter by weight

PARTICLE SIZE ANALYSIS METHODS

In order to obtain equivalent diameters with which to interpret the particle size of a powder it is necessary to carry out a size analysis using one or more different methods. Particle-size analysis methods can be divided into different categories based on several different criteria: size range of analysis; wet or dry methods; manual or automatic methods; speed of analysis. A summary of the different methods is presented below based on the salient features of each.

Sieve methods

Equivalent diameter

Sieve diameter, d_s – the particle dimension that passes through a square aperture (length = x) as shown in Figure 10.7.

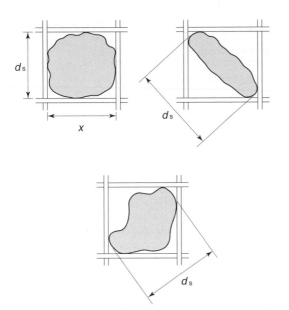

Fig. 10.7 Sieve diameter d_s for various shaped particles

Range of analysis

The International Standards Organization (ISO) sets a lowest sieve diameter of 45 μm and, as powders are usually defined as having a maximum diameter of 1000 μm, this could be considered to be the upper limit. In practice sieves can be obtained for size analysis over a range from 5 to 125 000 μm. These ranges are indicated diagrammatically in Figure 10.8.

Sample preparation and analysis conditions

Sieve analysis is usually carried out using dry powders, although for powders in liquid suspension or which agglomerate during dry sieving a process of wet sieving can be used.

Principle of measurement

Sieve analysis utilizes a woven, punched or electro-formed mesh, often in brass or stainless steel, with known aperture diameters which form a physical

barrier to particles. Most sieve analyses utilize a series, stack or 'nest' of sieves, which has the smallest mesh above a collector tray followed by meshes that become progressively coarser towards the top of the series. A sieve stack usually comprises 6–8 sieves with an aperture progression based on a $\sqrt{2}$ or $2\sqrt{2}$ change in diameter between adjacent sieves. Powder is loaded on to the coarsest sieve of the assembled stack and the nest is subjected to mechanical vibration. After a suitable time the particles are considered to be retained on the sieve mesh with an aperture corresponding to the sieve diameter. Sieving times should not be arbitrary and it is recommended that sieving be continued until less than 0.2% of material passes a given sieve aperture in any 5-minute interval.

Alternative techniques

Another form of sieve analysis, called air-jet sieving, uses individual sieves rather than a complete nest of sieves. Starting with the finest-aperture sieve and progressively removing the undersize particle fraction by sequentially increasing the apertures of each sieve, particles are encouraged to pass through each aperture under the influence of a partial vacuum applied below the sieve mesh. A reverse air jet circulates beneath the sieve mesh, blowing oversize particles away from the mesh to prevent blocking. Air-jet sieving is often more efficient and reproducible than using mechanically vibrated sieve analysis, although with finer particles agglomeration can become a problem.

Automatic methods

Sieve analysis is still largely a non-automated process, although an automated wet sieving technique has been described.

Microscope methods

Equivalent diameters

Projected area diameter, d_a; projected perimeter diameter d_p; Feret's diameter d_F and Martin's diameter d_M (see above).

Range of analysis

This is shown diagrammatically in Figure 10.9.

Sample preparation and analysis conditions

Specimens prepared for light microscopy must be adequately dispersed on a microscope slide to avoid

Fig. 10.8. Range of analysis for sieves

Fig. 10.9. Range of analysis for microscopy.

analysis of agglomerated particles Specimens for scanning electron microscopy are prepared by fixing to aluminium stubs before sputter coating with a film of gold a few nm in thickness. Specimens for transmission electron microscopy are often set in resin, sectioned by microtome and supported on a metal grid before metallic coating.

Principle of measurement

Size analysis by light microscopy is carried out on the two-dimensional images of particles which are generally assumed to be randomly oriented in three dimensions. In many cases this assumption is valid, although for dendrites, fibres or flakes it is very improbable that the particles will orient with their minimum dimensions in the plane of measurement. Under such conditions, size analysis is carried out accepting that they are viewed in their most stable orientation. This will lead to an overestimation of size, as the largest dimensions of the particle will be observed.

The two-dimensional images are analysed according to the desired equivalent diameter. Using a conventional light microscope, particle-size analysis can be carried out using a projection screen with screen distances related to particle dimensions by a previously derived calibration factor using a graticule. A graticule can also be used which has a series of opaque and transparent circles of different diameters, usually in a √2 progression. Particles are compared with the two sets of circles and are sized according to the circle that corresponds most closely to the equivalent particle diameter being measured. The field of view is divided into segments to facilitate measurement of different numbers of particles.

Alternative techniques

Alternative techniques to light microscopy include scanning electron microscopy (SEM) and transmission electron microscopy (TEM). Scanning electron microscopy is particularly appropriate when a three-dimensional particle image is required; in addition, the very much greater depth of field of an SEM compared to a light microscope may also be beneficial. Both SEM and TEM analysis allow the lower particle-sizing limit to be greatly extended over that possible with a light microscope.

Automatic methods

Semiautomatic methods of microscope analysis use some form of precalibrated variable distance to split particles into different size ranges. One technique, called a particle comparator, utilizes a variable diameter light spot projected on to a photomicrograph or electron photomicrograph of a particle under analysis. The variable iris controlling the light spot diameter is linked electronically to a series of counter memories, each corresponding to a different size range (Fig. 10.10). Alteration of the iris diameter causes the particle count to be directed into the appropriate counter memory following activation of a switch by the operator.

A second technique uses a double-prism arrangement mounted in place of the light microscope eyepiece. The image from the prisms is usually displayed on a video monitor. The double-prism arrangement allows light to pass through to the monitor unaltered, where the usual single particle image is pro-

Fig. 10.10 Particle comparator.

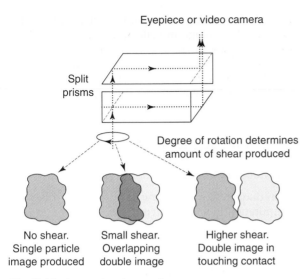

Eyepiece or video camera

Split prisms

Degree of rotation determines amount of shear produced

No shear. Single particle image produced

Small shear. Overlapping double image

Higher shear. Double image in touching contact

Fig. 10.11 Image-shearing eyepiece.

duced. When the prisms are sheared against one another a double image of each particle is produced and the separation of the split images corresponds to the degree of shear between the prisms (Fig. 10.11). Particle-size analysis can be carried out by shearing the prisms until the two images of a single particle make touching contact. The prism shearing mechanism is linked to a precalibrated micrometer scale from which the equivalent diameter can be read directly. Alternatively, a complete size distribution can be obtained more quickly by subjecting the prisms to a sequentially increased and decreased shear distance between two preset levels corresponding to a known size range. All particles whose images separate and overlap sequentially under a given shear range are considered to fall in this size range, and are counted by operating a switch which activates the appropriate counter memory. Particles whose images do not overlap in either shear sequence are undersize and particles whose images do not separate in either shear mode are oversize and will be counted in a higher size range.

Although semiautomatic size analysis methods remove some of the objectivity and fatigue associated with manual microscopic analysis, fully automatic size analysis has the advantage of being more objective, very much faster, and also enables a much wider variety of size and shape parameters to be processed.

Automatic microscopy is usually associated with microprocessor-controlled manipulation of an analogue signal derived from some form of video monitor used to image particles directly from a light microscope or from photomicrographs of particles.

Alternatively, the signal from an electron microscope can in some cases be processed directly without an intermediate video imaging system.

Automatic microscopy allows both image analysis and image processing to be carried out.

Electrical stream sensing zone method (Coulter counter)

Equivalent diameter

Volume diameter, d_v.

Range of analysis

This is shown in Figure 10.12

Sample preparation and analysis conditions

Powder samples are dispersed in an electrolyte to form a very dilute suspension, which is usually subjected to ultrasonic agitation for a period to break up any particle agglomerates. A dispersant may also be added to aid particle deagglomeration.

Principle of measurement

The particle suspension is drawn through an aperture (Fig. 10.13) accurately drilled through a sapphire crystal set into the wall of a hollow glass tube. Electrodes situated on either side of the aperture and surrounded by an electrolyte solution, monitor the change in electrical signal that occurs when a particle

Electrical stream sensing zone method

0.001 0.01 0.1 1 10 100 1000

Particle diameter (μm)

Fig. 10.12 Range of analysis for electrical stream sensing zone method.

Particle in orifice

Orifice tube wall

Fig. 10.13 Particle passing through the measuring aperture of an electrical stream sensing zone apparatus.

momentarily occupies the orifice and displaces its own volume of electrolyte. The volume of suspension drawn through the orifice is determined by the suction potential created by a mercury thread rebalancing in a convoluted U-tube (Fig. 10.14). The volume of electrolyte fluid which is displaced in the orifice by the presence of a particle causes a change in electrical resistance between the electrodes that is proportional to the volume of the particle. The change in resistance is converted into a voltage pulse which is amplified and processed electronically. Pulses falling within precalibrated limits or thresholds are used to split the particle size distribution into many different size ranges. In order to carry out size analysis over a wide diameter range it will be necessary to change the orifice diameter used, to prevent coarser particles blocking a small-diameter orifice. Conversely, finer particles in a large-diameter orifice will cause too small a relative change in volume to be accurately quantified.

Alternative techniques

Since the Coulter principle was first described there have been some modifications to the basic method such as use of alternative orifice designs and hydrodynamic focusing, but in general the particle detection technique remains the same.

Another type of stream sensing analyser utilizes the attenuation of a light beam by particles drawn through the sensing zone. Some instruments of this type use the change in reflectance, whereas others use the change in transmittance of light. It is also possible to use ultrasonic waves generated and monitored by a piezoelectric crystal at the base of a flowthrough tube containing particles in fluid suspension.

Laser light scattering methods

Equivalent diameters

Area diameter, d_a, volume diameter d_v following computation in some instruments.

Range of analysis

This is shown in Figure 10.15.

Sample preparation and analysis conditions

Depending on the type of measurement to be carried out and the instrument used, particles can be presented either in liquid or in air suspension.

Principles of measurement

Both the large-particle and small-particle analysers are based on the interaction of laser light with particles.

Fig. 10.14 Diagram of electrical stream sensing zone apparatus.

Fig. 10.15   Range of analysis for laser light scattering methods.

Fig. 10.17   Schematic diagram of laser diffraction pattern particle sizer.

Fraunhofer diffraction   For particles that are much larger than the wavelength of light, any interaction with particles causes light to be scattered in a forward direction with only a small change in angle. This phenomenon is known as Fraunhofer diffraction, and produces light intensity patterns that occur at regular angular intervals and are proportional to the particle diameter producing the scatter (Fig. 10.16). The composite diffraction pattern produced by different diameter particles may be considered to be the sum of all the individual patterns produced by each particle in the size distribution.

Light emitted by a helium–neon laser is incident on the sample of particles and diffraction occurs. In some cases the scattered light is focused by a lens directly on to a photodetector, which converts the signals into an equivalent area diameter. In other cases the scattered light is directed by a lens on to a rotating filter, which is used to convert equivalent area diameters into volume diameters which are quantified by final focusing on to a photodetector using a second lens. The light flux signals occurring on the photodetector are converted into electrical current, which is digitized and processed into size distribution data using a microprocessor (Fig. 10.17).

Small particle sizes can be analysed based on light diffraction or by photon correlation spectroscopy.

In the former case Fraunhofer diffraction theory is still useful for the particle fraction that is significantly larger than the wavelength of laser light. As particles approach the dimension of the wavelength of the light, some light is still scattered in the forward direction, according to Mie scatter theory, but there is also some side scatter at different wavelengths and polarizations. Use of the Mie theory requires a knowledge of the refractive index of the sample material for calculation of particle size distributions.

Photon-correlation spectroscopy   In the case of photon-correlation spectroscopy (PCS) the principle of Brownian motion is used to measure particle size. Brownian motion is the random movement of a small particle or macromolecule caused by collisions with the smaller molecules of the suspending fluid. It is independent of external variations except viscosity of fluid and temperature, and as it randomizes particle orientations any effects of particle shape are minimized. Brownian motion is independent of the suspending medium, and although increasing the viscosity does slow down the motion, the amplitude of the movements is unaltered. Because the suspended small particles are always in a state of motion, they undergo diffusion. Diffusion is governed by the mean free path of a molecule or particle, which is the average distance of travel before diversion by collision with another molecule. PCS analyses the constantly changing patterns of laser light scattered or diffracted by particles in Brownian motion and monitors the rate of change of scattered light during diffusion.

Particle movement during Brownian diffusion, D, is a three-dimensional random walk where the mean distance travelled, $\bar{x}$, does not increase

Fig. 10.16   Diffraction pattern intensity distribution.

linearly with time, t, but according to the following relationship:

$$\bar{x} = \sqrt{Dt}$$

A basic property of molecular kinetics is that each particle or macromolecule has the same average thermal or kinetic energy, E, regardless of mass, size or shape:

$$E = kT$$

where k is Boltzmann's constant and T is absolute temperature (Kelvin).

Thus at $T = 0$ K, molecules possess zero kinetic energy and therefore do not move. E can also be equated with the driving force, F, of particle motion:

$$F = \frac{E}{x}$$

At equilibrium

$$F = F_D$$

where F_D is the drag force resisting particle motion. According to Stokes' theory, discussed below,

$$F_D = 3\pi d_h \cdot \eta \cdot v_{st} \qquad (10.7)$$

where d_h is the hydrodynamic diameter, v_{st} the Stokes velocity of the particle and η the fluid viscosity, i.e.

$$E = F\bar{x} = 3\pi d_h \cdot \eta \cdot v_{st}$$

but

$$\bar{x}^2 = Dt$$

and

$$v_{st} = \bar{x}/t$$

Substituting, $E = 3\pi d_h \cdot \eta \cdot D$

Since $E = kt$,

$$D = \frac{kT \times 10^7}{3\pi \eta d_n}$$

or

$$D = \frac{1.38 \times 10^{-12}\ T}{3\pi\ \eta\ d}\ \mathrm{m^2 s^{-1}} \qquad (10.8)$$

Equation 10.8 is known as the Stokes–Einstein equation and is the basis for calculation of particle diameters using photon-correlation spectroscopy.

Alternative techniques

There is a wide variety of different instruments based on laser Doppler anemometry or velocimetry, and diffraction measurements. The instruments vary according to their ability to characterize different particle-size ranges, produce complete size distributions, measure both solid and liquid particles, and

determine molecular weights, diffusion coefficients, zeta potential or electrophoretic mobility.

Automatic methods

Most of the instruments based on laser light scattering produce a full particle-size analysis automatically. The data are often presented in graphical and tabular form, but in some instruments only a mean diameter is produced.

Sedimentation methods

Equivalent diameters

d_{fd}, frictional drag diameter, a sphere having an equivalent drag force to a particle of the same diameter in the same fluid at the same velocity; d_{st}, Stokes diameter, the diameter of a particle measured during sedimentation at constant rate in laminar flow conditions.

Range of analysis

This is represented in Figure 10.18.

Sample preparation and analysis conditions

Particle-size distributions can be determined by examining the powder as it sediments out. In cases where the powder is not uniformly dispersed in a fluid it can be introduced as a thin layer on the surface of the liquid. If the powder is hydrophobic it may be necessary to add a dispersing agent to aid wetting. In cases where the powder is soluble in water it will be necessary to use non-aqueous liquids, or carry out the analysis in a gas.

Principles of measurement

Techniques of size analysis by sedimentation can be divided into two main categories according to the method of measurement used. One type is based on

Fig. 10.18   Range of analysis for sedimentation methods.

measurement of particles in a retention zone; a second type uses a non-retention measurement zone.

An example of a non-retention zone measurement method is known as the pipette method. In this method, known volumes of suspension are drawn off and the concentration differences are measured with respect to time.

One of the most popular of the pipette methods was that developed by Andreasen and Lundberg and commonly called the Andreasen pipette (Fig. 10.19). The Andreasen fixed-position pipette consists of a 200 mm graduated cylinder which can hold about 500 mL of suspension fluid. A pipette is located centrally in the cylinder and is held in position by a ground-glass stopper so that its tip coincides with the zero level. A three-way tap allows fluid to be drawn into a 10 mL reservoir, which can then be emptied into a beaker or centrifuge tube. The amount of powder can be determined by weight following drying or centrifuging; alternatively, chemical analysis of the particles can be carried out. The largest size present in each sample is then calculated from Stokes' equation. Stokes' law is an expression of the drag factor in a fluid and is linked to the flow conditions characterized by a Reynolds number. Drag is one of three forces acting on a particle sedimenting in a gravitational field. A drag force, F_d, acts upwards, as does a buoyancy force, F_b; a third force is gravity, F_g, which acts as the driving force of sedimentation. At the constant terminal velocity, which is rapidly achieved by sedimenting particles, the drag force becomes synonymous with particle motion. Thus for a sphere of diameter d and density ρ_s, falling in a fluid of density ρ_f, the equation of motion is:

$$F_d = \frac{\pi}{6}(\rho_s - \rho_f)F_g \cdot d^3$$

Three-way tap

10 ml sampling reservoir

Upper set limit

Pipette

Lower set limit

Fig. 10.19 Diagram of Andreasen pipette.

According to Stokes (Eqn. 10.7):

$$F_d = 3\pi d \eta v_{st}$$

where v_{st} is the Stokes terminal velocity, i.e. sedimentation rate. That is,

$$v_{st} = \frac{(\rho_s - \rho_f)F_g d^2}{18\eta} \qquad (10.9)$$

as $v_{st} = h/t$ where h is sedimentation height or distance and t is sedimentation time. By rearrangement, Stokes' equation is obtained:

$$d_{st} = \frac{18\eta h}{(\rho_s - \rho_f)F_g t} \qquad (10.10)$$

Stokes' equation for determining particle diameters is based on the following assumptions: near-spherical particles; motion equivalent to that in a fluid of infinite length; terminal velocity conditions; low settling velocity so that inertia is negligible; large particle size relative to fluid molecular size, so that diffusion is negligible; no particle aggregation; laminar flow conditions, characterized by particle Reynolds numbers ($\rho u d_{particle}/\eta$) of less than approximately 0.2.

The second type of sedimentation size analysis, using retention zone methods, also uses Stokes' law to quantify particle size. One of the most common retention zone methods uses a sedimentation balance. In this method the amount of sedimented particles falling on to a balance pan suspended in the fluid is recorded. The continual increase in weight of sediment is recorded with respect to time.

Alternative techniques

One of the limitations of gravitational sedimentation is that below a diameter of approximately 5 μm particle settling becomes prolonged and is subject to interference from convection, diffusion and Brownian motion. These effects can be minimized by increasing the driving force of sedimentation by replacing gravitational forces with a larger centrifugal force. Once again, sedimentation can be monitored by retention or non-retention methods, although the Stokes equation requires modification because particles are subjected to different forces according to their distance from the axis of rotation. To minimize the effect of distance on the sedimenting force, a two-layer fluid system can be used. A small quantity of concentrated suspension is introduced on to the surface of a bulk sedimentation liquid known as spin fluid. Using this technique of disc centrifugation, all particles of the same size are

Table 10.4 Summary of particle size analysis instrument characteristics

Analysis method		Sample measurement environment				Size data			Approximate size range (μm)				Initial cost	
		Gas	Aqueous liquid	Non-aqueous liquid	Replica	Other functions	Rapid analysis	printout available	0.001–10	1–10	10–100	100–1000	High	Low
Sieve		✓	✓	✓							✓	✓		✓
Microscope Light	Manual	✓	✓	✓						✓	✓	✓		✓✓
	Semi-automatic	✓	✓	✓						✓	✓	✓		
	Automatic	✓	✓	✓						✓	✓	✓	✓✓	
Electron					✓	✓	✓	✓	✓	✓			✓	
Electrical stream sensing zone			✓				✓	✓		✓	✓		✓	
Laser light scattering	Diffraction	✓✓	✓✓	✓✓		✓✓	✓✓	✓✓	✓	✓✓	✓✓	✓✓	✓✓✓	
	Doppler anemometry										✓	✓	✓	
Sedimentation	Gravitational	✓	✓	✓			✓	✓	✓	✓	✓			✓
	Centrifugal		✓	✓			✗✓✗	✗✓✗	✓	✓			✓	

in the same position in the centrifugal field and hence move with the same velocity.

Automatic methods

In general, gravity sedimentation methods tend to be less automated than those using centrifugal forces. However, an adaptation of a retention zone gravity sedimentation method is known as a Micromerograph and measures sedimentation of particles in a gas rather than a fluid. The advantages of this method are that sizing is carried out relatively rapidly and the analysis is virtually automatic.

SELECTION OF A PARTICLE SIZE ANALYSIS METHOD

The selection of a particle size analysis method may be constrained by the instruments already available in a laboratory, but wherever possible the limitations on the choice of method should be governed by the properties of the powder particles and the type of size information required. For example, size analysis over a very wide range of particle diameters may preclude the use of a gravity sedimentation method; alternatively, size analysis of aerosol particles would probably not be carried out using an electric sensing zone method. As a general guide it is often most appropriate to determine the particle size distribution of a powder in an environment that most closely resembles the conditions in which the powder will be processed or handled. There are many different factors influencing the selection of an analysis method: these are summarized in Table 10.4 and may be used together with information from a preliminary microscopic analysis and any other known physical properties of the powder, such as solubility, density, cohesivity, in addition to analysis requirements such as speed of measurement, particle size data processing or the physical separation of different particle-size powders for subsequent processing.

BIBLIOGRAPHY

Allen, T. (1981) *Particle Size Measurement*, 3rd edn, Chapman and Hall, London and New York.

Barnett, M.I. and Nystrom, C. (1982) Coulter counters and microscopes for the measurement of particles in the sieve range. *Pharm. Tech.*, **6** (Mar), 49–50.

Kay, B.H. (1981) *Direct Characterization of Fine Particles*, John Wiley & Sons, New York and Chichester.

11

Particle-size reduction

John Staniforth

Objectives of size reduction

The significance of particle size has been discussed in Chapter 10 and some of the reasons for carrying out a size-reduction operation will already have been noted. In addition, the function of size reduction may be to aid efficient processing of solid particles by facilitating powder mixing or the production of suspensions. There are also some special functions of size reduction, such as exposing cells prior to extraction or reducing the bulk volume of a material to improve transportation efficiency.

INFLUENCE OF MATERIAL PROPERTIES ON SIZE REDUCTION

Crack propagation and toughness

Size reduction or comminution is carried out by a process of crack propagation, whereby localized stresses produce strains in the particles which are large enough to cause bond rupture and thus propagate the crack. In general, cracks are propagated through regions of a material that possess the most flaws or discontinuities, and is related to the strain energy in specific regions according to Griffith's theory. The stress in a material is concentrated at the tip of a crack and the stress multiplier can be calculated from an equation developed by Inglis:

$$\sigma_K = 1 + 2\left(\frac{L}{2r}\right) \qquad (11.1)$$

where σ_K is the multiplier of the mean stress in a material around a crack, L is the length of the crack and r is the radius of curvature of the cracks tip. For a simple geometric figure such as a circular discontinuity $L = 2r$ and the stress multiplier σ_K will have a value of 3. In the case of the thin disc-shaped crack shown in cross-section in Figure 11.1, the crack was

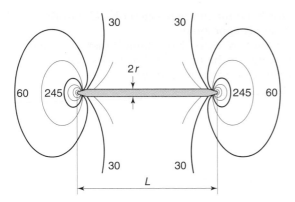

Fig. 11.1 Stress concentrations at the edges of a disc-shaped crack; *r* is the radius of curvature of the crack tip; *L* is the crack length.

considered to have occurred at molecular level between atomic surfaces separated by a distance of 2×10^{-10} m for a crack 3 μm long, which gives a stress multiplier of approximately 245. The stress concentration diminishes towards the mean stress according to the distance from the crack tip (Fig. 11.1). Once a crack is initiated the crack tip propagates at a velocity approaching 40% of the speed of sound in the solid. This crack propagation is so rapid that excess energy from strain relaxation is dissipated through the material and concentrates at other discontinuities, where new cracks are propagated. Thus a cascade effect occurs and an almost instantaneous brittle fracture occurs.

Not all materials exhibit this type of brittle behaviour and can resist fracture at much larger stresses. This occurs because these tougher materials can undergo plastic flow, which allows strain energy relaxation without crack propagation. When plastic flow occurs, atoms or molecules slip over one another and this process of deformation requires energy. Brittle materials can also exhibit plastic flow and Irwin and Orowan suggested a modification of Griffiths' crack theory to take this into account; the new relationship has a fracture stress which varies inversely with the square root of crack length:

$$\sigma = \frac{Ep}{C} \qquad (11.2)$$

where *Ep* is the energy required to form unit area of double surface.

It can therefore be seen that the ease of comminution depends on the brittleness or plasticity of the material and their relationship with crack initiation and propagation.

Surface hardness

In addition to the toughness of the material described above, size reduction may also be influenced by surface hardness. The hardness of a material can be described by its position in a scale devised by a German mineralogist called Mohs. Mohs' scale is a table of materials, at the top of which is diamond with Mohs hardness >7, which has a surface so hard that it can scratch anything below it; at the bottom of the table with Mohs hardness <3 is talc, which is soft enough to be scratched by anything above it.

A more quantitative measurement of surface hardness was devised by Brinell; such determinations of hardness may prove useful as a guide to the ease with which size reduction can be carried out: in general, harder materials are more difficult to comminute and can lead to abrasive wear of metal mill parts, which then cause product contamination. Conversely, materials with a large elastic component, such as rubber, are extremely soft yet difficult to size reduce.

Materials such as rubber which are soft under ambient conditions, waxy substances such as stearic acid which soften when heated, and 'sticky' materials such as gums are capable of absorbing large amounts of energy through elastic and plastic deformation without crack initiation and propagation. This type of polymeric material, which resists comminution at ambient or elevated temperatures, can be more easily size reduced by lowering the temperature below the glass transition point of the material. When this is carried out the material undergoes a transition from plastic to brittle behaviour and crack propagation is facilitated.

Other factors that influence the process of size reduction include the moisture content of the feed material. In general, a moisture content below 5% is suitable for dry grinding and greater than 50% if wet grinding is to be carried out.

Energy requirements of size reduction process

Only a very small amount of the energy put into a comminution operation actually effects size reduction. This has been estimated to be as little as 2% of the total energy consumption, the remainder being lost in many ways, including elastic deformation of particles, plastic deformation of particles without fracture, deformation to initiate cracks that cause fracture, deformation of metal machine parts, interparticle friction, particle–machine wall friction, heat, sound and vibration.

A number of hypotheses and theories have been proposed in an attempt to relate energy input to the degree of size reduction produced. Rittinger's hypothesis is usually interpreted according to the energy, E, used in a size-reduction process, which is proportional to the new surface area produced, S_n, or:

$$E = \kappa_R (S_n - S_i) \qquad (11.3)$$

where S_i is the initial surface area and κ_R is Rittinger's constant of energy per unit area.

Kick's theory states that the energy used in deforming or fracturing a set of particles of equivalent shape is proportional to the ratio of the change in size, or:

$$E = \kappa_K \log \frac{d_i}{d_n} \qquad (11.4)$$

where κ_K is Kick's constant of energy per unit mass, d_i is the initial particle diameter and d_n the new particle diameter.

Bond's theory states that the energy used in crack propagation is proportional to the new crack length produced, which is often related to the change in particle dimensions according to the following equation:

$$E = 2\kappa_B \left(\frac{1}{d_n} - \frac{1}{d_i} \right) \qquad (11.5)$$

κ_B is known as Bond's work index and represents the variation in material properties and size-reduction methods with dimensions of energy per unit mass.

Walker proposed a generalized differential form of the energy–size relationship which can be shown to link the theories of Rittinger and Kick, and in some cases that of Bond:

$$\partial E = -\kappa \frac{\partial d}{d^n} \qquad (11.6)$$

where d is a size function that can be characterized by an integrated mean size or by a weight function, n is an exponent – when $n = 1$ for particles defined by a weight function, integration of Walker's equation corresponds to a Kick-type theory; when $n = 2$ a Rittinger-type solution results; and when $n = 3/2$ Bond's theory is given.

When designing a milling process for a given particle, the most appropriate energy relationship will be required in order to calculate energy consumptions. It has been considered that the most appropriate values for n are 1 for coarse particles > 1 μm where Kick-type behaviour occurs, and 2 for Rittinger-type milling of particles <1 μm. The third value of $n = 3/2$ is the average of these two extremes and indicates a possible solution where neither Kick's nor Rittinger's theory is appropriate.

Other workers have found that n cannot be assumed to be constant, but varies according to a particle size function, so that:

$$n = f(d)$$

or

$$E = -\kappa \frac{d}{d^{f(d)}} \qquad (11.7)$$

As the particle size increases $f(d)$ tends to 1, and as the size reduces $f(d)$ tends to 2.

INFLUENCE OF SIZE REDUCTION ON SIZE DISTRIBUTION

In Chapter 10, several different size distributions were discussed and these were based on either a normal or a log-normal distribution of particle sizes. During a size-reduction process the particles of feed material will be broken down and particles in different size ranges undergo different amounts of breakage. This uneven milling leads to a change in the size distribution, which is superimposed on the general movement of the normal or log-normal curve towards smaller particle diameters. Changes in size distributions that occur as milling proceeds were demonstrated experimentally by Heywood, who showed that an initial normal particle size distribution was transformed through a size-reduced bimodal population into a much finer powder with a positively skewed, leptokurtic particle population (Fig. 11.2) as milling continued. The initial, approximately normal, size distribution was transformed into a size-reduced bimodal population through

Fig. 11.2 Changes in particle size distributions with increased milling time.

Fig. 11.3 Transformation of approximate normal particle size distribution into finer bimodal population following milling.

Fig. 11.4 Transformation of a fine bimodal particle population into a finer unimodal distribution following prolonged milling.

differences in the fracture behaviour of coarse and fine particles (Fig. 11.3). If milling is continued a unimodal population reappears, as the energy input is not great enough to cause further fracture of the finest particle fraction (Fig. 11.4). The lower particle-size limit of a milling operation is dependent on the energy input and on material properties. Below particle diameters of approximately 5 μm, interactive forces generally predominate over comminution stresses which are distributed over increasing surface areas, and particle agglomeration then opposes particle fracture and size reduction ceases. In some cases particle agglomeration occurs to such a degree that subsequent milling actually causes size enlargement.

SIZE REDUCTION METHODS

There are many different types of size reduction techniques but the milling equipment used can be classified according to the principal method employed. Examples of each type will be given and the approximate size-reduction range provided, although it should be remembered that the extent of size reduction is always related to milling time.

Cutting methods

Size reduction range

This is indicated in Figure 11.5.

Principle of operation

A cutter mill (Fig. 11.6) consists of a series of knives attached to a horizontal rotor which act against a series of stationary knives attached to the mill casing. During milling, size reduction occurs by fracture of particles between the two sets of knives, which have a clearance of a few millimetres. A screen is fitted in the base of the mill casing and acts to retain material in the mill until a sufficient degree of size reduction has been effected.

The high shear rates present in cutter mills are useful in producing a coarse degree of size reduction of dried granulations prior to tableting and of fibrous crude drugs such as roots, peels or barks prior to extraction.

Fig. 11.5 Size reduction range for cutting methods.

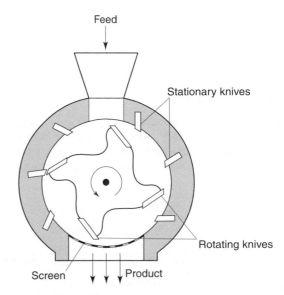

Fig. 11.6 Cutter mill.

169

Compression methods

Size reduction range

These are indicated in Figure 11.7.

Principle of operation

Size reduction by compression can be carried out on a small scale using a mortar and pestle. End-runner and edge-runner mills are mechanized forms of mortar and pestle-type compression comminution (Fig. 11.7). In the end-runner mill a weighted pestle is turned by the friction of material passing beneath it as the mortar rotates under power; the edge-runner mill has the pestle equivalent mounted horizontally and rotating against a bed of powder, so that size reduction occurs by attrition as well as compression. Such techniques are now rarely used in pharmaceutical production.

Alternative techniques

Another form of compression mill uses two cylindrical rolls mounted horizontally and rotated about their long axes. In roller mills, one of the rolls is driven directly while the second is rotated by friction as material is drawn through the gap between the rolls. This form of roller mill should not be confused with the type used for milling ointments, where both rolls are driven but at different speeds, so that size reduction occurs by attrition.

Impact methods

Size reduction range

These are shown in Figure 11.8.

Principle of operation

Size reduction by impact is carried out using a hammer mill (Fig. 11.9). Hammer mills consist of a series of four or more hammers, hinged on a central shaft which is enclosed within a rigid metal case.

Fig. 11.7 Size reduction range for compression methods.

Fig. 11.8 Size reduction range for impact methods.

During milling the hammers swing out radially from the rotating central shaft. The angular velocity of the hammers produces strain rates up to 80 s^{-1}, which are so high that most particles undergo brittle fracture. As size reduction continues the inertia of particles hitting the hammers reduces markedly and subsequent fracture is less probable, so that hammer mills tend to produce powders with narrow size distributions. Particles are retained within the mill by a screen, which allows only adequately comminuted particles to pass through. Particles passing through a given mesh can be much finer than the mesh apertures, as particles are carried around the mill by the hammers and approach the mesh tangentially. For this reason square, rectangular or herringbone slots are often used. According to the purpose of the operation, the hammers may be square-faced, tapered to a cutting edge or have a stepped form.

Alternative techniques

An alternative to hammer milling which produces size reduction is vibration milling (Fig. 11.10). Vibration mills are filled to approximately 80% total volume with porcelain or steel balls. During milling the whole body of the mill is vibrated and size reduction occurs by repeated impaction. Comminuted particles fall through a screen at the base of the mill.

Fig. 11.9 Hammer mill.

Fig. 11.10 Vibration mill.

The efficiency of vibratory milling is greater than that for conventional ball milling described below.

Attrition methods

Size reduction range

This is indicated in Figure 11.11.

Principle of operation

Roller mills use the principle of attrition to produce size reduction of solids in suspensions, pastes or ointments. Two or three porcelain or metal rolls are mounted horizontally with an adjustable gap, which can be as small as 20 μm. The rollers rotate at different speeds so that the material is sheared as it passes through the gap and is transferred from the slower to the faster roll, from which it is removed by means of a scraper.

Combined impact and attrition methods

Size reduction range

This is indicated in Figure 11.12.

Principle of operation

A ball mill is an example of a comminution method which produces size reduction by both impact and

Fig. 11.11 Size reduction range for attrition methods.

Fig. 11.12 Size reduction range for combined impact and attrition methods.

attrition of particles. Ball mills consist of a hollow cylinder mounted such that it can be rotated on its horizontal longitudinal axis (Fig. 11.13). Cylinder diameters can be greater than 3 m, although much smaller sizes are used pharmaceutically. The cylinder contains balls that occupy 30–50% of the total volume, ball size being dependent on feed and mill size; for example, a mill 1 m in diameter might contain balls with a diameter of 75 mm. Mills usually contain balls with many different diameters owing to self-attrition, and this helps to improve the product as the large balls tend to break down the coarse feed materials and the smaller balls help to form the fine product by reducing void spaces between balls.

The amount of material in a mill is of considerable importance: too much feed produces a cushioning effect and too little causes loss of efficiency and abrasive wear of the mill parts. The factor of greatest importance in the operation of the ball mill is the speed of rotation. At low angular velocities (Fig. 11.13(a)) the balls move with the drum until the force due to gravity exceeds the frictional force of the bed on the drum, and the balls then slide back *en masse* to the base of the drum. This sequence is repeated, producing very little relative movement of balls so that size reduction is minimal. At high angular velocities (Fig. 11.13(b)) the balls are thrown out on to the mill wall by centrifugal force and no size reduction occurs. At about two-thirds of the critical angular velocity where centrifuging occurs (Fig. 11.13(c)), a cascading action is produced. Balls are lifted on the rising side of the drum until their dynamic angle of repose is exceeded. At this point they fall or roll back to the base of the drum in a cascade across the diameter of the mill. By this means, the maximum size reduction occurs by impact of the particles with the balls and by attrition. The optimum rate of rotation is dependent on mill diameter but is usually of the order of 0.5 s^{-1}.

Alternative techniques

Fluid energy milling is another form of size-reduction method which acts by particle impaction and

171

Fig. 11.13   Ball mill in operation, showing correct cascade action.

attrition. A typical form of fluid energy or jet mill is shown in Fig. 11.14. This type of mill or 'micronizer' consists of a hollow toroid which has a diameter of 20–200 mm, depending on the height of the loop, which may be up to 2 m. A fluid, usually air, is injected as a high-pressure jet through nozzles at the bottom of the loop. The high velocity of the air gives rise to zones of turbulence into which solid particles are fed. The high kinetic energy of the air causes the particles to impact **with other particles** with sufficient momentum for fracture to occur. Turbulence ensures that the level of particle–particle collisions is high enough to produce substantial size reduction by impact and some attrition. A particle-

size classifier is incorporated in the system so that particles are retained in the toroid until sufficiently fine and remain entrained in the air stream that is exhausted from the mill.

Other types of fluid energy mill replace the turbulence zone technique with horizontally opposed air jets through which the feed material is forced; alternatively, a single air jet is used to feed particles directly on to a target plate, where impaction causes fracture.

In addition to ball mills and fluid energy mills, there are other methods of comminution that act by producing particle impact and attrition. These include pin mills, in which two discs with closely spaced pins rotate against one another at high speeds (Fig. 11.15). Particle-size reduction occurs by impaction with the pins and by attrition between pins as the particles travel outwards under the influence of centrifugal force.

SELECTION OF PARTICLE SIZE-REDUCTION METHOD

Different mills give differing products from the same starting material; for example, particle shape may vary according to whether size reduction occurs as a

Fig. 11.14   Fluid energy mill.

Fig. 11.15   Pin mill.

Table 11.1   Selection of size reduction mills according to particle properties and product size required

Mohs' 'hardness'	Tough	Sticky	Abrasive	Friable
(a) Fine powder product (< 50 μm)				
1–3 (soft)	Ball, vibration (under liquid nitrogen)	Ball, vibration		Ball, vibration, pin, fluid energy
3–5 (intermediate)	Ball, vibration			Ball, vibration, fluid energy
5–10 (hard)	Ball, vibration, fluid energy		Ball, vibration, fluid energy	
(b) Coarse powder product (50–1000 μm)				
1–3 (soft)	Ball, vibration, roller, pin, hammer, cutter (all under liquid nitrogen)	Ball, pin		Ball, roller, pin, hammer, vibration
3–5 (intermediate)	Ball, roller, pin, hammer, vibration, cutter			Ball, roller, pin, vibration, hammer
5–10 (hard)	Ball, vibration		Ball vibration, roller	
(c) Very coarse product (> 1000 μm)				
1–3 (soft)	Cutter, edge runner	Roller, edge runner, hammer		Roller, edge runner, hammer
3–5 (intermediate)	Edge runner, roller, hammer			Roller, hammer
5–10 (hard)	Roller		Roller	

result of impact or attrition. In addition, the proportion of fines in the product may vary, so that other properties of the powder will be altered.

The use to which a powder will be put usually controls the degree of size reduction, but in some cases the precise particle size required is not critical. In these circumstances the important factor is that, in general, the cost of size reduction increases as particle size decreases, so that it is economically undesirable to mill particles to a finer degree than necessary. Once the particle size required has been established the selection of mills capable of producing that size may be modified from a knowledge of the particle properties, such as hardness, toughness etc. The influences of various process and material variables on selection of a size reduction method are summarized in Table 11.1.

BIBLIOGRAPHY

Austin, L.G. and Brame, K. (1983) A comparison of the bond method for sizing wet tumbling ball mills with a size-mass balance simulation model. *Powder Technol.*, **34**, 261–274.

Lachman, L., Lieberman, H.A. and Kanig, J.L. In *Theory and Practice of Industrial Pharmacy*, Lea and Febiger, Philadelphia.

Mecham, W.J., Jardine, L.J., Reedy, G.T. and Steindler, M.J. (1983) General statistical description of the fracture particulates formed by mechanical impacts of brittle materials. *Ind. Engng. Chem. Fund.*, **22**, 384–391.

Paramanathan, B.K. and Bridgwater, J. (1983) Attrition of solids, Pts I & II. *Chem. Engng Sci.*, **38**, 197–224.

Voller, V.R. (1983) A note on energy-size reduction relationships in communition. *Powder Technol.*, **36**, 281–286.

Wheeler, D.A. (1982) Size reduction. *Processing* (Dec), 55–58.

12

Particle-size separation

John Staniforth

OBJECTIVES OF SIZE SEPARATION

The significance of particle size and the principles involved in differentiating a powder into fractions of known particle size and in reducing particle dimensions have been considered in Chapters 10 and 11. In this chapter the methods by which size separation can be achieved will be discussed, together with the standards that are applied to powders for pharmaceutical purposes.

Solid separation is a process by which powder particles are removed from gases or liquids, and has two main aims:

1. to recover valuable products or byproducts;
2. to prevent environmental pollution.

Although size separation uses many similar techniques to those used in solid separation it has a different aim, which is to classify powders into separate particle size ranges or 'cuts', and is therefore linked to particle-size analysis. However, an important difference exists between size separation, and size analysis: following size separation, powder in a given particle size range is available for separate handling or subsequent processing. This means that whereas a particle-size analysis method such as microscopy would be of no use as a size-separation method, the principle of sieving could be used for both purposes.

Size-separation efficiency

The efficiency with which a powder can be separated into different particle size ranges is related to the particle and fluid properties and the separation method used. Separation efficiency is determined as a function of the effectiveness of a given process in separating particles into oversize and undersize fractions.

In a continuous size-separation process the production of oversize and undersize powder streams from a single feed stream can be represented by the following equation:

$$f_F = f_o + f_u \qquad (12.1)$$

where f_F, f_o and f_u are functions of the mass flow rates of the feed material, oversize product and undersize product streams, respectively. If the separation process is 100% efficient then all oversize material will end up in the oversize product stream and all undersize material will end up in the undersize product stream. Invariably, industrial separation processes produce an incomplete size separation, so that some undersize material is retained in the oversize stream and some oversize material may find its way into the undersize stream.

Considering the oversize material, a given powder feed stream will contain a certain proportion of true oversize material, δ_F; the oversize product stream will contain a fraction, δ_o, of true oversize particles, and the undersize stream will contain a fraction, δ_u, of true oversize material (Fig. 12.1)

The efficiency of the separation of oversize material, can be determined by considering the relationship between mass flow rates of feed and product streams and the fractional contributions of true size grade in the streams. For example, the efficiency E_o

of a size-separation process for oversize material in the oversize stream is given by:

$$E_o = \frac{f_o \cdot \delta_o}{f_F \delta_F} \qquad (12.2)$$

and the separation efficiency for undersize material in the undersize stream is given by:

$$E_u = \frac{f_u(1-\delta_u)}{f_F(1-\delta_F)} \qquad (12.3)$$

The total efficiency, E_t, for the whole size separation process is given by:

$$E_t = E_u \cdot E_o \qquad (12.4)$$

Separation efficiency determination can be applied to each stage of a complete size classification and is often referred to as 'grade efficiency'. In some cases a knowledge of grade efficiency is insufficient, for example where a precise particle size cut is required. A 'sharpness index' can be used to quantify the sharpness of cut-off in a given size range. A sharpness index, S, can be determined in several different ways, for example by taking the percentage values from a grade efficiency curve at the 25 and 75% levels (L):

$$S_{25/75} = \frac{L_{25}}{L_{75}} \qquad (12.5)$$

or at other percentile points, such as the 10 and 90% levels:

$$S_{10/90} = \frac{L_{10}}{L_{90}} \qquad (12.6)$$

SIZE-SEPARATION METHODS

Size separation by sieving

Separation ranges

These are shown in Figure 12.2.

Sieve aperture diameter, d_A

f_F

f_o

f_u

(a)

δ_o

δ_f

δ_u

d_A
Sieve diameter

(b)

Fig. 12.1 Size separation efficiency determination. (a) Separation operation; (b) size distributions of feed, oversize and undersize material to obtain values for δ_o, δ_f and δ_u.

Maximum available range

Pharmacopoeial range

0.1   1   10   100   1000   10 000
Particle diameter (μm)

Fig. 12.2 Separation range for sieving.

175

Principles of operation

The principles of sieving in order to achieve particle-size analysis were described in Chapter 10. There may be some differences in the methods used to achieve size separation rather than size analysis. The wire mesh used for the construction of British Standard sieves should be of uniform circular cross-section, and the sieve mesh should possess adequate strength to avoid distortion and should also be resistant to chemical action with any of the material to be sifted. Commonly used materials for the construction of test sieve meshes for size analysis are brass and bronze, but it is probably more common and more suitable to use stainless steel meshes in process sieves used for size separation.

The use of sieving in size separation usually requires processing of larger volumes of powder than are commonly found in size analysis operations. For this reason, the sieves used for size separation are often larger in area than those used for size analysis. There are several techniques for encouraging particles to separate into their appropriate size fractions efficiently. In dry sieving processes these are based on mechanical disturbances of the powder bed and include the following.

Agitation methods Size separation is achieved by electrically induced oscillation or mechanically induced vibration of the sieve meshes, or alternatively by gyration, in which sieves are fitted to a flexible mounting which is connected to an out-of-balance flywheel. The eccentric rotation of the flywheel imparts a rotary movement of small amplitude and high intensity to the sieve and causes the particles to spin, thereby continuously changing their orientation and increasing their potential to pass through a given sieve aperture. The output from gyratory sieves is often considerably greater than that obtained using oscillation or vibration methods.

Agitation methods can be made continuous by inclination of the sieve and the use of separate outlets for the undersize and oversize powder streams.

Brushing methods A brush is used to reorientate particles on the surface of a sieve and prevent apertures becoming blocked. A single brush can be rotated about the midpoint of a circular sieve or, for large-scale processing, a horizontal cylindrical sieve, is employed, with a spiral brush rotating about its longitudinal axis.

Centrifugal methods Particles are thrown outwards on to a vertical cylindrical sieve under the action of a high-speed rotor inside the cylinder. The current of air created by the rotor movement also assists in sieving, especially where very fine powders are being processed.

Wet sieving can also be used to effect size separation and is generally more efficient than dry sieving methods.

Standards for powders based on sieving

Standards for powders used pharmaceutically are provided in pharmacopoeiae, which indicate that 'the degree of coarseness or fineness of a powder is differentiated and expressed by reference to the nominal mesh aperture size of the sieves used'. Five grades of powder are specified and defined in, for example, the BP and these are shown in Table 12.1.

Some pharmacopoeiae define another size fraction, known as 'ultrafine powder'. In this case it is required that the maximum diameter of at least 90% of the particles must be no greater than 5 μm and that none of the particles should have diameters greater than 50 μm.

It should be noted that the term 'sieve number' has been used as a method of quantifying particle size in Pharmacopoeia. However, various monographs use the term differently and in order to avoid confusion it is always advisable to refer to particle sizes according to the appropriate equivalent diameters expressed in micrometres.

Size separation by fluid classification

Sedimentation methods

Separation ranges

These are shown in Figure 12.3.

Table 12.1 Powder grades specified in British Pharmacopoeia		
Description of grade of powder	Coarsest sieve diameter (μm)	Sieve diameter through which no more than 40% of powder must pass (μm)
Coarse	1700	355
Moderately coarse	710	250
Moderately fine	355	180
Fine	180	—
Very fine	125	—

Fig. 12.3 Separation range for sedimentation techniques.

Principles of operation

The principles of liquid classification using sedimentation methods are described in Chapter 10. Size separation by sedimentation utilizes the differences in settling velocities of particles with different diameters, and these can be related according to Stokes' equations, see Eqns 10.9 and 10.10.

One of the simplest forms of sedimentation classification uses a chamber containing a suspension of solid particles in a liquid, which is usually water. After predetermined times, particles less than a given diameter can be recovered using a pipette placed a fixed distance below the surface of the liquid. Size fractions can be collected continuously using a pump mechanism in place of a pipette.

Alternatively, a single separation can be carried out simply by removing the upper layer of suspension fluid after the desired time. Disadvantages of these simple methods are that they are batch processes and discrete particle fractions cannot be collected, as samples contain every particle diameter up to the limiting diameter and not specific size ranges.

Alternative techniques

An alternative technique is to use a continuous settling chamber so that particles in suspension enter a shallow container, as shown in Figure 12.4. The particle Reynolds' number of the system ($\rho u d_{particle}/\eta$) is below approximately 0.2, so that streamline flow occurs. Particles entering at the top of the chamber are acted upon by a driving force which can be divided into two components: a horizontal component of particle velocity which is equal to the suspension fluid velocity, and a vertical component which corresponds to Stokes' settling velocity and is different for each particle size. These two components are constant for each particle, so that the settling path will be given by a curve whose slope depends on particle diameter. The coarsest particles will have the steepest settling paths and will sediment closest to the inlet, whereas the finest particles with low Stokes velocity component will have the shallowest settling paths and will sediment furthest from the fluid suspension feed stream (Fig. 12.4). Particles separated into the different hopper-type discharge points can be removed continuously.

Very fine particles will not sediment efficiently under the influence of gravity due to Brownian diffusion. In order to increase the driving force of sedimentation, centrifugal methods can be used to separate particles of different sizes in the submicrometre region.

Simple cylindrical centrifuges can be used to remove single size cuts from a fluid stream, but where separation is required over a wider number of size ranges multiple-chamber centrifuges can be used. In this type of centrifuge there are a number of spinning cylinders of different diameters set inside a closed chamber (Fig. 12.5). Fine particles in liquid suspension are fed in through the top of the inner or central cylinder. As in continuous-flow gravity sedimentation the particles are acted on by two component forces, one due to fluid flow and, in this case, one due to centrifugal force. The coarsest particles will have the shallowest trajectories and will be carried to the walls of the inner cylinder (Fig. 12.6); all other particles remain entrained in the liquid and flow out at the base of the cylinder and via a baffle or weir into the top of the next cylinder out, where the centrifugal force is higher. This sequence continues so that only the finest particles reach the outermost spinning cylinder.

Another type of sedimentation method is based on separation from particles dispersed in air and is known as ***mechanical air classification***.

Standards for powders based on sedimentation separation

There are no general pharmacopoeial standards for size separation based on sedimentation. However, tests are applied to Light Kaolin in order to limit the coarseness of the powder. Light Kaolin must consist of fine particles, partially because it is used in the

Fig. 12.4 Continuous settling chamber showing vectors of particle movement for different sizes.

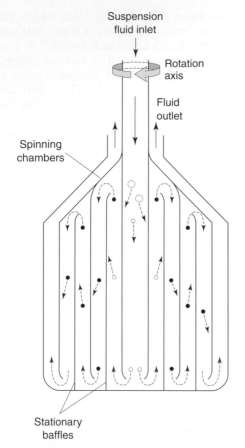

Fig. 12.5 Multiple-chamber separation centrifuge.

Fig. 12.6 Influence of particle size on particle movement in multiple-chamber centrifuge.

form of a suspension, but also because it is used therapeutically for its adsorptive properties, which are dependent on surface area and therefore on particle size. The test described in the *British Pharmacopoeia*,

for example, uses an adaptation of the batch sedimentation chamber method described above.

Elutriation methods

Separation ranges

These are shown in Figure 12.7.

Principles of operation

In sedimentation methods the fluid is stationary and the separation of particles of various sizes depends solely on particle velocity. Therefore, the division of particles into size fractions depends on the **time** of sedimentation.

Elutriation is a technique in which the fluid flows in an opposite direction to the sedimentation movement, so that in gravitational elutriators particles move vertically downwards while the fluid travels vertically upwards. If the upward velocity of the fluid is less than the settling velocity of the particle, sedimentation occurs and the particle moves downwards against the flow of fluid. Conversely, if the settling velocity of the particle is less than the upward fluid velocity, the particle moves upwards with the fluid flow. Therefore, in the case of elutriation, particles are divided into different size fractions depending on the **velocity** of the fluid. Elutriation and sedimentation are compared in Figure 12.8, where the arrows are vectors, that is, they show the direction and magnitude of particle movement. This figure indicates that if particles are suspended in a fluid moving up a column, there will be a clear cut into two fractions of particle size. In practice this does not occur, as there is a distribution of velocities across the tube in which a fluid is flowing – the highest velocity is found in the centre of the tube and the lowest velocity at the tube walls. Therefore, the size of particles that will be separated depends on their position in the tube, the largest particles in the centre, the smallest towards the outside. In practice, particles can be seen to rise

Fig. 12.7 Separation ranges for elutriation methods.

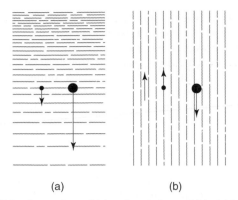

Fig. 12.8 Comparison of (a) sedimentation and (b) elutriation

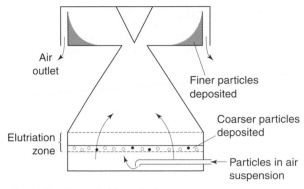

Fig. 12.10 Upward airflow elutriator.

with the fluid and then to move outwards to the tube wall, where the velocity is lower and they start to fall. A separation into two size fraction occurs, but the size cut will not be clearly defined. Assessing the sharpness of size cuts is discussed in more detail above.

Separation of powders into several size fractions can be effected by using a number of elutriators connected in series. The suspension is fed into the bottom of the narrowest column, overflowing from the top into the bottom of the next widest column and so on (Fig. 12.9). Because the mass flow remains the same, as the column diameter increases the fluid velocity decreases and therefore particles of decreasing size will be separated.

Alternative techniques

Air may be used as the counterflow fluid in place of water for elutriation of soluble particles into differ-

ent size ranges. There are several types of air elutriator, which differ according to the airflow patterns used. An example of an upward airflow elutriator is shown in Figure 12.10. Particles are held on a supporting mesh through which air is drawn. Classification occurs within a very short distance of the mesh and any particles remaining entrained in the air stream are accelerated to a collecting chamber by passage through a conical section of tube. Further separation of any fine particles still entrained in the air flow may be carried out subsequently using different air velocities.

It may be required to separate finer particles than can be achieved using gravitational elutriation, and in these cases counterflow centrifugal methods can be used. Particles in air suspension are fed into a rotating hollow torus at high speed, tangential to the outer wall. Coarse particles move outwards to the walls against the inwardly spiralling air flow, which leaves the elutriator in the centre. The desired particle size fraction can be separated by selecting the appropriate airflow rate and rotor speed.

Cyclone methods

Separation range

This is shown in Figure 12.11.

Fig. 12.9 Multistage elutriator. Particle outlets 1 to 4 collect fractions of decreasing particle size.

Fig. 12.11 Separation ranges for cyclone methods.

Principle of operation

Cyclone separation can take the form of a centrifugal elutriation process similar to the one described above, or a centrifugal sedimentation process in which particles sediment out of a helical gas or liquid stream.

Probably the most common type of cyclone used to separate particles from fluid streams is the reverse-flow cyclone (Fig. 12.12). In this system, particles in air or liquid suspension are often introduced tangentially into the cylindrical upper section of the cyclone, where the relatively high fluid velocity produces a vortex that throws solid particles out on to the walls of the cyclone. The particles are forced down the conical section of the cyclone under the influence of the fluid flow – gravity interactions are a relatively insignificant mechanism in this process. At the tip of the conical section the vortex of fluid is above the critical velocity at which it can escape through the narrow outlet and forms an inner vortex which travels back up the cyclone and out through a central outlet or vortex finder. Coarser particles separate from the fluid stream and fall out of the cyclone through the dust outlet, whereas finer particles remain entrained in the fluid stream and leave the cyclone through the vortex finder. In some cases, the outer vortex is allowed to enter a collector connected to the base of the cyclone, but the coarser particles still appear to separate from the fluid stream and remain in the collector. A series of cyclones having different flow rates or different dimensions could be used to separate a powder into different particle-size ranges.

SELECTION OF A SIZE SEPARATION PROCESS

Selection of a specific size separation may be limited by pharmacopoeial requirements, but for general cases the most efficient method should be selected based on particle properties. Of these, size is particularly important as each separation method is most efficient over a particular size range, as indicated in the foregoing text.

Particles that have just undergone size reduction will already be in suspension in a fluid, whether air or water, and can be separated quickly by elutriation or cyclone separation methods, so that oversize material can be returned to the mill.

Alternatively, many powders used pharmaceutically are soluble in water and size separation may have to be restricted to air classification methods.

Fig. 12.12 Reverse-flow cyclone separation.

Fluid outlet

Vortex finder

Particles in suspension

Outer vortex of particles and fluid

Inner vortex of fluid

Particle outlet

BIBLIOGRAPHY

Allen, T. (1981) *Particle Size Measurement*, 3rd edn, Chapman and Hall, London and New York.
Svarovsky, L. (1981) *Solid Gas Separation (Handbook of Powder Technology*, Vol. 3), Elsevier, Amsterdam.

13
Mixing

Andrew Twitchell

MIXING PRINCIPLES

The importance of mixing

There are very few pharmaceutical products that contain only one component. In the vast majority of cases several ingredients are needed so that the required dosage form functions as required. If, for example, a pharmaceutical company wishes to produce a tablet dosage form containing a drug which is active at a dose of 1 mg, other components (e.g. diluents, binders, disintegrants and lubricants) will be needed both to enable the product to be manufactured and for it to be handled by the patient. Whenever a product contains more than one component a mixing or blending stage will be required in the manufacturing process. This may be in order to ensure an even distribution of the active component(s), to ensure an even appearance, or to ensure that the dosage form releases the drug at the correct site and at the desired rate. The unit operation of mixing is therefore involved at some stage in the production of practically every pharmaceutical preparation. This is illustrated below by the list of products that invariably utilize mixing processes of some kind:

- Tablets, capsules, sachets and dry powder inhalers – mixtures of solid particles (powder mixing)
- Linctuses – mixtures of miscible liquids
- Emulsions and creams – mixtures of immiscible liquids
- Pastes and suspensions – dispersions of solid particles.

This chapter considers the objectives of the mixing operation, how mixing occurs, and the ways in which a satisfactory mix can be produced and maintained.

Definition and objectives of mixing

Mixing may be defined as a unit operation that aims to treat two or more components, initially in an unmixed or partially mixed state, so that each unit (particle, molecule etc.) of the components lies as nearly as possible in contact with a unit of each of the other components.

If this is achieved it produces a theoretical 'ideal' situation, i.e. a **perfect mix**. As will be shown, however, this situation is not normally practicable, is frequently unnecessary and is sometimes undesirable (e.g. mixing of lubricants with tablet granules; see Chapter 27).

How closely it is attempted to approach the 'ideal' situation depends on the product being manufactured and the objective of the mixing operation. For example, if a small amount of a potent drug is being mixed in a powder then the degree of mixing must be of a high order to ensure a consistent dose. Similarly, when dispersing two immiscible liquids, or dispersing a solid in a liquid, a well-mixed product is required to ensure product stability. In the case of mixing lubricants during tablet production, however, there is a danger of overmixing and the subsequent production of a weak tablet with an increased disintegration time.

Types of mixtures

Mixtures may be categorized into three types.

Positive mixtures

Positive mixtures are formed from materials such as gases or miscible liquids which mix **spontaneously** and **irreversibly** by diffusion, and tend to approach a perfect mix. There is no input of energy required with positive mixtures if the time available for mixing is unlimited, although it will shorten the time required to obtain the desired degree of mixing. In general materials that mix by positive mixing present no problems during product manufacture.

Negative mixtures

With negative mixtures the components will tend to separate out. If this occurs quickly, then energy must be continuously input to keep the components adequately dispersed, e.g. with a suspension formulation, such as calamine lotion, where there is a dispersion of solids in a liquid of low viscosity. With other negative mixtures the components tend to separate very slowly, e.g. emulsions, creams and viscous suspensions. Negative mixtures are generally more difficult to form and maintain and require a higher degree of mixing efficiency than do positive mixtures.

Neutral mixtures

Neutral mixtures are said to be static in behaviour, i.e. the components have no tendency to mix spontaneously or segregate spontaneously once work has been input to mix them. Examples of this type of mixture include mixed powders, pastes and ointments.

It should be noted that the type of mixture might change during processing. For example, if the viscosity increases the mixture may change from a negative to a neutral mixture. Similarly, if the particle size, degree of wetting or liquid surface tension changes the mixture type may also change.

The mixing process

To discuss the principles of the mixing process, a situation will be considered where there are equal quantities of two powdered components of the same size, shape and density that are required to be mixed, the only difference between them being their colour. This situation will not of course occur practically, but it will serve to simplify the discussion of the mixing process and allow some important considerations to be illustrated with the help of statistical analysis.

If the components are represented by coloured cubes, then a two-dimensional representation of the initial unmixed or completely segregated state can be produced, as shown in Figure 13.1(a).

From the definition of mixing, the ideal situation or '**perfect mix**' in this case would be produced when each particle lay adjacent to a particle of the other component (i.e. each particle lies as closely as possible in contact with a particle of the other component). This is shown in Figure 13.1(b), where it can be seen that the components are as evenly distributed as possible. If this mix were viewed in three dimensions then behind and in front of each grey particle would be a white particle, and vice versa.

Powder mixing, however, is a 'chance' process, and although the situation shown in Figure 13.1(b) could arise, the odds against it are so great that for practical purposes it can be considered impossible. For example, if there are only 200 particles present the chance of a perfect mix occurring is approximately 1 in 10^{60} and is similar to the chance of the situation in Figure 13.1(a) occurring after prolonged mixing. In practice, the best type of mix likely to be obtained will have the components under consideration distributed as indicated in Figure 13.1(c). This is referred to as a **random mix**, which is defined as a mix where the **probability** of selecting a particular type of particle is the **same** at all positions in the mix, and is equal to the **proportion** of such particles in the total mix.

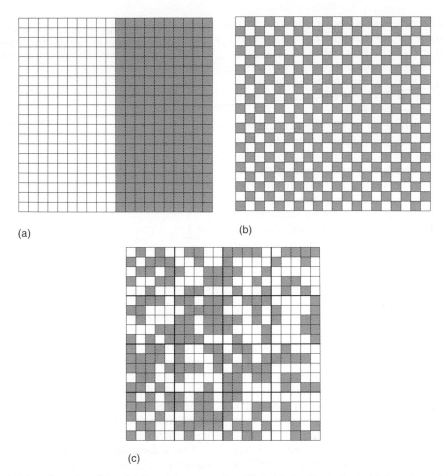

Fig. 13.1 Different states of powder mixing. (a) Complete segregation. (b) An ideal or 'perfect' mix. (c) A random mix.

If any two adjacent particles are selected from the random mix shown:

the chance of picking two grey particles = 1 in 4 (25%)

the chance of picking two white particles = 1 in 4 (25%)

and the chance of picking one of each = 2 in 4 (50%).

If any two adjacent particles are selected from the perfect mix shown, there will always be one grey and one white particle.

Thus if the samples taken from a random mix contain only two particles, then in 25% of cases the sample will contain no white particles and in 25% it will contain no grey particles.

It can be seen that in practice the components will not be perfectly evenly distributed, i.e. there will not be full mixing. However, if an overall view is taken the components can be described as being mixed, as in the total sample (Fig. 13.1c) the amounts of each component are approximately similar (48.8% grey and 51.2% white). If, however, Figure 13.1(c) is con-

sidered as 16 different blocks of 25 particles, then it can be seen that the number of grey particles in the blocks varies from 6 to 19 (i.e. 24–76% of the total number of particles in each block). Careful examination of Figure 13.1(c) shows that as the number of particles in the sample increases then the closer will be the proportion of each component to that which would occur with a perfect mix. This is a very important consideration in powder mixing, and is discussed in more detail in the sections that follow.

Scale of scrutiny

Often a mixing process produces a large 'bulk' of mixture that is subsequently subdivided into individual dose units (e.g. a tablet, capsule or 5 mL spoonful) and it is important that each dosage unit contains the correct amount/concentration of active component(s). It is the weight/volume of the *dosage unit* that dictates how closely the mix must be examined/analysed to ensure it contains the correct dose/concentration. This weight/volume is known as the *scale of scrutiny* and is the amount of material within which the quality of mixing is important. For example, if the unit weight of a tablet is 200 mg then a 200 mg sample from the mix needs to be analysed to see if mixing is adequate; the scale of scrutiny is therefore 200 mg.

The number of *particles* in the scale of scrutiny will depend on the sample weight, particle size and particle density, and will increase as the sample weight increases and the particle size and density decrease. This number should be sufficient to ensure minimal deviation in the required dose in the dosage forms.

Another important factor to consider when carrying out a mixing process is the proportion of the active component in the dosage form/scale of scrutiny. This is illustrated in Figure 13.2 and in Table 13.1, the latter also demonstrating the importance of the number of particles in the scale of scrutiny.

Figure 13.2 shows a random mix containing only 10% grey particles. If the blocks of 25 particles are examined it can be seen that the number of grey particles varies from 0 to 8, or 0–32%. Thus, the number of grey particles as a percentage of the theoretical content varies from 0 to 320%. This is considerably greater than the range of 48–152% when the proportion of grey particles was 0.5 or 50% (Fig. 13.1(c)).

Table 13.1 shows how the content of a minor active constituent (present in a proportion of one part in a 1000, i.e. 0.1%) typically varies with the number of particles in the scale of scrutiny when sampling a random mix. In the example shown, when there are 1000 particles in scale of scrutiny three samples contain no active constituent and two have twice the amount that should be present. With 10 000 particles

Table 13.1 Number of particles of a minor active constituent present in samples taken from a 1:1000 random powder mix with different numbers of particles in the scale of scrutiny

Sample number	Number of particles in scale of scrutiny		
	1000	10 000	100 000
1	1	7	108
2	0	10	91
3	1	15	116
4	2	8	105
5	0	13	84
6	1	10	93
7	1	6	113
8	2	5	92
9	0	12	104
10	1	13	90

The figures in the table are the numbers of particles of the minor constituent in the samples.

in the scale of scrutiny the deviation is reduced, but samples may still deviate from the theoretical content of 10 particles by ±50%. Even with 100 000 particles deviation from the theoretical content may be ±15%, which is unacceptable for a pharmaceutical mixture. The difficulty in mixing potent substances can be appreciated if it is realized that there may only be approximately 75 000 particles of diameter 150 μm in a tablet weighing 200 mg.

The information in Figures 13.1 and 13.2 and Table 13.1 leads to two important conclusions:

1. The lower the proportion of active component present in the mixture the more difficult it is to achieve an acceptably low deviation in active content.
2. The more particles there are present in a unit dose/scale of scrutiny the lower the deviation in content.

One way of reducing the deviation, therefore, would be to increase number of particles in the scale of scrutiny by reducing particle size. This may, however, lead to particle aggregation owing to the increased cohesion that occurs with smaller particles, which in turn may reduce the ease of mixing.

It should be noted that with liquids even very small samples are likely to contain many million 'particles'. Deviation in content is therefore likely to be very small with miscible liquids, even if they are randomly mixed. Diffusion effects in miscible liquids arising from the existence of concentration gradients in an unmixed system mean they tend to approach a perfect mix.

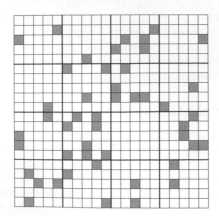

Fig. 13.2 Particle distribution in a representative random mix containing 10% active ingredient.

Mathematical treatment of the mixing process

It must be appreciated that there will always be some variation in the composition of samples taken from a random mix. The aim during formulation and processing is to minimize this variation to acceptable levels by selecting an appropriate scale of scrutiny, particle size and mixing procedure (choice of mixer, rotation speed etc). The following section uses a simplified statistical approach to illustrate some of the factors that influence dose variation within a batch of a dosage form, and demonstrates the difficulties encountered with drugs that are active in low doses (i.e. potent drugs).

Consider the situation where samples are taken from a random mix in which the particles are all of the same size, shape and density. The variation in the proportion of a component in samples taken from the random mix can be calculated from:

$$SD = \sqrt{\frac{p(1-p)}{n}} \qquad (13.1)$$

where SD is the standard deviation in the proportion of the component in the samples (content sample deviation), p is the proportion of the component in the total mix and n is the total number of particles in the sample.

Equation 13.1 shows that as the number of particles present in the sample increases the content standard deviation decreases (i.e. there is less variation in sample content), as illustrated previously by the data in Figure 13.2 and Table 13.1. The situation with respect to the effect of the proportion of the active component in the sample is not as clear from Eqn 13.1. As p is decreased the value of the content standard deviation decreases, which may lead to the incorrect conclusion that it is beneficial to have a low proportion of the active component. A more useful parameter to determine is the percentage coefficient of variation (%CV), which indicates the average deviation as a percentage of the mean amount of active component in the samples. Thus, %CV = (content standard deviation/mean content) × 100. The value of %CV will increase as p decreases, as illustrated below.

Consider the situation where n = 100 000 and p = 0.5. Using Eqn 13.1, it can be calculated that SD = 1.58×10^{-3} and %CV = $(1.58 \times 10^{-3}/0.5) \times 100$ = 0.32%. Thus on average the content will deviate from the mean content by 0.32%, which is an acceptably low value for a pharmaceutical product.

However, if p is reduced to 0.001 and n remains at 100 000 there is a reduction in SD to 9.99×10^{-5}, but the %CV = $(9.99 \times 10^{-5}/0.001) \times 100$ = 10%.

Thus in this latter case the content will deviate from theoretical content on average by 10%, which would be unacceptable for a pharmaceutical product.

It might be considered that the variation in content could be reduced by increasing the sample size (scale of scrutiny), as this would increase the number of particles in each sample. The dose of a drug will, however, be fixed, and any increase in the sample size will cause a reduction in the proportion of the active component. The consequence of increasing the sample size depends on the initial proportion of the active component. If p is relatively high initially, increasing the sample size causes the %CV in content to increase. If p is small, increasing the sample size has little effect. Inserting the appropriate values into Eqn 13.1 can substantiate this.

In a true random mix the content of samples taken from the mix will follow a normal distribution. With a normal distribution, 68.3% of samples will be within ±1 SD of the overall proportion of the component (p), 95.5% will be within ±2 SD of p, and 99.7% of samples will be within ±3 SD of p. For example, if p = 0.5 and the standard deviation in content is 0.02, then for 99.7% of samples the proportion of the component will be between 0.44 and 0.56. In other words, if 1000 samples were analysed, 997 would contain between 44% and 56% of drug (mean = 50%).

A typical specification for a pharmaceutical product is that the active component should not deviate by more than ±5% of the mean or specified content, i.e. the acceptable deviation = $p \times (5/100)$ or $p \times 0.05$. (NB: this is not the same as a standard deviation of 5%.)

If a product contains an active component which makes up half of the weight of the dosage form (p = 0.5) and it is required that the content of 99.7% of samples is within ±5% of p, then the number of particles required in the product can be estimated as described below.

As 99.7% of samples will be within ±3 SD and ±5% of p, then Eqn 13.2 can be used to calculate the standard deviation required:

$$3 \times SD = p \times (\% \text{ acceptable deviation}/100) \qquad (13.2)$$

In this case, $3 \times SD = 0.5 \times 0.05$

so
$$\frac{0.5 \times 0.05}{3} = \sqrt{\frac{p(1-p)}{n}}$$
$$6.94 \times 10^{-5} = 0.5 \ (1 - 0.5)/n$$

and therefore n = 3600.

The above calculation indicates that 3600 particles are required in each sample or dosage form in order to be 99.7% sure that the content is within ±5% of the theoretical amount.

If, however, the product contains a potent drug where $p = 1 \times 10^{-3}$, the number of particles needed to meet the same criteria can be estimated to be 3.6×10^6.

Estimation of particle size required when formulating a dosage form

Using the above information it is possible to estimate the particle size required so that a formulation may meet a desired specification. For example, imagine a tablet weighing 50 mg which contains 50 μg of a potent steroid needs to be produced, and that the product specification requires 99.7% of tablets to contain between 47.5 μg and 52.5 μg of steroid. If the mean particle density of the components is 1.5 g/cm^3 (1500 kg/m^3), what particle size should the steroid and the excipients be?

As there is 50 μg of the steroid in a 50 mg tablet, the proportion of active component (p) is 1×10^{-3}. The specification allows the content to vary by ± 2.5 μg, and so the percentage deviation allowed is $(2.5/50) \times 100 = 5\%$. Under these circumstances the previous section showed that, provided a random mix is achieved, the number of particles required in the tablet is 3.6×10^6. The 50 mg tablet must therefore contain at least 3.6×10^6 particles and each particle must weigh less than $50/3.6 \times 10^6$ mg = 1.39 $\times 10^{-5}$ mg = 1.39×10^{-11} kg. Because the density of a particle is equal to particle mass/particle volume, the volume of each particle must be less than $1.39 \times 10^{-11}/1500$ m^3 = 9.27×10^{-15} m^3.

The volume of a particle (assuming it is spherical) is $4\pi r^3/3$, and so

$$r^3 \text{ must be } <9.27 \times 10^{-15} \times 3/4\pi,$$
$$r^3 < 2.21 \times 10^{-15} \text{ m}^3 \text{ and}$$
$$r < 1.30 \times 10^{-5} \text{ m } (d < 26 \text{ } \mu m).$$

This calculation therefore indicates that in order to meet the product specification, the particle size of the components needs to be of the order of 26 μm. There would therefore be practical difficulties in making this product, as particles of this size tend to become very cohesive, flow poorly (see Chapter 14), and are difficult to mix.

In order to appreciate the effect of changing the scale of scrutiny, it is suggested that the reader calculates what particle size would be required if the tablet weight was increased to 250 mg. It should be remembered that the tablet weight or scale of scrutiny will affect both the number of particles present and the proportion of active component.

In summary, the above calculations illustrate the difficulty of mixing potent (low-dose) substances

and the importance of both the number of particles in the scale of scrutiny and the proportion of the active component.

Evaluation of the degree of mixing

Manufacturers require some means of monitoring a mixing process for a variety of reasons; these could include:

- To indicate the degree/extent of mixing
- To follow a mixing process
- To indicate when sufficient mixing has occurred
- To assess the efficiency of a mixer
- To determine the mixing time required for a particular process.

Many evaluation methods involve the generation of a ***mixing index***, which compares the content standard deviation of samples taken from a mix under investigation (S_{ACT}) with that of samples from a fully random mix (S_R). Comparison with a random mix is made because this is theoretically likely to be the best mix that is practically achievable. The simplest form of a mixing index (M) can be calculated as:

$$M = \frac{S_R}{S_{ACT}} \qquad (13.3)$$

At the start of the mixing process the value of S_{ACT} will be high and that for M will be low. As mixing proceeds S_{ACT} will tend to decrease as the mix approaches a random mix (Fig. 13.3). If the mix becomes random, $S_{ACT} = S_R$ and $M = 1$. There is typically an exponential decrease in S_{ACT} as the mixing time or number of mixer rotations increases, although the shape of the curve will depend on the powder properties and mixer design and use. Other more complicated equations for calculating the mixing index have been used, but all tend to rely on similar principles to those described.

In order to evaluate a mixing process in this way there are two basic requirements. First, a sufficient number of samples which are representative of the mix as a whole must be removed and analysed. A minimum of 10 samples is usually taken, these being removed from different depths into the mixer and from the middle and sides. Samples are often taken with a 'sampling thief', which is a device that can be inserted into the mix and samples withdrawn with minimum disruption to the powder bed. Second, a suitable analytical technique must be available so that the value of S_{ACT} is a true reflection of the variation in content in the samples and not due to variation arising from the method of analysis.

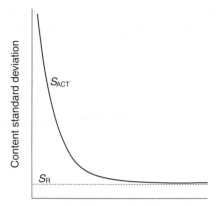

Fig. 13.3 The reduction in content standard deviation as a random mix is approached. S_{ACT} represents the content standard deviation of samples taken from the mix and S_R the standard deviation expected from a random mix.

Fig. 13.4 The reduction in mixing time possible if a random mix is not required. S_{ACT} represents the content standard deviation of samples taken from the mix, S_E the estimated acceptable standard deviation and S_R the standard deviation expected from a random mix.

When mixing formulations where the proportion of active component is high it is possible to achieve an acceptably low variation in content without obtaining a random mix. Thus it may be possible to stop the mixing process before a random mix is achieved and thereby reduce manufacturing costs. Equation 13.2 can be used to generate an estimated acceptable standard deviation value (S_E) that will allow the product to meets its specification. For example, if the proportion of active component present in the formulation is 0.5 and the acceptable variation from the mean content is ±5% for 99.7% of samples, then:

$$S_E = \frac{0.5 \times \left(5/100\right)}{3} = 8.3 \times 10^{-3}$$

Therefore, if when the mix is analysed the content standard deviation in the proportion of the active component is $< 8.3 \times 10^{-3}$ (%CV < 1.67), the product should meet the specification. This approach is illustrated in Figure 13.4.

MECHANISMS OF MIXING AND DEMIXING

Powders

In order that powders may be mixed, the powder particles need to move relative to each other. There are three main mechanisms by which powder mixing occurs, namely *convection*, *shear* and *diffusion*.

Convective mixing arises when there is the transfer of relatively large groups of particles from one part of the powder bed to another, as might occur when a mixer blade or paddle moves through the mix, for example. This type of mixing contributes mainly to the macroscopic mixing of powder mixtures and tends to produce a large degree of mixing fairly quickly (as evidenced by a rapid drop in S_{ACT}). Mixing does not, however, occur *within* the group of particles moving together as a unit, and so in order to achieve a random mix an extended mixing time is required.

Shear mixing occurs when a 'layer' of material moves/flows over another 'layer'. This might be due to the removal of a mass by convective mixing creating an unstable shear/slip plane, which causes the powder bed to collapse. It may also occur in high-shear mixers or tumbling mixers, where the action of the mixer induces velocity gradients within the powder bed and hence 'shearing' of one layer over another.

In order to achieve a true random mix, movement of individual particles is required. This occurs with diffusive mixing.

When a powder bed is forced to move or flow it will 'dilate', i.e. the volume occupied by the bed will increase. This is because the powder particles will become less tightly packed and there is an increase in the air spaces or voids between them. Under these circumstances there is the potential for the particles to fall under gravity, through the voids created. Mixing of individual particles in this way is referred to as diffusive mixing. Diffusive mixing, although having the potential to produce a random mix, generally results in a low rate of mixing.

All three mixing mechanisms are likely to occur in a mixing operation. Which one predominates and the extent to which each occurs will depend on the mixer type, mixing process conditions (mixer load, speed etc.) and the flowability of the powder components.

Liquids

The three main mechanisms by which liquids are mixed are **bulk transport**, **turbulent mixing** and **molecular diffusion**.

Bulk transport is analogous to the convective mixing of powders and involves the movement of a relatively large amount of material from one position in the mix to another, e.g. due to a mixer paddle. It too tends to produce a large degree of mixing fairly quickly, but leaves the liquid within the moving material unmixed.

Turbulent mixing arises from the haphazard movement of molecules when forced to move in a turbulent manner. The constant changes in speed and direction of movement means that induced turbulence is a highly effective mechanism for mixing. Within a turbulent fluid there are, however, small groups of molecules moving together as a unit, referred to as eddies. These eddies tend to reduce in size and eventually break up, being replaced by new eddies. Turbulent mixing alone may therefore leave small unmixed areas within the eddies and in areas near the container surface which will exhibit streamlined flow (see Chapter 4). Mixing of individual molecules in these regions will occur by the third mechanism, which is molecular diffusion (analogous to diffusive mixing in powders). This will occur with miscible fluids wherever a concentration gradient exists and will eventually produce a well-mixed product, although considerable time may be required if this is the only mixing mechanism. In most mixers all three mechanisms will occur, bulk transport and turbulence arising from the movement of a stirrer or mixer paddle set at a suitable speed.

Powder segregation (demixing)

Segregation is the opposite effect to mixing, i.e. components tend to separate out. This is very important in the preparation of pharmaceutical products, because if it occurs, a mix may change from being random to being non-random, or a random mix may never be achieved. Care must be taken to avoid segregation during handling after powders have been mixed, e.g. during transfer to filling machines, or in the hopper of a tablet/capsule/sachet-filling machine.

Segregation will cause an increase in content variation in samples taken from the mix and may cause a batch to fail a uniformity of content test. If segregation of granules occurs in the hopper of a filling machine an unacceptable variation in weight may result.

Segregation arises because powder mixes encountered practically are not composed of mono-sized spherical particles, but contain particles that differ in size, shape and density. These variations mean that particles will tend to behave differently when forced to move and hence, tend to separate. Particles exhibiting similar properties tend to congregate together, giving regions in the powder bed which have a higher concentration of a particular component. Segregation is more likely to occur, or may occur to a greater extent, if the powder bed is subjected to vibration and when the particles have greater flowability.

Particle-size effects

A difference in the particle sizes of components of a formulation is the main cause of segregation in powder mixes in practice. Smaller particles tend to fall through the voids between larger ones and so move to the bottom of the mass. This is known as **percolation segregation**. It may occur in static powder beds if the percolating particles are so small that they can fall into the void spaces between larger particles, but occurs to a greater extent as the bed 'dilates' on being disturbed. Domestically, percolation segregation is often observed in cereal packets or jars of coffee, where the smaller 'particles' congregate towards the bottom of the container.

Percolation can occur whenever a powder bed containing particles of different size is disturbed in such a way that particle rearrangement occurs, e.g. during vibration, stirring or pouring.

During mixing, larger particles will tend to have greater kinetic energy imparted to them (owing to their larger mass) and therefore move greater distances than smaller particles before they come to rest. This may result in the separation of particles of different size, an effect referred to as **trajectory segregation**. This effect, along with percolation segregation, accounts for the occurrence of the larger particles at the edge of a powder heap when it is poured from a container.

During mixing, or when a material is discharged from a container, very small particles ('dust') in a mix may tend to be 'blown' upwards by turbulent air currents as the mass tumbles, and remain suspended in the air. When the mixer is stopped or material discharge is complete, these particles will sediment and subsequently form a layer on top of the coarser particles. This is called *elutriation segregation* and is also referred to as '*dusting out*'.

Particle-density effects

If components are of different density, the more dense material will have a tendency to move downwards even if the particle sizes are similar. Trajectory segregation may also occur with particles of the same size but different densities, owing to their difference in mass. The effect of density on percolation segregation may be potentiated if the more dense particles are also smaller. Alternatively, size and density effects may cancel each other out if the larger particles are more dense. Often materials used in pharmaceutical formulations have similar density values and density effects are not generally too important. An exception to this is in fluidized beds, where density differences are often more serious than particle size differences.

Particle-shape effects

Spherical particles exhibit the greatest flowability and are therefore more easily mixed, but they also segregate more easily than non-spherical particles. Irregularly or needle-shaped particles may become interlocked, reducing the tendency to segregate once mixing has occurred. Non-spherical particles will also have a greater surface area to weight ratio (specific surface area), which will tend to decrease segregation by increasing any cohesive effects (greater contact surface area), but will also increase the likelihood of 'dusting out'.

It should be remembered that the particle size distribution and particle shape may change during processing (owing to attrition, aggregation etc.), and therefore the tendency to segregate may also change.

Non-segregating mixes will improve with continued increases in mixing time, as shown in Figure 13.3. This may not, however, occur for segregating mixes, where there is often an optimum mixing time. This is because the factors causing segregation generally require longer to take effect than the time needed to produce a reasonable degree of mixing. During the initial stages of the process the rate of mixing is greater than the rate of demixing. After a period of time, however, the rate of demixing may predominate until eventually an equilibrium situation will be reached

Fig. 13.5 Possible effect of extended mixing time on the content standard deviation of samples taken from a mix prone to segregation. S_{ACT} represents the content standard deviation of samples taken from the mix, S_E the estimated acceptable standard deviation and S_R the standard deviation expected from a random mix.

where the two effects are balanced. This is illustrated in Figure 13.5, which demonstrates that, if factors exist that might cause segregation, a random mix will not be achieved and there may be both an optimum mixing time and a time range over which an acceptable mix can be produced.

If segregation is a problem with a formulation there are a number of approaches that may be attempted to rectify the situation. These include:

- Selection of particular size fractions (e.g. by sieving to remove fines or lumps) to achieve drug and excipients of the same narrow particle size range;
- Milling of components (size reduction) either to reduce the particle size range (this may need to be followed by a sieving stage to remove fines) or to ensure that all particles are below approximately 30 μm – at which size segregation does not tend to cause serious problems (but may give rise to aggregation);
- Controlled crystallization during production of the drug/excipients to give components of a particular crystal shape or size range;
- Selection of excipients which have a density similar to the active component(s); there is usually a range of excipients that will produce a product with the required properties;
- Granulation of the powder mix (size enlargement) so that large numbers of different particles are evenly distributed in each segregating 'unit'/granule; (see Fig. 25.1).

- Reduce the extent to which the powder mass is subjected to vibration or movement after mixing;
- Use filling machine hoppers designed so that powder residence time is minimized;
- Use equipment where several operations can be carried out without transferring the mix, e.g. a fluidized-bed drier or a high-speed mixer/granulator for mixing and granulating;
- Production of an 'ordered' mix.

This latter technique, which may also be referred to as **adhesive** or **interactive** mixing, is described in greater detail below.

Ordered mixing

It would be expected that a mix comprised of very small and much larger particles would segregate because of the size differences. Sometimes, however, if one powder is sufficiently small (micronized) it may become adsorbed on to the 'active sites' on the surface of a larger 'carrier' particle and exhibit great resistance to being dislodged. This has the effect of minimizing segregation while maintaining good flow properties. It was first noticed during the mixing of micronized sodium bicarbonate with sucrose crystals, when the mixture was found to exhibit minimal segregation. The phenomenon is referred to as ordered mixing, as the particles are not independent of each other and there is a degree of order to the mix. If a carrier particle is removed then some of the adsorbed smaller particles will automatically be removed with it. Ordered mixing has also been used in the production of dry antibiotic formulations to which water is added before use to form a liquid or syrup product. In these cases the antibiotic in fine powder form is blended with, and adsorbed on to, the surface of larger sucrose or sorbitol particles (Nikolakakis and Newton 1989).

Ordered mixing probably occurs to a certain extent in every pharmaceutical powder mix, owing to interactions and cohesive/adhesive forces between constituents. It is most likely to occur when smaller particles exist, as these have a high specific surface area and so the attractive forces holding the particles to the adsorption site are more likely to be greater than the gravitational forces trying to separate the components.

Pharmaceutical mixes are therefore likely to be partly ordered and partly random, the extent of each depending on the component properties. With an ordered mix it may be possible to achieve a degree of mixing which is superior to that of a random mix, which may be beneficial for potent drugs.

Ordered mixing has been shown to be important in direct compression formulations (see Chapter 27) in preventing the segregation of drug from direct compression bases.

Dry powder inhaler formulations also use ordered mixing to deliver drugs to the lungs (see Chapter 31). In this case the drug needs to be in a micronized form in order to reach its site of action. By adsorbing the drug on to larger carrier particles (usually lactose) it is possible to manufacture a product that will provide an even dosage on each inhalation.

Segregation in ordered mixes

Although ordered mixes can reduce or prevent segregation, it may still occur if:

1. **The carrier particles vary in size**. Different-sized particles will have different surface area to weight ratios and will contain different amounts of adsorbed material per unit mass. If the different-sized carrier particles separate (e.g. by percolation segregation), drug-rich areas where the smaller carrier particles congregate may result. This is referred to as **ordered unit segregation**.
2. **There is competition for the active sites on the carrier particle**. If another component competes for sites on the carrier it may displace the original adsorbed material, which may then segregate owing to its small size. This is known as **displacement segregation**, and has been shown to occur under certain circumstances with the addition of the lubricant magnesium stearate to tablet formulations.
3. **There are insufficient carrier particles**. Each carrier particle can only accommodate a certain amount of adsorbed material on its surface. If there is any excess small-sized material that is not adsorbed on to the carrier particles this may quickly separate. This is referred to as **saturation segregation**, and may limit the proportion of the active component that can be used in the formulation.

With an ordered mix particles may be dislodged if the mix is subjected to excessive vibration. The extent to which this occurs depends on the forces of attraction between the components and therefore on how tightly the adsorbed particles are attached to the surface. The orientation of the particles is also important, those protruding from the surface being more likely to be dislodged than those lying parallel to it.

MIXING OF POWDERS

Practical considerations

When mixing formulations where there is a relatively low proportion of active ingredient(s) a more even distribution may be obtained by building up the amount of material in the mixer sequentially. This may be achieved by initially mixing the active component(s) with an approximately equal volume of diluent(s). Further amounts of diluents, equal to the amount of material in the mixer, can then be added and mixed, the process being continued until all material has been added. It may be more appropriate to pre-blend the active component with a diluent in a smaller mixer prior to transferring it to the main mixer in cases where the amount of active ingredient is very small.

Care must be taken to ensure that the volume of powder in the mixer is appropriate, as both over and underfilling may significantly reduce mixing efficiency. In the case of overfilling, for example, sufficient bed dilation may not take place for diffusive mixing to occur to the required extent, or the material may not be able to flow in a way that enables shear mixing to occur satisfactorily. Similarly, underfilling may mean the powder bed does not move in the required manner in the mixer, or that an increased number of mixing operations may be needed for a batch of material.

The mixer used should produce the mixing mechanisms appropriate for the formulation. For example, diffusive mixing is generally preferable for potent drugs, and high shear is needed to break up aggregates of cohesive materials and ensure mixing at a particulate level. The impact or attrition forces generated if too-high shear forces are used may, however, damage fragile material and so produce fines.

The mixer design should be such that it is dust-tight, can be easily cleaned, and the product can be fully discharged. These reduce the risk of cross-contamination between batches and protect the operator from the product.

In order to determine the appropriate mixing time, the process should be checked by removing and analysing representative samples after different mixing intervals. This may also indicate whether segregation is occurring in the mixer, and whether problems occur if the mixing time is extended.

When particles rub past each other as they move within the mixer, static charges will be produced. These tend to result in 'clumping' and a reduction in diffusive mixing, and cause material to adhere to machine or container surfaces. To avoid this, mixers should be suitably earthed to dissipate the static charge and the process should be carried out at a relative humidity greater than approximately 40%.

Powder mixing equipment

Tumbling mixers/blenders

Tumbling mixers are commonly used for the mixing/blending of granules or free-flowing powders. There are many different designs of tumbling mixer, e.g. double-cone mixers, twin-shell mixers, cube mixers, Y-cone mixers and drum mixers, some of which are shown diagrammatically in Figure 13.6. It is now common to use **intermediate bulk containers** (IBCs) both as the mixer bowl and to either feed the hopper of a tablet or capsule machine or as the hopper itself. The shape of an IBC used for this purpose is illustrated in Figure 13.7.

Mixing containers are generally mounted so that they can be rotated about an axis. When operated at the correct speed, the tumbling action indicated in Figure 13.8 is achieved. Shear mixing will occur as a velocity gradient is produced, the top layer moving with the greatest velocity and the velocity decreasing as the distance from the surface increases. When the bed tumbles it dilates, allowing particles to move

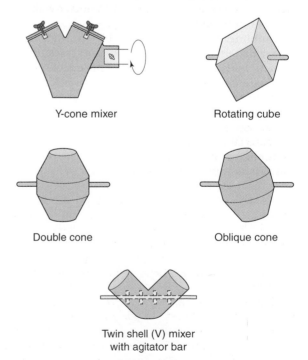

Y-cone mixer   Rotating cube

Double cone   Oblique cone

Twin shell (V) mixer
with agitator bar

Fig. 13.6 Different designs of tumbling mixers.

Fig. 13.7 Typical intermediate bulk container.

downwards under gravity, and so diffusive mixing occurs. Too high a rotation speed will cause the material to be held on the mixer walls by centrifugal force, and too low a speed will generate insufficient bed expansion and little shear mixing. The addition of 'prongs', baffles or rotating bars will also cause convective mixing, for example the V-mixer with agitator bar in Figure 13.6.

Tumbling mixers are available to mix from approximately 50 g, e.g. for laboratory-scale development work, to over 100 kg at a production scale. The material typically occupies about a half to two-thirds of the mixer volume. The rate at which the product is mixed will depend on mixer design and rotation speed, as these influence the movement of the material in the mixer.

Tumbling mixers are good for free-flowing powders/granules but poor for cohesive/poorly flowing powders, because the shear forces generated are usually insufficient to break up any aggregates. Care must also be taken if there are significant differences in particle size present, as segregation is likely to occur. A common use of tumbling mixers is in the blending of lubricants, glidants or external disintegrants with granules prior to tableting.

Tumbling mixers can also be used to produce ordered mixes, although the process is often slow because of the cohesiveness of the adsorbing particles.

The Turbula shaker-mixer (WAB, Switzerland) is a more sophisticated form of tumbling mixer that uses inversional motion in addition to the rotational and translational motion of traditional tumbling mixers. This leads to more efficient mixing and makes it less likely that materials of different sizes and densities will segregate.

High-speed mixer–granulators

In pharmaceutical product manufacture it is often preferable to use one piece of equipment to carry out more than one function. An example of this is the use of a mixer–granulator (one design of which is shown diagrammatically in Figure 13.9). As the name suggests, it can both mix and granulate a product, thereby removing the need to transfer the product between pieces of equipment and so reducing the opportunity for segregation to occur.

The centrally mounted impeller blade at the bottom of the mixer rotates at high speed, throwing the material towards the mixer bowl wall by centrifugal force. The material is then forced upwards before dropping back down towards the centre of the mixer. The particulate movement within the bowl tends to mix the components quickly owing to high shear forces (arising from the high velocity) and the expansion in bed volume that allows diffusive mixing. Once mixed, granulating agent can be added and granules formed in situ using a slower impeller speed and the action of the side-mounted chopper blade. Further details of granule production using this method can be found in Chapter 25.

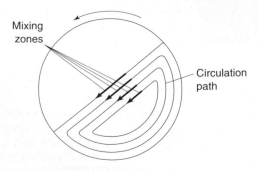

Fig. 13.8 Movement of the powder bed in a tumbling mixer.

Fig. 13.9 Diagrammatic representation of a high-speed mixer–granulator.

Because of the high-speed movement within a mixer–granulator, care must be taken if material fractures easily. This, and the problems associated with overmixing of lubricants, means that this type of mixer is not normally used for blending lubricants.

Fluidized-bed mixers

The main use of fluidized-bed equipment is in the drying of granules (Chapter 26) or the coating of multiparticulates (Chapter 28). Fluidized-bed equipment can, however, be used to mix powders prior to granulation in the same bowl. This is discussed in detail in Chapter 25.

Agitator mixers

This type of mixer depends on the motion of a blade or paddle through the product, and hence the main mixing mechanism is convection. Examples include the ribbon mixer (Fig. 13.10), the planetary mixer (Fig. 13.11) and the Nautamixer (Fig. 13.12). In the first, mixing is achieved by the rotation of helical blades in a hemispherical trough. 'Dead spots' are difficult to eliminate in this type of mixer and the shearing action caused by the movement of the

Fig. 13.12   Nautamixer (courtesy of Nautamixer Ltd).

blades may be insufficient to break up drug aggregates. The mixer does, however, mix poorly flowing material and is less likely to cause segregation than a tumbling mixer. The Nautamixer consists of a conical vessel fitted at the base with a rotating screw, which is fastened to the end of a rotating arm at the upper end. The screw conveys the material to near the top, where it cascades back into the mass. The mixer thus combines convective mixing (as the material is raised by the helical conveyor) and shear and diffusive mixing (as the material cascades downwards).

Scale-up of powder mixing

The extent of mixing achieved at a small laboratory scale during development work may not necessarily be mirrored when the same formulation is mixed at a full production scale, even if the same mixer design is used for both. Often, mixing efficiency and the extent of mixing is improved on scale-up owing to increased shear forces. This is likely to be beneficial in most cases, although when blending lubricants care is needed to avoid overlubrication, which may for example lead to soft tablets and delayed disintegration and dissolution.

Problems associated with a deficiency of some of the components of a formulation, which have been encountered at a production scale but not in development work, have been traced to adsorption of a

Fig. 13.10   Ribbon agitator powder mixer.

Fig. 13.11   Planetary mixer – top view, showing path of paddle.

minor constituents (e.g a drug or colourant) on to the mixer wall or mixing blade.

Drug particle characteristics may also change when the drug is manufactured on a large scale. This may in turn affect the movement of the particles in the mixer or the interaction with other components, and hence the tendency to mix and segregate.

The optimum mixing time and conditions should therefore be established and validated at a production scale, so that the appropriate degree of mixing is obtained without segregation, overlubrication or damage to component particles. Minimum and maximum mixing times that give a satisfactory product should be determined if appropriate, so that the 'robustness' of the mixing process is established.

Fig. 13.13 Propeller mixer with (a) unbaffled tank and (b) baffled tank.

MIXING OF MISCIBLE LIQUIDS AND SUSPENSIONS

Mobile liquids with a low viscosity are easily mixed with each other. Similarly, solid particles are readily suspended in mobile liquids, although the particles are likely to settle rapidly when mixing is discontinued. Viscous liquids are more difficult to stir and mix, but they reduce the sedimentation rate of suspended particles (see Chapter 23).

Propeller mixers

A common arrangement for medium-scale fluid mixing is a propeller-type stirrer which may be clamped to the edge of a vessel. A propeller has angled blades, which cause the fluid to circulate in both an axial and a radial direction. An off-centre mounting discourages the formation of a vortex, which may occur when the stirrer is mounted centrally. A vortex forms when the centrifugal force imparted to the liquid by the propeller blades causes it to back up around the sides of the vessel and create a depression at the shaft. As the speed of rotation is increased air may be sucked into the fluid by the formation of a vortex; this can cause frothing and possible oxidation (Figure 13.13(a)). Another method of suppressing a vortex is to fit vertical baffles into the vessel. These divert the rotating fluid from its circular path into the centre of the vessel, where the vortex would otherwise form (Figure 13.13(b)).

The ratio of the diameter of a propeller stirrer to that of the vessel is commonly 1:10–1:20, and it typically operates at speeds of 1–20 rps. The propeller stirrer depends for its action on a satisfactory axial and radial flow pattern, which will not occur if the fluid is sufficiently viscous. There must be a fast flow of fluid towards the propeller, which can only occur if the fluid is mobile.

Turbine mixers

A turbine mixer may be used for more viscous fluids and a typical construction is shown in Figure 13.14. The impeller has four flat blades surrounded by perforated inner and outer diffuser rings. The rotating impeller draws the liquid into the mixer 'head' and forces the liquid through the perforations with considerable radial velocity, sufficient to overcome the viscous drag of the bulk of the fluid. One drawback is the absence of an axial component, but a different head with the perforations pointing upwards can be fitted if this is desired.

As the liquid is forced through the small orifices of the diffuser rings at high velocity large shear forces are produced. When mixing immiscible liquids, if the orifices are sufficiently small and velocity sufficiently high, the shear forces produced enable the generation of droplets of the dispersed phase which are small enough to produce stable dispersions (water-in-oil or oil-in-water). Turbine mixers of this type are therefore often fitted to vessels used for the large-scale production of emulsions and creams.

Turbine-type mixes will not cope with liquids of very high viscosity, as the material will not be drawn into the mixer head. These liquids are best treated as semisolids and handled in the same equipment as used for such materials.

Fig. 13.14 Turbine mixer.

Inline mixers

As an alternative to mixing fluids in batches in vessels, mobile miscible components may be fed through an 'inline' mixer designed to create turbulence in a flowing fluid stream. In this case a continuous mixing process is possible.

MIXING OF SEMISOLIDS

The problems that arise during the mixing of semi-solids (ointments and pastes) stem from the fact that, unlike powders and liquids, semisolids will not flow easily. Material that finds its way to 'dead' spots will remain there. For this reason, suitable mixers must have rotating elements with narrow clearances between themselves and the mixing vessel wall and they must produce a high degree of shear mixing, as diffusion and convection cannot occur.

Mixers for semisolids

Planetary mixers

This type of mixer is commonly found in the domestic kitchen (e.g. Kenwood-type mixers) and larger machines which operate on the same principle are used in industry.

The mixing blade is set off-centre and is carried on a rotating arm. It therefore travels round the circumference of the mixing bowl while simultaneously rotating around its own axis (as Fig. 13.11). This is therefore a double rotation similar to that of a spinning planet rotating around the sun – hence the name.

A small clearance between the vessel and the paddle gives shear, but 'scraping down' several times is necessary to mix the contents well as some materials are forced to the top of the bowl. Planetary mixers are also sometimes used to mix powders, particularly if a wet mass for granulation is required (see Chapter 25).

Sigma-blade mixer

This robust mixer will deal with stiff pastes and ointments and depends for its action on the close intermeshing of the two blades which resemble the Greek letter Σ in shape. The clearance between the blades and the mixing trough is kept small by the shape shown in Figure 13.15.

It is very difficult using primary mixers to completely disperse powder particles in a semisolid base so that they are invisible to the eye. The mix is usually subjected to the further action of a roller mill or colloid mill, so as to 'rub out' these particles by the intense shear generated by rollers or cones set with a very small clearance between them.

Fig. 13.15 Sigma blade mixer.

REFERENCE

Nikolakakis, N. and Newton, M. (1989) *J. Pharm. Pharmacol.*, **41**, 145.

BIBLIOGRAPHY

Kaye, B.H. (1997) *Powder Mixing*. Chapman & Hall, London.

Miyanami, K. (1991) Mixing. In: Linoya, K., Gotoh, K. and Higashitani, K. (eds) *Powder Technology Handbook*. Marcel Dekker, New York, p 595–612.

Rothman, H. (1981) High speed mixing in the pharmaceutical industry. *Manuf. Chemist Aerosol News*, **52(4)**, 47–49.

Rumpf, H. (1990) *Particle Technology*. Chapman & Hall, London.

Staniforth, J.N. (1982) Advances in powder mixing and segregation in relation to pharmaceutical processing. *Int. J. Pharmaceut. Tech. Product Manuf.*, 3(Suppl), 1–12.

Williams, J.C. (1990) Mixing and segregation of powders. In: Rhodes, M.J. (ed) *Principles of Powder Technology*. John Wiley, Chichester, Ch 4, p 71–90.

14

Powder flow

John Staniforth

Powders are generally considered to be composed of solid particles of the same or different chemical compositions having equivalent diameters less than 1000 μm. However, the term 'powder' will also be used here to describe groups of particles formed into granules which may have overall dimensions greater than 1000 μm.

The largest use of powders pharmaceutically is to produce tablets and capsules. Together with mixing and compression properties, the flowability of a powder is of critical importance in the production of pharmaceutical dosage forms. Some of the reasons for producing free-flowing pharmaceutical powders include:

1. uniform feed from bulk storage containers or hoppers into the feed mechanisms of tabletting or capsule-filling equipment, allowing uniform particle packing and a constant volume-to-mass ratio which maintains tablet weight uniformity;
2. reproducible filling of tablet dies and capsule dosators, which improves weight uniformity and allows tablets to be produced with more consistent physicomechanical properties;
3. uneven powder flow can result in excess entrapped air within powders, which in some high-speed tabletting conditions may promote capping or lamination;
4. uneven powder flow can result from excess fine particles in a powder, which increase particle–die-wall friction, causing lubrication problems, and increase dust contamination risks during powder transfer.

There are many industrial processes that require powders to be moved from one location to another and this is achieved by many different methods, such as gravity feeding, mechanically assisted feeding, pneumatic transfer, fluidization in gases and liquids and hydraulic transfer. In each of these examples powders are required to flow and, as with other operations described earlier, the efficiency with which

197

they do so is dependent on both process design and particle properties.

PARTICLE PROPERTIES

Adhesion and cohesion

The presence of molecular forces produces a tendency for solid particles to stick to themselves and to other surfaces. Adhesion and cohesion can be considered as two parts of the same phenomenon: cohesion occurs between like surfaces, such as component particles of a bulk solid, whereas adhesion occurs between two unlike surfaces, for example between a particle and a hopper wall.

Cohesive forces acting between particles in a powder bed are composed mainly from short-range non-specific van der Waals forces which increase as particle size decreases and vary with changes in relative humidity. Other attractive forces contributing to interparticle cohesion may be produced by surface tensional forces between adsorbed liquid layers at the particle surfaces and electrostatic forces arising from contact or frictional charging, which may have short half-lives but increase cohesion through improving interparticle contacts and hence increasing the quantity of van der Waals interactions. Cohesion provides a useful method of characterizing the drag or frictional forces acting within a powder bed to prevent powder flow.

Measurement of adhesive/cohesive properties

Adhesive/cohesive forces acting between a single pair of particles or a particle and substrate surface can be accurately determined using a specially adapted ultracentrifuge to apply very high forces strong enough to separate the two surfaces.

However, it is more usual when studying powder flow to characterize adhesion/cohesion in a bed of powder.

Shear strength   Cohesion can be defined as the stress (force per unit area) necessary to shear a powder bed under conditions of zero normal load. Using this criterion, the shear strength of a powder can be determined from the resistance to flow caused by cohesion or friction and can be measured using a shear cell.

The shear cell (Fig. 14.1) is a relatively simple piece of apparatus which is designed to measure shear stress, τ, at different values of normal stress, σ. There are several types of shear cell, such as the

Fig. 14.1   Diagrammatic representation of Jenike shear cell.

Jenike and the Portishead, which use different methods of applying the stresses and measuring the shear strengths. In order to carry out a shear strength determination, powder is packed into the two halves of the cell. Weights are placed on the lid of the assembled cell, or some other method may be used to apply the normal stress. A system of a cord connected from the lid of the cell, by a pulley, to weights, or other means are used to apply a shearing stress across the two halves of the cell. The shear stress is found by dividing the shear force by the cross-sectional area of the powder bed and will increase as the normal stress increases. One of the most convenient, informative and widely used methods of presenting this stress interrelationship is provided by plotting a Mohr diagram.

A Mohr diagram is constructed by plotting the normal stress, τ, as the ordinate and the stress, σ, as the abscissa. For two values of shear stress on the abscissa, at which failure occurs and the cell is sheared, σ_1 and σ_2 are used as the diameter of a Mohr circle with radius $\frac{\sigma_1 + \sigma_2}{2}$ (Fig. 14.2). A series of Mohr semicircles can be constructed in this way with different pairs of shear stresses causing failure (Fig. 14.3). A line is constructed to touch all of the Mohr semicircles and define the critical combinations of normal and shearing stresses at which failure occurs. The line is called the yield locus and is a characteristic of the powder under given conditions. Several different properties of the powder can be obtained from the complete Mohr diagram, and some of these are shown in Table 14.1.

Fig. 14.2   Mohr circle

Fig. 14.3 Mohr diagram

In order to calculate the cohesion in a powder bed using the shear cell method, the yield locus is extrapolated back to zero normal stress; the shear stress at zero normal stress is, by definition, equal to the cohesion of the powder. For a non-cohesive powder the extrapolated yield locus will pass through the origin, equivalent to zero shear stress. In rheological terms the stress due to cohesion along the yield locus may be called the yield stress and the powder termed a plastic solid.

Tensile strength   The tensile strength of a powder bed is a characteristic of the internal friction or cohesion of the particles, but unlike shear strength determinations, the powder bed is caused to fail in tension by splitting, rather than failing in shear by sliding. The powder is packed into a split plate, one half of which is fixed and the other half free to move by means of small wheels or ball bearings that run in tracks in a table (Fig. 14.4). The table is then tilted towards the vertical until the angle is reached at which the powder cohesion is overcome and the mobile half-plate breaks away from the static half-plate. The tensile strength, σ_t, of the powder can then be determined from Eqn 14.1.

$$\sigma_t = \frac{M \sin \theta}{A} \times 10^5 \ \text{Pa} \qquad (14.1)$$

where M is the mass of the mobile half plate + powder, θ the angle of the tilted table to the horizon-

Fig. 14.4   Measurement of tensile strength of a powder bed using tilting table method

---

Table 14.1   Some properties relating to powder cohesion and flowability which can be obtained from Mohr diagrams

Measurement	Property measured	Powder characteristics
1 Acute angle of the extrapolated yield locus at the shear stress axis	Angle of internal friction, ϕ	Difficulty of maintaining constant volume flow
2 Tan ϕ or slope of the yield locus	Coefficient of friction	Indirect measurement of powder flowability
3 Diameter of circle with tangent to t linking minor stress at $\sigma = 0$ to major unconfined yield stress σ_u	Stress equilibrium in powder arch when no flow occurs	Minimum opening dimensions to prevent arching
4 Extrapolation of yield locus to cut normal stress axis	σ_a, apparent tensile strength of powder bed	Resistance to failure in tension
5 Shear stress, t_e, at zero normal stress, σ_o	Cohesion coefficient	Cohesion, when powder is non-cohesive, yield locus passes through origin and shear stress = 0

tal at the point of failure, and A is the cross-sectional area of the powder bed.

The tensile strength values of different powders have been found to correlate reasonably well with another measurement of powder cohesion, angle of repose.

Angle of repose From the previous discussion it will be realized that an object, such as a particle, will begin to slide when the angle of inclination is large enough to overcome frictional forces. Conversely, an object in motion will stop sliding when the angle of inclination is below that required to overcome adhesion/cohesion. This balance of forces causes a powder poured from a container on to a horizontal surface to form a heap: initially the particles stack until the approach angle for subsequent particles joining the stack is large enough to overcome friction, and they slip and roll over each other until the gravitational forces balance the interparticle forces. The sides of the heap formed in this way make an angle with the horizontal which is called the angle of repose and is a characteristic of the internal friction or cohesion of the particles. The value of the angle of repose will be high if the powder is cohesive and low if the powder is non-cohesive. If the powder is very cohesive the heap may be characterized by more than one angle of repose. Initially the interparticle cohesion causes a very steep cone to form, but on the addition of further powder this tall stack may suddenly collapse, causing air to be entrained between particles and partially fluidizing the bed, making it more mobile. The resulting heap has two angles of repose: a large angle remaining from the initial heap and a shallower angle formed by the powder flooding from the initial heap (Fig. 14.5).

In order to overcome this problem, it has been suggested that determinations of angles of repose be carried out using different concentrations of very

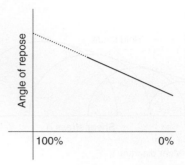

Fig. 14.6 Determination of angle of repose for very cohesive powders.

cohesive powders and non-cohesive powders. The angles of repose are plotted against mixture concentration and extrapolated to 100% cohesive powder content so as to obtain the appropriate angle of repose (Fig. 14.6).

Particle properties and bulk flow

In the discussion concerning adhesion/cohesion it has become clear that an equilibrium exists between forces responsible for promoting powder flow and those preventing powder flow, i.e. at equilibrium:

$$\Sigma f(\text{driving forces}) = \Sigma f(\text{drag forces}) \quad (14.2)$$

that is,

Σf(gravitational force, particle mass, angle of inclination of powder bed, static head of powder, mechanical force ...) = Σf(adhesive forces, cohesive forces, other surface forces, mechanical interlocking...).

$$(14.3)$$

Some of these forces are modified or controlled by external factors related to particle properties.

Particle-size effects

Because cohesion and adhesion are phenomena that occur at surfaces, particle size will influence the flowability of a powder. In general, fine particles with very high surface to mass ratios are more cohesive than coarser particles which are influenced more by gravitational forces. Particles larger than 250 μm are usually relatively free flowing, but as the size falls below 100 μm powders become cohesive and flow problems are likely to occur. Powders having a particle size less than 10 μm are usually extremely cohesive and resist flow under gravity, except possibly as large agglomerates.

Fig. 14.5 Cohesive powder poured in a heap and showing different angles of repose: σ_m maximum angle formed by cohesive particles σ_s shallowest angle formed by collapse of cohesive particle heap, resulting in flooding. In some cases a third angle, σ_i is identifiable as an intermediate slope produced by cohesive particles stacking on flooded powder.

Particle shape

Powders with similar particle sizes but dissimilar shapes can have markedly different flow properties owing to differences in interparticle contact areas. For example, a group of spheres has minimum interparticle contact and generally optimal flow properties, whereas a group of particle flakes or dendritic particles has a very high surface-to-volume ratio and poorer flow properties.

Particle density (true density)

Because powders normally flow under the influence of gravity, dense particles are generally less cohesive than less dense particles of the same size and shape.

Packing geometry

A set of particles can be filled into a volume of space to produce a powder bed which is in static equilibrium owing to the interaction of gravitational and adhesive/cohesive forces. By slight vibration of the bed, particles can be mobilized so that if the vibration is stopped, the bed is once more in static equilibrium but occupies a different spatial volume than before. The change in bulk volume has been produced by rearrangement of the packing geometry of the particles. In general, such geometric rearrangements result in a transition from loosely packed particles to more tightly packed ones, so that the equilibrium balance moves from left to right in Eqn 14.2 and cohesion increases. This also means that more tightly packed powders require a higher driving force to produce powder flow than more loosely packed particles of the same powder.

Characterization of packing geometry by porosity and bulk density

A set of monosized spherical particles can be arranged in many different geometric configurations. At one extreme, when the spheres form a cubic arrangement, the particles are most loosely packed and have a porosity of 48% (Fig. 14.7(a)). At the other extreme, when the spheres form a rhombohedral arrangement, they are most densely packed and have a porosity of only 26% (Fig. 14.7(b)). The porosity used to characterize packing geometry is linked to the bulk density of the powder. Bulk density, ρ_B, is a characteristic of a powder rather than individual particles and is given by the mass, M, of powder occupying a known volume, V, according to the relationship:

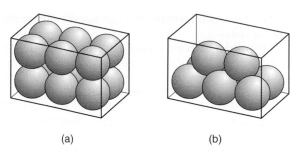

Fig. 14.7 Different geometric packings of spherical particles: (a) cubic packing; (b) rhombohedral packing.

$$\rho_B = \frac{M}{V} \text{ kg m}^{-3} \qquad (14.4)$$

The bulk density of a powder is always less than the true density of its component particles because the powder contains interparticle pores or voids. This statement reveals that whereas a powder can only possess a single true density it can have many different bulk densities, depending on the way in which the particles are packed and the bed porosity. However, a high bulk density value does not necessarily imply a close-packed low-porosity bed, as bulk density is directly proportional to true density.

bulk density α true density

i.e.   bulk density = k true density   (14.5)

or

$$k = \frac{\text{bulk density}}{\text{true density}} \qquad (14.6)$$

The constant of proportionality, k, is known as the **packing fraction** or **fractional solids content**. For example, the packing fraction for dense, randomly packed spheres is approximately 0.63, whereas the packing fraction for a set of dense, randomly packed discs is 0.83.

Also:

$$1 - k = e \qquad (14.7)$$

where e is the fractional voidage of the powder bed, which is usually expressed as a percentage and termed the bed porosity. Another way of expressing fractional voidage is to use the ratio of particle volume V_P to bulk powder volume V_B, i.e.

$$e = \frac{1 - V_P}{V_B} \qquad (14.8)$$

A simple ratio of void volume V_v to particle volume V_P represents the voids ratio:

$$\frac{V_v}{V_p} = \frac{e}{(1-e)} \qquad (14.9)$$

which provides information about the stability of the powder mass.

For powders having comparable true densities an increase in bulk density causes a decrease in porosity. This increases the number of interparticle contacts and contact areas and causes an increase in cohesion. In very coarse particles this may still be insufficient to overcome the gravitational influence on particles. Conversely, a decrease in bulk density may be associated with a reduction in particle size and produce a loose-packed powder bed which, although porous, is unlikely to flow because of the inherent cohesiveness of the fine particles. The use of porosity as a means of characterizing packing geometrics can sometimes be misleading. For example, monosize cubic crystals could be considered to be loosely packed with a porosity of 20%, as the closest packed cubic arrangement would have a porosity close to 0%. By comparison, a system of spheronized crystals of the same size with a porosity of 30% could be considered to be more closely packed, as the closest packed spherical arrangement has a porosity of 26%. In this example the powder with the higher porosity is relatively more closely packed than that with the lower porosity.

In powders where the particle shape or cohesiveness promotes arch or bridge formation, two equilibrium states could have similar porosities but widely different packing geometries. In such conditions, interparticle pore-size distributions can be useful for comparing packing geometry.

For example, Fig. 14.8(a) shows a group of particles in which arching has occurred and Fig. 14.8(b) shows a similar group of particles in which arch formation is absent. The total porosity of the two systems can be seen to be similar but the pore size distributions (Fig. 14.9) reveal that the powder in which arch formation has occurred is generally more tightly packed than that in which arching is absent.

Fig. 14.9 (a) Interparticle pore size distribution corresponding to close-packed bed containing a powder arch. (b) Interparticle pore size distribution corresponding to loosely packed bed.

Factors affecting packing geometry

1 *Particle size and size distribution*: void spaces between coarse particles may become filled with finer particles in a powder with a wide size range, resulting in a more closely packed cohesive powder.

2 *Particle shape and texture*: these influence the minimum porosity of the powder bed. Arches or bridges within the powder bed will be formed more readily through the interlocking of non-isometric, highly textured particles.
   This tendency for irregular particles to produce open structures supported by small or large powder arches causes them to have a larger difference in porosity between loose packing and tight packing geometries than more regularly shaped particles.

3 *Surface properties*: the presence of electrostatic forces can add to interparticle attractions and promote closer particle packing, resulting in increased cohesion.

4 *Handling and processing conditions*: the way in which a powder has been handled prior to flow or packing influences the type of packing geometry.

PROCESS CONDITIONS: HOPPER DESIGN

Flow through an orifice

There are many examples of this type of flow to be found in the manufacture of pharmaceutical solid dosage forms, for example when granules or powders flow through the opening in a hopper or bin used to feed powder to tabletting machines, capsule-filling machines or sachet-filling machines. Because of the importance of such flow in producing unit

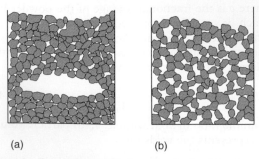

(a)   (b)

Fig. 14.8 Two equidimensional powders having the same porosity but different packing geometries.

doses containing the same or very similar powder masses, and the importance of flow behaviour in other industries, the behaviour of particles being fed through orifices has been extensively studied.

A hopper or bin can be modelled as a tall cylindrical container having a closed orifice in the base and initially full of a free-flowing powder which has a horizontal upper surface (Fig. 14.10(a)). When the orifice at the base of the container is opened, flow patterns develop as the powder discharges. (Fig. 14.10(a)–(f)).

The observed sequence is as follows:

1 On opening the orifice there is no instantaneous movement at the surface, but particles just above the orifice fall freely through it (Fig. 14.10(b)).
2 A depression forms at the upper surface and spreads outwards to the sides of the hopper (Fig. 14.10(c) and (d)).
3 Provided that the container is tall and not too narrow, the flow pattern illustrated in Fig. 14.10(e) and shown schematically in Figure 14.11 is rapidly established. Particles in zone A move rapidly over the slower moving

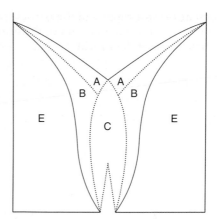

Fig. 14.11 Fully developed flow of a free-flowing powder through an orifice.

particles in zone B, whereas those in zone E, remain stationary. The particles in zone A feed into zone C, where they move quickly downwards and out through the orifice. The more slowly moving particles in zone B do not enter zone C.

4 Both powder streams in zones B and C converge to a 'tongue' just above the orifice, where the

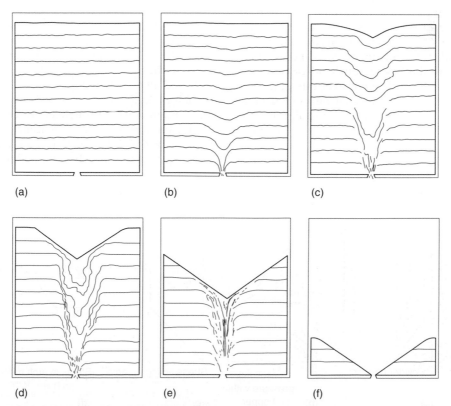

(a) (b) (c)

(d) (e) (f)

Fig. 14.10 Development of flow through an orifice. The horizontal lines are formed by indicator particles to show the course of the discharge.

movement is most rapid and the particle packing is least dense. In a zone just above the orifice, the particles are in free flight.

Important practical consequences of this flow pattern are that if a square-bottomed hopper or bin is repeatedly refilled and partially emptied, the particles in a zone towards the base and sides of the container (Fig. 14.10(f)) will not be discharged and may degrade; alternatively, this static zone may provide a segregation potential for previously homogeneous powders.

Factors affecting flow rates through orifices

The flow patterns described above, together with powder flow rates through orifices, are dependent on many different factors, some of which are particle related and some process related. Particle-related effects, notably particle size, are discussed above. Process-related effects include the following.

Orifice diameter Flow rate α D_o^A. The rate of powder flow through an orifice is proportional to a function of orifice diameter, D_o (A is a constant with a value of approx, 2.6). Provided that the height of the powder bed, called the head of powder, remains considerably greater than the orifice diameter, flow rate is virtually independent of powder head. This situation is unlike that relating to liquid flow through an orifice, where the flow rate falls off continuously as the head diminishes. The constant rate of flow for powders is a useful property as it means that if a bulk powder is filled into dies, sachets, capsules or other enclosures, they will receive equal weights if filled for equal times.

Hopper width At different positions within a powder bed the consolidating stresses and shear or tensile strengths are different (Fig. 14.12(b)). If the bed strength at a given point in the hopper is great enough to resist the driving forces promoting flow, then a stable arch will be formed. At all other points in the powder the bed strength will not be high enough to support an arch against the stresses within it, and flow will occur. The stresses acting on a stable arch are proportional to the width of the container and vary with diameter, as exemplified in Figure 14.12(a) and (b). The relationship between the stress on the arch and the arch strength, resulting in part from consolidating pressures at different points in the hopper (Fig. 14.12(c)), shows that with the exception of a region close to the hopper outlet and another at the point where the cylindrical section meets the conical section of the hopper, powder arches are weaker than the stresses on them. This suggests that powder flow will occur in all other regions (Fig. 14.12(d)) and allows the hopper design to be adjusted so that the minimum hopper widths are always large enough to produce arch stresses greater than arch strengths, and thereby ensure continuous, uniform powder flow.

Head size Figure 14.12(b) shows the way in which solids' pressure changes with powder head size (powder depth). The pressure below the upper free surface increases to a constant governed by frictional factors. The pressure again falls off towards the hopper outlet and drops below atmospheric at the orifice, causing air to be drawn up into the region close to the base so as to equalize this negative pressure and allow flow to continue.

Hopper wall angle It was noted above in the description of flow through an orifice, that a flat-bottomed bin retains a certain volume of powder in the form of a drained cone centred on the orifice. In order to prevent this behaviour and to ensure that all the powder is discharged from a hopper, the walls are frequently angled inwards as the outlet is

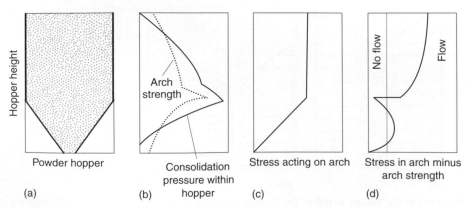

(a) Powder hopper

(b) Consolidation pressure within hopper — Arch strength

(c) Stress acting on arch

(d) Stress in arch minus arch strength — No flow / Flow

Hopper height

Fig. 14.12 Influence of stress interactions within a hopper on powder flow.

approached. The wall angle that is required to ensure that powder empties freely is determined by the particle–wall adhesion component of friction within powders, and is characterized by a wall-friction angle, ϕ. Powders with very low wall-friction angles will empty freely, even from hoppers with very shallow slopes, whereas powders with very high wall-friction angles will empty poorly even from steep-walled hoppers. In between these two extremes powder discharge characteristics will be determined by the relationship between wall friction and hopper angle, as shown in Figure 14.13.

Mass flow and funnel flow

Powder that discharges freely from a hopper is said to undergo mass flow when particles that enter the hopper first leave it first. This first-in–first-out sequence holds throughout the bed, so that powder can be considered to leave in near-horizontal bands which move down the hopper *en masse* (Fig. 14.14(a)).

Powders which do not discharge freely, due either to high adhesion/cohesion or to hopper angles which are too shallow, may undergo funnel flow (Fig. 14.14(b)). Particles which are loaded into the hopper last are among the first to leave, forming a 'pipe', 'rat-hole' or 'funnel', extending from the upper free powder surface to the hopper outlet and producing uneven erratic flow. Another problem associated with funnel flow may occur when the rat-hole collapses. This produces a sudden rapid discharge of powder which can entrain relatively large volumes of air, causing the particles to partially fluidize and flood out of the hopper. This 'flooding' or 'flushing' may be succeeded by periods when the bed is quiescent and flow is slow or interrupted.

In general, most powders will discharge by mass flow from hoppers with θ angles of about 20°, and by

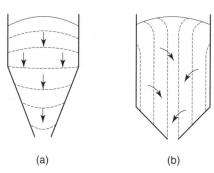

Fig. 14.14 (a) Mass flow hopper, (b) funnel flow hopper.

funnel flow from hoppers with angles of approximately 50°.

Mass flow rate

Throughout this section it has been shown that specific particle properties and individual design criteria influence powder flow. However, in a given practical situation powder flowability is the resultant of the relative influences of all these factors. An equation has been derived which relates some particulate properties, such as bulk density, ρ_B, and angle of repose, α, and hopper design criteria such as orifice diameter, D_o, and a discharge coefficient, C, to mass flow rate of powder, M:

$$M = \pi/4 \; C\rho_B\rho \; [(g \, D^5{}_o)/2 \tan \alpha]^{\frac{1}{2}} \quad (14.10)$$

where g is acceleration due to gravity.

CHARACTERIZATION OF POWDER FLOW

When examining the flow properties of a powder it is useful to be able to quantify the type of behaviour and many different methods have been described, either directly using dynamic or kinetic methods, or indirectly, generally by measurements carried out on static beds.

Indirect methods

Angle of repose

Angles of repose have been used as indirect methods of quantifying powder flowability, because of their relationship with interparticle cohesion. There are many different methods of determining angles of repose and some of these are shown in Table 14.2.

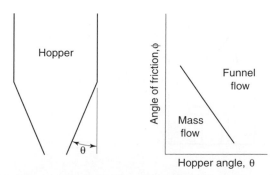

Fig. 14.13 Influence of hopper wall angle and particle-wall friction on powder flow.

The different methods may produce different values for the same powder, although these may be self-consistent. It is also possible that different angles of repose could be obtained for the same powder, owing to differences in the way the samples were handled prior to measurement. For these reasons, angles of repose tend to be variable and are not always representative of flow under specific conditions.

Table 14.2	Methods of measuring angle of repose					
Apparatus		Method	Angle defined	Apparatus	Method	Angle defined
		Fixed height cone	Angle of repose		Ledge	Drained angle of repose
		Fixed base cone	Angle of repose		Crater	Drained angle of repose
		Tilting table	Angle of repose		Platform	Drained angle of repose
		Rotating cylinder	Dynamic angle of repose			

As a general guide, powders with angles of repose greater than 50° have unsatisfactory flow properties, whereas minimum angles close to 25° correspond to very good flow properties.

Shear cell determinations

It is possible to characterize flowability indirectly from the behaviour of powder in a shear cell. A flow factor, f.f., can be obtained by determining the reciprocal slope of a curve or tangent to a curve of unconfined yield stress σ_u, plotted against the maximum normal stress on a yield locus, σ_m (Fig. 14.15(a)). The unconfined yield stresses are those in Mohr semi-circles constructed through the origin; the maximum normal stresses have a semicircle passing through the largest normal stress (Fig. 14.15(b)). By plotting a series of different yield loci, several values can be obtained for σ_u and σ_m.

The relationship between flow factors and powder flowability is shown in Table 14.3.

Bulk density measurements

The bulk density of a powder is dependent on particle packing and changes as the powder consolidates. A consolidated powder is likely to have a greater arch strength than a less consolidated one and may therefore be more resistant to powder flow. The ease with which a powder consolidates can be used as an indirect method of quantifying powder flow.

Figure 14.16 shows a mechanical tapping device or jolting volumeter which can be used to follow the change in packing volume that occurs when void space diminishes and consolidation occurs. The powder contained in the measuring cylinder is mechanically tapped by means of a constant velocity rotating cam and increases from an initial bulk

Table 14.3 Relationship between flow factors (f.f.) and powder flowability

f.f. value	Flow descriptor
>10	Free flowing
4–10	Easy flowing
1.6–4	Cohesive
<1.6	Very cohesive

Fig. 14.16 Mechanical tapping device (Jolting Volumeter).

density D_o (also known as fluff or poured bulk density) to a final bulk density D_f (also known as equilibrium, tapped or consolidated bulk density) when it has attained its most stable, i.e. unchanging arrangement.

Hausner found that the ratio D_f/D_o was related to interparticle friction and, as such, could be used to predict powder flow properties. He showed that powders with low interparticle friction, such as coarse spheres, had ratios of approximately 1.2, whereas more cohesive, less free-flowing powders such as flakes have Hausner ratios greater than 1.6.

Another indirect method of measuring powder flow from bulk densities was developed by Carr. The percentage compressibility of a powder is a direct measure of the potential powder arch or bridge strength and stability and is calculated according to Eqn 14.11.

Fig. 14.15 (a) Plot of unconfined yield stress, σ_u, against maximum stress, σ_m, with a slope corresponding to the flow factor, f.f. (b) Example of Mohr diagram used to obtain one pair of values for σ_u and σ_m.

$$\% \text{ compressibility} = \frac{D_f - D_o}{D_f} \times 100 \qquad (14.11)$$

Table 14.4   Relationship between powder flowability and % compressibility

% Compressibility range	Flow description
5–15	Excellent (free-flowing granules)
12–16	Good (free flowing powdered granules)
18–21	Fair (powdered granules)
23–28	Poor (very fluid powders)
28–35	Poor (fluid cohesive powders)
35–38	Very poor (fluid cohesive powders)
>40	Extremely poor (cohesive powders)

Table 14.4 shows the generalized relationship between descriptions of powder flow and percent compressibility, according to Carr.

Critical orifice diameter

In order to carry out measurements of critical orifice diameter, powder is filled into a shallow tray to a uniform depth with near-uniform packing. The base of the tray is perforated with a graduated series of holes, which are blocked either by resting the tray on a plane surface or by the presence of a simple shutter. The critical orifice diameter is the size of the smallest hole through which powder discharges when the tray is lifted or the shutter removed. Sometimes repetition of the experiment produces different critical orifice diameters, and in these cases maximum and minimum values are sometimes quoted.

Critical orifice diameter is a direct measure of powder cohesion and arch strength since:

$$\tan \alpha = \frac{r}{x} \qquad (14.12)$$

where r is the particle radius and x is the orifice radius, and

$$\tan F' = \frac{\tan \phi}{1 - \tan \phi \dfrac{r}{x} - \dfrac{r^2}{x^2}} \qquad (14.13)$$

where F' is the angle of form, which is the obtuse angle between the contracting powder dome and the horizontal, and $\tan \phi$ is a coefficient of friction.

An alternative critical orifice method for determining powder flowability uses a cylinder with a series of interchangeable base plate discs having different diameter orifices. Using this system, flowability indices related to orifice diameters have been used as a method of specifying materials for use in filling given capsule sizes or producing particular tablet sizes at a specified rate.

Direct methods

Hopper flow rate

The simplest method of determining powder flowability directly is to measure the rate at which powder discharges from a hopper. A simple shutter is placed over the hopper outlet and the hopper filled with powder. The shutter is then removed and the time taken for the powder to discharge completely is recorded. By dividing the discharged powder mass by this time, a flow rate is obtained which can be used for quantitative comparison of different powders.

Hopper or discharge tube outlets should be selected to provide a good model for a particular flow application. For example, if a powder discharges well from a hopper into a tablet machine feed frame, but does not flow reproducibly into the tablet die, then it is likely that more useful information will be generated by selecting experimental conditions to model those occurring in flow from the feeder to the die rather than those in flow from the hopper to the feeder.

Recording flowmeter

A recording flowmeter is essentially similar to the method described above except that powder is allowed to discharge from a hopper or container on to a balance.

In the case of analogue balances a chart recorder is used to produce a permanent record of the increase in powder mass with time. In some systems the signal from the balance is digitized and processed by a microcomputer. Recording flowmeters allow mass flow rates to be determined and also provide a means of quantifying uniformity of flow.

IMPROVEMENT OF POWDER FLOWABILITY

Alteration of particle size and size distribution

Because coarse particles are generally less cohesive than fine particles and an optimum size for free flow exists, there is a distinct disadvantage in using a finer grade of powder than is necessary.

The size distribution can also be altered to improve flowability by removing a proportion of the fine particle fraction or by increasing the proportion of coarser particles, such as occurs through granulation.

Alteration of particle shape or texture

In general, for a given particle size more spherical particles have better flow properties than more irregular particles. The process of spray-drying can be used to produce near-spherical excipients, such as spray-dried lactose. Under certain circumstances, drug particles that are normally acicular can be made more spherical by temperature-cycling crystallization.

The texture of particles may also influence powder flowability, as particles with very rough surfaces will be more cohesive and have a greater tendency to interlock than smooth-surfaced particles. The shape and texture of particles can also be altered by control of production methods, such as crystallization conditions.

Alteration of surface forces

Reduction of electrostatic charges can improve powder flowability and this can be achieved by altering process conditions to reduce frictional contacts. For example, where powder is poured down chutes or conveyed along pipes pneumatically, the speed and length of transportation should be minimized. Electrostatic charges in powder containers can be prevented or discharged by efficient earth connections.

The moisture content of particles is also of importance to powder flowability, as adsorbed surface moisture films tend to increase bulk density and reduce porosity. In cases where moisture content is excessive powders should be dried and, if hygroscopic, stored and processed under low-humidity conditions.

Formulation additives: flow activators

Flow activators are commonly referred to pharmaceutically as 'glidants', although some also have lubricant or antiadherent properties. Flow activators improve the flowability of powders by reducing adhesion and cohesion.

Some commonly used glidants include talc, maize starch and magnesium stearate, which may have their effect by reducing or altering electrostatic interactions. A flow activator with an exceptionally high specific surface area is colloidal silicon dioxide, which may act by reducing the bulk density of tightly packed powders. Colloidal silicon dioxide also improves flowability of formulations, even those containing other glidants, although in some cases it can cause flooding.

Where powder flowability is impaired through increased moisture content, a small proportion of very fine magnesium oxide may be used as a flow activator. Used in this way, magnesium oxide appears to disrupt the continuous film of adsorbed water surrounding the moist particles.

The use of silicone-treated powder, such as silicone-coated talc or sodium bicarbonate, may also be beneficial in improving the flowability of moist or hygroscopic powder.

Alteration of process conditions

Use of vibration-assisted hoppers

In cases where the powder arch strength within a bin or hopper is greater than the stresses in it, due to gravitational effects, powder flow will be interrupted or prevented. If the hopper cannot be redesigned to provide adequate stresses and if the physical properties of the particles cannot be adjusted or the formulation altered, then extreme measures are required. One method of encouraging powder flow where arching or bridging has occurred within a hopper, is to add to the stresses due to gravitational interactions by vibrating the hopper mechanically. Both the amplitude and the frequency of vibration can be altered to produce the desired effect, and may vary from a single cycle or shock produced by a compressed-air device or hammer, to higher frequencies produced, for example, by out-of-balance electric motors mounted on a hopper frame.

Use of force feeders

The flow of powders that discharge irregularly or flood out of hoppers can be improved by fitting vibrating baffles, known as live-bottom feeders, at the base of the conical section within a hopper.

The outflowing stream from a hopper can be encouraged to move towards its required location using a slightly sloping moving belt, or in the case of some tabletting machines, the use of mechanical force feeders. Force feeders are usually made up of a single or two counter-rotating paddles at the base of the hopper just above the die table in place of a feed frame. The paddles presumably act by preventing powder arching over dies, and thereby improve die filling especially at high turret speeds.

Caution!

In most pharmaceutical technology operations it is difficult to alter one process without adversely influencing another. For example, increasing compression pressure to produce stronger tablets may also impair disintegration and prolong dissolution; increasing mixing times of drugs with excipients in the presence of magnesium stearate, to improve homogeneity, may also impair tablet strength.

In the case of alterations made in order to improve powder flow, relative particle motion will be promoted and can lead to demixing or segregation. *In extremis*, improving powder flow to improve weight uniformity may reduce content uniformity through increased segregation.

BIBLIOGRAPHY

Gioia, A. (1980) Intrinsic flowability. A new technology for powder-flowability classification. *Pharm. Techn.*, **4** (Feb.), 65–68.

Lieberman, H.A. and Lachman, L. (eds) (1981) *Pharmaceutical Dosage Forms*, Volume 2, Marcel Dekker Inc., New York and Basel.

McNaughton, K. (ed.) (1981) *Solids Handling*, McGraw-Hill Publications Co., New York.

Sadek, H.M., Olsen, J.L., Smith, H.L. and Onay, S. (1982) A systematic approach to glidant selection. *Pharm. Tech.*, **6** (Feb.), 42–44, 46, 50, 52, 54, 56, 59–60, 62.

Shahinpoor, M. (ed.) (1983) *Advances in the Mechanics and the Flow of Granular Materials*, Volumes 1 and 2. Gulf Publishing Co., Houston and London.

Singley, M.E. and Chaplin, R.V. (1982) Flow of particulate materials, *Trans. ASAE*, **25**, 1360–1373.

Taubmann, H.J. (1982) The influence of flow activators on the flow behaviour of powders. *Aufbereitungs-Technik*, **23**, 423–428.

BIOPHARMACEUTICAL PRINCIPLES OF DRUG DELIVERY

PART THREE

BIOPHARMACEUTICAL PRINCIPLES OF DRUG DELIVERY

15

Introduction to biopharmaceutics

Marianne Ashford

WHAT IS BIOPHARMACEUTICS?

Biopharmaceutics can be defined as the study of how the physicochemical properties of drugs, dosage forms and routes of administration affect the rate and extent of drug absorption.

The relationship between the drug, its dosage form and the route by which it is administered governs how much of the drug and how fast it enters the systemic circulation. For a drug to be effective, enough of it needs to reach its site(s) of action and stay there long enough to be able to exert its pharmacological effect. This depends upon the route of administration, the form in which it is administered and the rate at which it is delivered.

Background

Apart from the intravenous route, where a drug is introduced directly into the bloodstream, all other routes of administration where a systemic action is required, involve the absorption of the drug into the blood from the route of administration. Once the drug reaches the bloodstream it partitions between the plasma and the red blood cells, the erythrocytes. Drug in the plasma partitions between the plasma proteins (mainly albumin) and the plasma water. It is this free or unbound drug in plasma water, and not the drug bound to the proteins, that can pass out of the plasma through the capillary endothelium and reach other body fluids and tissues and hence the site(s) of action.

A dynamic equilibrium exists between the concentration of the drug in the blood plasma and the drug at its site(s) of action. This is termed *distribution*, the degree of which will depend largely on the physicochemical properties of the drug, in particular its lipophilicity. As it is often difficult to access the drug at its site(s) of action, its concentration in the plasma is often taken as a surrogate for its concentration at its site(s) of action. Even though the unbound drug in the plasma would give a better estimate of the concentration of the drug at its site(s) of action, this requires a much more complex and sensitive assay than a measurement of the total concentration of the drug (i.e. the sum of the bound and unbound drug) within the blood plasma. Thus it is this total drug concentration within the plasma that is usually measured for clinical purposes. Therefore, plasma protein binding is a critical parameter to consider when investigating the therapeutic effect of a drug molecule.

The concentration of the drug in blood plasma depends on numerous factors. These include the amount of an administered dose that is **absorbed** and reaches the systemic circulation; the extent of **distribution** of the drug between the systemic circulation and other tissues and fluids (which is usually a rapid and reversible process); and the rate of **elimination** of the drug from the body. The drug can either be eliminated unchanged or be enzymatically cleaved or biochemically transformed, in which case it is said to have been **metabolized**. The study and characterization of the time course of drug **a**bsorption, **d**istribution, **m**etabolism and **e**limination (ADME) is termed **pharmacokinetics**. Pharmacokinetics is used in the clinical setting to enhance the safe and effective therapeutic management of individual patients.

Figure 15.1 illustrates some of the factors that can influence the concentration of the drug in the blood plasma and also at its site(s) of action. Biopharmaceutics is concerned with the first stage, getting the drug from its route of administration to the blood.

THE CONCEPT OF BIOAVAILABILITY

If a drug is given intravenously it is administered directly into the blood, and therefore we can be sure that all the drug reaches the systemic circulation. The drug is therefore said to be 100% **bioavailable**. However, if a drug is given by another route there is no guarantee that the whole dose will reach the systemic circulation intact. The fraction of an administered dose of the drug that reaches the systemic circulation in the unchanged form is known as the **bioavailable dose**. The relative amount of an administered dose of a particular drug that reaches the systemic circulation intact and the rate at which this occurs is known as the **bioavailability**. Bioavailability is therefore defined as the rate and extent of drug absorption. The bioavailability exhibited by a drug is thus very important in determining whether a therapeutically effective concentration will be achieved at the site(s) of action.

In defining bioavailability in these terms it is assumed that the intact drug is the therapeutically active form. This definition would not be valid in the

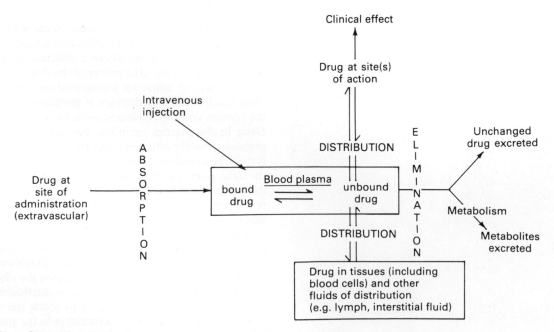

Fig. 15.1 Schematic representation of drug absorption, distribution and elimination.

case of prodrugs, whose therapeutic action normally depends on their being converted into a therapeutically active form prior to or on reaching the systemic circulation. It should also be noted that, in the context of bioavailability, the term systemic circulation refers primarily to venous blood (excluding the hepatic portal vein, which carries blood from the gastrointestinal tract to the liver in the absorption phase) and the arterial blood, which carries the intact blood to the tissues.

Therefore, for a drug which is administered orally to be 100% bioavailable, the entire dose must move from the dosage form to the systemic circulation. The drug must therefore be:

- completely released from the dosage form
- fully dissolved in the gastrointestinal fluids.
- stable in solution in the gastrointestinal fluids
- pass through the gastrointestinal barrier into the mesenteric circulation without being metabolized
- pass through the liver into the systemic circulation unchanged.

Anything which adversely affects either the release of the drug from the dosage form, its dissolution into the gastrointestinal fluids, its permeation through and stability in the gastrointestinal barrier or its stability in the hepatic portal circulation will influence the bioavailability exhibited by that drug from the dosage form in which it was administered.

THE CONCEPT OF BIOPHARMACEUTICS

Many factors have been found to influence the rate and extent of absorption, and hence the time course of a drug in the plasma and therefore at its site(s) of action. These include the foods eaten by the patient, the effect of the disease state on drug absorption, the age of the patient, the site(s) of absorption of the administered drug, the coadministration of other drugs, the physical and chemical properties of the administered drug, the type of dosage form, the composition and method of manufacture of the dosage form, the size of the dose and the frequency of administration.

Thus, a given drug may exhibit differences in its bioavailability if it is administered:

- in the same type of dosage form by different routes of administration, e.g. an aqueous solution of a given drug administered by the oral and intramuscular routes;

- by the same routes of administration but different types of dosage form, e.g. a tablet, a hard gelatin capsule and an aqueous suspension administered by the peroral route;
- in the same type of dosage form by the same route of administration but with different formulations of the dosage form, e.g. different formulations of an oral aqueous suspensions.

Variability in the bioavailability exhibited by a given drug from different formulations of the same type of dosage form, or from different types of dosage forms, or by different routes of administration, can cause the plasma concentration of the drug to be too high and therefore cause side effects, or too low and therefore the drug will be ineffective. Figure 15.2 shows the plasma concentration–time curve following a single oral dose of a drug, indicating the parameters associated with a therapeutic effect.

Poor biopharmaceutical properties often result in:

- poor and variable bioavailability
- difficulties in toxicological evaluation
- difficulties with bioequivalence of formulations
- multi-daily dosing
- the requirement for a non-conventional delivery system
- long and costly development times.

a–b rate of drug absorption > rate of drug elimination
c–d rate of drug elimination > rate of drug absorption

Fig. 15.2 A typical blood plasma concentration–time curve obtained following the peroral administration of a single dose of a drug in a tablet.

CONCLUDING COMMENTS

The following chapters (Chapters 16 and 17) deal in more detail with the physiological factors, dosage form factors and intrinsic properties of drugs that influence the rate and extent of absorption. Chapter 18 looks at means of assessing the biopharmaceutical properties of compounds.

A thorough understanding of the biopharmaceutical properties of a candidate drug are important both in the discovery setting, where potential drug candidates are being considered, and in the development setting, where it is important to anticipate formulation problems and assess whether the drug is a candidate for a controlled-release formulation.

BIBLIOGRAPHY

Dressman J.B., Lennernäs, H. (2000), *Oral Drug Absorption, Prediction & Assessment*, Marcel Dekker, New York.

Gibaldi, M. (1991). *Biopharmaceutics and Clinical Pharmacokinetics*, 4th edn, Lea & Febiger, Philadelphia.

Johnson, L.R. (1994). *Physiology of the Gastro-intestinal Tract*, Volume 2, 3rd edn. Raven Press, New York.

Macheras, P., Reppas, C. & Dressman, J.B. (1995) *Biopharmaceutics of Orally Administered Drugs*, Ellis Horwood, London.

Washington, N. and Wilson, C. (2000) *Physiological Pharmaceutics* 2nd edn. Taylor and Francis, London.

16

The gastrointestinal tract – physiology and drug absorption

Marianne Ashford

The factors that influence the rate and extent of absorption depend upon the route of administration. As stated in Chapter 15, the intravenous route offers direct access to the systemic circulation and the total dose administered via this route is available in the plasma for distribution into other body tissues and the site(s) of action of the drug. Other routes will require an absorption step before the drug reaches the systemic circulation. Factors affecting this absorption will depend on the physiology of the administration site(s) and the membrane barriers present at those site(s), that the drug needs to cross in order to reach the systemic circulation. A summary of some of the properties of each route of administration is given in Chapter 1.

The GI tract is discussed in detail in this chapter and a detailed description of the physiology of some of the other more important routes of administration is given in Part 4. The oral route of delivery is by far the most popular, mainly because it is natural and convenient for the patient and because it is relatively easy to manufacture oral dosage forms. Oral dosage forms do not need to be sterilized, are compact, and can be produced in large quantities by automated machines. This chapter and the next will therefore be confined to discussing the biopharmaceutical factors (that is, physiological, dosage form and drug factors) that influence oral drug absorption.

PHYSIOLOGICAL FACTORS INFLUENCING ORAL DRUG ABSORPTION

The gastrointestinal tract is complex. Figure 16.1 shows a diagram of the gastrointestinal tract, outlining some of the key structures involved in and key physiological parameters that affect oral drug absorption. In order to gain an insight into the numerous factors that can potentially influence the

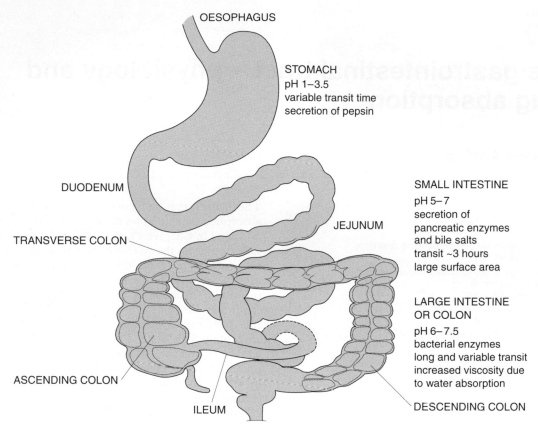

OESOPHAGUS

STOMACH
pH 1–3.5
variable transit time
secretion of pepsin

DUODENUM

SMALL INTESTINE
pH 5–7
secretion of
pancreatic enzymes
and bile salts
transit ~3 hours
large surface area

JEJUNUM

TRANSVERSE COLON

LARGE INTESTINE
OR COLON
pH 6–7.5
bacterial enzymes
long and variable transit
increased viscosity due
to water absorption

ASCENDING COLON

ILEUM

DESCENDING COLON

Fig. 16.1 The gastrointestinal tract.

rate and extent of drug absorption into the systemic circulation, a schematic illustration of the steps involved in the release and absorption of a drug from a tablet dosage form is presented in Figure 16.2. It can be seen from this that the rate and extent of appearance of intact drug in the systemic circulation depends on a succession of kinetic processes.

The slowest step in this series, which is known as the *rate-limiting step*, controls the overall rate and extent of appearance of intact drug in the systemic circulation. The particular rate-limiting step will vary from drug to drug. For a drug which has a very poor aqueous solubility the rate at which it dissolves in the gastrointestinal fluids is often the slowest step, and the bioavailability of that drug is said to be *dissolution-rate limited*. In contrast, for a drug that has a high aqueous solubility its dissolution will be rapid and the rate at which the drug crosses the gastrointestinal membrane may be the rate-limiting step (permeability limited). Other potential rate-limiting steps include the rate of release of the drug from the dosage form (this can be by design in the case of controlled-release dosage forms), the rate at which the

stomach empties the drug into the small intestine, the rate at which the drug is metabolized by enzymes in the intestinal mucosal cells during its passage through them into the mesenteric blood vessels, and the rate of metabolism of drug during its initial passage through the liver, often termed the *'first-pass' effect*.

PHYSIOLOGY OF THE GASTROINTESTINAL TRACT

The gastrointestinal tract is a muscular tube approximately 6 m in length with varying diameters. It stretches from the mouth to the anus and consists of four main anatomical areas: the oesophagus, the stomach, the small intestine and the large intestine or colon. The luminal surface of the tube is not smooth but very rough, thereby increasing the surface area for absorption.

The wall of the gastrointestinal tract is essentially similar in structure along its length, consisting of four principal histological layers (Fig. 16.3):

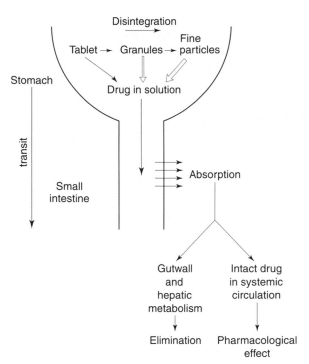

Fig. 16.2 Steps involved prior to a pharmacological effect after administration of a rapidly disintegrating tablet.

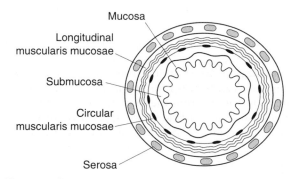

Fig. 16.3 Cross-section through the gastrointestinal tract.

1. The serosa, which is an outer layer of epithelium and supporting connective tissue;
2. The muscularis externa, which contains two layers of smooth muscle tissue, a thinner outer layer which is longitudinal in orientation, and a thicker inner layer, whose fibres are oriented in a circular pattern. Contractions of these muscles provide the forces for movement of gastrointestinal contents;
3. The submucosa, which is a connective tissue layer containing some secretory tissue and which is richly supplied with blood and lymphatic vessels. A network of nerve cells, known as the submucous plexus, is also located in this layer;

4. The mucosa, which is essentially composed of three layers, the muscularis mucosa, which can alter the local conformation of the mucosa, a layer of connective tissue known as the lamina propria, and the epithelium.

The majority of the gastrointestinal epithelium is covered by a layer of mucus. This is a viscoelastic translucent aqueous gel that is secreted throughout the gastrointestinal tract, acting as a protective layer and a mechanical barrier. Mucus is a constantly changing mix of many secretions and exfoliated epithelial cells. It has a large water component (~95%). Its other primary components, which are responsible for its physical and functional properties, are large glycoproteins called mucins. Mucins consist of a protein backbone approximately 800 amino acids long and oligosaccharide side chains that are typically up to 18 residues in length.

The mucus layer ranges in thickness from 5 μm to 500 μm along the length of the gastrointestinal tract, with average values of around 80 μm. The layer is thought to be continuous in the stomach and duodenum, but may not be so in the rest of the small and large intestines.

Mucus is constantly being removed from the luminal surface of the gastrointestinal tract through abrasion and acidic and enzymatic breakdown, and is continually replaced from beneath. Turnover time has been estimated at 4–5 hours, but this may well be an underestimate and is liable to vary along the length of the tract.

The oesophagus

The mouth is the point of entry for most drugs (so-called peroral – via the mouth – administration). At this point contact with the oral mucosa is usually brief. Linking the oral cavity with the stomach is the oesophagus. This is composed of a thick muscular layer approximately 250 mm long and 20 mm in diameter. It joins the stomach at the gastro-oesophageal junction, or cardiac orifice as it is sometimes known.

The oesophagus, apart from the lowest 20 mm which is similar to the gastric mucosa, contains a well differentiated squamous epithelium of non-proliferative cells. Epithelial cell function is mainly protective: simple mucous glands secrete mucus into the narrow lumen to lubricate food and protect the lower part of the oesophagus from gastric acid. The pH of the oesophageal lumen is usually between 5 and 6.

Materials are moved down the oesophagus by the act of swallowing. After swallowing, a single peristaltic wave of contraction, its amplitude linked to the size of the material being swallowed, passes down the length of the oesophagus at the rate of 20–60 mm per second, speeding up as it progresses. When swallowing is repeated in quick succession, the subsequent swallows interrupt the initial peristaltic wave and only the final wave proceeds down the length of the oesophagus to the gastrointestinal junction, carrying material within the lumen with it. Secondary peristaltic waves occur involuntarily in response to any distension of the oesophagus and serve to move sticky lumps of material or refluxed material to the stomach. In the upright position the transit of materials through the oesophagus is assisted by gravity. The oesophageal transit of dosage forms is extremely rapid, usually of the order of 10–14 seconds.

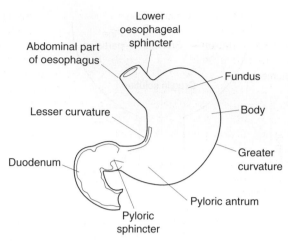

Fig. 16.4 The anatomy of the stomach.

The stomach

The next part of the gastrointestinal tract to be encountered by both food and pharmaceuticals is the stomach. The two major functions of the stomach are:

- to act as a temporary reservoir for ingested food and to deliver it to the duodenum at a controlled rate;
- to reduce ingested solids to a uniform creamy consistency, known as chyme, by the action of acid and enzymatic digestion. This enables better contact of the ingested material with the mucous membrane of the intestines and thereby facilitates absorption.

Another, perhaps less obvious, function of the stomach is its role in reducing the risk of noxious agents reaching the intestine.

The stomach is the most dilated part of the gastrointestinal tract and is situated between the lower end of the oesophagus and the small intestine. Its opening to the duodenum is controlled by the pyloric sphincter. The stomach can be divided into four anatomical regions (Fig. 16.4), namely the fundus, the body, the antrum and the pylorus.

The stomach has a capacity of approximately 1.5 L, although under fasting conditions it usually contains no more than 50 mL of fluid, which is mostly gastric secretions. These include:

- acid secreted by the parietal cells, which maintains the pH of the stomach between 1 and 3.5 in the fasted state;
- the hormone gastrin, which itself is a potent stimulator of gastric acid production. The release

of gastrin is stimulated by peptides, amino acids and distension of the stomach;
- pepsins, which are secreted by the peptic cells in the form of its precursor pepsinogen. Pepsins are peptidases which break down proteins to peptides at low pH. Above pH 5 pepsin is denatured;
- mucus, which is secreted by the surface mucosal cells and lines the gastric mucosa. In the stomach the mucus protects the gastric mucosa from autodigestion by the pepsin–acid combination.

Contrary to popular belief very little drug absorption occurs in the stomach owing to its small surface area compared to the small intestine. The rate of gastric emptying can be a controlling factor in the onset of drug absorption from the major absorptive site, the small intestine. Gastric emptying will be discussed under gastrointestinal transit later in this chapter.

The small intestine

The small intestine is the longest (4–5 m) and most convoluted part of the gastrointestinal tract, extending from the pyloric sphincter of the stomach to the ileocaecal junction where it joins the large intestine. Its main functions are:

- digestion: the process of enzymatic digestion, which began in the stomach, is completed in the small intestine.
- absorption: the small intestine is the region where most nutrients and other materials are absorbed.

The small intestine is divided into the duodenum, which is 200–300 mm in length, the jejunum, which is approximately 2 m in length, and the ileum, which is approximately 3 m in length.

The wall of the small intestine has a rich network of both blood and lymphatic vessels. The gastrointestinal circulation is the largest systemic regional vasculature and nearly a third of the cardiac output flows through the gastrointestinal viscera. The blood vessels of the small intestine receive blood from the superior mesenteric artery via branched arterioles. The blood leaving the small intestine flows into the hepatic portal vein, which carries it via the liver to the systemic circulation. Drugs that are metabolized by the liver are degraded before they reach the systemic circulation: this is termed hepatic presystemic clearance, or first-pass metabolism.

The wall of the small intestine also contains lacteals, which contain lymph and are part of the lymphatic system. The lymphatic system is important in the absorption of fats from the gastrointestinal tract. In the ileum are areas of lymphoid tissue close to the epithelial surface which are known as Peyer's patches. These cells play a key role in the immune response as they transport macromolecules and are involved in antigen uptake.

The surface area of the small intestine is increased enormously, by about 600 times that of a simple cylinder, to approximately 200 m^2 in an adult, by several adaptations which render the small intestine such a good absorption site:

- Folds of Kerckring: these are submucosal folds which extend circularly most of the way around the intestine and are particularly well developed in the duodenum and jejunum. They are several millimetres in depth.
- Villi: these have been described as finger-like projections into the lumen (approximately 0.5–1.5 mm in length and 0.1 mm in diameter). They are well supplied with blood vessels. Each villus contains an arteriole, a venule and a blind-ending lymphatic vessel (lacteal). The structure of a villus is shown in Figure 16.5.
- Microvilli: approximately 600–1000 of these brush-like structures (~ 1 μm in length and 0.1 μm in width) cover each villus, providing the largest increase in surface area. These are covered by a fibrous substance known as glycocalyx.

The luminal pH of the small intestine increases to between about 6 and 7.5. The sources of the secretions that produce these pH values in the small intestine are:

- Brunner's glands, which are located in the duodenum and are responsible for the secretion of bicarbonate which neutralizes the acid emptied from the stomach;

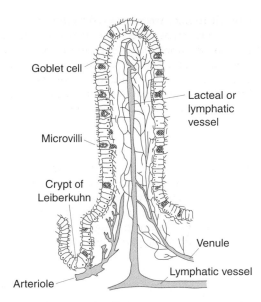

Fig. 16.5 Structure of a villus.

Goblet cell

Lacteal or lymphatic vessel

Microvilli

Crypt of Leiberkuhn

Venule

Arteriole

Lymphatic vessel

- intestinal cells, which are present throughout the small intestine and secrete mucus and enzymes. The enzymes, hydrolases and proteases, continue the digestive process;
- pancreatic secretions. The pancreas is a large gland which secretes about 1–2 L of pancreatic juice per day into the small intestine via a duct. The components of pancreatic juice are sodium bicarbonate and enzymes. The enzymes consist of proteases, principally trypsin, chymotrypsin and carboxypeptidases, which are secreted as inactive precursors or zymogens and converted to their active forms in the lumen by the enzyme enterokinase. Lipase and amylase are both secreted in their active forms. The bicarbonate component is largely regulated by the pH of chyme delivered into the small intestine from the stomach;
- bile, which is secreted by hepatocytes in the liver into bile canaliculi, concentrated in the gallbladder and hepatic biliary system by the removal of sodium ions, chloride and water, and delivered to the duodenum. Bile is a complex aqueous mixture of organic solutes (bile acids, phospholipids, particularly lecithin, cholesterol and bilirubin) and inorganic compounds (plasma electrolytes; sodium and potassium). Bile pigments, the most important of which is bilirubin, are excreted in the faeces, but the bile acids are absorbed by an active process in the terminal ileum. They are returned to the liver via the hepatic portal vein and, as they have a high

hepatic clearance, are resecreted in the bile. This process is known as enterohepatic recirculation. The main functions of the bile are promoting the efficient absorption of dietary fat, such as fatty acids and cholesterol, by aiding its emulsification and micellar solubilization, and the provision of excretory pathways for degradation products.

The colon

The colon is the final part of the gastrointestinal tract. It stretches from the ileocaecal junction to the anus and makes up approximately the last 1.5 m of the 6 m of the gastrointestinal tract. It is composed of the caecum (~85 mm in length), the ascending colon (~200 mm), the hepatic flexure, the transverse colon (usually greater than 450 mm), the splenic flexure, the descending colon (~300 mm), the sigmoid colon (~400 mm) and the rectum, as shown in Figure 16.6. The ascending and descending colons are relatively fixed, as they are attached via the flexures and the caecum. The transverse and sigmoid colons, however, are much more flexible.

The colon, unlike the small intestine has no specialized villi. However, the microvilli of the absorptive epithelial cells, the presence of crypts, and the irregularly folded mucosae serve to increase the surface area of the colon by 10–15 times that of a simple cylinder. The surface area nevertheless remains approximately 1/30th that of the small intestine.

The main functions of the colon are:

- the absorption of sodium ions, chloride ions and water from the lumen in exchange for bicarbonate and potassium ions. Thus the colon has a significant homeostatic role in the body.
- the storage and compaction of faeces.

The colon is permanently colonized by an extensive number (about 10^{12} per gram of contents) and variety of bacteria. This large bacterial mass is capable of several metabolic reactions, including hydrolysis of fatty acid esters and the reduction of inactive conjugated drugs to their active form. The bacteria rely upon undigested polysaccharides in the diet and the carbohydrate components of secretions such as mucus for their carbon and energy sources. They degrade the polysaccharides to produce short-chain fatty acids (acetic, proprionic and butyric acids), which lower the luminal pH, and the gases hydrogen, carbon dioxide and methane. Thus the pH of the caecum is around 6–6.5. This increases to around 7–7.5 towards the distal parts of the colon.

Recently there has been much interest in the exploitation of the enzymes produced by these bacteria with respect to targeted drug delivery to this region of the gastrointestinal tract.

THE TRANSIT OF PHARMACEUTICALS IN THE GASTROINTESTINAL TRACT

As the oral route is the one by which the majority of pharmaceuticals are administered, it is important to know how these materials behave during their passage through the gastrointestinal tract. It is known that the small intestine is the major site of drug absorption, and thus the time a drug is present in this part of the gastrointestinal tract is extremely significant. If sustained- or controlled-release drug delivery systems are being designed, it is important to consider factors that will affect their behaviour and, in particular, their transit times through certain regions of the gastrointestinal tract.

In general, most dosage forms, when taken in an upright position, transit through the oesophagus quickly, usually in less than 15 seconds. Transit through the oesophagus is dependent both upon the dosage form and posture.

Tablets/capsules taken in the supine position, especially if taken without water, are liable to lodge in the oesophagus. Adhesion to the oesophageal wall can occur as a result of partial dehydration at the site of contact and the formation of a gel between the formulation and the oesophagus. The chances of adhesion will depend on the shape, size and type of formulation. Transit of liquids, for example, has always been observed to be rapid, and in general faster than that of solids. A delay in reaching the stomach may well delay a drug's onset of action or

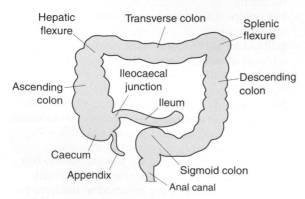

Fig. 16.6 The anatomy of the colon.

cause damage or irritation to the oesophageal wall, e.g. potassium chloride tablets.

Gastric emptying

The time a dosage form takes to traverse the stomach is usually termed the *gastric residence time, gastric emptying time* or *gastric emptying rate*.

Gastric emptying of pharmaceuticals is highly variable and is dependent on the dosage form and the fed/fasted state of the stomach. Normal gastric residence times usually range between 5 minutes and 2 hours, although much longer times (over 12 hours) have been recorded, particularly for large single units. In the fasted state the electrical activity in the stomach – the interdigestive myoelectric cycle, or migrating myoelectric complex (MMC) as it is known – governs its activity and hence the transit of dosage forms. It is characterized by a repeating cycle of four phases.

Phase I is a relatively inactive period of 40–60 minutes with only rare contractions occurring. Increasing numbers of contractions occur in phase II, which has a similar duration to phase I. Phase III is characterized by powerful peristaltic contractions which open the pylorus at the base and clear the stomach of any residual material. This is sometimes called the *housekeeper wave*. Phase IV is a short transitional period between the powerful activity of phase III and the inactivity of phase I. The cycle repeats itself every 2 hours until a meal is ingested and the fed state or motility is initiated. In this state, two distinct patterns of activity have been observed. The proximal stomach relaxes to receive food and gradual contractions of this region move the contents distally. Peristalsis – contractions of the distal stomach – serve to mix and break down food particles and move them towards the pyloric sphincter. The pyloric sphincter allows liquids and small food particles to empty while other material is retropulsed into the antrum of the stomach and caught up by the next peristaltic wave for further size reduction before emptying.

Thus in the fed state liquids, pellets and disintegrated tablets will tend to empty with food, yet large sustained or controlled release dosage forms can be retained in the stomach for long periods of time. In the fasted state the stomach is less discriminatory between dosage form types, with emptying appearing to be an exponential process and being related to the point in the MMC at which the formulation is ingested.

Many factors influence gastric emptying, as well as the type of dosage form and the presence of food: these include the postural position, the composition of the food, the effect of drugs and disease state. In general, food, particularly fatty foods, delays gastric emptying and hence the absorption of drugs. Therefore, a drug will reach the small intestine most rapidly if it is administered with water to a patient whose stomach is empty. Metoclopramide, which is a drug that increases gastric emptying rate, has been shown to increase the rate of absorption of paracetamol, whereas proprantheline, a drug which delays gastric emptying, has been shown to delay its rate of absorption (Nimmo et al 1973).

Small intestinal transit

There are two main types of intestinal movement, propulsive and mixing. The propulsive movements primarily determine the intestinal transit rate and hence the residence time of the drug or dosage form in the small intestine. As this is the main site of absorption in the gastrointestinal tract for most drugs, the small intestinal transit time (that is, the time of transit between the stomach and the caecum) is an important factor with respect to drug bioavailability.

Small intestinal transit has been found to be relatively constant, at around 3 hours. In contrast to the stomach, the small intestine does not discriminate between solids and liquids, and hence between dosage forms, or between the fed and the fasted state.

Small intestinal residence time is particularly important for dosage forms that release their drug slowly (e.g. controlled- sustained- prolonged-release systems) as they pass along the length of the gastrointestinal tract; enteric-coated dosage forms which release drug only when they reach the small intestine; drugs that dissolve slowly in intestinal fluids; and drugs that are absorbed by intestinal carrier-mediated transport systems.

Colonic transit

The colonic transit of pharmaceuticals is long and variable and depends on the type of dosage form, diet, eating pattern and disease state.

Contractile activity in the colon can be divided into two main types:

- Propulsive contractions or mass movements, which are associated with the aboral (away from the mouth) movement of contents;
- Segmental or haustral contractions, which serve to mix the luminal contents and result in only small aboral movements. Segmental contractions are brought about by contraction of the circular

muscle and predominate, whereas the propulsive contractions, which are due to contractions of the longitudinal muscle, occur only 3–4 times daily in normal individuals.

Colonic transit is thus characterized by short bursts of activity followed by long periods of stasis. Movement is mainly aboral, i.e. towards the anus. Colonic transit can vary from anything between 2 and 48 hours. In most individuals mouth-to-anus transit times are longer than 24 hours.

BARRIERS TO DRUG ABSORPTION

Some of the barriers to absorption that a drug may encounter once it is released from its dosage form and has dissolved into the gastrointestinal fluids are shown in Figure 16.7. The drug needs to remain in solution and not become bound to food or other material within the gastrointestinal tract. It needs to be chemically stable in order to withstand the pH of the gastrointestinal tract, and it must be resistant to enzymatic degradation in the lumen. The drug then needs to diffuse across the mucous layer, without binding to it, across the unstirred water layer, and subsequently across the gastrointestinal membrane, its main cellular barrier. After passing through this cellular barrier the drug encounters the liver before it reaches the systemic circulation. Any of these bar-

riers can prevent some or all of the drug reaching the systemic circulation, and can therefore have a detrimental effect on its bioavailability.

The environment within the lumen

The environment within the lumen of the gastrointestinal tract has a major effect on the rate and extent of drug absorption.

Gastrointestinal pH

The pH of fluids varies considerably along the length of the gastrointestinal tract. Gastric fluid is highly acidic, normally exhibiting a pH within the range 1–3.5 in healthy people in the fasted state. Following the ingestion of a meal the gastric juice is buffered to a less acidic pH, which is dependent on meal composition. Typical gastric pH values following a meal are in the range 3–7. Depending on meal size the gastric pH returns to the lower fasted-state values within 2–3 hours. Thus only a dosage form ingested with or soon after a meal will encounter these higher pH values. This may be an important consideration in terms of the chemical stability of a drug, or in achieving drug dissolution or absorption.

Intestinal pH values are higher than gastric pH values owing to the neutralization of the gastric acid with bicarbonate ions secreted by the pancreas into the small intestine. There is a gradual rise in pH along the length of the small intestine from the duo-

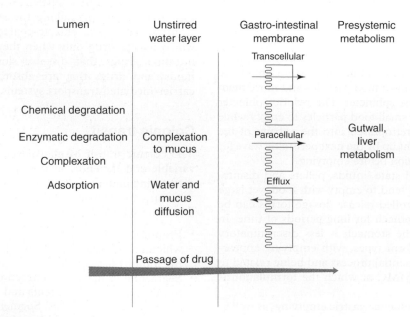

Fig. 16.7 Barriers to absorption.

Table 16.1 pH in the small intestine in healthy humans in the fasted and fed states		
Location	Fasted state pH	Fed state pH
Mid-distal duodenum	4.9	5.2
	6.1	5.4
	6.3	5.1
	6.4	
Jejunum	4.4–6.5	5.2–6.0
	6.6	6.2
Ileum	6.5	6.8–7.8
	6.8–8.0	6.8–8.0
	7.4	7.5

Data from Gray and Dressman 1996.

denum to the ileum. Table 16.1 summarizes some of the literature values recorded for small intestinal pH in the fed and fasted states. The pH drops again in the colon, as the bacterial enzymes, which are localized in the colonic region, break down undigested carbohydrates into short-chain fatty acids; this lowers the pH in the colon to around 6.5.

The gastrointestinal pH may influence the absorption of drugs in a variety of ways. It may influence the chemical stability of the drug in the lumen, its dissolution or its absorption, if the drug is a weak electrolyte.

Chemical degradation due to pH-dependent hydrolysis can occur in the gastrointestinal tract. The result of this instability is incomplete bioavailability, as only a fraction of the administered dose reaches the systemic circulation in the form of intact drug. The extent of degradation of penicillin G (benzylpenicillin), the first of the penicillins, after oral administration depends on its residence time in the stomach and gastric pH. This gastric instability tends to preclude its oral use. The antibiotic erythromycin and proton pump inhibitors (e.g. omeprazole) degrade rapidly at acidic pH values and therefore have to be formulated as enteric-coated dosage forms to ensure good bioavailability (see Chapter 17).

The effects of pH on the drug dissolution and absorption processes are also discussed in Chapter 17.

Luminal enzymes

The primary enzyme found in gastric juice is pepsin. Lipases, amylases and proteases are secreted from the pancreas into the small intestine in response to ingestion of food. These enzymes are responsible for most of nutrient digestion. Pepsins and the proteases are responsible for the degradation of protein and

peptide drugs in the lumen. Other drugs that resemble nutrients, such as nucleotides and fatty acids, may also be susceptible to enzymatic degradation. The lipases may also affect the release of drugs from fat/oil-containing dosage forms. Drugs that are esters can also be susceptible to hydrolysis in the lumen.

Bacteria, which are mainly localized within the colonic region of the gastrointestinal tract, also secrete enzymes which are capable of a range of reactions. These enzymes have been utilized when designing drugs or dosage forms to target the colon. Sulphasalazine, for example, is a prodrug of 5-aminosalicylic acid linked via an azo bond to sulphapyridine. The sulphapyridine moiety makes the drug too large and hydrophilic to be absorbed in the upper gastrointestinal tract, and thus permits its transport intact to the colonic region, where the bacterial enzymes reduce the azo bond and release the active drug, 5-aminosalycylic acid, for local action in colonic diseases such as inflammatory bowel disease.

Influence of food in the gastrointestinal tract

The presence of food in the gastrointestinal tract can influence the rate and extent of absorption, either directly or indirectly via a range of mechanisms.

Complexation of drugs with components in the diet Drugs are capable of binding to components within the diet. In general this only becomes an issue (with respect to bioavailability) where an irreversible or an insoluble complex is formed. In such cases the fraction of the administered dose that becomes complexed is unavailable for absorption. Tetracycline, for example, forms non-absorbable complexes with calcium and iron, and thus it is advised that patients do not take products containing calcium or iron, such as milk, iron preparations or indigestion remedies, at the same time of day as the tetracycline. However, if the complex formed is water soluble and readily dissociates to liberate the 'free' drug, then there may be little effect on drug absorption.

Alteration of pH In general, food tends to increase stomach pH by acting as a buffer. This is liable to decrease the rate of dissolution and subsequent absorption of a weakly basic drug and increase that of a weakly acidic one.

Alteration of gastric emptying As already mentioned, some foods, particularly those containing a high proportion of fat, and some drugs, tend to reduce gastric emptying and thus delay the onset of action of certain drugs.

Stimulation of gastrointestinal secretions Gastrointestinal secretions (e.g. pepsin) produced in response to food may result in the degradation of drugs that are susceptible to enzymatic metabolism, and hence in a reduction in their bioavailability. The ingestion of food, particularly fats, stimulates the secretion of bile. Bile salts are surface active agents and can increase the dissolution of poorly soluble drugs, thereby enhancing their absorption. However, bile salts have been shown to form insoluble and hence non-absorbable complexes with some drugs, such as neomycin, kanamycin and nystatin.

Competition between food components and drugs for specialized absorption mechanisms In the case of those drugs that have a chemical structure similar to nutrients required by the body for which specialized absorption mechanisms exist, there is a possibility of competitive inhibition of drug absorption.

Increased viscosity of gastrointestinal contents The presence of food in the gastrointestinal tract provides a viscous environment which may result in a reduction in the rate of drug dissolution. In addition, the rate of diffusion of a drug in solution from the lumen to the absorbing membrane lining the gastrointestinal tract may be reduced by an increase in viscosity. Both of these effects tend to decrease the bioavailability of drug.

Food-induced changes in presystemic metabolism Certain foods may increase the bioavailability of drugs that are susceptible to presystemic intestinal metabolism by interacting with the metabolic process. Grapefruit juice, for example, is capable of inhibiting the intestinal cytochrome P450 (CYP3A family) and thus, taken with drugs that are susceptible to CYP3A metabolism, is likely to result in their increased bioavailability. Clinically relevant interactions exist between grapefruit juice and the antihistamine terfenadine, the immunosuppresant cyclosporin, the protease inhibitor saquinavir and the calcium channel blocker verapamil.

Food-induced changes in blood flow Blood flow to the gastrointestinal tract and liver increases shortly after a meal, thereby increasing the rate at which drugs are presented to the liver. The metabolism of some drugs (e.g. propranolol, hydralazine, dextropropoxyphene) is sensitive to their rate of presentation to the liver: the faster the rate of presentation the larger the fraction of drug that escapes first-pass metabolism. This is because the enzyme systems responsible for their metabolism become saturated by the increased rate of presentation of the drug to the site of biotransformation. For this reason, the effects of food serve to increase the bioavailability of some drugs that are susceptible to first-pass metabolism.

It is evident that food can influence the absorption of many drugs from the gastrointestinal tract by a variety of mechanisms. Drug–food interactions are often classified into five categories: those that cause reduced, delayed, increased and accelerated absorption, and those on which food has no effect. The reader is referred to reviews by Fleischer et al. (1999), Welling (1996) and Evans (2000) for more detailed information on the effect of food on the rate and extent of drug absorption.

Disease state and physiological disorders

Disease states and physiological disorders associated with the gastrointestinal tract are likely to influence the absorption and hence the bioavailability of orally administered drugs. Local diseases can cause alterations in gastric pH that can affect the stability, dissolution and/or absorption of the drug. Gastric surgery can cause drugs to exhibit differences in bioavailability than that in normal individuals. For example, partial or total gastrectomy results in drugs reaching the duodenum more rapidly than in normal individuals. This increased rate of presentation to the small intestine may result in an increased overall rate of absorption of drugs that are primarily absorbed in the small intestine. However, drugs that require a period of time in the stomach to facilitate their dissolution may show reduced bioavailability in such patients.

The unstirred water layer

The unstirred water layer or aqueous boundary layer is a more or less stagnant layer of water, mucus and glycocalyx adjacent to the intestinal wall. It is thought to be created by incomplete mixing of the luminal contents near the intestinal mucosal surface, and to be around 30–100 μm in thickness. This layer can provide a diffusion barrier to drugs. Some drugs are also capable of complexing with mucus, thereby reducing their availability for absorption.

The gastrointestinal membrane

The structure of the membrane

The gastrointestinal membrane separates the lumen of the stomach and intestines from the systemic circulation. It is the main cellular barrier to the absorption of drugs from the gastrointestinal tract. The membrane is complex in nature, being composed of lipids, proteins, lipoproteins and polysaccharides, and has a bilayer structure (Fig. 16.8). The barrier has the characteristics of a semipermeable membrane, allowing the rapid transit of some materials and impeding

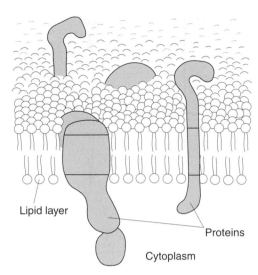

Fig. 16.8   Structure of the membrane.

1 – Transcellular   3 – Carrier mediated
2 – Paracellular   4 – Transcytosis

Fig. 16.9   Mechanisms of permeability (absorptive).

or preventing the passage of others. It is permeable to amino acids, sugars, fatty acids and other nutrients, and impermeable to plasma proteins. The membrane can be viewed as a semipermeable lipoidal sieve, which allows the passage of lipid-soluble molecules across it and the passage of water and small hydrophilic molecules through its numerous aqueous pores. In addition there are a number of transporter proteins or carrier molecules that exist in the membrane and which, with the help of energy, transport materials back and forth across it.

Mechanisms of transport across the membrane

There are two main mechanisms of drug transport across the gastrointestinal epithelium: transcellular, i.e. across the cells, and paracellular, i.e. between the cells. The transcellular pathway is further divided into simple passive diffusion, carrier-mediated transport (active transport and facilitated diffusion) and endocytosis. These pathways are illustrated in Figure 16.9.

Transcellular pathways

Passive diffusion   This is the preferred route of transport for relatively small lipophilic molecules and thus many drugs. In this process, drug molecules pass across the lipoidal membrane via passive diffusion from a region of high concentration in the lumen to a region of lower concentration in the blood. This lower concentration is maintained primarily by blood flow. The rate of transport is determined by the physicochemical properties of the drug, the nature of the membrane and the concen-

tration gradient of the drug across the membrane. The process initially involves the partitioning of the drug between the aqueous fluids within the gastrointestinal tract and the lipoidal-like membrane of the lining of the epithelium. The drug in solution in the membrane then diffuses across the epithelial cell/cells within the gastrointestinal barrier to blood in the capillary network in the lamina propria. Upon reaching the blood the drug will be rapidly distributed, so maintaining a much lower concentration than that at the absorption site. If the cell membranes and fluid regions making up the gastrointestinal–blood barrier can be considered as a single membrane, then the stages involved in gastrointestinal absorption could be represented by the model shown in Figure 16.10.

Passive diffusion of drugs across the gastrointestinal–blood barrier can often be described mathematically by Fick's first law of diffusion. This states that the rate of diffusion across a membrane (dC/dt) is proportional to the difference in concentration on each side of that membrane. Therefore, the rate of appearance of drug in the blood at the absorption site is given by:

$$dC/dt = k(C_g - C_b) \qquad (16.1)$$

where dC/dt is the rate of appearance of drug in the blood at the site of absorption, k is the proportionality constant, C_g is the concentration of drug in solution in the gastrointestinal fluid at the absorption site, and C_b is the concentration of drug in the blood at the site of absorption.

The proportionality constant k incorporates the diffusion coefficient of the drug in the gastrointestinal membrane (D), and the thickness (h) and surface area of the membrane (A).

$$k = \frac{DA}{h} \qquad (16.2)$$

These equations indicate that the rate of gastrointestinal absorption of a drug by passive diffusion depends on the surface area of the membrane that is

Fig. 16.10   Diagrammatic representation of absorption via passive diffusion.

available for drug absorption. Thus the small intestine, primarily the duodenum, is the major site of drug absorption, owing principally to the presence of villi and microvilli which provide such a large surface area for absorption (see earlier).

Equation 16.1 also indicates that the rate of drug absorption depends on a large concentration gradient of drug existing across the gastrointestinal membrane. This concentration gradient is influenced by the apparent partition coefficients exhibited by the drug with respect to the gastrointestinal membrane/fluid interface and the gastrointestinal membrane/blood interface. It is important that the drug has sufficient affinity (solubility) for the membrane phase that it can partition readily into the gastrointestinal membrane. In addition, after diffusing across the membrane the drug should exhibit sufficient solubility in the blood such that it can partition readily out of the membrane phase into the blood.

On entering the blood in the capillary network in the lamina propria, the drug will be carried away from the site of absorption by the rapidly circulating gastrointestinal blood supply and will become diluted by distribution into a large volume of blood (i.e. the systemic circulation), distribution into body tissues and other fluids, and by metabolism and excretion. In addition, the drug may bind to plasma proteins in the blood which will further lower the concentration of free (i.e. diffusable) drug in the blood. Consequently, the blood acts as a 'sink' for absorbed drug and ensures that the concentration of drug in the blood at the site of absorption is low in relation to that in the gastrointestinal fluids at the site of absorption, i.e. $C_g \gg C_b$. The 'sink' conditions provided by the systemic circulation ensure that a large concentration gradient is maintained across the gastrointestinal membrane during the absorption process.

The passive absorption process is driven solely by the concentration gradient of the diffusable species of the drug that exists across the gastrointestinal–blood barrier. Thus Eqns 16.1 and 16.2 can be combined and written as:

$$dC / dt = \frac{DAC_g}{h}$$ (16.3)

and because for a given membrane D, A and h can be regarded as constants, Eqn 16.3 becomes:

$$dC/dt = kC_g$$ (16.4)

Equation 16.4 is an expression for a first-order kinetic process (see Chapter 7) and indicates that the rate of passive absorption will be proportional to the concentration of absorbable drug in solution in the gastrointestinal fluids at the site of absorption, and therefore that the gastrointestinal absorption of most drugs follows first-order kinetics.

It has been assumed in this description that the drug exists solely in one single absorbable species. Many drugs, however, are weak electrolytes that exist in aqueous solution as two species, namely the unionized species and the ionized species. Because it is the unionized form of a weak electrolyte drug that exhibits greater lipid solubility compared to the corresponding ionized form, the gastrointestinal membrane is more permeable to the unionized species. Thus the rate of passive absorption of a weak electrolyte is related to the fraction of total drug that exists in the unionized form in solution in the gastrointestinal fluids at the site of absorption. This fraction is determined by the dissociation constant of the drug (i.e. its pK_a value) and by the pH of the aqueous environment, in accordance with the Henderson–Hasselbalch equations for weak acids and bases (see Chapters 3 and 8). The gastrointestinal absorption of a weak electrolyte drug is enhanced when the pH at the site of absorption favours the formation of a large fraction of the drug in aqueous solution that is unionized. This forms the basis of the pH-partition hypothesis (see Chapter 17).

Carrier-mediated transport As already stated, the majority of drugs are absorbed across cells (i.e. transcellularly) via passive diffusion. However, certain compounds and many nutrients are absorbed transcellularly by a carrier-mediated transport mechanism, of which there are two main types, **active transport** and **facilitated diffusion** or **transport**.

Active transport In contrast to passive diffusion, active transport involves the active participation by the apical cell membrane of the columnar absorption cells. A carrier or membrane transporter is responsible for binding a drug and transporting it across the membrane by a process illustrated in Figure 16.11.

Carrier-mediated absorption is often explained by assuming a shuttling process across the epithelial membrane. The drug molecule or ion forms a complex with the carrier/transporter in the surface of the apical cell membrane of a columnar absorption cell; the drug–carrier complex then moves across the membrane and liberates the drug on the other side of the membrane. The carrier (now free) returns to its initial position in the surface of the cell membrane adjacent to the gastrointestinal tract, to await the arrival of another drug molecule or ion.

Active transport is a process whereby materials can be transported against a concentration gradient across a cell membrane, i.e. transport can occur from a region of lower concentration to one of higher concentration. Therefore, active transport is an energy-consuming process. The energy arises either from the hydrolysis of ATP or from the transmembranous sodium gradient and/or electrical potential.

There are a large number of carrier-mediated active transport systems or membrane transporters in the small intestine, which can be present either on the apical (brush border) or on the basolateral membrane. These include the peptide transporters, the nucleoside transporters, the sugar transporters, the bile acid transporters, the amino acid transporters, the organic anion transporters and the vitamin transporters.

Many nutrients, such as amino acids, sugars, electrolytes (e.g. sodium, potassium, calcium, iron, chloride, bicarbonate), vitamins (thiamine (B_1), nicotinic acid, riboflavin (B_2), pyroxidine (B_6) and B_{12}) and bile salts are actively transported. Each carrier system is generally concentrated in a specific segment of the gastrointestinal tract. The substance that is transported by that carrier will thus be absorbed preferentially in the location of highest carrier density. For example, the bile acid transporters are only found in the lower part of the small intestine, the ileum. Each carrier/transporter has its own substrate specificity with respect to the chemical structure of the substance that it will transport. Some carriers/transporters have broader specificity than others. Thus if a drug structurally resembles a natural substance which is actively transported, then the drug is also likely to be transported by the same carrier mechanism.

Many peptide-like drugs, such as the penicillins, cephalosporins, angiotensin-converting enzyme inhibitors (ACE) inhibitors and renin inhibitors, rely on the peptide transporters for their efficient absorption. Nucleosides and their analogues for antiviral and anticancer drugs depend on the nucleoside transporters for their uptake. L-dopa and α-methyldopa are transported by the carrier-mediated process for amino acids. L-dopa has a much faster

Fig. 16.11 Diagrammatic representation of active transport of a drug across a cell membrane.

permeability rate than methyldopa, which has been attributed to the lower affinity of methyldopa for the amino acid carrier.

Unlike passive absorption, where the rate of absorption is directly proportional to the concentration of the absorbable species of the drug at the absorption site, active transport proceeds at a rate that is proportional to the drug concentration only at low concentrations. At higher concentrations the carrier mechanism becomes saturated and further increases in drug concentration will not increase the rate of absorption, i.e. the rate of absorption remains constant. Absorption rate–concentration relationships for active and passive processes are compared in Figure 16.12.

Competition between two similar substances for the same transfer mechanism, and the inhibition of absorption of one or both compounds, are other characteristics of carrier-mediated transport. Inhibition of absorption may also be observed with agents such as sodium fluoride, cyanide or dinitrophenol, which interfere with cell metabolism.

Some substances may be absorbed by simultaneous carrier-mediated and passive transport processes. For example, certain pyrimidines, such as uracil and thymine, are absorbed both passively and via a carrier-mediated process. The contribution of the carrier-mediated process to the overall absorption rate decreases with concentration, and at a sufficiently high concentration is negligible.

In summary, active transport mechanisms:

- must have a carrier molecule;
- must have a source of energy;
- can be inhibited by metabolic inhibitors such as dinitrophenol;

Fig. 16.12 Relationship between rate of absorption and concentration at the absorption site for active and passive processes.

- show temperature dependence;
- can be competitively inhibited by substrate analogues.

Active transport also plays an important role in the intestinal, renal and biliary excretion of many drugs.

Facilitated diffusion or transport This carrier-mediated process differs from active transport in that it cannot transport a substance against a concentration gradient of that substance. Therefore, facilitated diffusion does not require an energy input but does require a concentration gradient for its driving force, as does passive diffusion. When substances are transported by facilitated diffusion they are transported down the concentration gradient but at a much faster rate than would be anticipated based on the molecular size and polarity of the molecule. The process, like active transport, is saturable and is subject to inhibition by competitive inhibitors. In terms of drug absorption, facilitated diffusion seems to play a very minor role.

More information on carrier-mediated transport of drugs within the intestines can be obtained from reviews by Oh et al. (1999), Tsuji and Tamia (1996) and Yang et al. (1999).

Endocytosis Endocytosis is the process by which the plasma membrane of the cell invaginates and the invaginations become pinched off, forming small intracellular membrane-bound vesicles that enclose a volume of material. Thus material can be transported into the cell. After invagination the material is often transferred to other vesicles or lysosomes and digested. Some material will escape digestion and migrate to the basolateral surface of the cell, where it is exocytosed. This uptake process is energy dependent. Endocytosis can be further subdivided into four main processes: fluid-phase endocytosis or pinocytosis; receptor-mediated endocytosis; phagocytosis; and transcytosis. Endocytosis is thought to be the primary mechanism of transport of macromolecules. The process and pathways of endocytosis are complex.

Pinocytosis Fluid-phase endocytosis or pinocytosis is the engulfment of small droplets of extracellular fluid by membrane vesicles. The cell will internalize material regardless of its metabolic importance to that cell. The efficiency of this process is low. The fat-soluble vitamins A, D, E and K are absorbed via pinocytosis.

Receptor-mediated endocytosis Many cells within the body have receptors on their cell surfaces that are capable of binding with suitable ligands to form ligand–receptor complexes on the cell surface. These complexes cluster on the cell surface and then invaginate and break off from the membrane to form coated vesicles. The binding process between the ligand and the receptor on the cell surface is thought to trigger a conformational change in the membrane to allow this process to occur. Once within the cytoplasm of the cell the coated vesicles rapidly lose their coat, and the resulting uncoated vesicles will promptly deliver their contents to early endosomes. Within the endosomes the ligands usually dissociate from their receptors many of which are then recycled to the plasma membrane. The dissociated ligands and solutes are next delivered to prelysosomes and finally to lysosomes, the end-stage of the endocytic pathway. Lysosomes are spherical or oval cell organelles surrounded by a single membrane. They contain digestive enzymes which break down bacteria and large molecules, such as protein, polysaccharides and nucleic acids, which have entered the cell via endocytosis.

Phagocytosis Phagocytosis can be defined as the engulfment by the cell membrane of particles larger than 500 nm. This process is important for the absorption of polio and other vaccines from the gastrointestinal tract.

Transcytosis Transcytosis is the process by which the material internalized by the membrane domain is transported through the cell and secreted on the opposite side.

Paracellular pathway

The paracellular pathway differs from all the other absorption pathways as it is the transport of materials in the aqueous pores between the cells rather than across them. The cells are joined together via closely fitting tight junctions on their apical side. The intercellular spaces occupy only about 0.01% of the total surface area of the epithelium. The tightness of these junctions can vary considerably between different epithelia in the body. In general, absorptive epithelia, such as that of the small intestine, tend to be leakier than other epithelia. The paracellular pathway decreases in importance down the length of the gastrointestinal tract, and as the number and size of pores between the epithelial cells decrease.

The paracellular route of absorption is important for the transport of ions such as calcium and for the transport of sugars, amino acids and peptides at concentrations above the capacity of their carriers. Small hydrophilic and charged drugs that do not distribute into cell membranes cross the gastrointestinal epithelium via the paracellular pathway. The molecular weight cut-off for the paracellular route is usually considered to be 200 Da, although some larger drugs have been shown to be absorbed via this route.

The paracellular pathway can be divided into a convective ('solvent drag') and diffusive component.

The convective component is the rate at which the compound is carried across the epithelium via the water flux.

Efflux of drugs from the intestine

It is now known that there are countertransport efflux proteins that expel specific drugs back into the lumen of the gastrointestinal tract after they have been absorbed. One of the key countertransport proteins is P-glycoprotein. P-glycoprotein is expressed at high levels on the apical surface of columnar cells (brush border membrane) in the jejunum. It is also present on the surface of many other epithelia and endothelia in the body, and on the surface of tumour cells. P-glycoproteins were originally discovered because of their ability to cause multidrug resistance in tumour cells by preventing the intracellular accumulation of many cytotoxic cancer drugs by pumping the drugs back out of the tumours. Certain drugs with wide structural diversity (Table 16.2) are susceptible to efflux from the intestine via P-glyocprotein. Such efflux may have a detrimental effect on drug bioavailability. These countertransport efflux proteins pump

Table 16.2 Examples of transport mechanisms of commonly used drugs across the gastrointestinal absorptive epithelia (adapted from Brayden 1997)

Route	Examples	Therapeutic class
Transcellular passive diffusion	Propranol	β-Blocker
	Testosterone	Steroid
	Ketoprofen	Non-steroidal anti-inflammatory
	Cisapride	Antispasmodic
	Oestradiol	Sex hormone
	Naproxen	Non-steroidal anti-inflammatory
Paracellular	Cimetidine	H₂ antagonist
	Loperamide	Antidiarrhoeal
	Atenolol	β-Blocker
	Mannitol	Sugar used as paracellular marker
	Tiludronate	Bisphosphonate
Carrier mediated	Cephalexin	Anti-bacterial
	Captopril	ACE inhibitor
	Bestatin	Anticancer
	Levodopa	Dopaminergic
	Foscarnet	Antiviral
Transcellular diffusion subject to P-glycoprotein efflux	Cyclosporine	Immunosuppressant
	Nifedipine	Calcium channel blocker
	Verapamil	Calcium channel blocker
	Paclitaxel	Anticancer
	Celiprolol	β-Blocker
	Digoxin	Cardiac glycoside

drugs out of cells in a similar way to which nutrients, and drugs are actively absorbed across the gastrointestinal membrane. This process therefore requires energy, can work against a concentration gradient, can be competitively inhibited by structural analogues or be inhibited by inhibitors of cell metabolism, and is a saturable process.

Table 16.2 summarizes the main mechanisms of drug transport across the gastrointestinal epithelia for a number of commonly used drugs.

Presystemic metabolism

As well as having the ability to cross the gastrointestinal membrane by one of the routes described, drugs also need to be resistant to degradation/metabolism during this passage. All drugs that are absorbed from the stomach, small intestine and upper colon pass into the hepatic portal system and are presented to the liver before reaching the systemic circulation. Therefore, if the drug is going to be available to the systemic circulation it must also be resistant to metabolism by the liver. Hence, an oral dose of drug could be completely absorbed but incompletely available to the systemic circulation because of *first-pass* or *presystemic* metabolism by the gut wall and/or liver.

Gut-wall metabolism

It is only relatively recently that the full extent of gut-wall metabolism has been recognized. Watkins and co-workers were the first to report that a major cytochrome P450 enzyme, CYP3A, that is present in the liver and is responsible for the hepatic metabolism of many drugs, is present in the intestinal mucosa and that intestinal metabolism may be important for substrates of this enzyme (Watkins et al. 1987, Kolars et al. 1992). This effect can also be known as *first-pass metabolism* by the intestine. One drug that is susceptible to extensive gut metabolism that results in a significant reduction in its bioavailability is cyclosporin (Benet et al, 1996).

Hepatic metabolism

The liver is the primary site of drug metabolism and thus acts as a final barrier for oral absorption. This first pass of absorbed drug through the liver may result in extensive metabolism of the drug, and a significant portion may never reach the systemic circulation, resulting in a low bioavailability of those drugs which are rapidly metabolized by the liver. The bioavailability of a susceptible drug may be reduced to such an extent as to render the gastrointestinal route of administration ineffective, or to necessitate an oral dose which is many times larger than the intravenous dose, e.g. propranolol. Although propranolol is well absorbed, only about 30% of an oral dose is available to the systemic circulation owing to the first-pass effect. The bioavailability of sustained-release propranolol is even less as the drug is presented via the hepatic portal vein more slowly than from an immediate-release dosage form, and the liver is therefore capable of extracting and metabolizing a larger portion. Other drugs which are susceptible to a large first-pass effect are the anaesthetic lidocaine, the tricyclic antidepressant imipramine and the analagesic pentazocine.

SUMMARY

There are many physiological factors that influence the rate and extent of drug absorption; these are initially dependent on the route of administration. For the oral route the physiological and environmental factors of the gastrointestinal tract, the gastrointestinal membrane and presystemic metabolism can all influence drug bioavailability.

REFERENCES AND BIBLIOGRAPHY

Benet, L.Z., Wu, C., Hevert, M. Wacher V.J. (1996) Intestinal drug metabolism and antitransport processes: a potential paradigm shift in oral drug delivery. *J. Cont. Rel.* **39**, 139–143.

Brayden, D. (1997) Human intestinal epithelial monolayers as prescreens for oral drug delivery. *Pharmaceutical News*, **4** (1), 11–13.

Evans A.M. (2000) Influence of dietary components on the gastrointestinal metabolism and transport of drugs. **22**, 131–136.

Fleisher, D. Cheng, L. Zhou, Y. Li-Heng, P and Karim, A (1999) Drug, meal and formulation interactions influencing drug absorption after oral administration. *Clin Pharmacokinet*, **36**, 233–254.

Gray, V. and Dressman J. (1996) Simulated intestinal fluid TS – Change to pH 6.8. *Pharmacopeial Forum* **22**, 1943–1945.

Kolars, J.C., Schmiedlin-Ren, P., Schuetz, J.D., Fang, C. and Watkins, P.B. (1992) Identification of rifampicin-inducible P450IIIA4 (CYP 3A4) in human bowel enterocytes. *J. Clin. Invest.* **90**, 1871–1878.

Lennernas, H. (1998) Human intestinal permeability. *J. Pharm Sci.*, **87**, 403–410.

Nimmo, J. Heading, R.C., Tothill, P. and Prescott, L.F. (1973) Pharmacological modification of gastric emptying: effects of propantheline and metoclopramide on paracetamol absorption. *Br. Med. J.* **1**, 587–589.

Oh, D.M. Han, H.K. and Amidon, G.L. (1999) Drug transport and targeting. *Intest. Transport Pharml. Biotech.* **12**, 59–88.

Tsuji, A. and Tamia, I. (1996) Carrier-mediated intestinal transport of drugs. *Pharm. Res.* **13**, 963–977.

Watkins, P.B., Wrighton, S.A., Schuetz, E.G., Molowa, D.T. and Guzelian, P.S. (1987) Identification of glucocorticoid-inducible cytochromes P-450 in intestinal mucosa of rats and man. *J. Clin. Invest.* **80**, 1029–1036.

Welling, P.G. (1996) Effects of food on drug absorption. *Annu. Rev. Nutr.*, **16**, 383–414.

Yang, C.Y., Dantzig, A H, Pidgeon, C. (1999) *Pharm. Res.* **16**, 1331–43.

17

Bioavailability – physicochemical and dosage form factors

Marianne Ashford

As discussed in Chapter 16, the rate and extent of absorption are influenced by the physiological factors associated with the structure and function of the GI tract. This chapter discusses the physicochemical properties of the drug and dosage form factors that influence bioavailability. For a drug to be absorbed it needs to be in solution and, secondly, to pass across the membrane; in the case of orally administered drugs this is the gastrointestinal epithelium. The physicochemical properties of the drug that will influence its passage into solution and transfer across membranes include its dissolution rate, pK_a, lipid solubility, chemical stability and complexation potential.

PHYSICOCHEMICAL FACTORS INFLUENCING BIOAVAILABILITY

Dissolution and solubility

Solid drugs need to dissolve before they can be absorbed. The dissolution of drugs can be described by the Noyes–Whitney equation (Eqn 17.1). This equation, first proposed in 1897, describes the rate of dissolution of spherical particles when the dissolution process is diffusion controlled and involves no chemical reaction:

$$dC/dt = \frac{DA(C_s - C)}{h} \tag{17.1}$$

where dC/dt is the rate of dissolution of the drug particles, D is the diffusion coefficient of the drug in solution in the gastrointestinal fluids, A is the effective surface area of the drug particles in contact with the gastrointestinal fluids, h is the thickness of the diffusion layer around each drug particle, C_s is the saturation solubility of the drug in solution in the diffusion layer and C is the concentration of the drug in the gastrointestinal fluids.

Table 17.1   Physicochemical and physiological factors affecting drug dissolution in the gastrointestinal tract (adapted from Dressman et al, 1998)

Factor	Physicochemical parameter	Physiological parameter
Effect surface area of drug	Particle size, wettability	Surfactants in gastric juice and bile
Solubility in diffusion layer	Hydrophilicity, crystal structure, solubilization	pH, buffer capacity, bile, food components
Amount of drug already dissolved		Permeability, transit
Diffusivity of drug	Molecular size	Viscosity of luminal contents
Boundary layer thickness		Motility patterns and flow rate
Volume of solvent available		Gastrointestinal secretions, co-administered fluids

The limitations of the Noyes–Whitney equation in describing the dissolution of drug particles are discussed in Chapter 2. Despite these limitations, the equation serves to illustrate and explain how various physicochemical and physiological factors can influence the rate of dissolution in the gastrointestinal tract. These are summarized in Table 17.1 and are discussed in more detail in the next section.

Figure 17.1 illustrates the dissolution of a spherical drug particle in the gastrointestinal fluids.

Physiological factors affecting the dissolution rate of drugs

The environment of the gastrointestinal tract can affect the parameters of the Noyes–Whitney equation (Eqn 17.1) and hence the dissolution rate of a drug. For instance, the diffusion coefficient, D, of the drug in the gastrointestinal fluids may be decreased by the presence of substances that increase the viscosity of the fluids. Hence the presence of food in the gastrointestinal tract may cause a decrease in dissolution rate of a drug by reducing the rate of diffusion of the drug molecules away from the diffusion layer surrounding each undissolved drug particle. Surfactants in gastric juice and bile salts will affect both the wettability of the drug, and hence the effective surface area, A, exposed to gastrointestinal fluids, and the solubility of the drug in the gastrointestinal fluids via micellization. The thickness of the diffusion layer, h, will be influenced by the degree of agitation experienced by each drug particle in the

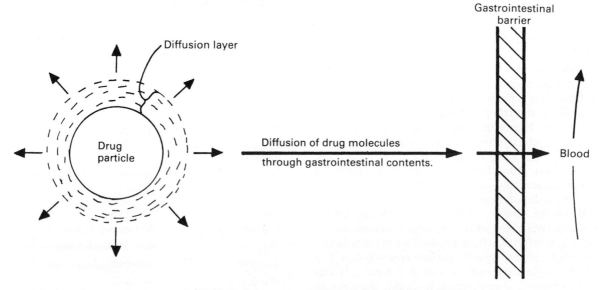

Fig. 17.1   Schematic representation of the dissolution of a drug particle in the gastrointestinal fluids.

235

gastrointestinal tract. Hence an increase in gastric and/or intestinal motility may increase the dissolution rate of a sparingly soluble drug by decreasing the thickness of the diffusion layer around each drug particle. The concentration, C, of drug in solution in the bulk of the gastrointestinal fluids will be influenced by such factors as the rate of removal of dissolved drug by absorption through the gastrointestinal–blood barrier, and by the volume of fluid available for dissolution, which will be dependent on the position of the drug in the gastrointestinal tract and the timing with respect to meal intake. In the stomach the volume of fluid will be influenced by the intake of fluid in the diet. According to the Noyes–Whitney equation a low value of C will favour more rapid dissolution of the drug by virtue of increasing the value of the term $(C_s - C)$. In the case of drugs whose absorption is dissolution-rate limited, the value of C is normally kept very low by absorption of the drug. Hence dissolution occurs under sink conditions, that is, under conditions such that the value of $(C_s - C)$ approximates to C_s. Thus for the dissolution of a drug from the gastrointestinal tract under sink conditions the Noyes–Whitney equation can be expressed as:

$$dC / dt = \frac{DAC_S}{h} \qquad (17.2)$$

Drug factors affecting dissolution rate

Drug factors that can influence the dissolution rate are the particle size, the wettability, the solubility and the form of the drug (whether a salt or a free form, crystalline or amorphous).

Surface area and particle size According to Eqn 17.1, an increase in the total surface area of drug in contact with the gastrointestinal fluids will cause an increase in dissolution rate. Provided that each particle of drug is intimately wetted by the gastrointestinal fluids, the effective surface area exhibited by the drug will be directly proportional to the particle size of the drug. Hence the smaller the particle size, the greater the effective surface area exhibited by a given mass of drug, and the higher the dissolution rate. Particle size reduction is thus likely to result in increased bioavailability, provided the absorption of the drug is dissolution-rate limited.

One of the classic examples of particle size effects on the bioavailability of poorly soluble compounds is that of griseofulvin, where a reduction of particle size from about 10 μm (specific surface area = 0.4 m^2 g^{-1}) to 2.7 μm (specific surface area = 1.5 m^2 g^{-1}) was shown to produce approximately double the amount of drug absorbed in humans. Many poorly soluble, slowly dissolving drugs are routinely presented in micronized form to increase their surface area.

Examples of drugs where a reduction in particle size has been shown to improve the rate and extent of oral absorption and hence bioavailability are shown in Table 17.2. Such improvements in bioavailability can result in an increased incidence of side-effects, thus for certain drugs it is important that the particle size is well controlled, and many Pharmacopoeia state the requirements of particle size.

For some drugs, particularly those that are hydrophobic in nature, micronization and other dry particle size-reduction techniques can result in aggregation of the material, with a consequent reduction in the effective surface area exposed to the gastrointestinal fluids and hence their dissolution rate and bioavailability. Aspirin, phenacetin and phenobarbitone are all prone to aggregation during particle size reduction; one approach that may overcome this problem is to micronize or mill the drug with a wetting agent or hydrophilic carrier. To overcome aggregation and to achieve particle sizes in the nanosize region, wet milling in the presence of stabilizers has been used. The relative bioavailability of danazol has been increased 400% by administering particles in the nano- rather than the micrometre size range.

As well as milling with wetting agents the effective surface area of hydrophobic drugs can be increased by the addition of a wetting agent to the formulation. The presence of polysorbate-80 in a fine suspension of phenacetin (particle size less than 75 μm) greatly improved the rate and extent of absorption of the phenacetin in human volunteers compared to the

Table 17.2 Examples of drugs where a reduction in particle size has led to improvements in bioavailability

Drug	Therapeutic class
Digoxin	Cardiac glycoside
Nitrofurantoin	Antifungal
Medoxyprogesterone acetate	Hormone
Danazol	Steroid
Tolbutamide	Antidiabetic
Aspirin	Analgesic
Sulphadiazine	Antibacterial
Naproxen	Non-steroidal anti-inflammatory
Ibuprofen	Non-steroidal anti-inflammatory
Phenacetin	Analgesic

same-size suspension without a wetting agent. Polysorbate-80 helps by increasing the wetting and solvent penetration of the particles and by minimizing aggregation of suspended particles, thereby maintaining a large effective surface area. Wetting effects are highly drug specific.

If an increase in the effective surface area of a drug does not increase its absorption rate it is likely that the dissolution process is not rate limiting. For drugs such as penicillin G and erythromycin, which are unstable in gastric fluids, their chemical degradation will be minimized if they remain in the solid state. Thus particle size reduction would not only serve to increase their dissolution rate, but would also increase chemical degradation and therefore reduce the amount of intact drug available for absorption.

Solubility in the diffusion layer, C_S The dissolution rate of a drug under sink conditions, according to the Noyes–Whitney equation, is directly proportional to its intrinsic solubility in the diffusion layer surrounding each dissolving drug particle, C_s. The aqueous solubility of a drug is dependent on the interactions between molecules within the crystal lattice, intermolecular interactions with the solution in which it is dissolving, and the entropy changes associated with fusion and dissolution. In the case of drugs that are weak electrolytes, their aqueous solubilities are dependent on pH (see Chapter 2). Hence in the case of an orally administered solid dosage form containing a weak electrolyte drug, the dissolution rate of the drug will be influenced by its solubility and the pH in the diffusion layer surrounding each dissolving drug particle. The pH in the diffusion layer – the microclimate pH – for a weak electrolyte will be affected by the pK_a and solubility of the dissolving drug and the pK_a and solubility of the buffers in the bulk gastrointestinal fluids. Thus

differences in dissolution rate will be expected in different regions of the gastrointestinal tract.

The solubility of weakly acidic drugs increases with pH, and so as a drug moves down the gastrointestinal tract from the stomach to the intestine, its solubility will increase. Conversely, the solubility of weak bases decreases with increasing pH, i.e. as the drug moves down the gastrointestinal tract. It is important therefore for poorly soluble weak bases to dissolve rapidly in the stomach, as the rate of dissolution in the small intestine will be much slower. The antifungal drug ketoconazole, a weak base, is particularly sensitive to gastric pH. Dosing ketoconazole 2 hours after the administration of the H_2 blocker cimetidine, which reduces gastric acid secretion, results in a significantly reduced rate and extent of absorption (van der Meer et al 1980). Similarly, in the case of the antiplatelet dipyrimidole, pretreatment with the H_2 blocker famotidine reduces the peak plasma concentration by a factor of up to 10 (Russell et al 1994).

Salts The dissolution rate of a weakly acidic drug in gastric fluid (pH 1–3.5) will be relatively low. If the pH in the diffusion layer could be increased, then the solubility, C_s, exhibited by the acidic drug in this layer, and hence its dissolution rate in gastric fluids, would be increased even though the bulk pH of gastric fluids remained at the same low value. The pH of the diffusion layer would be increased if the chemical nature of the weakly acidic drug were changed from that of the free acid to a basic salt, for example the sodium or potassium form of the free acid. The pH of the diffusion layer surrounding each particle of the salt form would be higher (e.g. 5–6) than the low bulk pH (1–3.5) of the gastric fluids because of the neutralizing action of the strong anions (Na$^+$ or K$^+$) ions present in the diffusion layer (Fig. 17.2).

Fig. 17.2 Schematic representation of the dissolution process of a salt form of a weakly acidic drug in gastric fluid.

Because the salt form of the weakly acidic drug has a relatively high solubility at the elevated pH in the diffusion layer, dissolution of the drug particles will take place at a faster rate. When dissolved drug diffuses out of the diffusion layer into the bulk of the gastric fluid, where the pH is lower than that in the diffusion layer, precipitation of the free acid form is likely to occur. This will be a result of the overall solubility exhibited by the drug at the lower bulk pH. Thus the free acid form of the drug in solution, which is in excess of its solubility at the bulk pH of gastric fluid, will precipitate out, leaving a saturated (or near-saturated) solution of free acid in gastric fluid. Often this precipitated free acid will be in the form of very fine, non-ionized wetted particles which exhibit a very large total effective surface area in contact with gastric fluids. This large total effective surface area will facilitate rapid redissolution of the precipitated particles of free acid when additional gastric fluid becomes available as a consequence of either dissolved drug being absorbed, additional fluid accumulating in the stomach, or the fine precipitated particles being emptied from the stomach to the intestine. This rapid redissolution will ensure that the concentration of free acid in solution in the bulk of the gastric fluids will be at or near to saturation.

Thus the oral administration of a solid dosage form containing a strong basic salt of a weakly acidic drug would be expected to give a more rapid rate of drug dissolution and (in the case of drugs exhibiting dissolution rate limited absorption) a more rapid rate of drug absorption than the free acid form of the drug.

Many examples can be found of the effects of salts improving the rate and extent of absorption. The dissolution rate of the oral hypoglycaemic tolbutamide sodium in 0.1 M HCl is 5000 times faster than that of the free acid. Oral administration of a non-disintegrating disc of the more rapidly dissolving sodium salt of tolbutamide produced a very rapid decrease in blood sugar level (a consequence of the rapid rate of drug absorption), followed by a rapid recovery. In contrast, a non-disintegrating disc of the tolbutamide free acid produced a much slower rate of decrease of blood sugar (a consequence of the slower rate of drug absorption) that was maintained over a longer period of time. The barbiturates are often administered in the form of sodium salts to achieve a rapid onset of sedation and provide more predictable effects.

The non-steroidal anti-inflammatory drug naproxen was originally marketed as the free acid for the treatment of rheumatoid and osteoarthritis. However, the sodium salt (naproxen sodium) is absorbed faster and is more effective in newer indications, such as mild to moderate pain (Sevelius et al 1980).

Conversely, strongly acidic salt forms of weakly basic drugs, for example chlorpromazine hydrochloride, dissolve more rapidly in gastric and intestinal fluids than do the free bases (e.g. chlorpromazine). The presence of strongly acidic anions (e.g. Cl^- ions) in the diffusion layer around each drug particle ensures that the pH in that layer is lower than the bulk pH in either the gastric or the intestinal fluid. This lower pH will increase the solubility of the drug C_s in the diffusion layer. The oral administration of a salt form of a weakly basic drug in a solid oral dosage form generally ensures that dissolution occurs in the gastric fluid before the drug passes into small intestine, where pH conditions are unfavourable. Thus the drug should be delivered to the major absorption site, the small intestine, in solution. If absorption is fast enough, precipitation of the dissolved drug is unlikely to significantly affect bioavailability. It is important to be aware that hydrochloride salts may experience a common ion effect owing to the presence of chloride ions in the stomach (see Chapter 8). The in vitro dissolution of a sulphate salt of an HIV protease inhibitor analogue is significantly greater in hydrochloric acid than that of the hydrochloride salt. The bioavailability of the sulphate salt is more than three times greater than that of the hydrochloride salt. These observations are attributed to the common ion effect of the hydrochloride (Loper et al 1999).

The sodium salts of acidic drugs and the hydrochloride salts of basic drugs are by far the most common. However, many other salt forms are increasingly being employed (see Chapter 8). Some salts have a lower solubility and dissolution rate than the free form, for example aluminium salts of weak acids and palmoate salts of weak bases. In these cases insoluble films of either aluminium hydroxide or palmoic acid are found to coat the dissolving solids when the salts are exposed to a basic or an acidic environment, respectively. In general, poorly soluble salts delay absorption and may therefore be used to sustain the release of the drug. A poorly soluble salt form is generally employed for suspension dosage forms.

Although salt forms are often selected to improve bioavailability, other factors, such as chemical stability, hygroscopicity, manufacturability and crystallinity, will all be considered during salt selection and may preclude the choice of a particular salt. The sodium salt of aspirin, sodium acetylsalicylate, is much more prone to hydrolysis than is aspirin, acetylsalicylic acid, itself. One way to overcome chemical instabilities or other undesirable features of salts is to form the salt in situ or to add basic/acidic excipients to the formulation of a weakly acidic or weakly basic drug. The presence of the basic excipients in the formulation of acidic drugs ensures that a relatively basic diffusion layer is formed around each dissolving particle. The inclusion of the basic ingredients aluminium dihydroxyaminoacetate and magnesium carbonate in aspirin tablets was found to increase their dissolution rate and bioavailability.

Crystal form

Polymorphism Many drugs can exist in more than one crystalline form, e.g. chloramphenicol palmitate, cortisone acetate, tetracyclines and sulphathiazole. This property is referred to as **polymorphism** and each crystalline form is known as a polymorph (see Chapter 9). As discussed in Chapter 2, a metastable polymorph usually exhibits a greater dissolution rate than the corresponding stable polymorph. Consequently, the metastable polymorphic form of a poorly soluble drug may exhibit an increased bioavailability compared to the stable polymorphic form.

A classic example of the influence of polymorphism on drug bioavailability is provided by chloramphenicol palmitate. This drug exists in three crystalline forms designated A, B and C. At normal temperature and pressure A is the stable polymorph, B is the metastable polymorph and C is the unstable polymorph. Polymorph C is too unstable to be included in a dosage form, but polymorph B, the metastable form, is sufficiently stable. The plasma profiles of chloramphenicol from orally administered suspensions containing varying proportions of the polymorphic forms A and B were investigated. The extent of absorption of chloramphenicol increases as the proportion of the polymorphic form B of chloramphenicol palmitate is increased in each suspension. This was attributed to the more rapid in vivo rate of dissolution of the metastable polymorphic form, B, of chloramphenicol palmitate. Following dissolution, chloramphenicol palmitate is hydrolysed to give free chloramphenicol in solution, which is then absorbed. The stable polymorphic form A of chloramphenicol palmitate dissolves so slowly and consequently is hydrolysed so slowly to chloramphenicol in vivo that this polymorph is virtually ineffective. The importance of polymorphism to the gastrointestinal bioavailability of chloramphenicol palmitate is reflected by a limit being placed on the content of the inactive polymorphic form, A, in Chloramphenicol Palmitate Mixture.

Amorphous solids In addition to different polymorphic crystalline forms, a drug may exist in an amorphous form (see Chapter 9). Because the amorphous form usually dissolves more rapidly than the corresponding crystalline form(s), the possibility exists that there will be significant differences in the bioavailabilities exhibited by the amorphous and crystalline forms of drugs that show dissolution-rate limited bioavailability.

A classic example of the influence of amorphous versus crystalline forms of a drug on its gastrointestinal bioavailability is provided by that of the antibiotic novobiocin. The more soluble and rapidly dissolving amorphous form of novobiocin was readily absorbed following oral administration of an aqueous suspension to humans and dogs. However, the less soluble and slower-dissolving crystalline form of novobiocin was not absorbed to any significant extent. The crystalline form was thus therapeutically ineffective. A further important observation was made in the case of aqueous suspensions of novobiocin. The amorphous form of novobiocin slowly converts to the more thermodynamically stable crystalline form, with an accompanying loss of therapeutic effectiveness. Thus unless adequate precautions are taken to ensure the stability of the less stable, more therapeutically effective amorphous form of a drug in a dosage form, then unacceptable variations in therapeutic effectiveness may occur.

Several delivery technologies for poorly soluble drugs rely on stabilizing the drug in its amorphous form to increase its dissolution and bioavailability.

Solvates Another variation in the crystalline form of a drug can occur if the drug is able to associate with solvent molecules to produce crystalline forms known as solvates. When water is the solvent, the solvate formed is called a hydrate. Generally the greater the solvation of the crystal, the lower are the solubility and dissolution rate in a solvent identical to the solvation molecules. As the solvated and non-solvated forms usually exhibit differences in dissolution rates, they may also exhibit differences in bioavailability, particularly in the case of poorly soluble drugs that exhibit dissolution-rate limited bioavailability.

A valuable example is that of the antibiotic ampicillin: the faster-dissolving anhydrous form of ampicillin was absorbed to a greater extent from both hard gelatin capsules and an aqueous suspension than was the slower-dissolving trihydrate form. The anhydrous form of the hydrochloride salt of an HIV protease inhibitor, an analogue of indinavir, has a much faster dissolution rate than the hydrated form in water; this is reflected by a significantly greater rate and extent of absorption and overdoubling of the bioavailability of the anhydrous form (Loper et al 1999).

Factors affecting the concentration of drug in solution in the gastrointestinal fluids

The rate and extent of absorption of a drug depend on the effective concentration of that drug, i.e. the concentration of drug in solution in the gastrointestinal fluids which is in an absorbable form. Complexation, micellar solubilization, adsorption and chemical stability are the principal physicochemical properties that can influence the effective drug concentration in the gastrointestinal fluids.

Complexation Complexation of a drug may occur within the dosage form and/or in the gastrointestinal fluids, and can be beneficial or detrimental to absorption.

Mucin, a normal component of gastrointestinal fluids, complexes with some drugs. The antibiotic streptomycin binds to mucin, thereby reducing the available concentration of the drug for absorption. It is thought that this may contribute to its poor bioavailability. Another example of complexation is that between drugs and dietary components, as in the case of the tetracyclines, which is discussed in Chapter 16.

The bioavailability of some drugs can be reduced by the presence of excipients within the dosage forms. The presence of calcium (e.g. from the diluent dicalcium phosphate) in the dosage form of tetracycline reduces its bioavailability via the formation of a poorly soluble complex. Other examples of complexes that reduce drug bioavailability are those between amphetamine and sodium carboxymethylcellulose, and between phenobarbitone and polyethylene glycol 4000. Complexation between drugs and excipients probably occurs quite often in liquid dosage forms.

Complexation is sometimes used to increase drug solubility, particularly of poorly water-soluble drugs. One class of complexing agents that is increasingly being employed is the cyclodextrin family. Cyclodextrins are enzymatically modified starches. They are composed of glucopyranose units which form a ring of either six (α-cyclodextrin), seven (β-cyclodextrin) or eight (γ-cyclodextrin) units. The outer surface of the ring is hydrophilic and the inner cavity is hydrophobic. Lipophilic molecules can fit into the ring to form soluble inclusion complexes. The ring of β-cyclodextrin is the correct size for the majority of drug molecules, and normally one drug molecule will associate with one cyclodextrin molecule to form reversible complexes, although other stoichiometries are possible. For example the antifungal miconazole shows poor oral bioavailability owing to its poor solubility. However, in the presence of cyclodextrin the solubility and dissolution rate of miconazole are significantly enhanced (by up to 55- and 255-fold, respectively). This enhancement of dissolution rate resulted in a more than doubling of the oral bioavailability in a study in rats (Terjarla et al 1998). There are numerous examples in the literature of drugs whose solubility and hence bioavailability have been increased by the use of cyclodextrins: they include piroxicam, itraconazole, indamethacin, pilocarpine, naproxen, hydrocortisone, diazepam and digitoxin. The first product on the UK market containing a cyclodextrin is the poorly soluble antifungal itraconazole, which has been formulated as a liquid dosage form with the more soluble derivative of β-cyclodextrin, hydroxypropyl-β-cyclodextrin.

Micellar solubization Micellar solubilization can also increase the solubility of drugs in the gastrointestinal tract. The ability of bile salts to solubilize drugs depends mainly on the lipophilicity of the drug (Naylor et al 1995). Further information on solubilization and complex formation can be found in Florence and Attwood (1998).

Adsorption The concurrent administration of drugs and medicines containing solid adsorbents (e.g. antidiarrhoeal mixtures) may result in the adsorbents interfering with the absorption of drugs from the gastrointestinal tract. The adsorption of a drug on to solid adsorbents such as kaolin or charcoal may reduce its rate and/or extent of absorption, owing to a decrease in the effective concentration of the drug in solution available for absorption. A consequence of the reduced concentration of free drug in solution at the site of absorption will be a reduction in the rate of drug absorption. Whether there is also a reduction in extent of absorption will depend on whether the drug–absorbent interaction is readily reversible. If the absorbed drug is not readily released from the solid absorbent in order to replace the free drug that has been absorbed from the gastrointestinal tract, there will also be a reduction in the extent of absorption from the gastrointestinal tract.

Examples of drug–adsorbent interactions that give reduced extents of absorption are promazine–charcoal and linomycin–kaopectate. The adsorbent properties of charcoal have been exploited as an antidote in drug intoxification.

Care also needs to be taken when insoluble excipients are included in dosage forms to check that the drug will not adsorb to them. Talc, which can be included in tablets as a glidant, is claimed to interfere with the absorption of cyanocobalamin by virtue of its ability to adsorb this vitamin.

Further details of the biopharmaceutical implications of adsorption can be found in Florence and Attwood (1998).

Chemical stability of the drug in the gastrointestinal fluids If the drug is unstable in the gastrointestinal fluids the amount of drug that is available for absorption will be reduced and its bioavailability reduced. Instability in gastrointestinal fluids is usually caused by acidic or enzymatic hydrolysis. When a drug is unstable in gastric fluid its extent of degradation would be minimized (and hence its bioavailability improved) if it exhibited minimal dissolution in gastric fluid but still rapid dissolution in intestinal fluid. The concept of delaying the dissolution of a drug until it reaches the small intestine has been employed to improve the bioavailability of erythromycin in the gastrointestinal tract. Enteric coating of tablets containing the free base erythromycin is one method that has been used to protect this drug from gastric fluid. The enteric coating resists gastric fluid but disrupts or dissolves at the less acid pH range of the small intestine (see later and Chapter 28). An alternative method of protecting a susceptible drug from gastric fluid, which has been employed in the case of erythromycin, is the administration of chemical derivatives of the parent drug. These derivatives, or prodrugs, exhibit limited solubility (and hence minimal dissolution) in gastric fluid but, once in the small intestine, liberate the parent drug to be absorbed. For instance, erythromycin stearate, after passing through the stomach undissolved, dissolves and dissociates in the intestinal fluid, yielding the free base erythromycin that is absorbed.

Instability in gastrointestinal fluids is one of the reasons why many peptide-like drugs are poorly absorbed when delivered via the oral route.

Poorly soluble drugs

Poorly water-soluble drugs are increasingly becoming a problem in terms of obtaining the satisfactory dissolution within the gastrointestinal tract that is necessary for good bioavailability. It is not only existing drugs that cause problems, but it is the challenge of medicinal chemists to ensure that new drugs are not only active pharmacologically but have enough solubility to ensure fast-enough dissolution at the site of administration, often the gastrointestinal tract. This is a particular problem for certain classes

of drugs, such as the HIV protease inhibitors, the glycoprotein IIb/IIIa inhibitors, and many anti-infective and anticancer drugs. Medicinal chemists are using approaches such as introducing ionizable groups, reducing melting points, changing polymorphs or introducing prodrugs to improve solubility. Further information on these approaches can be obtained from reviews by Lipinski et al (1997) and Panchagnula and Thomas (2000). Pharmaceutical scientists are also applying a wide range of formulation approaches to improve the dissolution rate of poorly soluble drugs. These include formulating in the nano-size range; formulating in a solid solution or dispersion or self-emulsifying drug delivery system; stabilizing the drug in the amorphous form or formulating with cyclodextrins. Many drug delivery companies thrive on technologies designed to improve the delivery of poorly soluble drugs.

Drug absorption

Once the drug has successfully passed into solution it is available for absorption. In Chapter 16 many physiological factors were shown to influence drug absorption. Absorption, and hence the bioavailability of a drug once in solution, is also influenced by many drug factors, in particular its pK_a, lipid solubility, molecular weight, the number of hydrogen bonds in the molecule and its chemical stability.

Drug dissociation and lipid solubility

The dissociation constant and lipid solubility of a drug, and the pH at the absorption site, often influence the absorption characteristics of a drug throughout the gastrointestinal tract. The interrelationship between the degree of ionization of a weak electrolyte drug (which is determined by its dissociation constant and the pH at the absorption site) and the extent of absorption is embodied in the pH-partition hypothesis of drug absorption, first proposed by Overton in 1899. Although it is an oversimplification of the complex process of absorption, the pH-partition hypothesis provides a useful framework for understanding the transcellular passive route of absorption, which is that favoured by the majority of drugs.

pH-partition hypothesis of drug absorption According to the pH-partition hypothesis, the gastrointestinal epithelia acts as a lipid barrier towards drugs which are absorbed by passive diffusion, and those that are lipid soluble will pass across the barrier. As most drugs are weak electrolytes, the unionized form of weakly acidic or basic drugs (i.e. the lipid-soluble form) will pass across the gastrointestinal epithelia, whereas the gastrointestinal epithelia is impermeable to the ionized (i.e. poorly lipid-soluble) form of such drugs. Consequently, according to the pH-partition hypothesis, the absorption of a weak electrolyte will be determined chiefly by the extent to which the drug exists in its unionized form at the site of absorption.

The extent to which a weakly acidic or basic drug ionizes in solution in the gastrointestinal fluid may be calculated using the appropriate form of the Henderson–Hasselbalch equation (see Chapter 3). For a weakly acidic drug having a single ionizable group (e.g. aspirin, phenylbutazone, salicylic acid) the equation takes the form of:

$$\log \frac{\left[A^-\right]}{\left[HA\right]} = pH - pK_a \qquad (17.3)$$

where pK_a is the negative logarithm of the acid dissociation constant of the drug, and [HA] and [A⁻] are the respective concentrations of the unionized and ionized forms of the weakly acidic drug, which are in equilibrium and in solution in the gastrointestinal fluid. pH refers to the pH of the environment of the ionized and unionized species, i.e. the gastrointestinal fluids.

For a weakly basic drug possessing a single ionizable group (e.g. chlorpromazine) the analogous equation is:

$$\log \frac{\left[BH^+\right]}{\left[B\right]} = pK_a - pH \qquad (17.4)$$

where [BH⁺] and [B] are the respective concentrations of the ionized and unionized forms of the weak basic drug, which are in equilibrium and in solution in the gastrointestinal fluids.

Therefore, according to these equations a weakly acidic drug, pK_a 3.0, will be predominantly unionized in gastric fluid at pH 1.2 (98.4%) and almost totally ionized in intestinal fluid at pH 6.8 (99.98%), whereas a weakly basic drug, pK_a 5, will be almost entirely ionized (99.98%) at gastric pH of 1.2 and predominantly unionized at intestinal pH of 6.8 (98.4%). This means that, according to the pH-partition hypothesis, a weakly acidic drug is more likely to be absorbed from the stomach where it is unionized, and a weakly basic drug from the intestine where it is predominantly unionized. However, in practice, other factors need to be taken into consideration.

Limitations of the pH-partition hypothesis The extent to which a drug exists in its unionized form is not the only factor determining the rate and extent of absorption of a drug molecule from the gastrointestinal tract. Despite their high degree of ionization,

weak acids are still quite well absorbed from the small intestine. In fact, the rate of intestinal absorption of a weak acid is often higher than its rate of absorption in the stomach, even though the drug is unionized in the stomach. The significantly larger surface area that is available for absorption in the small intestine more than compensates for the high degree of ionization of weakly acidic drugs at intestinal pH values. In addition, a longer small intestinal residence time and a microclimate pH, that exists at the surface of the intestinal mucosa and is lower than that of the luminal pH of the small intestine, are thought to aid the absorption of weak acids from the small intestine.

The mucosal unstirred layer is another recognized component of the gastrointestinal barrier to drug absorption that is not accounted for in the pH-partition hypothesis. During absorption drug molecules must diffuse across this layer and then on through the lipid layer. Diffusion across this layer is liable to be a significant component of the total absorption process for those drugs that cross the lipid layer very quickly. Diffusion across this layer will also depend on the relative molecular weight of the drug.

The pH-partition hypothesis cannot explain the fact that certain drugs (e.g. quaternary ammonium compounds and tetracyclines) are readily absorbed despite being ionized over the entire pH range of the gastrointestinal tract. One suggestion for this is that the gastrointestinal barrier is not completely impermeable to ionized drugs. It is now generally accepted that ionized forms of drugs are absorbed in the small intestine but at a much slower rate than the unionized form. Another possibility is that such drugs interact with endogenous organic ions of opposite charge to form an absorbable neutral species – an *ion pair* – which is capable of partitioning into the lipoidal gastrointestinal barrier and be absorbed via passive diffusion.

Another, physiological, factor that causes deviations from the pH-partition hypothesis is *convective flow* or *solvent drag*. The movement of water molecules into and out of the gastrointestinal tract will affect the rate of passage of small water-soluble molecules across the gastrointestinal barrier. Water movement occurs because of differences in osmotic pressure between blood and the luminal contents, and differences in hydrostatic pressure between the lumen and the perivascular tissue. The absorption of water-soluble drugs will be increased if water flows from the lumen to the blood, provided that the drug and water are using the same route of absorption; this will have greatest effect in the jejunum, where water movement is at its greatest. Water flow also effects the absorption of lipid-soluble drugs. It is thought that this is because the drug becomes more concentrated as water flows out of the intestine, thereby favouring a greater drug concentration gradient and increased absorption.

Lipid solubility A number of drugs are poorly absorbed from the gastrointestinal tract despite the fact that their unionized forms predominate. For example, the barbiturates, barbitone and thiopentone, have similar dissociation constants – pK_a 7.8 and 7.6, respectively – and therefore similar degrees of ionization at intestinal pH. However, thiopentone is absorbed much better than barbitone. The reason for this difference is that the absorption of drugs is also affected by the lipid solubility of the drug. Thiopentone, being more lipid soluble than barbitone, exhibits a greater affinity for the gastrointestinal membrane and is thus far better absorbed.

An indication of the lipid solubility of a drug, and therefore whether that drug is liable to be transported across membranes, is given by its ability to partition between a lipid-like solvent and water or an aqueous buffer. This is known as the drug's **partition coefficient**, and is a measure of its lipophilicity. The value of the partition coefficient P is determined by measuring the drug partitioning between water and a suitable solvent at constant temperature. As this ratio normally spans several orders of magnitude it is usually expressed as the logarithmn. The organic solvent that is usually selected to mimic the biological membrane, because of its many similar properties, is octanol.

$$\text{Partition coefficient} = \frac{\text{concentration of drug in organic phase}}{\text{concentration in aqueous phase}} \quad (17.5)$$

The effective partition coefficient, taking into account the degree of ionization of the drug, is known as the **distribution coefficient** and again is normally expressed as the logarithm (log D); it is given by the following equations for acids and bases:

For acids:

$$D = \frac{[HA]_{org}}{[HA]_{aq} + [A^-]_{aq}} \quad (17.6)$$

$$\log D = \log P - [1 + \text{antilog} (pH - pK_a)] \quad (17.7)$$

For bases:

$$D = \frac{[B]_{org}}{[B]_{aq} + [BH^+]_{aq}} \quad (17.8)$$

$$\log D = \log P - [1 + \text{antilog} (pK_a - pH)] \quad (17.9)$$

The lipophilicity of a drug is critical in the drug discovery process. Polar molecules, i.e. those that are poorly lipid soluble (log $P < 0$) and relatively large, such as gentamicin, ceftriaxone, heparin and streptokinase, are poorly absorbed after oral administration and therefore have to be given by injection. Smaller molecules that are poorly lipid soluble, i.e. hydrophilic in nature, such as the β-blocker atenolol, can be absorbed via the paracellular route. Lipid-soluble drugs with favourable partition coefficients (i.e. log $P > 0$) are usually absorbed after oral administration. Drugs which are very lipid soluble (log $P > 3$) tend to be well absorbed but are also more likely to be susceptible to metabolism and biliary clearance. Although there is no general rule that can be applied across all drug molecules, within a homologous series drug absorption usually increases as the lipophilicity rises. This has been shown for a series of barbiturates by Schanker (1960) and for a series of β-blockers by Taylor et al (1985).

Sometimes, if the structure of a compound cannot be modified to yield lipid solubility while maintaining pharmacological activity, medicinal chemists may investigate the probability of making lipid prodrugs to improve absorption. A prodrug is a chemical modification, frequently an ester of an existing drug, which converts back to the parent compound as a result of metabolism by the body. A prodrug has no pharmacological activity itself. Examples of prodrugs which have been successfully used to improve the lipid solubility and hence absorption of their parent drugs are shown in Table 17.3.

Molecular size and hydrogen bonding Two other drug properties that are important in permeability are the number of hydrogen bonds within the molecule and the molecular size

For paracellular absorption the molecular weight should ideally be less than 200 Da; however, there are examples where larger molecules (up to molecular weights of 400 Da) have been absorbed via this

Table 17.3 Prodrugs with improved lipid solubility and oral absorption

Parent drug	Prodrug	Ester
Ampicillin	Pivampicillin	Pivaloyloxymethyl
Ampicillin	Bacampicillin	Carbonate
Carbenicillin	Indanylcarbenicillin	Indanyl
Cefuroxime	Cefuroxime axetil	Acetylethyl
Enalaprilat	Enalapril	Ester of 1-carboxylic acid
Terbutaline	Ibuterol	Dibutyl

route. Shape is also an important factor for paracellular absorption.

In general, for transcellular passive diffusion a molecular weight of less than 500 Da is preferable. Drugs with molecular weights above this may be absorbed less efficiently. There are few examples of drugs with molecular weights above 700 Da being well absorbed.

Too many hydrogen bonds within a molecule are detrimental to its absorption. In general, no more than five hydrogen bond donors and no more than 10 hydrogen bond acceptors (the sum of nitrogen and oxygen atoms in the molecule is often taken as a rough measure of hydrogen bond acceptors) should be present if the molecule is to be well absorbed. The large number of hydrogen bonds within peptides is one of the reasons why peptide drugs are poorly absorbed.

Summary

There are many properties of the drug itself that will influence its passage into solution in the gastrointestinal tract and across the gastrointestinal membrane, and hence its overall rate and extent of absorption.

DOSAGE FORM FACTORS INFLUENCING BIOAVAILABILITY

Introduction

The rate and/or extent of absorption of a drug from the gastrointestinal tract have been shown to be influenced by many physiological factors and by many physicochemical properties associated with the drug itself. The bioavailability of a drug can also be influenced by factors associated with the formulation and production of the dosage form. Increasingly many dosage forms are being designed to affect the release and absorption of drugs, for example controlled-release systems (see Chapter 20) and delivery systems for poorly soluble drugs. This section focuses on summarizing how the type of dosage form and the excipients used in conventional oral dosage forms can affect the rate and extent of drug absorption.

Influence of the type of dosage form

The type of dosage form and its method of preparation or manufacture can influence bioavailability. Thus, whether a particular drug is incorporated and administered in the form of a solution, a suspension or solid dosage form can influence its rate and/or extent of absorption from the gastrointestinal tract. The type of oral dosage form will influence the number of possible intervening steps between administration and the appearance of dissolved drug in the gastrointestinal fluids, i.e. the type of dosage form will influence the release of drug into solution in the gastrointestinal fluids (Fig. 17.3).

In general, drugs must be in solution in the gastrointestinal fluids before absorption can occur. Thus the greater the number of intervening steps, the greater will be the number of potential obstacles to absorption and the greater will be the likelihood of that type of dosage form reducing the bioavailability

Fig. 17.3 Schematic outline of the influence of the dosage form on the appearance of drug in solution in the gastrointestinal tract.

exhibited by the drug. Hence the bioavailability of a given drug tends to decrease in the following order of types of dosage form: aqueous solutions > aqueous suspensions > solid dosage forms (e.g. hard gelatin capsules or tablets). Although this ranking is not universal, it does provide a useful guideline. In general, solutions and suspensions are the most suitable for administering drugs intended to be rapidly absorbed. However, it should be noted that other factors (e.g. stability, patient acceptability etc.) can also influence the type of dosage form in which a drug is administered via the gastrointestinal route.

Aqueous solutions

For drugs that are water soluble and chemically stable in aqueous solution, formulation as a solution normally eliminates the in vivo dissolution step and presents the drug in the most readily available form for absorption. However, dilution of an aqueous solution of a poorly water-soluble drug whose aqueous solubility had been increased by formulation techniques such as cosolvency, complex formation or solubilization can result in precipitation of the drug in the gastric fluids. Similarly, exposure of an aqueous solution of a salt of a weak acidic compound to gastric pH can also result in precipitation of the free acid form of the drug. In most cases the extremely fine nature of the resulting precipitate permits a more rapid rate of dissolution than if the drug had been administered in other types of oral dosage forms, such as aqueous suspension, hard gelatin capsule or tablet. However, for some drugs this precipitation can have a major effect on bioavailability. The same dose of an experimental drug was given to dogs in three different solution formulations, a polyethlyene glycol solution and two different concentrations of hydroxypropyl-β-cyclodextrin. Bioavailabilities of 19%, 57% and 89% were obtained for polyethylene glycol, the lower concentration and the higher concentration of hydroxypropyl-β-cyclodextrin, respectively. The difference in bioavailability of the three solutions was attributed to the difference in precipitation rates of the candidate drug from the three solutions on dilution. The experimental drug was observed to precipitate most quickly from the polyethylene glycol solution, and slowest from the most concentrated hydroxypropyl-β-cyclodextrin solution.

Factors associated with the formulation of aqueous solutions that can influence drug bioavailability include:

- The chemical stability exhibited by the drug in aqueous solution and the gastrointestinal fluids;

- Complexation, i.e. the formation of a complex between the drug and an excipient included to increase the aqueous solubility, the chemical stability of the drug or the viscosity of the dosage form;
- Solubilization, i.e. the incorporation of the drug into micelles in order to increase its aqueous solubility;
- The viscosity of a solution dosage form, particularly if a viscosity-enhancing agent has been included.

Information concerning the potential influence of each of the above factors was given earlier. Further details concerning the formulation of oral solution dosage forms are given in Chapter 21.

Aqueous suspensions

An aqueous suspension is a useful dosage form for administering an insoluble or poorly water-soluble drug. Usually the absorption of a drug from this type of dosage form is dissolution-rate limited. The oral administration of an aqueous suspension results in a large total surface area of dispersed drug being immediately presented to the gastrointestinal fluids. This facilitates dissolution and hence absorption of the drug. In contrast to powder-filled hard gelatin capsule and tablet dosage forms, dissolution of all drug particles commences immediately on dilution of the suspension in the gastrointestinal fluids. A drug contained in a tablet or hard gelatin capsule may ultimately achieve the same state of dispersion in the gastrointestinal fluids, but only after a delay. Thus a well formulated, finely subdivided aqueous suspension is regarded as being an efficient oral drug delivery system, second only to a non-precipitating solution-type dosage form.

Factors associated with the formulation of aqueous suspension dosage forms that can influence the bioavailabilities of drugs from the gastrointestinal tract include:

- The particle size and effective surface area of the dispersed drug;
- The crystal form of the drug;
- Any resulting complexation, i.e. the formation of a non-absorbable complex between the drug and an excipient such as the suspending agent;
- The inclusion of a surfactant as a wetting, flocculating or deflocculating agent;
- The viscosity of the suspension.

Information concerning the potential influence of the above factors on drug bioavailability is given in earlier sections. Further information concerning the formulation and uses of suspensions as dosage forms is given in Chapter 23.

Liquid-filled capsules

Liquids can be filled into capsules made from soft or hard gelatin. Both types combine the convenience of a unit dosage form with the potentially rapid drug absorption associated with aqueous solutions and suspensions. Drugs encapsulated in liquid-filled capsules for peroral administration are dissolved or dispersed in non-toxic, non-aqueous vehicles. Such vehicles may be water immiscible (i.e. lipophilic) or water miscible (i.e. hydrophilic). Vegetable oils are popular water-immiscible vehicles, whereas polyethylene glycols and certain non-ionic surfactants (e.g. polysorbate-80) are water miscible. Sometimes the vehicles have thermal properties such that they can be filled into capsules while hot, but are solids at room temperature.

The release of the contents of gelatin capsules is effected by dissolution and splitting of the flexible shell. Following release, a water-miscible vehicle disperses and/or dissolves readily in the gastrointestinal fluids, liberating the drug (depending on its aqueous solubility) as either a solution or a fine suspension, which is conducive to rapid absorption. In the case of gelatin capsules containing drugs in solution or suspension in water-immiscible vehicles, release of the contents will almost certainly be followed by dispersion in the gastrointestinal fluids. Dispersion is facilitated by emulsifiers included in the vehicle, and also by bile. Once dispersed, the drug may end up as an emulsion, a solution, a fine suspension or a nano/microemulsion. Well formulated liquid-filled capsules aimed at improving the absorption of poorly soluble drugs will ensure that no precipitation of drug occurs from the nano- or microemulsion in the gastrointestinal fluids. If the lipophilic vehicle is a digestible oil and the drug is highly soluble in the oil, it is possible that the drug will remain in solution in the dispersed oil phase and be absorbed (along with the oil) by fat absorption processes. For a drug that is less lipophilic or is dissolved in a non-digestible oil, absorption probably occurs following partitioning of the drug from the oily vehicle into the aqueous gastrointestinal fluids. In this case the rate of drug absorption appears to depend on the rate at which drug partitions from the dispersed oil phase. The increase in interfacial area of contact resulting from dispersion of the oily vehicle in the gastrointestinal fluids will facilitate partition of the drug across the oil/aqueous interface. For drugs suspended in an oily vehicle release may involve dissolution in the vehicle, diffusion to the oil/aqueous interface and partition across the interface.

Many poorly water-soluble drugs have been found to exhibit greater bioavailabilities from liquid-filled capsule formulations. The cardiac glycoside digoxin, when formulated as a solution in a mixture of polyethylene glycol, ethanol and propylene glycol in a soft gelatin capsule, has been shown to be absorbed faster than the standard commercial tablets.

More recently, far more complex capsule formulations have been investigated to improve the absorption of poorly soluble drugs. Cyclosporin is a hydrophobic drug with poor solubility in gastrointestinal fluids. It showed low and variable oral bioavailability from its original liquid-filled soft gelatin capsule formulation (Sandimmun) and was particularly sensitive to the presence of fat in diet and bile acids. In its new formulation (Sandimmun Neoral), which is a complex mixture of hydrophilic and lipophilic phases, surfactants, cosurfactants and a cosolvent, it forms a non-precipitating microemulsion on dilution with gastrointestinal fluids. It has a significantly improved bioavailability with reduced variability that is independent of the presence of food (Drewe et al 1992).

Many protease inhibitors (antiviral drugs) are peptidomimetic in nature. They have high molecular weights and low aqueous solubility, are susceptible to degradation in the lumen and extensive hepatic metabolism, and consequently have poor bioavailability (Barry et al 1997). Saquinavir has recently been reformulated from a powder-filled hard gelatin capsule (Invirase) to a complex soft gelatin formulation (Fortovase). The latter shows a significant improvement in bioavailability (3–4 times) over the standard hard gelatin formulation, and as a consequence, a significantly greater viral load reduction (Perry and Noble 1998)

Factors associated with the formulation of liquid-filled gelatin capsules which can influence the bioavailabilities of drugs from this type of dosage form include:

- the solubility of the drug in the vehicle (and gastrointestinal fluids);
- the particle size of the drug (if suspended in the vehicle);
- the nature of the vehicle, i.e. hydrophilic or lipophilic (and whether a lipophilic vehicle is a digestible or a non-digestible oil);
- the inclusion of a surfactant as a wetting/emulsifying agent in a lipophilic vehicle or as the vehicle itself;
- the inclusion of a suspending agent (viscosity-enhancing agent) in the vehicle;
- the complexation, i.e. formation, of a non-absorbable complex between the drug and any excipient.

Powder-filled capsules

Generally the bioavailability of a drug from a well formulated powder-filled hard gelatin capsule dosage form will be better than or at least equal to that from the same drug in a compressed tablet. Provided the hard gelatin shell dissolves rapidly in the gastrointestinal fluids and the encapsulated mass disperses rapidly and efficiently, a relatively large effective surface area of drug will be exposed to the gastrointestinal fluids, thereby facilitating dissolution. However, it is incorrect to assume that a drug formulated as a hard gelatin capsule is in a finely divided form surrounded by a water-soluble shell, and that no bioavailability problems can occur. The overall rate of dissolution of drugs from capsules appears to be a complex function of the rates of different processes, such as the dissolution rate of the gelatin shell, the rate of penetration of the gastrointestinal fluids into the encapsulated mass, the rate at which the mass deaggregates (i.e. disperses) in the gastrointestinal fluids, and the rate of dissolution of the dispersed drug particles.

The inclusion of excipients (e.g. diluents, lubricants and surfactants) in a capsule formulation can have a significant effect on the rate of dissolution of drugs, particularly those that are poorly soluble and hydrophobic. Figure 17.4 shows that a hydrophilic diluent (e.g. sorbitol, lactose) often serves to increase the rate of penetration of the aqueous gastrointestinal fluids into the contents of the capsule, and to aid the

Hard gelatin capsule containing only hydrophobic drug particles

Hard gelatin capsule containing hydrophobic drug particles (o) and hydrophilic diluent particles (●)

In gastrointestinal fluids, hard gelatin capsule shell dissolves, thereby exposing contents to fluids

Contents remain as a capsule-shaped plug. Hydrophobic nature of contents impedes penetration of gastrointestinal fluids

Particles of hydrophilic diluent dissolve in gastrointestinal fluids leaving a porous mass of drug

Gastrointestinal fluids can penetrate porous mass

Dissolution of drug occurs only from surface of plug-shaped mass. Relatively low rate of dissolution

Effective surface area of drug and hence dissolution rate is increased

Fig. 17.4 Diagrammatic representation of how a hydrophilic diluent can increase the rate of dissolution of a poorly soluble, hydrophobic drug from a hard gelatin capsule.

dispersion and subsequent dissolution of the drug in these fluids. However, the diluent should exhibit no tendency to adsorb or complex with the drug, as either can impair absorption from the gastrointestinal tract.

Both the formulation and the type and conditions of the capsule-filling process can affect the packing density and liquid permeability of the capsule contents. In general, an increase in packing density (i.e. a decrease in porosity) of the encapsulated mass will probably result in a decrease in liquid permeability and dissolution rate, particularly if the drug is hydrophobic, or if a hydrophilic drug is mixed with a hydrophobic lubricant such as magnesium stearate. If the encapsulated mass is tightly packed and the drug is hydrophobic in nature, then a decrease in dissolution rate with a concomitant reduction in particle size would be expected, unless a surfactant had been included to facilitate liquid penetration.

In summary, formulation factors that can influence the bioavailabilities of drugs from hard gelatin capsules include:

- the surface area and particle size of the drug (particularly the effective surface area exhibited by the drug in the gastrointestinal fluids);
- the use of the salt form of a drug in preference to the parent weak acid or base;
- the crystal form of the drug;
- the chemical stability of the drug (in the dosage form and in gastrointestinal fluids);
- the nature and quantity of the diluent, lubricant and wetting agent;
- drug–excipient interactions (e.g. adsorption, complexation);
- the type and conditions of the filling process;
- the packing density of the capsule contents;
- the composition and properties of the capsule shell (including enteric capsules);
- interactions between the capsule shell and its contents.

Tablets

Uncoated tablets Tablets are the most widely used dosage form. When a drug is formulated as a compressed tablet there is an enormous reduction in the effective surface area of the drug, owing to the granulation and compression processes involved in tablet making. These processes necessitate the addition of excipients, which serve to return the surface area of the drug back to its original precompressed state. Bioavailability problems can arise if a fine, well dispersed suspension of drug particles in the gastrointestinal fluids is not generated following the

administration of a tablet. Because the effective surface area of a poorly soluble drug is an important factor influencing its dissolution rate, it is especially important that tablets containing such drugs should disintegrate rapidly and completely in the gastrointestinal fluids if rapid release, dissolution and absorption are required. The overall rate of tablet disintegration is influenced by several interdependent factors, which include the concentration and type of drug, diluent, binder, disintegrant, lubricant and wetting agent, as well as the compaction pressure (see Chapter 27).

The dissolution of a poorly soluble drug from an intact tablet is usually extremely limited because of the relatively small effective surface area of drug exposed to the gastrointestinal fluids. Disintegration of the tablet into granules causes a relatively large increase in effective surface area of drug and the dissolution rate may be likened to that of a coarse, aggregated suspension. Further disintegration into small, primary drug particles produces a further large increase in effective surface area and dissolution rate. The dissolution rate is probably comparable to that of a fine, well dispersed suspension. Disintegration of a tablet into primary particles is thus important, as it ensures that a large effective surface area of a drug is generated in order to facilitate dissolution and subsequent absorption.

However, simply because a tablet disintegrates rapidly this does not necessarily guarantee that the liberated primary drug particles will dissolve in the gastrointestinal fluids, and that the rate and extent of absorption are adequate. In the case of poorly soluble drugs the rate-controlling step is usually the overall rate of dissolution of the liberated drug particles in the gastrointestinal fluids. The overall dissolution rate and bioavailability of a poorly soluble drug from an uncoated conventional tablet is influenced by many factors associated with the formulation and manufacture of this type of dosage form. These include:

- the physicochemical properties of the liberated drug particles in the gastrointestinal fluids, e.g. wettability, effective surface area, crystal form, chemical stability;
- the nature and quantity of the diluent, binder, disintegrant, lubricant and any wetting agent;
- drug–excipient interactions (e.g. complexation), the size of the granules and their method of manufacture;
- the compaction pressure and speed of compression used in tabletting;
- the conditions of storage and age of the tablet.

Because drug absorption and hence bioavailability are dependent upon the drug being in the dissolved state, suitable dissolution characteristics can be an important property of a satisfactory tablet, particularly if it contains a poorly soluble drug. On this basis, specific in vitro dissolution test conditions and dissolution limits are included in the *British Pharmacopoeia* for tablets (and hard gelatin capsules) containing certain drugs, e.g. digoxin. That a particular drug product meets the requirements of a compendial dissolution standard provides a greater assurance that the drug will be released satisfactorily from the formulated dosage form in vivo and be absorbed adequately (see also Chapter 18).

Coated tablets Tablet coatings may be used simply for aesthetic reasons to improve the appearance of a tablet or to add a company logo, or may be employed to mask an unpleasant taste or odour or to protect an ingredient from decomposition during storage. Currently the most common type of tablet coat is film; however, several older preparations, such as vitamins and ibuprofen, still have sugar coats. The presence of a coating presents a physical barrier between the tablet core and the gastrointestinal fluids: coated tablets therefore not only possess all the potential bioavailability problems associated with uncoated conventional tablets, but are subject to the additional potential problem of being surrounded by a physical barrier. In the case of a coated tablet which is intended to disintegrate and release drug rapidly into solution in the gastrointestinal fluids, the coating must dissolve or disrupt before these processes can occur. The physicochemical nature and thickness of the coating can thus influence how quickly a drug is released from a tablet.

In the process of sugar coating the tablet core is usually sealed with a thin continuous film of a poorly water-soluble polymer such as shellac or cellulose acetate phthalate. This sealing coat serves to protect the tablet core and its contents from the aqueous fluids used in the subsequent steps of the sugar-coating process. Hence the presence of this water-impermeable sealing coat can potentially retard drug release from sugar-coated tablets. In view of this potential problem, annealing agents such as polyethylene glycols or calcium carbonate, which do not substantially reduce the water impermeability of the sealing coat during sugar coating, but which dissolve readily in gastric fluid, may be added to the sealer coat in order to reduce the barrier effect to rapid drug release.

The coating of a tablet core by a thin film of a water-soluble polymer, such as hydroxypropyl methycellulose, should have no significant effect on the rate of disintegration of the tablet core and subsequent drug dissolution, provided that the film coat dissolves rapidly and independently of the pH of the gastrointestinal fluids. However, if hydrophobic water-insoluble film-coating materials, such as ethylcellulose or certain acrylic resins, are used (see Chapter 28), the resulting film coat acts as a barrier which delays and/or reduces the rate of drug release. Thus these types of film-coating materials form barriers which can have a significant influence on drug absorption. Although the formation of such barriers would be disadvantageous in the case of film-coated tablets intended to provide rapid rates of drug absorption, the concept of barrier coating has been used (along with other techniques) to obtain more precise control over drug release than is possible with conventional uncoated tablets (see Chapter 20). In this context, film coating has been used to provide limited control over the site at which a drug is released from a tablet into the gastrointestinal tract.

Enteric-coated tablets The use of barrier coating to control the site of release of an orally administered drug is well illustrated by enteric-coated tablets. An enteric coat is designed to resist the low pH of gastric fluids but to disrupt or dissolve when the tablet enters the higher pH of the duodenum. Polymers such as cellulose acetate phthalate, hydroxypropyl methylcellulose phthalate, the copolymers of methacrylic acid and their esters and polyvinyl acetate phthalate, can be used as enteric coatings. These materials do not dissolve over the gastric pH range but dissolve rapidly at the less acid pH (about 5) values associated with the small intestine. Enteric coating should preferably begin to dissolve at pH5 in order to ensure the availability of drugs which are absorbed primarily in the proximal region of the small intestine. Enteric coating thus provides a means of delaying the release of a drug until the dosage form reaches the small intestine. Such delayed release provides a means of protecting drugs which would otherwise be destroyed if released into gastric fluid. Hence, enteric coating serves to improve the oral bioavailability exhibited by such drugs from uncoated conventional tablets. Enteric coating also protects the stomach against drugs which can produce nausea or mucosal irritation (e.g. aspirin, ibuprofen) if released at this site.

In addition to the protection offered by enteric coating, the delayed release of drug also results in a significant delay in the onset of the therapeutic response of a drug. The onset of the therapeutic response is largely dependent on the residence time of the enteric-coated tablet in the stomach. Gastric emptying of such tablets is an all-or-nothing process, i.e. the tablet is either in the stomach or in the duodenum. Consequently, drug is either not being released or being released. The residence time of an intact enteric-coated tablet in the stomach can vary from about 5 minutes to several hours (see Chapter 16).

Hence there is considerable intra- and intersubject variation in the onset of therapeutic action exhibited by drugs administered as enteric-coated tablets.

The formulation of an enteric-coated product in the form of small individually enteric-coated granules or pellets (multiparticulates) contained in a rapidly dissolving hard gelatin capsule or a rapidly disintegrating tablet, largely eliminates the dependency of this type of dosage form on the all-or-nothing gastric emptying process associated with intact (monolith) enteric coated tablets. Provided the coated granules or pellets are sufficiently small (less than 1 mm diameter), they will be able to empty from the stomach with liquids. Hence enteric-coated granules and pellets exhibit a gradual but continual release from the stomach into the duodenum. This type of release also avoids the complete dose of drug being released into the duodenum, as occurs with an enteric-coated tablet. The intestinal mucosa is thus not exposed locally to a potentially toxic concentration of drug.

Further information on coated tablets and multiparticulates is given in Chapter 28.

Influence of excipients for conventional dosage forms

Drugs are almost never administered alone but rather in the form of dosage forms that generally consist of a drug (or drugs) together with a varying number of other substances (called **excipients**). Excipients are added to the formulation in order to facilitate the preparation, patient acceptability and functioning of the dosage form as a drug delivery system. Excipients include disintegrating agents, diluents, lubricants, suspending agents, emulsifying agents, flavouring agents, colouring agents, chemical stabilizers etc. Although historically excipients were considered to be inert in that they themselves should exert no therapeutic or biological action, or modify the biological action of the drug present in the dosage form, they are now regarded as having the ability to influence the rate and/or extent of absorption of the drug. For instance, the potential influence of excipients on drug bioavailability has already been illustrated by virtue of the formation of poorly soluble, non-absorbable drug–excipient complexes between tetracyclines and dicalcium phosphate, amphetamine and sodium carboxymethylcellulose, and phenobarbitone and polyethylene glycol 4000.

Diluents

The classic example of the influence that excipients employed as diluents can have on drug bioavail-

ability is provided by the Australian outbreak of phenytoin intoxication which occurred in epileptic patients as a consequence of the diluent in sodium phenytoin capsules being changed. Many epileptic patients who had been previously stabilized with sodium phenytoin capsules containing calcium sulphate dihydrate as the diluent, developed clinical features of phenytoin overdosage when given sodium phenytoin capsules containing lactose as the diluent even though the quantity of drug in each capsule formulation was identical. It was later shown that the excipient calcium sulphate dihydrate had been responsible for decreasing the gastrointestinal absorption of phenytoin, possibly because part of the administered dose of drug formed a poorly absorbable calcium–phenytoin complex. Hence, although the size of dose and frequency of administration of the sodium phenytoin capsules containing calcium sulphate dihydrate gave therapeutic blood levels of phenytoin in epileptic patients, the efficiency of absorption of phenytoin had been lowered by the incorporation of this excipient in the hard gelatin capsules. Hence, when the calcium sulphate dihydrate was replaced by lactose without any alteration in the quantity of drug in each capsule, or in the frequency of administration, an increased bioavailability of phenytoin was achieved. In many patients the higher plasma levels exceeded the maximum safe concentration for phenytoin and produced toxic side-effects.

Surfactants

Surfactants are often used in dosage forms as emulsifying agents, solubilizing agents, suspension stabilizers or wetting agents. However, surfactants in general cannot be assumed to be 'inert' excipients as they have been shown to be capable of either increasing, decreasing or exerting no effect on the transfer of drugs across biological membranes.

Surfactant monomers can potentially disrupt the integrity and function of a biological membrane. Such an effect would tend to enhance drug penetration and hence absorption across the gastrointestinal barrier, but may also result in toxic side-effects. Inhibition of absorption may occur as a consequence of a drug being incorporated into surfactant micelles. If such surfactant micelles are not absorbed, which appears usually to be the case, then solubilization of a drug may result in a reduction of the concentration of 'free' drug in solution in the gastrointestinal fluids that is available for absorption. Inhibition of drug absorption in the presence of micellar concentrations of surfactant would be expected to occur in the case of drugs that are normally soluble in the gastrointestinal fluids, i.e. in the absence of surfactant. Conversely, in the case of poorly soluble drugs whose absorption is dissolution-rate limited, the increase in saturation solubility of the drug by solubilization in surfactant micelles could result in more rapid rates of dissolution and hence absorption.

The release of poorly soluble drugs from tablets and hard gelatin capsules may be increased by the inclusion of surfactants in their formulations. The ability of a surfactant to reduce the solid/liquid interfacial tension will permit the gastrointestinal fluids to wet the solid more effectively, and thus enable it to come into more intimate contact with the solid dosage forms. This wetting effect may thus aid the penetration of gastrointestinal fluids into the mass of capsule contents that often remains when the hard gelatin shell has dissolved, and/or reduce the tendency of poorly soluble drug particles to aggregate in the gastrointestinal fluids. In each case, the resulting increase in the total effective surface area of drug in contact with the gastrointestinal fluids would tend to increase the dissolution and absorption rates of the drug. It is interesting to note that the enhanced gastrointestinal absorption of phenacetin in humans resulting from the addition of polysorbate-80 to an aqueous suspension of this drug was attributed to the surfactant preventing aggregation and thus increasing the effective surface area and dissolution rate of the drug particles in the gastrointestinal fluids.

The possible mechanisms by which surfactants can influence drug absorption are varied and it is likely that only rarely will a single mechanism operate in isolation. In most cases the overall effect on drug absorption will probably involve a number of different actions of the surfactant (some of which will produce opposing effects on drug absorption), and the observed effect on drug absorption will depend on which of the different actions is the overriding one. The ability of a surfactant to influence drug absorption will also depend on the physicochemical characteristics and concentration of the surfactant, the nature of the drug and the type of biological membrane involved.

Lubricants

Both tablets and capsules require lubricants in their formulation to reduce friction between the powder and metal surfaces during their manufacture. Lubricants are often hydrophobic in nature. Magnesium stearate is commonly included as a lubri-

cant during tablet compression and capsule-filling operations. Its hydrophobic nature often retards liquid penetration into capsule ingredients, so that after the shell has dissolved in the gastrointestinal fluids a capsule-shaped plug often remains, especially when the contents have been machine-filled as a consolidated plug (Chapter 29). Similar reductions in dissolution rate may be observed when magnesium stearate is included in tablets. However, these effects can usually be overcome by the simultaneous addition of a wetting agent (i.e. a water-soluble surfactant) and the use of a hydrophilic diluent.

Disintegrants

Disintegrants are required to break up capsules, tablets and granules into primary powder particles in order to increase the surface area of the drug exposed to the gastrointestinal fluids. A tablet that fails to disintegrate or disintegrates slowly may result in incomplete absorption or a delay in the onset of action of the drug. The compaction force used in tablet manufacture can affect disintegration: in general, the higher the force the slower the disintegration time. Even small changes in formulation may result in significant effects on dissolution and bioavailability. A classic example is that of tolbutamide, where two formulations, the commercial product and the same formulation but with half the amount of disintegrant, were administered to healthy volunteers. Both tablets disintegrated in vitro within 10 minutes meeting pharmacopoeial specifications, but the commercial tablet had a significantly greater bioavailability and hypoglycaemic response.

Viscosity-enhancing agents

Viscosity-enhancing agents are often employed in the formulation of liquid dosage forms for oral use in order to control such properties as palatability, ease of pouring and, in the case of suspensions, the rate of sedimentation of the dispersed particles. The viscosity-enhancing agent is often a hydrophilic polymer.

There are a number of mechanisms by which a viscosity-enhancing agent may produce a change in the gastrointestinal absorption of a drug. Complex formation between a drug and a hydrophilic polymer could reduce the concentration of drug in solution that is available for absorption. The administration of viscous solutions or suspensions may produce an increase in viscosity of the gastrointestinal contents. This could lead to a decrease in dissolution rate and/or a decrease in the rate of movement of drug molecules to the absorbing membrane.

Normally, a decrease in the rate of dissolution would not be applicable to solution dosage forms unless dilution of the administered solution in the gastrointestinal fluids caused precipitation of the drug.

In the case of suspensions containing drugs with bioavailabilities that are dissolution-rate dependent, an increase in viscosity could also lead to a decrease in the rate of dissolution of the drug in the gastrointestinal tract.

Summary

As well as physiological and drug factors, the dosage form can play a major role in influencing the rate and extent of absorption. Often this is by design. However, even with conventional dosage forms it is important to consider whether changing the dosage form or excipients will affect the bioavailability of the drug. Some drugs will be more susceptible to changes in rate and extent of absorption through dosage form changes than others: this will depend on the biopharmaceutical properties of the drug (see Chapter 18).

estimate the solubility and permeability in drug discovery and development settings. *Adv. Drug Del. Rev.* **23**, 3–29.

Loper, A., Hettrick, L., Novak, L., Landis, E., Yeh, S., Asgharnejad, M., Gehret, J. and Ostovic, D. (1999) Factors influencing the absorption of an HIV protease inhibitor analogue of indinavir in beagle dogs. *AAPS Pharm. Sci.*, 4243.

Naylor, L.J. et al. (1995) Dissolution of steroids in bile salt and lecithin solutions, with references to bile salt concentrations in the GI tract. *Eur. J. Pharm. Biopharm.*, **41**, 346–353.

Panchagnula, R. and Thomas, N.S. (2000) Biopharmaceutics and pharmacokinetics in drug research. *Int. J. Pharm.*, **201**, 131–150.

Perry, C.M. Noble, S. (1998) Saquinavir soft-gel capsule formulation. A review of its use in patients with HIV infection. *Drugs* (3) 461–486.

Russell T.L. et al (1994). Influence of gastric pH and emptying on dipyridamole absorption. *Pharm. Res.*, **11**; 136–143.

Sevelius, H. et al. (1980); Bioavailability of naproxen sodium and its relationship to clinical analgesic effects. *Br. J. Clin. Pharmacol.*, **10**, 259.

Taylor, D.C., Pownall, R., Burke, W. (1985). Absorption of beta-adrenoceptor antagonists in the rat in situ small intestine. *J. Pharm. Pharmacol.*, **37**, 280–283.

Terjarla, S., Puranjoti, P., Kasina, P., Mandal, J. (1998) Preparation, characterisation and evaluation of miconazole–cyclodextrin complexes for improved oral and topical delivery. *J. Pharm. Sci.*, **87**; 425–429.

REFERENCES

Barry, M., Gribous, Back D., Mulcahy F. (1997) Protease inhibitors in patients with HIV disease. Clinically important pharmacokinetic considerations. *Clin Pharmacokinet* **32** (3) 194–209.

Dressman, J.B., Amidon, G.L., Reppas, C., Shah, V.P. (1998). Dissolution testing as a prognostic tool for oral drug absorption; immediate release dosage forms. *Pharm. Res*, **15**, 11–22.

Drewe, J., Meier, R., Vonderscher, J., Kiss, D., Posanki, U., Kissel, T., Gyr, K. (1992). *Br. J. Clin. Pharmacol.*, **34**, 60.

Florence, A.T. and Attwood, D. (1998). Physicochemical principles of Pharmacy, 3rd edn. Macmillan Press.

Lipinski, C.A., Lombardo, F., Dominy, B.W. and Feeney, P.J. (1997) Experimental and computational approaches to

BIBLIOGRAPHY

Brayden, D. (1997) Human intestinal epithelial monolayers as prescreens for oral drug delivery. *Pharm. News*, **4** (1). 11–13.

Dressman, J.B., Amidon, G.L., Reppas, C., Shah, V.P. (1998). Dissolution testing as a prognostic tool for oral drug absorption; immediate release dosage forms. *Pharm. Res*, **15**, 11–22.

Lennernäs, H. (1998) Human intestinal permeability. *J. Pharm. Sci.*, **87**, 403–410.

vander Meer, J.W., Keuning, J.J., Scheijgrond, H.W., Heykants, J., Van Cutsem J., Brugmans, J. (1980) The influence of gastric acidity on the bioavailability of ketoconazole. *Antimicrob. Chemother,* **6** (4). 552–554.

18

Assessment of biopharmaceutical properties

Marianne Ashford

INTRODUCTION

Biopharmaceutics is involved with factors that influence the rate and extent of drug absorption. As discussed in Chapters 16 and 17, the factors that affect the release of a drug from its dosage form, its dissolution into physiological fluids, its stability within those fluids, its permeability across the relevant biological membranes and its presystemic metabolism will all influence its rate and extent of absorption (Fig. 18.1). Once the drug is absorbed into the systemic circulation, its distribution within the body tissues (including to its site of action), its metabolism and elimination are described by the pharmacokinetics of the compound. The pharmacokinetics of the compound influence the length and magnitude of the therapeutic effect or the response of the compound, i.e. its pharmacodynamics (see Chapter 15).

The key biopharmaceutical properties that can be quantified and therefore give an insight into the absorption of a drug are its:

- release from its dosage form into solution at the absorption site;
- stability in physiological fluids;
- permeability;
- susceptibility to presystemic clearance.

As most drugs are delivered via the mouth, these properties will be discussed with respect to the peroral route. The bioavailability of a compound is an overall measure of its availability in the systemic circulation, and so the assessment of bioavailability will also be discussed. Other methods of assessing the performance of dosage forms in vivo will also be briefly mentioned. The Biopharmaceutical Classification Scheme, which classifies drugs according to two of their key biopharmaceutical properties, solubility and permeability, is outlined.

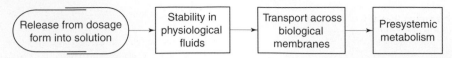

Fig. 18.1   Key biopharmaceutical properties affecting drug absorption.

MEASUREMENT OF KEY BIOPHARMACEUTICAL PROPERTIES

Release of drug from its dosage form into solution

As discussed in the Chapter 17 and Part 4 of this book, a dosage form is normally formulated to aid the release of drug from it. For example, for an immediate-release tablet, the tablet needs to disintegrate to give the primary drug particles. Further, a suspension should not be so thick that it impedes the diffusion of dissolving drug away from the solid particles.

The solubility of a drug across the gastrointestinal pH range will be one of the first indicators as to whether dissolution is liable to be rate limiting in the absorption process. A knowledge of the solubility across the gastrointestinal pH range can be determined by measuring the equilibrium solubility in suitable buffers or by using an acid or a base titration method.

Methods of measuring the dissolution rate of both a drug itself (intrinsic dissolution rate) and of various dosage forms are discussed in Chapters 8 and 2, respectively.

The aim of dissolution testing is to find an in vitro characteristic of a potential formulation that reflects its in vivo performance. Historically, dissolution tests have been developed mainly for quality control purposes and as a guide in the development of new formulations, rather than to predict the in vivo performance of the product. The tests tend to be carried out with standard procedures (volumes, agitation rates etc.) and under sink conditions. These conditions are not representative of physiological conditions and are therefore liable to correlate poorly with the in vivo situation.

When designing a dissolution test to assess drug release from a biopharmaceutical perspective, it is important to mimic as closely as possible the conditions of the gastrointestinal tract. Clinical scientists increasingly want to rely on dissolution tests to establish in vitro/in vivo correlations between the release of drug from the dosage form and its absorption. If this can be successfully achieved, it is possible that the dissolution test could replace some of the in vivo studies that need to be performed during product development and registration. Such correlations should have the benefit of reducing both the

use of animals to evaluate formulations and the size and number of costly clinical studies to assess bioavailability.

An in vitro/in vivo correlation may only be possible for those drugs where dissolution is the rate-limiting step in the absorption process. Determining full dissolution profiles of such drugs in a number of different physiologically representative media will aid the understanding of the factors affecting the rate and extent of dissolution. The profiles can also be used to generate an in vitro/in vivo correlation. To achieve this, at least three batches that differ in their in vivo as well as their in vitro behaviour should be available. The differences in the in vivo profiles need to be mirrored by the formulations in vitro. Normally, the in vitro test conditions can be modified to correspond with the in vivo data to achieve a correlation. Very often a well designed in vitro dissolution test is found to be more sensitive and discriminating than the in vivo test. From a quality assurance perspective a more discriminative dissolution method is preferred because the test will indicate possible changes in the product before the in vivo performance is affected.

A dilute hydrochloric acid-based solution at pH 1.2 can simulate gastric fluid, and phosphate-buffered solution at pH 6.8 can mimic intestinal fluid. However, dissolution media more closely representing physiological conditions may well provide more relevant conditions. Dressman et al (1998) studied in detail a range of physiological parameters and suggested four more appropriate media for simulated gastric and intestinal conditions in the fed and fasted states. Each of these media takes into account not only the pH of the fluids in the different states, but their ionic composition, surface tension, buffer capacity and bile and lecithin contents. The proposed composition for gastric fluid in the fasted state and intestinal fluids in the fed and fasted states are shown in Tables 18.1–18.3.

In the fed state the conditions in the stomach are highly dependent on the composition of the meal eaten and therefore difficult to simulate. In trying to produce an in vitro/in vivo correlation it has been suggested that a more appropriate way of simulating the fed-state gastric fluids is to homogenize the meal to be used in clinical studies and then dilute it with

Table 18.1 Dissolution medium to simulate gastric conditions in the fasted state (proposed by Dressman et al 1998)

Component	Concentration/amount
Hydrochloric acid	0.01–0.05 M
Sodium lauryl sulphate	2.5 g
Sodium chloride	2 g
Distilled water	qs to 1000 mL

Table 18.2 Dissolution medium to simulate intestinal conditions in the fasted state (proposed by Dressman et al 1998)

Component	Concentration/amount
Potassium dihydrogen phosphate	0.029 M
Sodium hydroxide	qs to pH 6.8
Sodium taurocholate (bile salt)	5 mM
Lecithin	1.5 mM
Potassium chloride	0.22 M
Distilled water	qs to 1000 mL

pH = 6.8, osmolarity = 280–310 mOSm.
Buffer capacity = 10 ± 2 mEq/L/pH.

Table 18.3 Dissolution medium to simulate intestinal conditions in the fed state (proposed by Dressman et al 1998)

Component	Concentration/amount
Acetic acid	0.144 M
Sodium hydroxide	qs to pH 5
Sodium taurocholate (bile salt)	15 mM
Lecithin	4 mM
Potassium chloride	0.19 M
Distilled water	qs to 1000 mL

pH = 5, osmolarity = 485–535 mOSm.
Buffer capacity = 76 ± 2 mEq/L/pH

diction of the permeability properties of the drug is beneficial. If, for example, the drug is absorbed from the upper intestine and is likely to be dosed in the fasted state, the most appropriate dissolution conditions may be a short test (~ 15–30 minutes) in a medium simulating gastric fluid in the fasted state (see Table 18.1). Alternatively, if it is advised that a drug should be administered with food, and it is known to be well absorbed throughout the length of the gastrointestinal tract, a far longer dissolution test, perhaps several hours in duration, with a range of media such as, initially, simulated gastric fluid for the fed state, simulated intestinal fluid for the fed and then the fasted states, may be more appropriate.

The volumes in, and agitation of, the stomach and intestines vary enormously, particularly between the fed and the fasted states, and so it is difficult to choose a representative volume and degree of agitation. The latest Guidance for Industry on the dissolution testing of immediate-release solid oral dosage forms from the Food and Drug Administration (1997) suggests volumes of 500, 900 or 1000 mL and gentle agitation conditions.

Stability in physiological fluids

The stability of drugs in physiological fluids (in the case of orally administered drugs, the gastrointestinal fluids) depends on two factors: the chemical stability of the drug across the gastrointestinal pH range, i.e. the drug's pH–stability profile between pH 1 and pH 8, and its susceptibility to enzymatic breakdown by the gastrointestinal fluids. Means of assessing the chemical stability of a drug are discussed in Chapters 7 and 8. The stability of a drug in gastrointestinal fluids can be assessed by simulated gastric and intestinal media or by obtaining gastrointestinal fluids from humans or animals. The latter provides a harsher assessment of gastrointestinal stability but is more akin to the in vivo setting. In general the drug is incubated with either real or simulated fluid at 37°C for a period of 3 hours and the drug content analysed. A loss of more than 5% of drug indicates potential instability. Many of the permeability methods described below can be used to identify whether gastrointestinal stability is an issue for a particular drug.

For drugs that will still be in the gastrointestinal lumen when they reach the colonic region, resistance to the bacterial enzymes present in this part of the intestine need to be considered. The bacterial enzymes are capable of a whole host of reactions. There may be a significant portion of a poorly soluble drug still in the gastrointestinal tract by the

water. Long-life milk has also been used to simulate gastric conditions in the fed state.

It has been proposed that the duration of the dissolution test should depend on the site of absorption of the drug and its timing of administration. Thus, in designing a dissolution test some knowledge or pre-time it reaches the colon. If the drug is absorbed along the length of the gastrointestinal tract, and is susceptible to degradation or metabolism by the bacterial enzymes within the tract, its absorption and hence its bioavailability is liable to be reduced. Similarly, for sustained- or controlled-release products that are designed to release their drug along the length of the gastrointestinal tract, the potential of degradation or metabolism by bacterial enzymes should be assessed. If the drug is metabolized to a metabolite which can be absorbed the potential toxicity of this metabolite should be considered.

Permeability

There is a wealth of techniques available for either estimating or measuring the rate of permeation across membranes that are used to gain an assessment of oral absorption in humans. These range from computational (in silico) predictions and both physicochemical and biological methods. The biological methods can be further subdivided into in vitro, in situ and in vivo methods. In general, the more complex the technique the more information that can be gained and the more accurate is the assessment of oral absorption in humans. The range of techniques is summarized in Table 18.4. Some of the more popular ones are discussed below.

Partition coefficients

One of the first properties of a molecule that can be predicted or measured is its partition coefficient between an oil and a water phase ($\log P$). This gives

Table 18.4 Some of the models available for predicting or measuring drug absorption

Model type	Model	Description
Computational	cLog$P$	Commercial software that calculates octanol/water partition coefficient based on fragment analysis, known as the Leo–Hansch method
	mLog$P$	Method of calculating log P, known as the Moriguchi method (see text)
Physicochemical	Partition coefficient	Measure of lipophilicity of drug, usually measured between octanol and aqueous buffer via a shake-flask method
	Immobilized artificial membrane	Measures partition into more sophisticated lipidic phase on an HPLC column
Cell culture	Caco-2 monolayer	Measures transport across monolayers of differentiated human colon adenocarcinoma cells
	HT-29	Measures transport across polarized cell monolayer with mucin-producing cells
Excised tissues	Cells	Measures uptake into cell suspensions, e.g. erythrocytes
	Freshly isolated cells	Measures uptake into enterocytes; however, the cells are difficult to prepare and are short-lived
	Membrane vesicles	Measures uptake into brush border membrane vesicles prepared from intestinal scrapings or isolated enterocytes
	Everted sacs	Measures uptake into intestinal segments/sacs
	Everted intestinal rings	Studies the kinetics of uptake into the intestinal mucosa
	Isolated sheets	Measures the transport across sheets of intestine
In situ studies	In-situ perfusion	Measures drug disappearance from either closed or open loop perfusate of segments of intestine of anaesthetized animals
	Vascularly perfused intestine	Measures drug disappearance from perfusate and its appearance in blood
In vivo studies	Intestinal loop	Measures drug disappearance from perfusate of loop of intestine in awake animal
Human data	Loc-I-Gut	Measures drug disappearance from perfusate of human intestine
	High-frequency capsule	Non-invasive method; measures drug in systemic circulation
	InteliSite capsule	Non-invasive method; measures drug in systemic circulation.
	Bioavailability	Deconvolution of pharmacokinetic data

a measure of the lipophilicity of a molecule, which can be used as a prediction as to how well it will be able to cross a biological membrane. As discussed in Chapter 17, octanol is usually chosen as the solvent for the oil phase as it has similar properties to biological membranes. If the aqueous phase is at a particular pH, the distribution coefficient at that pH is measured (log D), this then accounts for the ionization of the molecule at that pH. In the case of a weakly acidic or a weakly basic drug, the log D measured at an intestinal pH (e.g. 6.8) is liable to give a better prediction of the drug's ability to cross the lipid gastrointestinal membrane than its partition coefficient, log P, which does not take the degree of ionization into account.

One of the most common ways of measuring partition coefficients is to use the shake flask method. This relies on the equilibrium distribution of a drug between an oil and an aqueous phase. Prior to the experiment the aqueous phase should be saturated with the oil phase and vice versa. The experiment should be carried out at constant temperature. The drug should be added to the aqueous phase and the oil phase which, in the case of octanol, as it is less dense than water, will sit on top of the water. The system is mixed and then left to reach equilibrium (usually at least 24 hours). The two phases are separated and the concentration of drug is measured in each phase and a partition coefficient calculated (Fig. 18.2). As discussed in Chapter 17, within a homologous series increasing lipophilicity (log P/D) tends to result in greater absorption. A molecule is unlikely to cross a membrane (i.e. be absorbed via the transcellular passive route) if it has a log P less than 0.

Instead of measuring log P computational methods can be used to estimate it, and there are a number of software packages available to do this. There is a reasonably good correlation between the calculated and the measured values. Log P can be estimated by breaking down the molecule into fragments and calculating the contribution of each fragment to overall lipophilicity (often called the cLog$P$). Another method used to calculate log P is the Moriguchi method, which uses 13 parameters for hydrophobic and hydrophilic atoms, proximity effects, unsaturated bonds, intramolecular bonds, ring structures, amphoteric properties and several specific functionalities to obtain a value for the partition coefficient. This is often called the mLog$P$. The advantages of these methods are in drug discovery, where an estimate of the lipophilicity of many molecules can be obtained before they are actually synthesized.

Another more sophisticated physicochemical means of gaining a view as to how well a drug will partition into a lipophilic phase is by investigating how well the molecule can be retained on a high-performance liquid chromatography column (HPLC). HPLC columns can be simply coated with octanol to mimic octanol–aqueous partition, or more elaborately designed to mimic biological membranes, for example the Immobilized Artificial Membrane (IAM). This technique provides a measure of how well a solute (i.e. the drug) in the aqueous phase will partition into biological membranes (i.e. be retained on the column). Good correlations between these methods and biological in vitro methods of estimating transcellular passive drug absorption have been obtained.

Cell culture techniques

Cell culture techniques for measuring the intestinal absorption of molecules have been increasingly used over recent decades and are now a well accepted model for absorption.

The cell line that is most widely used is Caco-2. Caco-2 cells are a human colon carcinoma cell line that was first proposed and characterized as a model for oral drug absorption by Hidalgo in 1989. In culture, Caco-2 cells spontaneously differentiate to form a monolayer of polarized enterocytes. These enterocytes resemble those in the small intestine, in that they contain microvilli and many of the transport systems present in the small intestine, for example those for sugars, amino acids, peptides and the P-glycoprotein efflux transporter. Adjacent Caco-2 cells adhere through tight junctions. However, the tightness of these junctions is more like those of the colon than those of the leakier small intestine.

There are many variations on growing and carrying out transport experiments with Caco-2 monolayers. In general the cells are grown on porous supports, usually for a period of 15–21 days in typical cell

Fig. 18.2 Diagram of the shake-flask method for determining partition coefficient.

culture medium, Dulbecco's Modified Eagle Medium supplemented with 20% fetal bovine serum, 1% non-essential amino acids and 2mM L-glutamine. The cells are grown at 37°C in 10% carbon dioxide at a relative humidity of 95%. The culture medium is replaced at least twice each week. Transport experiments are carried out by replacing the culture medium with buffers, usually Hanks Balanced Salt Solution adjusted to pH 6.5 on the apical surface and Hanks Balanced Salt Solution adjusted to pH 7.4 on the basolateral surface (Fig. 18.3).

After a short incubation period – usually about 30 minutes – when the cells are maintained at 37°C in a shaking water bath, the buffers are replaced with fresh buffers and a dilute solution of drug is introduced to the apical chamber. At regular intervals the concentration of the drug in the basolateral chamber is determined. The apparent permeability coefficient across cells can be calculated as follows:

$$P_{app} = dQ/dt(1/C_0A) \qquad (18.1)$$

where P_{app} is the apparent permeability coefficient (cm/s), dQ/dt is the rate of drug transport (μg/s), C_0 is the initial donor concentration (μg/mL) and, A is the surface area of the monolayer (cm^2).

To check that the monolayer has maintained its integrity throughout the transport process, a marker for paracellular absorption, such as mannitol, which is often radiolabelled for ease of assay, is added to the apical surface. If less than 2% of this crosses the monolayer in an hour then the integrity of the monolayer has been maintained. Another way to check the integrity of the monolayer is by measuring the transepithelial resistance, or TEER.

To use the Caco-2 cells as an absorption model a calibration curve needs to be generated. This is done for compounds for which the absorption in humans is known. Figure 18.4 shows the general shape of the curve of fraction absorbed in humans versus the

Fig. 18.4 The relationship between the fraction absorbed in humans and the apparent permeability coefficient in Caco cells.

apparent permeability coefficient in Caco-2 cells. As cells are biological systems, and as small changes in their source, method of culture and the way in which the transport experiment is carried out will affect the apparent permeability of a drug, this curve can shift significantly to the right or left or alter its steepness. Therefore, when carrying out Caco-2 experiments it is important always to standardize the procedure within a particular laboratory, and ensure that this procedure is regularly calibrated with a set of standard compounds.

Caco-2 monolayers can also be used to elucidate the mechanism of permeability. If the apparent permeability coefficient is found to increase linearly with increasing concentration of drug (i.e. the transport is not saturated), is the same whether the drug transport is measured from the apical to basolateral or the basolateral to apical direction, and is independent of pH, it can be concluded that the transport is a passive and not an active process. If the transport in the basolateral to apical direction is significantly greater than that in the apical to basolateral direction, then it is likely that the drug is actively effluxed from the cells by a countermembrane transporter such as P-glycoprotein. If the transport of the drug is

Fig. 18.3 Diagram of a Caco-2 cell culture system for determining apparent permeability.

also inhibited by the presence of compounds that are known inhibitors of P-glycoprotein, such as verapamil, this gives a further indication that the drug is susceptible to P-glycoprotein efflux.

To help elucidate whether other membrane transporters are involved in the absorption of a particular drug, further competitive inhibition studies can be carried out with known inhibitors of the particular transporter. For example, the dipeptide glycosylsarcosine can be used to probe whether the dipeptide transporter is involved in the absorption of a particular drug.

To evaluate whether a compound is absorbed via the paracellular or the transcellular pathway, the tight junctions can be artificially opened with compounds such as EDTA, which chelates calcium. Calcium is involved in keeping the junctions together. If the apparent permeability of a compound is not affected by the opening of these junctions, which can be assessed by using a paracellular marker such as mannitol, one can assume the drug transport is via a transcellular pathway.

If the disappearance of drug on the apical side of the membrane is not mirrored by its appearance on the basolateral side, and/or the mass balance at the end of the transport experiment does not account for 100% of the drug, there may be a problem with binding to the membrane porous support. This will need investigation, or the drug may have a stability issue. The drug could be susceptible to enzymes secreted by the cells and/or to degradation by hydrolytic enzymes as it passes through the cells, or it may be susceptible to metabolism by cytochrome P450 within the cell. Thus the Caco-2 cells are not only capable of evaluating the permeability of drugs but have value in investigating whether two of the other potential barriers to absorption, stability and presystemic metabolism, are likely to affect the overall rate and extent of absorption.

Caco-2 cells are very useful tools for understanding the mechanism of absorption of drugs and have furthered significantly our knowledge of the absorption of a variety of drugs. Other advantages of Caco-2 cells are that they are a non-animal model, require only small amounts of compound for transport studies, can be used as a rapid screening tool to assess the permeability of large numbers of compounds in the discovery setting, and can be used to evaluate the potential toxicity of compounds to cells.

The main disadvantages of Caco-2 monolayers as an absorption model are that, because of the tightness of the monolayer, they are more akin to the paracellular permeability of the colon rather than that of the small intestine, and that they lack a mucus

layer. HT-29-18C1, a subclone of a human intestinal adenocarcinoma cell line, can differentiate in culture to produce both absorptive cells containing a microvillus structure and mucus secreting goblet cells. It also has a resistance similar to that of the small intestine, and so it can be argued that this cell line is preferable to Caco-2 in that it will give better information about the transcellular and paracellular routes of absorption. However, this cell line has yet to be well characterized as an absorption model, and therefore its use is not widespread.

Further information on the use of Caco-2 monolayers as an absorption model can be obtained from Artusson et al (1996).

Tissue techniques

A range of tissue techniques have been used as absorption models (Table 18.4). Two of the more popular ones are the use of isolated sheets of intestinal mucosa and of everted intestinal rings. These are discussed in more detail below.

Isolated sheets of intestinal mucosa are prepared by cutting the intestine into strips; the musculature is then removed and the sheet mounted and clamped in a diffusion chamber or an Ussing chamber filled with appropriate biological buffers (Fig. 18.5). The transepithelial resistance is measured across the tissue to check its integrity. The system is maintained at 37°C and stirred so that the thickness of the unstirred water layer is controlled and oxygen provided to the tissue. The drug is added to the donor chamber and

Fig. 18.5 Diagram of a diffusion chamber.

the amount accumulating in the receiver chamber is measured as a function of time. The permeability across the tissue can then be calculated.

Similar to cell monolayers, the two sides of the tissue can be sampled independently and thus fluxes from mucosal to serosal and from serosal to mucosal can be measured. Any pH dependence of transport can be determined by altering the pH of the buffers in the donor and/or receiver chambers. This system can also therefore be used to probe active transport.

One advantage of this technique over cell culture techniques is that permeability across different regions of the intestine can be assessed. It is particularly helpful to be able to compare permeabilities across intestinal and colonic tissue, especially when assessing whether a drug is suitable for a controlled-release delivery system. In addition, different animal tissues can be used, which permits an assessment of permeability in different preclinical models. The rat intestine is usually preferred for absorption studies as its permeability correlates well with that of human intestine. Human tissue and cell monolayers have also been used in this system.

Everted intestinal rings use whole intestinal segments rather than just sheets. The musculature is therefore intact. Intestinal segments are excised, again usually from rats; the segment is then tied at one end and carefully everted by placing it over a glass rod, and cut into small sections or rings. These rings are incubated in stirred oxygenated drug-containing buffer at 37°C. After a set period of time, drug uptake is quenched by quickly rinsing the ring with ice-cold buffer and carefully drying it. The ring is then assayed for drug content and the amount of drug taken up per gram of wet tissue over a specific period of time is calculated (mol g^{-1} time^{-1}). The advantage of using intestinal rings is that the test is relatively simple and quick to perform. A large number of rings can be prepared from each segment of intestine, which allows each animal to act as its own control. In addition, the conditions of the experiment can be manipulated and so provide an insight into the mechanisms of absorption.

The disadvantages of this system are that it is biological and that care must be taken to maintain the viability of the tissue for the duration of the experiment. As the drug is taken up into the ring, the tissue needs to be digested and the drug extracted from it before it is assayed, which results in lengthy sample preparation and complicates the assay procedure. In addition, as this is an uptake method no polarity of absorption can be assessed.

Both these absorption models can be calibrated with a standard set of compounds similar to the Caco-2 model. A similarly shaped curve for the percentage of drug absorbed in humans versus apparent permeability or uptake (mole per weight of tissue) for the isolated sheet and everted ring methods, respectively, is obtained.

Perfusion studies

Many variations of intestinal perfusion methods have been used as absorption models over the years. Again, in general, because of its relative ease of use and similarity to the permeability of the human intestine, the rat model is preferred. In situ intestinal perfusion models have the advantage that the whole animal is used, with the nerve, lymphatic and blood supplies intact, and therefore there should be no problem with tissue viability and all the transport mechanisms present in a live animal should be functional.

The animal is anaesthetized and the intestine exposed. In the open loop method a dilute solution of drug is pumped slowly through the intestine and the difference in drug concentration between the inlet and outlet concentrations is calculated (Fig. 18.6). An absorption rate constant or effective permeability coefficient across the intestine can be calculated as follows:

$$P_{eff} = Q \cdot \ln (C_i - C_0)/2\pi rl \qquad (18.2)$$

where P_{eff} is the effective permeability coefficient (cm/s), Q is the flow rate in mL/s, C_i is the initial drug concentration, C_0 is the final drug concentration, r is the radius of the intestinal loop (cm), and, l is the length of intestinal loop (cm).

In the closed loop method a dilute solution of drug is added to a section of the intestine and the

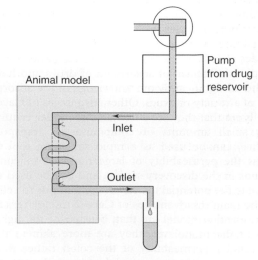

Fig. 18.6 Diagram of an in situ rat perfusion.

intestine closed. The intestine is then excised and drug content analysed immediately and after an appropriate time or time intervals, depending on the expected rate of absorption. Again, assuming a first-order rate process and hence an exponential loss of drug from the intestine, an absorption rate constant and effective permeability can be calculated. Like the intestinal ring method, the closed loop in situ perfusion model requires a lengthy digestion, extraction and assay procedure to analyse the drug remaining in the intestinal loop.

There is a lot of fluid moving in and out of the intestine, and so the drug concentrations in both these in situ perfusion methods need to be corrected for fluid flux. This is normally done by gravimetric means or by using a non-absorbable marker to assess the effect of fluid flux on the drug concentration. As with other absorption models, correlations have been made with standard compounds where the fraction absorbed in humans is known, and similar-shaped curves have been obtained (Fig. 18.4). In these models the 'absorption rate' is calculated by measuring the disappearance of the drug from the lumen and not its accumulation in the plasma. It is therefore important to check that the drug is not degraded in the lumen or intestinal wall, as drug that has disappeared will be erroneously assumed to have been absorbed.

More sophisticated techniques are those involving vascular perfusion. In these techniques, either a pair of mesenteric vessels supplying an intestinal segment or the superior mesenteric artery and portal vein perfusing almost the entire intestine are cannulated. The intestinal lumen and sometimes the lymph duct are also cannulated for the collection of luminal fluid and lymph, respectively. This model, although complicated, is very versatile as drug can be administered into the luminal or the vascular perfusate. When administered to the intestinal lumen, drug absorption can be evaluated from both its disappearance from the lumen and its appearance in the portal vein. Using this method both the rate and extent of absorption can be estimated, as well as carrier-mediated transport processes. Collection of the lymph allows the contribution of lymphatic absorption for very lipophilic compounds to be assessed. One of the other advantages of this system is the ability to determine whether any intestinal metabolism occurs before or after absorption.

A further extension of this model is to follow the passage of drugs from the intestine through the liver, and several adaptations of rat intestinal–liver perfusion systems have been investigated. Such a combined system gives the added advantage of assessing the first-pass or presystemic metabolism through the liver, and determining the relative importance of the intestine and liver in presystemic metabolism.

The disadvantages of these perfusion systems is that as they become more complex, a larger number of animals are required to establish suitable perfusion conditions and the reproducibility of the technique. However, in general, as the complexity increases so does the amount of information obtained.

Assessment of permeability in humans

Intestinal perfusion studies Until relatively recently the most common way to evaluate the absorption of drugs in humans was by performing bioavailability studies and deconvoluting the data available to calculate an absorption rate constant. This rate constant, however, is dependent on the release of the drug from the dosage form, and is affected by intestinal transit and presystemic metabolism. Therefore, very often it does not reflect the true intrinsic intestinal permeability of a drug.

Extensive studies have been carried out using a regional perfusion technique which has afforded a greater insight into human permeability (Loc-I-Gut). The Loc-I-Gut is a multichannel tube system with a proximal and a distal balloon (Fig. 18.7). These balloons are 100 mm apart and allow a segment of intestine 100 mm long to be isolated and perfused. Once the proximal balloon passes the ligament of Treitz both balloons are filled with air thereby preventing mixing of the luminal contents in the segment of interest with other luminal contents. A non-absorbable marker is used in the perfusion solution to check that the balloons work to occlude the region of interest. A tungsten weight is placed in front of the distal balloon to facilitate its passage down the gastrointestinal tract.

Drug absorption is calculated from the rate of disappearance of the drug from the perfused segment. This technique has afforded greater control in human intestinal perfusions, primarily because it isolates the

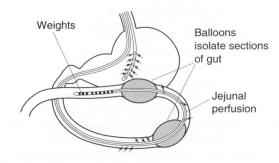

Fig. 18.7 Diagram of the Loc-I-Gut.

luminal contents of interest, and has greatly facilitated the study of permeability mechanisms and the metabolism of drugs and nutrients in the human intestine (Knutson et al 1989, Lennernas et al 1992).

Non-invasive approaches   There is concern that the invasive nature of perfusion techniques can affect the function of the gastrointestinal tract, in particular the fluid content, owing to the intubation process altering the absorption and secretion balance. To overcome this problem, several engineering-based approaches have been developed to evaluate drug absorption in the gastrointestinal tract. These include high-frequency (HF) capsules (Fuhr et al 1994) and the InteliSite capsule (Wilding 1997).

The transit of the high-frequency capsule down the gastrointestinal tract is followed by X-ray fluoroscopy. Once the capsule reaches its desired release site drug release is triggered by a high-frequency signal, which leads to rupturing of a latex balloon that has been loaded with drug. Concerns about X-ray exposure and the difficulties of loading the drug into the balloon have limited the use of this technique.

The InteliSite capsule is a more sophisticated system for measuring drug absorption. Either a liquid or a powder formulation can be filled into the capsule, the transit of which is followed by gamma-scintigraphy (see later). Once the capsule reaches its desired release site it is activated by exposure to a radiomagnetic field, which induces a small amount of heat in the capsule's electronic assembly. The heat causes some shape-memory alloys to straighten, rotating the inner sleeve of the capsule with respect to an outer sleeve and allowing a series of slots in the two sleeves to become aligned and the enclosed drug to be released. For both these systems blood samples need to be taken to quantify drug absorption.

Presystemic metabolism

Presystemic metabolism is the metabolism that occurs before the drug reaches the systemic circulation. Therefore, for an orally administered drug this includes the metabolism that occurs in the gut wall and the liver. As discussed above, perfusion models that involve both the intestines and the liver allow an evaluation of the presystemic metabolism in both organs. In other models it is sometimes possible to design mass balance experiments that will assess whether presystemic intestinal metabolism is likely to occur.

Intestinal cell fractions, such as brush border membrane preparations which contain an abundance of hydrolytic enzymes, and homogenized preparations of segments of rat intestine, can also be used to determine intestinal presystemic metabolism. Drugs are incubated with either brush border membrane preparations or gut wall homogenate at 37°C and the drug content analysed.

Various liver preparations, for example subcellular fractions such as microsomes, isolated hepatocytes and liver slices, are used to determine hepatic metabolism in vitro. Microsomes are prepared by high-speed centrifugation of liver homogenates (100 000 g) and are composed mainly of fragments of the endoplasmic reticulum. They lack cystolic enzymes and cofactors and are therefore only suitable to evaluate some of the metabolic processes the liver is capable of, known as phase I metabolism. Hepatocytes must be freshly and carefully prepared from livers and are only viable for a few hours. It is therefore difficult to obtain human hepatocytes. Hepatocytes are very useful for hepatic metabolism studies as it is possible to evaluate most of the metabolic reactions, i.e. both phase I and II metabolism. Whole liver slices again have the ability to evaluate both phase I and II metabolism. Because they are tissue slices rather than cell suspensions, and because they do not require enzymatic treatment in their preparation, this may be why a higher degree of in vivo correlation can be achieved with liver slices than with hepatocytes and microsomes. The reader is referred to a review by Carlile et al (1997).

ASSESSMENT OF BIOAVAILABILITY

The measurement of bioavailability gives the net result of the effect of the release of drug into solution in the physiological fluids at the site of absorption, its stability in those physiological fluids, its permeability and its presystemic metabolism on the rate and extent of drug absorption by following the concentration–time profile of drug in a suitable physiological fluid. The concentration–time profile also gives information on other pharmacokinetic parameters, such as the distribution and elimination of the drug. The most commonly used method of assessing the bioavailability of a drug involves the construction of a blood plasma concentration–time curve, but urine drug concentrations can also be used and are discussed below.

Plasma concentration–time curves

When a single dose of a drug is administered orally to a patient, serial blood samples are withdrawn and the plasma assayed for drug concentration at specific periods of time after administration, a plasma concentration–time curve can be constructed.

Figure 18.8 shows a typical plasma concentration–time curve following the administration of an oral tablet.

At zero time, when the drug is first administered, the concentration of drug in the plasma will be zero. As the tablet passes into the stomach and/or intestine it disintegrates, the drug dissolves and absorption occurs. Initially the concentration of drug in the plasma rises, as the rate of absorption exceeds the rate at which the drug is being removed by distribution and elimination. Concentrations continue to rise until a maximum (or peak) is attained. This represents the highest concentration of drug achieved in the plasma following the administration of a single dose, and is often termed the $C_{p_{max}}$. It is reached when the rate of appearance of drug in the plasma is equal to its rate of removal by distribution and elimination.

The ascending portion of the plasma concentration–time curve is sometimes called the **absorption phase**. Here the rate of absorption outweighs the rate of removal of drug by distribution and elimination. Drug absorption does not usually stop abruptly at the time of peak concentration, but may continue for some time into the descending portion of the curve. The early descending portion of the curve can thus reflect the net result of drug absorption, distribution, metabolism and elimination, but in this phase the rate of drug removal from the blood exceeds the rate absorption. Therefore, the concentration of the drug in the plasma declines.

Eventually drug absorption ceases when the bioavailable dose has been absorbed, and the concentration of drug in the plasma is now controlled only by its rate of elimination by metabolism and/or excretion. This is sometimes called the elimination phase of the curve. It should be appreciated, however, that elimination of a drug begins as soon as it appears in the plasma.

Several parameters based on the plasma concentration–time curve which are important in bioavailability studies are shown in Figure 18.9, and are discussed below.

Minimum effective (or therapeutic) plasma concentration It is generally assumed that some minimum concentration of drug must be reached in the plasma before the desired therapeutic or pharmacological effect is achieved. This is called the **minimum effective (or therapeutic) plasma concentration**. Its value not only varies from drug to drug but also from individual to individual, and with the type and severity of the disease state. In Figure 18.9 the minimum effective concentration is indicated by the lower line.

Maximum safe concentration The concentration of drug in the plasma above which side-effects or toxic effects occur is known as the maximum safe concentration.

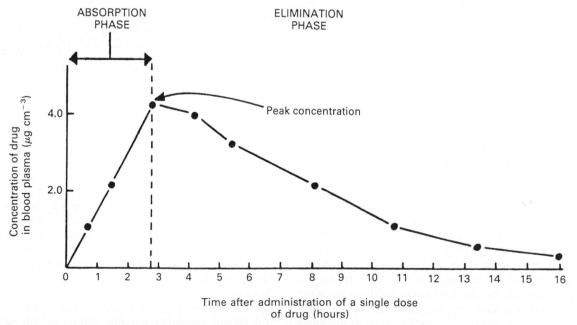

Fig. 18.8 A typical blood plasma concentration–time curve obtained following the peroral administration of a single dose of a drug in a tablet.

Fig. 18.9 Relationship between the plasma concentration–time curve obtained following a single extravascular dose of a drug and parameters associated with the therapeutic or pharmacological response.

Therapeutic range or window A range of plasma drug concentrations is also assumed to exist, over which the desired response is obtained yet toxic effects are avoided. This range is called the **therapeutic range** or **window**. The intention in clinical practice is to maintain plasma drug concentrations within this range.

Onset The onset may be defined as the time required to achieve the minimum effective plasma concentration following administration of the dosage form.

Duration The duration of the therapeutic effect of the drug is the period during which the concentration of drug in the plasma exceeds the minimum effective plasma concentration.

Peak concentration This represents the highest concentration of the drug achieved in the plasma, which is often referred to as the $C_{p_{max}}$.

Time of peak concentration This is the period of time required to achieve the peak plasma concentration of drug after the administration of a single dose. This parameter is related to the rate of absorption of the drug and can be used to assess that rate. It is often referred to as the T_{max}.

Area under the plasma concentration–time curve This is related to the total amount of drug absorbed into the systemic circulation following the administration of a single dose, and is often known as the AUC. However, changes in the area under the plasma concentration–time curve need not necessarily reflect changes in the total amount of drug absorbed, but can reflect modifications in the kinetics of distribution, metabolism and excretion.

The use of plasma concentration–time curves in bioavailability studies

In order to illustrate the usefulness of plasma concentration–time curves in bioavailability studies to assess the rate and extent of absorption, the administration of single equal doses of three different formulations, A, B and C, of the same drug to the same healthy individual by the same route of administration on three separate occasions can be considered. The assumption is made that sufficient time was allowed to elapse between the administration of each formulation such that the systemic circulation contained no residual concentration of drug and no residual effects from any previous administrations. It is also assumed that the kinetics and pattern of distribution of the drug, its binding phenomena, the kinetics of elimination and the experimental conditions under which each plasma concentration–time profile was obtained, were the same on each occasion. The plasma concentration–time profiles for the three formulations are shown in Figure 18.10. The differences between the three curves are attributed solely to differences in the rate and/or extent of absorption of the drug from each formulation.

The three plasma profiles in Figure 18.10 show that each of the three formulations (A, B and C) of the same dose of the same drug results in a different peak plasma concentration. However, the areas under the curves for formulation A and B are similar, and this indicates that the drug is absorbed to a similar extent from these two formulations. Consideration of the times at which the peak plasma concentrations occur for formulations A and B show that the drug is absorbed faster from A than from B, meaning that formulation A shows a fast onset of therapeutic action, but as its peak plasma concentration exceeds the maximum safe concentration it is likely that this formulation will result in toxic side-effects. Formulation B, which gives a slower rate of absorption than A, shows a slower therapeutic onset than A, but its peak plasma concentration lies within the therapeutic range. In addition, the duration of action of the therapeutic effect obtained with formulation B is longer than that obtained with A. Hence formulation B appears to be superior to formulation A from a clinical viewpoint, in that its peak plasma concentration lies within the therapeutic range of the drug and the duration of the therapeutic effect is longer.

Formulation C gives a much smaller area under the plasma concentration–time curve, indicating that a lower proportion of the dose has been absorbed.

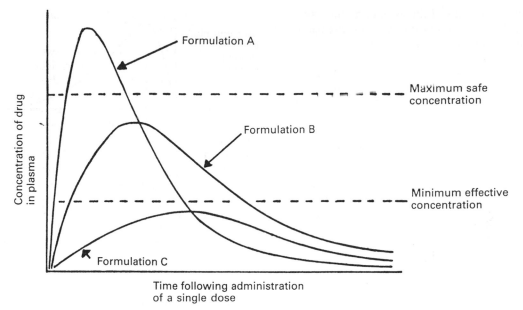

Fig. 18.10 Plasma concentration–time curves for three different formulations of the same drug administered in equal single doses by the same extravascular route.

This, together with the slower rate of absorption from formulation C (the time of peak concentration is longer than for formulations A and B), results in the peak plasma concentration not reaching the minimum effective concentration, i.e. formulation C does not produce a therapeutic effect and consequently is clinically ineffective as a single dose.

This simple hypothetical example illustrates how differences in bioavailability exhibited by a given drug from different formulations can result in a patient being either over, under, or correctly medicated.

It is important to realize that the study of bioavailability based on drug concentration measurements in the plasma (or urine or saliva) is complicated by the fact that such concentration–time curves are affected by factors other than the biopharmaceutical factors of the drug product itself. Factors such as body weight, sex and age of the test subjects, disease states, genetic differences in drug metabolism, excretion and distribution, food and water intake, concomitant administration of other drugs, stress and time of administration of the drug are some of the variables that can complicate the interpretation of bioavailability studies. As far as possible, studies should be designed to control these factors.

Although plots such those in as Figure 18.10 can be used to compare the relative bioavailability of a given drug from different formulations, they cannot be used indiscriminately to compare different drugs. It is quite usual for different drugs to exhibit differ-

ent rates of absorption, metabolism, excretion and distribution, different distribution patterns and differences in their binding phenomena, all of which would influence the concentration–time curve. Therefore it would be extremely difficult to attribute differences in the concentration–time curves obtained for different drugs presented in different formulations to differences in their bioavailabilities.

Cumulative urinary drug excretion curves

Measurement of the concentration of intact drug and/or its metabolite(s) in the plasma can also be used to assess bioavailability.

When a suitable specific assay method is not available for the intact drug in the urine, or the specific assay method available for the parent drug is not sufficiently sensitive, it may be necessary to assay the principal metabolite or intact drug plus its metabolite(s) in the urine to obtain an index of bioavailability. Measurements involving metabolite levels in the urine are only valid when the drug in question is not subject to metabolism prior to reaching the systemic circulation. If an orally administered drug is subject to intestinal metabolism or first-pass liver metabolism, then measurement of the principal metabolite, or of intact drug plus metabolites, in the urine would give an overestimate of the systemic availability of that drug. It should be remembered that the definition of bioavailability is in terms of the extent and the rate at which intact drug appears in the systemic circulation after the administration of a known dose.

The assessment of bioavailability by urinary excretion is based on the assumption that the appearance of the drug and/or its metabolites in the urine is a function of the rate and extent of absorption. This assumption is only valid when a drug and/or its metabolites are extensively excreted in the urine, and where the rate of urinary excretion is proportional to the concentration of the intact drug in the blood plasma. This proportionality does not hold if:

- the drug and/or its metabolites are excreted by an active transport process into the distal kidney tubule;
- the intact drug and/or its metabolites are weakly acidic or weakly basic (i.e. their rate of excretion is dependent on urine pH);
- the excretion rate depends on the rate of urine flow.

The important parameters in urinary excretion studies are the cumulative amount of intact drug and/or metabolites excreted, and the rate at which this excretion takes place. A cumulative urinary excretion curve is obtained by collecting urine samples (resulting from total emptying of the bladder) at known intervals after a single dose of the drug has been administered. Urine samples must be collected until all drug and/or its metabolites has been excreted (this is indicated by the cumulative urinary excretion curve becoming parallel to the abscissa) if a comparison of the extent of absorption of a given drug from different formulations or dosage forms is to be made. A typical cumulative urinary excretion curve and the corresponding plasma concentration–time curve obtained following the admission of a single dose of a given drug by the oral route to a subject is shown in Figure 18.11.

The initial segments (X–Y) of the curves reflect the 'absorption phase' (i.e. where absorption is the dominant process) and the slope of this segment of the urinary excretion curve is related to the rate of absorption of the drug into the blood. The total amount of intact drug (and/or its metabolite) excreted in the urine at point Z corresponds to the time at which the plasma concentration of intact drug is zero and essentially all the drug has been eliminated from the body. The total amount of drug excreted at point Z may be quite different from the total amount of drug administered (i.e. the dose), either because of incomplete absorption on because of the drug being eliminated by processes other than urinary excretion.

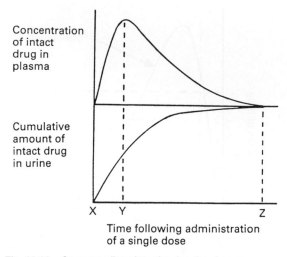

Fig. 18.11 Corresponding plots showing the plasma concentration–time curve (*upper curve*) and the cumulative urinary excretion curve (*lower curve*) obtained following the administration of a single dose of a drug by the peroral route

The use of urinary drug excretion curves in bioavailability studies

In order to illustrate how cumulative urinary excretion curves can be used to compare the bioavailabilities of a given drug from different formulations, let us consider the urinary excretion data that would have been obtained following the administration of single equal doses of the three different formulations, A, B and C, of the same drug to the same healthy individual by the same extravascular route on three different occasions, and giving the plasma concentration–time curves shown in Figure 18.10. The corresponding cumulative urinary excretion curves are shown in Figure 18.12.

The cumulative urinary excretion curves show that the rate at which drug appeared in the urine (i.e. the slope of the initial segment of each urinary excretion curve) from each formulation decreased in order A > B > C. Because the slope of the initial segment of the urinary excretion curve is related to the rate of drug absorption, the cumulative urinary excretion curves indicate that the rates of absorption of drug from the three formulations decrease in the order A > B > C. Inspection of the corresponding plasma concentration–time curves in Figure 18.10 shows that this is the case, i.e. peak concentration times (which are inversely related to the rate of drug absorption) for the three formulations increase in the order A > B > C. Although Figure 18.12 shows that the rate of appearance of drug in the urine from formulation A is faster than from B, the total amount of drug eventually

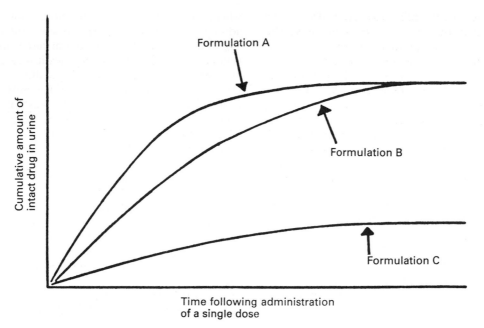

Fig. 18.12 Cumulative urinary excretion curves corresponding to the plasma concentration–time curves shown in Fig. 18.10 for three different formulations of the same drug administered in equal single doses by the same extravascular route.

excreted from these two formulations is the same, i.e. the cumulative urinary excretion curves for formulations A and B eventually meet and merge. As the total amount of intact drug excreted is assumed to be related to the total amount absorbed, the cumulative urinary excretion curves for formulations A and B indicate that the extent of drug absorption from these two formulations is the same. This is confirmed by the plasma concentration–time curves for formulations A and B in Figure 18.10, which exhibit similar areas under their curves.

Thus both the plasma concentration–time curves and the corresponding cumulative urinary excretion curves for formulations A and B show that the extent of absorption from these formulations is equal, despite being at different rates from the respective formulations.

Consideration of the cumulative urinary excretion curve for C shows that this formulation not only results in a slower rate of appearance of intact drug in the urine, but also that the total amount of drug that is eventually excreted is much less than from the other two formulations. Thus the cumulative urinary excretion curve suggests that both the rate and extent of drug absorption are reduced in the case of formulation C. This is confirmed by the plasma concentration–time curve shown in Figure 18.10 for formulation C, i.e. formulation C exhibits a longer peak concentration time and a smaller area under the

curve than do formulations A and B. Thus one can conclude that cumulative urinary excretion curves may be used to compare the rate and extent of absorption of a given drug presented in different formulations, provided that the conditions mentioned previously apply.

Absolute and relative bioavailability

Absolute bioavailability

The absolute bioavailability of a given drug from a dosage form is the fraction (or percentage) of the administered dose which is absorbed intact into the systemic circulation. Absolute bioavailability may be calculated by comparing the total amount of intact drug that reaches the systemic circulation after the administration of a known dose of the dosage form via a route of administration, with the total amount that reaches the systemic circulation after the administration of an equivalent dose of the drug in the form of an intravenous bolus injection. An intravenous bolus injection is used as a reference to compare the systemic availability of the drug administered via different routes, because when a drug is delivered intravenously the entire administered dose is introduced directly into the systemic circulation, i.e. it has no absorption barriers to cross and is therefore considered to be totally bioavailable.

The absolute bioavailability of a given drug using plasma data may be calculated by comparing the total areas under the plasma concentration–time curves obtained following the administration of equivalent doses of the drug via an absorption site and via the intravenous route in the same subject on different occasions. Typical plasma concentration–time curves obtained by administering equivalent doses of the same drug by the intravenous route (bolus injection) and the gastrointestinal route are shown in Figure 18.13.

For equivalent doses of administered drug:

$$\text{absolute bioavailability} = \frac{\left(\text{AUC}_T\right)_{abs}}{\left(\text{AUC}_T\right)_{iv}} \qquad (18.3)$$

where $(\text{AUC}_T)_{abs}$ is the total area under the plasma concentration–time curve following the administration of a single dose via an absorption site and $(\text{AUC}_T)_{iv}$ is the total area under the plasma concentration–time curve following administration by rapid intravenous injection.

If different doses of the drug are administered by both routes, a correction for the sizes of the doses can be made as follows:

$$\text{absolute bioavailability} = \frac{\left(\text{AUC}_T\right)_{abs} / D_{abs}}{\left(\text{AUC}_T\right)_{iv} / D_{iv}} \qquad (18.4)$$

where D_{abs} is the size of the single dose of drug administered via the absorption site, and D_{iv} is the size of the dose of the drug administered as an intravenous bolus injection. Sometimes it is necessary to use different dosages of drugs via different routes. Often the dose administered intravenously is lower to avoid toxic side-effects and for ease of formulation. Care should be taken when using different dosages to calculate bioavailability data, as sometimes the pharmacokinetics of a drug are non-linear and different doses will then lead to an incorrect figure for the absolute bioavailability calculated using a simple ratio, as in Eqn 18.4.

Absolute bioavailability using urinary excretion data may be determined by comparing the total cumulative amounts of unchanged drug ultimately excreted in the urine following administration of the drug via an absorption site and the intravenous route (bolus injection), respectively, on different occasions to the same subject.

For equivalent doses of administered drug:

$$\text{absolute bioavailability} = \frac{\left(X_u\right)_{abs}}{\left(X_u\right)_{iv}} \qquad (18.5)$$

where $(X_U)_{abs}$ and $(X_U)_{iv}$ are the total cumulative amounts of unchanged drug ultimately excreted in the urine following administration of equivalent

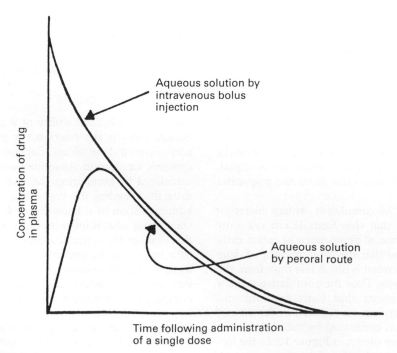

Fig. 18.13 Typical plasma concentration–time curves obtained by administering equivalent doses of the same drug by intravenous bolus injection and by the peroral route.

single doses of drug via an absorption site and as an intravenous bolus injection, respectively.

If different doses of drug are administered,

$$\text{absolute bioavailability } = \frac{\left(X_u\right)_{abs} / D_{abs}}{\left(X_u\right)_{iv} / D_{iv}} \quad (18.6)$$

The absolute bioavailability of a given drug from a particular type of dosage form may be expressed as a fraction or, more commonly, as a percentage.

Measurements of absolute bioavailability obtained by administering a given drug in the form of a simple aqueous solution (that does not precipitate on dilution with gastrointestinal fluids) by both the oral and the intravenous routes provide an insight into the effects that factors associated with the oral route may have on bioavailability, e.g. presystemic metabolism by the intestine or liver, the formation of complexes between the drug and endogenous substances (e.g. mucin) at the site of absorption and drug stability in the gastrointestinal fluids.

It should be noted that the value calculated for the absolute bioavailability will only be valid for the drug being examined if the kinetics of elimination and distribution are independent of the route and time of administration, and also of the size of dose administered (if different doses are administered by the intravenous route and absorption site). If this is not the case, one cannot assume that the observed differences in the total areas under the plasma concentration–time curves or in the total cumulative amounts of unchanged drug ultimately excreted in the urine are due entirely to differences in bioavailability.

Relative bioavailability

In the case of drugs that cannot be administered by intravenous bolus injection, the relative (or comparative) bioavailability is determined rather than the absolute bioavailability. In this case the bioavailability of a given drug from a 'test' dosage form is compared to that of the same drug administered in a 'standard' dosage form, which is either an orally administered solution (from which the drug is known to be well absorbed) or an established commercial preparation of proven clinical effectiveness. Hence relative bioavailability is a measure of the fraction (or percentage) of a given drug that is absorbed intact into the systemic circulation from a dosage form relative to a recognized (i.e. clinically proven) standard dosage form of that drug.

The relative bioavailability of a given drug administered as equal doses of a test dosage form and a recognized standard dosage form, respectively, by

the same route of administration to the same subject on different occasions, may be calculated from the corresponding plasma concentration–time curves as follows:

$$\text{relative bioavailability } = \frac{\left(\text{AUC}_T\right)_{test}}{\left(\text{AUC}_T\right)_{standard}} \quad (18.7)$$

where $(\text{AUC}_T)_{test}$ and $(\text{AUC}_T)_{standard}$ are the total areas under the plasma concentration–time curves following the administration of a single dose of the test dosage form and of the standard dosage form, respectively.

When different doses of the test and standard dosage forms are administered, a correction for the size of dose is made as follows:

$$\text{relative bioavailability } = \frac{\left(\text{AUC}_T\right)_{abs} / D_{test}}{\left(\text{AUC}_T\right)_{standard} / D_{standard}} \quad (18.8)$$

where D_{test} and $D_{standard}$ are the sizes of the single doses of the test and standard dosage forms, respectively.

Like absolute bioavailability, relative bioavailability may be expressed as a fraction or as a percentage.

Urinary excretion data may also be used to measure relative bioavailability as follows:

$$\text{relative bioavailability } = \frac{\left(X_u\right)_{test}}{\left(X_u\right)_{standard}} \quad (18.9)$$

where $(X_u)_{test}$ and $(X_u)_{standard}$ are the total cumulative amounts of unchanged drug ultimately excreted in the urine following the administration of single doses of the test dosage form and the standard dosage form, respectively.

If different doses of the test and standard dosage forms are administered on separate occasions, the total amounts of unchanged drug ultimately excreted in the urine per unit dose of drug must be used in the above equation.

It should be noted that measurements of relative and absolute bioavailability based on urinary excretion data may also be made in terms of either the total amounts of principal drug metabolite or of unchanged drug plus its metabolites ultimately excreted in the urine. However, the assessment of relative and absolute bioavailability in terms of urinary excretion data is based on the assumption that the total amount of unchanged drug (and/or its metabolites) ultimately excreted in the urine is a reflection of the total amount of intact drug entering the systemic circulation (as discussed in the earlier section on cumulative urinary excretion curves).

Relative bioavailability measurements are often used to determine the effects of dosage form differences on the systemic bioavailability of a given drug. Numerous dosage form factors can influence the bioavailability of a drug. These include the type of dosage form (e.g. tablet, solution, suspension, hard gelatin capsule), differences in the formulation of a particular type of dosage form, and manufacturing variables employed in the production of a particular type of dosage form. A more detailed account of the influence of these factors on bioavailability is given in Chapter 17.

Bioequivalence

An extension of the concept of relative bioavailability, which essentially involves comparing the total amounts of a particular drug that are absorbed intact into the systemic circulation from a test and a recognized standard dosage form, is that of determining whether test and standard dosage forms containing equal doses of the same drug are equivalent or not in terms of their rates and extents of absorption (i.e. systemic availabilities). This is called *bioequivalence*.

Two or more chemically equivalent products (i.e. products containing equal doses of the same therapeutically active ingredient(s) in identical types of dosage form which meet all the existing physicochemical standards in official compendia) are said to be bioequivalent if they do not differ significantly in their bioavailability characteristics when administered in the same dose under similar experimental conditions. Hence in those cases where bioavailability is assessed in terms of plasma concentration–time curves, two or more chemically equivalent drug products may be considered bioequivalent if there is no significant difference between any of the following parameters: maximum plasma concentrations (C_{max}), time to peak height concentration (T_{max}) and areas under the plasma concentration–time curves (AUC).

In conducting a bioequivalence study it is usual for one of the chemically equivalent drug products under test to be a clinically proven, therapeutically effective product which serves as a standard against which the other 'test' products may be compared. If a test product and this standard product are found to be bioequivalent then it is reasonable to expect that the test product will also be therapeutically effective, i.e. the test and the reference products are therapeutically equivalent. Bioequivalence studies are therefore important in determining whether chemically equivalent drug products manufactured by different companies are therapeutically equivalent, i.e. produce identical therapeutic responses in patients.

If two chemically equivalent drug products are absolutely bioequivalent, their plasma concentration–

time and/or cumulative urinary excretion curves would be superimposable. In such a case there would be no problem in concluding that these products were bioequivalent. Nor would there be a problem in concluding bioinequivalence if the parameters associated with the plasma concentration–time and/or cumulative urinary excretion profiles for the test differed from the standard product by, for instance, 50%. However, a problem arises in deciding whether the test and standard drug products are bioequivalent when such products show relatively small differences in their plasma concentration–time curves and/or cumulative urinary excretion curves.

The problem is how much of a difference can be allowed between two chemically equivalent drug products and still permit them to be considered bioequivalent. Should this be 10%, 20%, 30% or more? The magnitude of the difference that could be permitted will depend on the significance of such a difference on the safety and therapeutic efficacy of the particular drug. This will depend on such factors as the toxicity, the therapeutic range and the therapeutic use of the drug. In the case of a drug with a wide therapeutic range, the toxic effects of which occur only at relatively high plasma concentrations, chemically equivalent products giving quite different plasma concentration–time curves (Fig. 18.14) may still be considered satisfactory from a therapeutic point of view, although they are not strictly bioequivalent.

In the case of the hypothetical example shown in Figure 18.14, provided that the observed difference in the rates of absorption (as assessed by the times of peak plasma concentration), and hence in the times of onset, for formulations X and Y is not considered to be therapeutically significant, both formulations may be considered to be therapeutically satisfactory. However, if the drug in question was a hypnotic, in which case the time of onset for the therapeutic response is important, then the observed difference in the rates of absorption would become more important.

If the times of peak plasma concentration for formulations X and Y were 0.5 and 1.0 hour, respectively, it is likely that both formulations would still be deemed to be therapeutically satisfactory despite a 100% difference in their times of peak plasma concentration. However, if the times of peak plasma concentration for formulations X and Y were 2 and 4 hours, respectively, these formulations might no longer be regarded as being therapeutically equivalent even though the percentage difference in their peak plasma concentration was the same.

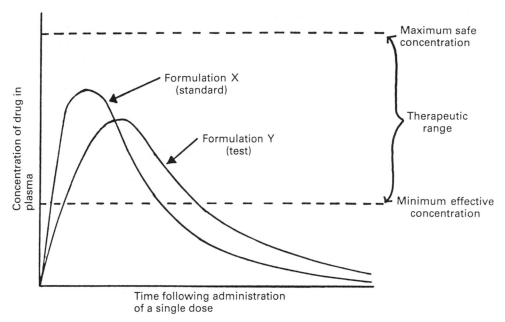

Fig. 18.14 Plasma concentration–time curves for two chemically equivalent drug products administered in equal single doses by the same extravascular route.

It is difficult to quote a universally acceptable percentage difference that can be tolerated before two chemically equivalent drug products are regarded as being bioinequivalent and/or therapeutically inequivalent. In the case of chemically equivalent drug products containing a drug which exhibits a narrow range between its minimum effective plasma concentration and its maximum safe plasma concentration (e.g. digoxin), the concept of bioequivalence is fundamentally important, as in such cases small differences in the plasma concentration–time curves of chemically equivalent drug products may result in patients being overmedicated (i.e. exhibiting toxic responses) or undermedicated (i.e. experiencing therapeutic failure). These two therapeutically unsatisfactory conditions are illustrated in Figure 18.15a & b respectively.

Despite the problems of putting a value on the magnitude of the difference that can be tolerated before two chemically equivalent drug products are deemed to be bioinequivalent, a value of 20% for the tolerated difference used to be regarded as suitable as a general criterion for determining bioequivalence. Thus if all the major parameters in either the plasma concentration–time or cumulative urinary excretion curves for two or more chemically equivalent drug products differed from each other by less than 20%, these products would have been judged to be bioequivalent. However, if any one or more of these parameters differed by more than 20% then there might have been a problem with the bioequivalence of the test product(s) with respect to the standard product. However, recently some regulatory authorities have been adopting more stringent requirements for bioequivalence, involving statistical models and considerations of average, population and individual pharmacokinetics.

A further crucial factor in establishing bioequivalence, or in determining the influence of the type of dosage form, the route of administration etc., have on the bioavailability of a given drug, is the proper design, control and interpretation of such experimental studies.

ASSESSMENT OF SITE OF RELEASE IN VIVO

There are many benefits of being able to assess the fate of a dosage form in vivo and the site and release pattern of the drug. Particularly for drugs that show poor oral bioavailability, or in the design and development of controlled- or sustained-release delivery systems, the ability to follow the transit of the dosage form and the release of drug from it is advantageous. The technique of gamma scintigraphy is now used extensively and enables a greater knowledge and understanding of the transit and fate

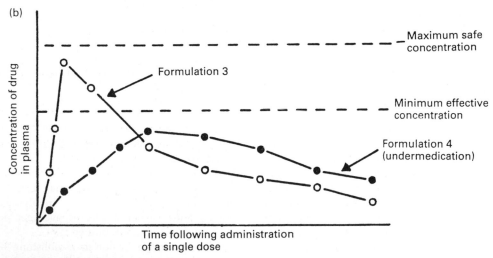

Fig. 18.15 Plasma concentration–time curves for chemically equivalent drug products administered in equal single doses by the same extravascular route, showing potential consequences of bioinequivalence for a drug having a narrow therapeutic range, i.e., (a) overmedication and (b), undermedication. (After Chodos and Di Santo 1973.)

of pharmaceuticals in the gastrointestinal tract to be gained.

Gamma scintigraphy is a versatile, non-invasive and ethically acceptable technique which is capable of obtaining information both quantitatively and continuously. The technique involves the radio-labelling of a dosage form with a gamma-emitting isotope of appropriate half-life and activity. Technetium-99m is often the isotope of choice for pharmaceutical studies because of its short half-life (6 hours). The radiolabelled dosage form is administered to a subject who is positioned in front of a gamma camera. Gamma radiation emitted from the isotope is focused by a collimator and detected by a scintillation crystal and its associated circuitry.

The signals are assembled by computer software to form a two-dimensional image of the dosage form in the gastrointestinal tract. The anatomy of the gastrointestinal tract can be clearly seen from liquid dosage forms, and the site of disintegration of solid dosage forms identified. The release of the radiolabel from the dosage form can be measured by following the intensity of the radiation. By co-administration of a radiolabelled marker and a drug in the same dosage form, and simultaneous imaging and taking of blood samples, the absorption site and release rate of a drug can be determined (for example with the InteliSite capsule; see earlier). When used in this way, the technique is often referred to as **_pharmacoscintigraphy_**.

THE BIOPHARMACEUTICAL CLASSIFICATION SCHEME

A biopharmaceutical classification scheme has been proposed which classifies drugs into four classes according to their solubility across the gastrointestinal pH range and their permeability across the gastrointestinal mucosa (Amidon et al 1995). Two of the four potential barriers to absorption are thus addressed by the scheme (see Fig. 18.1).

The scheme was originally proposed for the identification of immediate-release solid oral products for which in vivo bioequivalence tests may not be necessary, but it is also useful to classify drugs and predict bioavailability issues that may arise during the various stages of the development process. The four classes are:

- Class I: high solubility/low permeability
- Class II: low solubility/high permeability
- Class III: high solubility/low permeability
- Class IV: low solubility/low permeability.

A drug is considered to be highly soluble where the highest dose strength is soluble in 250 mL or less of aqueous media over the pH range 1–8. The volume is derived from the minimum volume anticipated in the stomach when a dosage form is taken in the fasted state with a glass of water. If the volume of aqueous media taken to dissolve the drug in pH conditions ranging from 1 to 8 is greater than 250 mL then the drug is considered to have low solubility. The classification therefore takes into account the dose of the drug as well as its solubility. A drug is considered to be highly permeable when the extent of absorption in humans is expected to be greater than 90% of the administered dose. Permeability can be assessed using one of the methods discussed earlier which has been calibrated with known standard compounds or by pharmacokinetic studies.

Class I drugs Class I drugs will dissolve rapidly when presented in immediate-release dosage forms, and are also rapidly transported across the gut wall. Therefore, unless they form insoluble complexes, are unstable in gastric fluids or undergo presystemic clearance, it is expected that such drugs will be rapidly absorbed and thus show good bioavailability. Examples of class I drugs are the β-blockers propranolol and metoprolol.

Class II drugs In contrast, for drugs in class II the dissolution rate is liable to be the rate-limiting step in oral absorption. For class II drugs, therefore, it should be possible to generate a strong correlation between in vitro dissolution and in vivo absorption (see earlier). Examples of class II drugs are the non-steroidal anti-inflammatory drug ketoprofen and the antiepileptic carbamazepine. This class of drug should be amenable to formulation approaches to improve the dissolution rate and hence oral bioavailability.

Class III drugs Class III drugs are those that dissolve rapidly but which are poorly permeable; examples are the H_2-antagonist ranitidine and the β-blocker atenolol. It is important that dosage forms containing class III drugs release them rapidly, in order to maximize the amount of time these drugs, which are slow to permeate the gastrointestinal epithelium, are in contact with it.

Class IV drugs Class IV drugs are those that are classed as poorly soluble and poorly permeable. These drugs are liable to have poor oral bioavailability, or the oral absorption may be so low that they cannot be given by the oral route. The diuretics hydrochlorothiazide and frusemide are examples of class IV drugs. Forming prodrugs of class IV compounds or finding an alternative route of delivery are approaches that have to be adopted to significantly improve their absorption into the systemic circulation.

SUMMARY

This chapter discusses the range of current approaches to assessing the biopharmaceutical properties of drugs that are intended for oral administration. Methods of measuring and interpreting bioavailability data are described. The concepts of bioequivalence and the biopharmaceutical classification of drugs are introduced. It is imperative that the biopharmaceutical properties of drugs are fully understood, both in the selection of candidate drugs during the discovery process and in the design and development of efficacious immediate- and controlled-release dosage forms.

REFERENCES

Amidon, G.L., Lennernäs, H., Shah, V.P. and Crison, J.R.A., (1995) Theoretical basis for a biopharmaceutic drug classification: the correlation of in vitro drug product dissolution and in vivo bioavailability. *Pharm. Res.*, **12**, 413–420.

Artusson, P., Palm, K., Luthman, K., (1996) Caco-2 monolayers in experimental and theoretical predictions of drug transport. *Adv. Drug Del. Rev.*, **22**, 67–84.

Carlile, D.J., Zomorodi, K., Houston, J.B. (1997) Scaling factors to relate drug metabolic clearance in heptaic microsomes, isolated hepatocytes and the intact liver –

studies with induced livers involving diazepam. *Drug Metab. Dispos.* **25**, 903–911.

Chodos, D.J. and Di Santo, A.R. (1973) *Basis of Bioavailability.* The Upjohn Company, Kalamazoo, Michigan.

Dressman, J.B., Amidon, G.L., Reppas, C. and Shah, V.P. (1998) Dissolution testing as a prognostic tool for oral drug absorption: immediate release dosage forms. *Pharm. Res.*, **15**, 11–22.

Fuhr U., Staib, A.N., Harder, S. et al. (1994) Absorption of ipsapirone along the human gastrointestinal. *Br. J. Clin. Pharmacol.*, **38**, 83–86.

Hidalgo, I.J., Raub, T.J., Borchardt, R.T. (1989) Characterization of the human colon carcinoma cell line (Caco-2) as a model system for intestinal epithelium permeability. *Gastroenterology*, **96**, 736–749.

Knutson, L., Odlind, B., Hallgren, R. (1989) A new technique for segmental jejunal perfusion in man. *Am. J. Gastroenterol.*, **84**, 1278–1284.

Lennernäs, H., Abrenstedt, O., Hallgren, R., Knutson L., Ryde, M., Paalzow, L.K. (1992) Regional jejunal perfusion, a new in vivo approach to study oral drug absorption in amn. *Pharm. Res.*, **9**, 1243–1251.

Wilding (1997) Non invasive techniques to study human drug absorption. *Eur. J. Pharm. Sci.*, **5** 518–519.

19

Dosage regimens

Stuart Proudfoot (updated by John Collett)

DOSAGE REGIMENS: THEIR INFLUENCE ON THE CONCENTRATION–TIME PROFILE OF A DRUG IN THE BODY

The subject of dosage regimens is concerned with the dose, time of administration and drug plasma levels factors associated with *multiple* dosing of a drug. The influence that physiological factors, the physicochemical properties of a drug and dosage form factors can have in determining whether a therapeutically effective concentration of a drug is achieved in the plasma following peroral administration of a *single* dose of drug has been discussed previously in Chapters 16, 17 and 18.

Some drugs, such as hypnotics, analgesics and antiemetics, may provide effective treatment following the administration of a single dose. However, the duration of most illnesses is longer than the therapeutic effect produced by the administration of a single dose of a drug in a conventional dosage form, i.e. a dosage form which is formulated to give rapid and complete drug release. In such cases doses are usually administered on a repetitive basis over a period of time determined by the nature of the illness. For instance, one 250 mg ampicillin capsule may be administered every 6 hours for a period of 5 days to treat a bacterial infection. Such a regimen, in which the total dose of drug (i.e. in this example 5 g) administered over 5 days is given in the form of multiple doses (i.e. each of 250 mg) at given intervals of time (i.e. every 6 hours) is known as a *multiple-dosage regimen*.

The proper selection of both the dose size and the frequency of administration is an important factor that influences whether a satisfactory therapeutic plasma concentration is achieved and maintained over the prescribed course of treatment. Thus the design of a multiple-dosage regimen is crucial to successful drug therapy.

ONE-COMPARTMENT OPEN MODEL OF DRUG DISPOSITION IN THE BODY

In order to understand how the design of a dosage regimen can influence the time course of a drug in the body, as measured by its plasma concentration–time curve, consider that the complex kinetic processes of drug input, output and distribution in the body may be represented by the pharmacokinetic model of drug disposition, the one-compartment open model, shown in Figure 19.1. In this case the drug is considered to be distributed instantly throughout the whole body following its release and absorption from the dosage form. Thus the body behaves as a single compartment in which absorbed drug is distributed so rapidly that a concentration equilibrium exists at any given time between the plasma, other body fluids, and the tissues into which the drug has become distributed.

To assume that the body behaves as one-compartment open model does not necessarily mean that the drug concentrations in all body tissues at any given time are equal. The model does assume, however, that any changes that occur in the plasma reflect quantitatively changes occurring in the concentration of drug at the site(s) of action.

Rate of drug input versus rate of drug output

In a one-compartment open model, the overall kinetic processes of drug input and drug output are described by first-order kinetics. In the case of a perorally administered dosage form, the process of drug input into the body compartment involves drug release from the dosage form and passage of the drug across the cellular membranes constituting the gastrointestinal barrier. The rate of input or absorption represents the net result of all these processes. The rate of input (absorption) at any given time is proportional to the concentration of drug, which is assumed to be in an absorbable form, in solution in the gastrointestinal fluids at the site(s) of absorption, i.e. the effective concentration, C_e, of drug at time t. Hence:

$$\text{rate of drug input at time } t \propto C_e \quad (19.1)$$

and

$$\text{rate of drug input at time } t = -k_a\, C_e \quad (19.2)$$

where k_a is the apparent absorption rate constant.

The negative sign in Eqn 19.2 indicates that the effective concentration of drug at the absorption site(s) decreases with time. The apparent absorption rate constant gives the proportion (or fraction) of drug that enters the body compartment per unit time. Its units are time^{-1}, e.g. h^{-1}.

Unlike the rate of drug input into the body compartment, the apparent absorption rate constant, k_a, is independent of the effective concentration of drug at the absorption site(s). Because the rate of drug input is proportional to the effective drug concentration, it will be maximal following the administration of a dose contained in a peroral dosage form which gives rapid and complete drug release. The rate of drug input will decrease gradually with time as a consequence of the effective drug concentration at the absorption site(s) decreasing progressively with time, chiefly as a result of absorption into the body compartment. Other processes, such as chemical degradation and movement of drug away from the absorption site(s), will also contribute to the gradual decrease in the effective drug concentration with time.

In the case of a one-compartment open model, the rate of drug output or elimination is a first-order process. Consequently, the magnitude of this parameter at any given time is dependent on the concentration of drug in the body compartment at that time. Immediately following administration of the first dose of a peroral dosage form, the rate of drug output from the body will be low as little of the drug will have been absorbed into the body compartment. However, as absorption proceeds – initially at a higher rate than the rate of drug output – the net concentration of drug in the body will increase with time. Likewise, the rate of drug output from the

Fig. 19.1   One-compartment open model of drug disposition for a perorally administered drug.

body compartment will also increase with time. As the rate of drug output is increasing with time while the rate of input into the body compartment is decreasing with time, the situation is eventually reached when the rate of drug output just exceeds that of drug input. Consequently, the net concentration of drug in the body compartment will reach a peak value and then begin to fall with time. The ensuing decreases in the net concentration of drug in the body will also cause the rate of drug output to decrease with time.

These changes in the rates of drug input and output relative to each other with time are responsible for the characteristic shape of the concentration–time course of a drug in the body shown in Figure 19.2 following peroral administration of a single dose of drug.

It is evident from the above discussion and Figure 19.2, that the greater the rate of drug input relative to that of drug output from the body compartment over the net absorption phase, the higher will be the peak concentration achieved in the body or plasma following peroral administration of a single dose of drug. This interplay explains why increases in dose size and formulation changes in dosage forms which produce increases in the effective concentration of drug at the absorption site(s), result in higher peak plasma and body concentrations being obtained for a given drug. It should also be noted that any unexpected decrease in the rate of drug output relative to that of drug input, which may occur as the result of renal impairment, is also likely to result in higher plasma and body concentrations of drug than expected, and the possibility of the patient exhibiting undesirable side-effects. The adjustment of dosage regimens in cases of patients having severe renal impairment is considered later in this chapter.

Elimination rate constant and biological half-life of a drug

In the case of a one-compartment open model the rate of elimination or output of a drug from the body compartment follows first-order kinetics (Chapter 7) and is related to the concentration of drug, C_t,

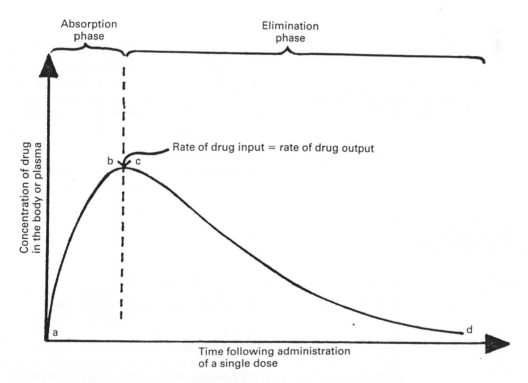

Fig. 19.2 Concentration–time course of a drug in the body following peroral administration of a single dose of drug which confers one-compartment open model characteristics on the body.

remaining in the body compartment at time t, by the following equation:

$$\text{rate of elimination at time } t = -k_e \, C_t \qquad (19.3)$$

where k_e is the apparent elimination rate constant. The negative sign in Eqn 19.3 indicates that elimination is removing drug **from** the body compartment.

The apparent elimination rate constant of a drug gives the proportion or fraction of that drug which is eliminated from the body per unit time. Its units are in terms of time^{-1}. The apparent elimination constant of a given drug therefore provides a quantitative index of the persistence of that drug in the body.

An alternative parameter used is the biological or elimination half-life of the drug, $t_{1/2}$. This is the time required for the body to eliminate 50% of the drug that it contained. Thus, the larger the biological half-life exhibited by a drug, the slower will be its elimination from the body or plasma.

For a drug whose elimination follows first-order kinetics, the value of its biological half-life is independent of the concentration of drug remaining in the body or plasma. Hence, if a single dose of a drug having a biological half-life of 4 hours was administered perorally, then after the peak plasma concentration had been reached the plasma concentration of drug would fall by 50% every 4 hours until all the drug had been eliminated or a further dose was administered. The relationship between the numbers of half-lives elapsed and the percentage of drug eliminated from the body following administration of a single dose is given in Table 19.1.

An appreciation of the relationship between the percentage of drug eliminated from the body and the number of biological half-lives elapsed is useful when considering how much drug is eliminated from

Table 19.2 The biological half-life ranges for phenobarbitone, digoxin and theophylline

Drug	Biological half-life (h)
Phenobarbitone	50–120
Digoxin	36–51
Theophylline	3–8

the body over the time interval between successive doses in a multiple-dosage regimen. Biological half-life varies from drug to drug and, even for a given drug, from patient to patient. Some biological half-lives for various drugs are given in Table 19.2.

For a drug whose elimination follows first-order kinetics, the biological half-life, $t_{1/2}$, is related to the apparent elimination rate constant, k_e, of that drug according to the following equation:

$$t_{1/2} = \frac{0.693}{k_e} \qquad (19.4)$$

Thus the biological half-life of a drug will be influenced by any factor that influences the apparent elimination rate constant of that drug. This explains why factors such as genetic differences between individuals, age and disease can affect the biological half-life exhibited by a given drug. Biological half-life is an important factor that influences the plasma concentration–time curve obtained following peroral administration of a multiple-dosage regimen.

Concentration–time curve of a drug in the body following the peroral administration of equal doses of a drug at fixed intervals of time

In discussing how the design of multiple peroral dosage regimen can influence the concentration–time course of a drug in the body, the following assumptions have been made:

1. The drug confers upon the body the characteristics of a one-compartment open model.
2. The values of the apparent absorption rate and apparent elimination rate constants for a given drug do not change during the period for which the dosage regimen is administered to a patient.
3. The fraction of each administered dose which is absorbed by the body compartment remains constant for a given drug.

Table 19.1 Relationship between the amount of drug eliminated and the number of half-lives elapsed

Number of half-lives elapsed	Percentage of drug eliminated
0.5	29.3
1.0	50.0
2.0	75.0
3.0	87.5
3.3	90.0
4.0	94.0
4.3	95.0
5.0	97.0
6.0	98.4
6.6	99.0
7.0	99.2

4. The aim of drug therapy is to achieve promptly and maintain a concentration of drug at the appropriate site(s) of action which is both clinically efficacious and safe for the desired duration of treatment. This aim is assumed to be achieved by the prompt attainment and maintenance of plasma concentrations of drug which lie within the therapeutic range of that drug.

If the interval between each perorally administered dose is longer than the time required for complete elimination of the previous dose, then the plasma concentration–time profile of a drug will exhibit a series of isolated single-dose profiles, as shown in Figure 19.3.

Consideration of the plasma concentration–time profile shown in Figure 19.3 in relation to the minimum effective and maximum safe plasma concentrations (MEC and MSC, respectively) for the drug reveals that the design of this particular dosage regimen is unsatisfactory. The plasma concentration only lies within the therapeutic concentration range of the drug for a relatively short period following the administration of each dose, and the patient remains undermedicated for relatively long periods. If the dosing time interval is reduced so that it is now shorter than the time required for complete elimina-

tion of the previous dose, then the resulting plasma concentration–time curve exhibits the characteristic profile shown in Figure 19.4.

Figure 19.4 shows that at the start of this multiple-dosage regimen the maximum and minimum plasma concentrations of drug observed during each dosing time interval tend to increase with successive doses. This increase is because the time interval between successive doses is less than that required for complete elimination of the previous absorbed dose. Consequently, the total amount of the drug remaining in the body compartment at any time after a dose is equal to the sum of that remaining from all the previous doses. The accumulation of drug in the body and plasma with successively administered doses does not continue indefinitely. Provided drug elimination follows first-order kinetics, the rate of elimination will increase as the average concentration of drug in the body (and plasma) rises. If the amount of drug supplied to the body compartment per unit dosing time interval remains constant, then a situation is eventually reached when the overall rate of elimination from the body over the dosing time interval becomes equal to the overall rate at which drug is being supplied to the body compartment over that interval, i.e. the overall rate of elimination has effectively caught up with the overall rate of supply. This effect

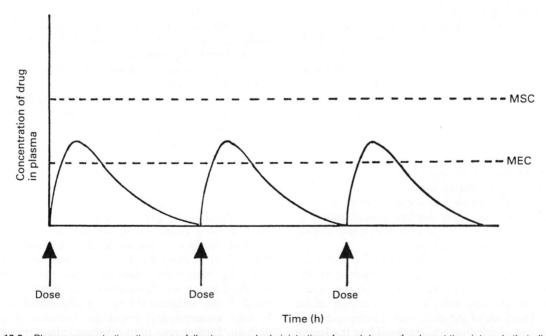

Fig. 19.3 Plasma concentration–time curve following peroral administration of equal doses of a drug at time intervals that allow complete elimination of the previous dose. (MSC, maximum safe plasma concentration of the drug; MEC, minimum effective plasma concentration of the durg.)

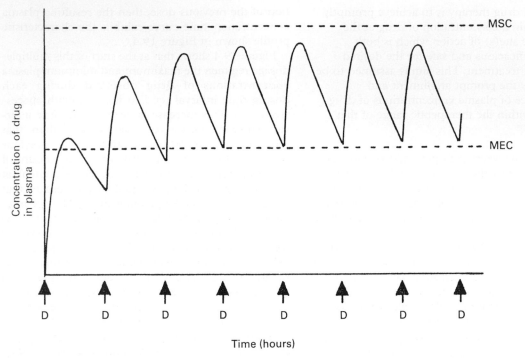

Fig. 19.4 Plasma concentration–time curve following peroral administration of equal doses, *D*, of a drug every 4 hours. (MSC, maximum safe plasma concentration of the drug; MEC, minimum effective plasma concentration of the drug.)

is due to the elimination rate increasing as the residual concentration of drug in the plasma rises (as elimination is first order here).

When the overall rate of drug supply equals the overall rate of drug output from the body compartment, a ***steady state*** is reached with respect to the average concentration of drug remaining in the body over each dosing time interval. At steady state, the amount of drug eliminated from the body over each dosing time interval is equal to the amount that was absorbed into the body compartment following administration of the previous dose.

Figure 19.5 shows that the amount of drug in the body, as measured by the plasma concentration, fluctuates between maximum and minimum values which remain more or less constant from dose to dose. At steady state the average concentration of drug in the plasma, $C^{ss}_{average}$, over successive dosing time intervals remains constant.

For a drug administered repetitively in equal doses and at equal time intervals, the time required for the average plasma concentration to attain the corresponding steady-state value is a function only of the biological half-life of the drug, and is independent of both the size of the dose administered and the length of the dosing time interval. The time required for the average plasma concentration to reach 95% of the

steady-state value corresponding to the particular multiple dosage regimen is 4.3 times the biological half-life of the drug. The corresponding figure for 99% is 6.6 times. Therefore, depending on the magnitude of the biological half-life of the drug being administered, the time taken to attain the average steady-state plasma concentration may range from a few hours to several days.

From a clinical viewpoint the time required to reach steady state is important, because for a properly designed multiple-dosage regimen the attainment of steady state corresponds to the achievement and maintenance of maximal clinical effectiveness of the drug in the patient.

It should be noted that for a drug such as phenytoin, whose elimination is not described by first-order kinetics, the peroral administration of equal doses at fixed intervals may not result in the attainment of steady-state plasma levels. If the concentration of such drug in the body rises sufficiently following repetitive administration, the pathway responsible for its elimination may become saturated. If this occurred the rate of elimination would become maximal and could not increase to cope with any further rises in the average concentration of drug in the body. Hence the overall rate of elimination would not become equal to the overall rate of

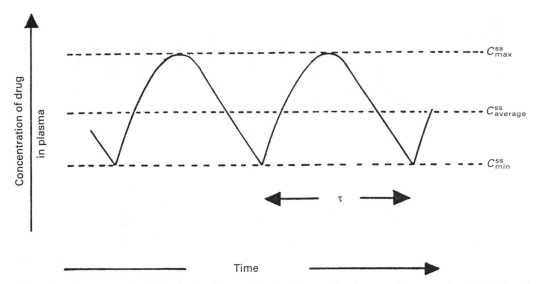

Fig. 19.5 Fluctuation of concentration of drug in the plasma at steady state resulting from repetitive peroral administration of equal doses, D, of drug at a fixed interval of time, τ. C_{max}^{ss}, C_{min}^{ss} and $C_{average}^{ss}$ represent the maximum, minimum and average plasma concentrations of drug, respectively, achieved at steady state.

supply over each dosing time interval, and the condition necessary for the attainment of steady state would not be achieved. If repetitive administration continued at the same rate, the average concentration of drug in the body and plasma would tend to continue to accumulate, rather than to reach a plateau.

IMPORTANT FACTORS INFLUENCING STEADY-STATE PLASMA DRUG CONCENTRATIONS

Dose size and frequency of administration

In designing a multiple-dosage regimen that balances patient convenience with the achievement and maintenance of maximal clinical effectiveness, only two parameters can be adjusted for a given drug: the size of dose and the frequency of administration. Consider how the maximum, minimum and average steady-state plasma concentrations of drug are influenced by these parameters.

Size of dose

Figure 19.6 illustrates the effects of changing the dose size on the concentration of drug in the plasma following repetitive administration of peroral doses at equal intervals of time. As the size

of the administered dose is increased, the higher are the corresponding maximum, minimum and average plasma drug levels, C_{max}^{ss}, C_{min}^{ss} and $C_{average}^{ss}$, respectively, achieved at steady state. What may not be so well appreciated is that the larger the dose the larger is the fluctuation between C_{max}^{ss} and C_{min}^{ss} during each dosing time interval. Large fluctuations between C_{max}^{ss} and C_{min}^{ss} can be hazardous, particularly with a drug such as digoxin, which has a narrow therapeutic range. In such cases, it is possible that C_{max}^{ss} could exceed the maximum safe plasma concentration. Figure 19.6 also illustrates that the time required to attain steady-state plasma concentrations is independent of the size of the administered dose.

Interval between successive equal doses

Figure 19.7 illustrates the effects of constant doses administered at various dosing intervals, which are multiples of the biological half-life of the drug $t_{1/2}$. The uppermost plasma concentration–time curve in Figure 19.7 shows that the repetitive administration of doses at a time interval which is less than the biological half-life of the drug results in higher steady-state plasma drug concentrations being obtained. This is a consequence of the extent of elimination of the drug from the body over a dosing time interval equal to $0.5\ t_{1/2}$ being smaller than that which is eliminated when the dosing time interval is equal to $t_{1/2}$ (see Table 19.1).

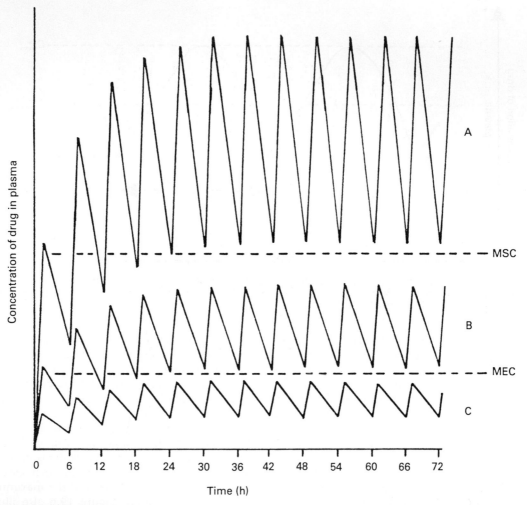

Fig. 19.6 Diagrammatic representation of the effect of dose size on the plasma concentration–time curve obtained following peroral administration of equal doses of a given fixed drug at fixed intervals of time equal to the biological half-life of the drug. Curve A, dose = 250 mg. Curve B, dose = 100 mg. Curve C, dose = 40 mg.

Figure 19.7 also shows that repetitive administration of doses at intervals greater than the biological half-life of the drug results in the lower steady-state plasma drug concentrations being obtained. This is a consequence of a greater proportion of the drug being eliminated over a dosing time interval equal to $2t_{1/2}$, compared to that which is eliminated when the dosing time interval is equal to $t_{1/2}$.

Summary of the effects of dose size and frequency of administration

Consideration of the effects of dose size and the dosage interval on the amount of a given drug achieved in the body, as measured by the plasma concentration, following repetitive peroral administration of equal doses, have revealed the following relationships:

1. The magnitude of the fluctuations between the maximum and minimum steady-state amounts of drug in the body is determined by the size of dose administered or, more accurately, by the amount of drug absorbed following each dose administered.

2. The magnitude of the fluctuations between the maximum and minimum steady-state plasma concentrations are an important consideration for any drug that has a narrow therapeutic range, e.g. digoxin. The more frequent administration of smaller doses is a means of

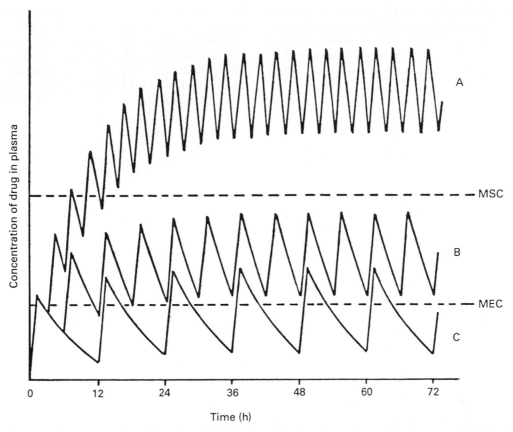

Fig. 19.7 Diagrammatic representation of the effect of changing the dosing time interval, τ, on the plasma concentration–time curve obtained following repetitive peroral administration of equal size doses of a given drug. Curve A, dosing time interval = 3 hours ($0.5t_{\frac{1}{2}}$). Curve B, dosing time interval = 6 hours ($t_{\frac{1}{2}}$). Curve C, dosing time = 12 hours ($2t_{\frac{1}{2}}$).

reducing the steady-state fluctuations without altering the average steady-state plasma concentration. For example, a 500 mg dose given every 6 hours will provide the same $C_{average}^{ss}$ value as a 250 mg dose of the same drug given every 3 hours, whereas the C_{max} and C_{min} fluctuation for the latter dose will be decreased by half.

3. The average maximum and minimum amounts of drug achieved in the body at steady state are influenced by either the dose size, the dosage time interval in relation to the biological half-life of the drug, or both. The greater the dose size and the smaller the dosage time interval relative to the biological half-life of the drug, the greater are the average, maximum and minimum steady-state amounts of drug in the body.

4. For a given drug, the time taken to achieve steady state is independent of dose size and dosage time interval.

5. If the maximum safe and minimum effective plasma drug concentrations are represented by the dashed lines shown in Figures 19.6 and 19.7, respectively, then it is evident that the proper selection of dose size and dosage time interval are important with respect to achieving and maintaining steady-state plasma concentrations that lie within the therapeutic range of the particular drug being administered.

It is evident from the preceding discussion that the proper selection of the dose size and the dosage time interval is crucial in ensuring that a multiple-dosage regimen provides steady-state concentrations of drug in the body which are both clinically efficacious and safe.

Mathematical relationships that predict the values of the various steady-state parameters achieved in the body following repetitive administration of doses at constant intervals of time have been used to assist the design of clinically acceptable multiple dosage regimens. For example, a useful equation for predicting the average amount of drug achieved in the body at steady state, $D_{average}^{ss}$, following repetitive peroral administration of equal doses, D, at a fixed time interval, τ is:

$$D_{average}^{ss} = \frac{F \cdot D \cdot t_{1/2} \cdot 1.44}{\tau} \quad (19.5)$$

where F is the fraction of drug absorbed following the administration of a dose, D, of drug; thus $F \cdot D$ is the bioavailable dose of drug, and $t_{1/2}$ is the biological half-life of that drug. The average amount of a given drug in the body at steady state, $D_{average}^{ss}$ is related to the corresponding average plasma concentration of the drug by the factor known as the *apparent volume of distribution*, i.e.:

$$D_{average}^{ss} = V_d \, C_{average}^{ss} \quad (19.6)$$

where V_d is the apparent volume of distribution of the drug and $C_{average}^{ss}$ is the average steady-state plasma concentration. Equation 19.5 can be rewritten in terms of the average steady-state plasma concentration of the drug as follows:

$$C_{average}^{ss} = \frac{F \cdot D \cdot t_{1/2} \cdot 1.44}{\tau \cdot V_d} \quad (19.7)$$

If the value of the average body amount or the average plasma concentration of a given drug at steady state which gives a satisfactory therapeutic response in a patient is known, then Eqns 19.5 or 19.7 can be used respectively to estimate either the size of dose that should be administered repetitively at a preselected constant dosage time interval, or the dosage time interval at which a preselected dose should be administered repetitively. In order to illustrate a dosage regimen calculation, based on the average steady-state plasma concentration of a drug, consider the following worked example.

An antibiotic is to be administered on a repetitive basis to a male patient weighing 76 kg. The antibiotic is commercially available in the form of tablets, each containing 250 mg of the drug. The fraction of the drug that is absorbed following peroral administration of one 250 mg tablet is 0.9. The antibiotic has been found to exhibit a biological half-life of 3 hours and the patient has an apparent volume of distribution of 0.2 L kg^{-1} of body weight. What dosage time interval should be selected to administer this drug on a repetitive basis so that a therapeutic average steady-state plasma concentration of 16 mg L^{-1} will be achieved?

Using Eqn 19.7:

$$C_{average}^{ss} = \frac{F \cdot D \cdot t_{1/2} \cdot 1.44}{\tau \cdot V_d} \quad (19.8)$$

where the average steady-state plasma concentration of drug, $C_{average}^{ss}$, is 16 mg L^{-1}, the fraction of each administered dose absorbed, $F = 0.9$, the size of administered dose, $D = 250$ mg, the biological half-life of the drug, $t_{1/2} = 3$ h, and the apparent volume of distribution, $V_d = 0.2$ L kg^{-1} of patient's body weight.

Hence, for a patient weighing 76 kg the value of

$$V_d = 0.2 \times 76 \text{ L}$$
$$= 15.2 \text{ L}.$$

To calculate the dosage time interval, τ, requires substitution of the above values into Eqn 19.7, which gives:

$$16 = \frac{0.9 \times 250 \times 3 \times 1.44}{\tau \times 15.2}$$

$$\tau = \frac{0.9 \times 250 \times 3 \times 1.44}{16 \times 15.2}$$

$$= \frac{972.0 \text{h}}{243.2}$$

$$\approx 4 \text{h}.$$

Thus one 250 mg tablet should be administered every 4 hours in order to achieve the required averaged average steady-state plasma concentration.

Mathematical equations which predict the maximum or minimum steady-state plasma concentrations of a drug achieved in the body followed by repetitive administration of equal doses at a fixed interval of time are also available for drugs whose time course in the body is described by the one-compartment open pharmacokinetic model.

The concept of 'loading doses'

As discussed earlier, the time required for a given drug to reach 95% of the average steady-state plasma concentration is 4.3 biological half-lives, when equal doses of the drug are administered repetitively at equal intervals of time. Thus, for a drug with a long half-life of 24 hours it would take more than 4 days for the average concentration in the plasma to reach 95% of its steady-state value. Because the attainment of steady-state plasma concentrations is normally associated with the attainment of maximal clinical effectiveness of the drug, it is conceivable that a number of days could elapse before a patient experienced the full therapeutic benefit of a drug having a long half-life. To reduce the time required for onset of the full therapeutic effect, a large single dose of the drug may be administered initially in order to achieve a peak plasma concentration that lies within the therapeutic range of the drug and is approximately equal to the value of C_{max}^{ss} required. This is known as the *loading dose* or *priming dose*.

Thereafter smaller, equal doses are administered repetitively at suitable fixed intervals so as to maintain the plasma concentrations of drug at the maximum, minimum and average state levels that provide the patient with the full therapeutic benefit. These are known as *maintenance doses*. As a general rule, the loading dose should be twice the size of the maintenance dose if the selected dosage time interval corresponds to the biological half-life of the drug.

Figure 19.8 illustrates how rapidly therapeutic steady-state plasma concentrations of drug are achieved when the dosage regimen consists of an initial loading dose followed by equal maintenance doses at fixed intervals, compared to a 'simple' multiple-dosage regimen consisting of doses that are equal in size and are administered at the same dosage time intervals as the maintenance doses.

Influence of changes in the apparent elimination rate constant of a drug: the problem of patients with renal impairment

Whereas the loading dose, maintenance dose and dosage time interval may be varied in order to design a clinically efficacious multiple dosage regimen, one factor cannot normally be adjusted. This is the apparent elimination rate constant exhibited by the particular drug being administered. However, the elimination rate constant of a given drug does vary from patient to patient, and is influenced by whether the patient has normal or impaired renal function.

Figure 19.9 indicates the effects produced by changes in the apparent elimination rate constant on the plasma concentration–time curve obtained following repetitive, peroral administration of equal doses of a given drug at equal intervals of time. Any reduction in the apparent elimination rate constant will produce a proportional increase in the biological half-life exhibited by the drug. This reduction, in turn, will result in a greater degree of accumulation of the drug in the body following repetitive administration

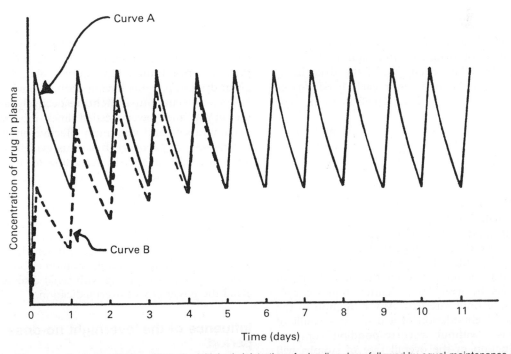

Fig. 19.8 Diagrammatic representation of how the initial administration of a loading dose followed by equal maintenance doses at fixed intervals of time ensure rapid attainment of steady-state plasma levels for a drug having a long biological half-life of 24 hours. Curve A represents the plasma concentration–time curve obtained following peroral administration of a loading dose of 500 mg followed by a maintenance dose of 250 mg every 24 hours. Curve B represents the plasma concentration–time curve obtained following peroral administration of a 250 mg dose every 24 hours.

Fig. 19.9 Diagrammatic representation of the effect of changing the biological half-life of a given drug on the plasma concentration–time curve exhibited by the drug following peroral administration of one 250 mg dose every 6 hours. Curve A, biological half-life of drug = 6 hours. Curve B, biological half-life of drug = 12 hours.

before steady-state drug levels are achieved. The greater degree of drug accumulation is a consequence of a smaller proportion of the drug being eliminated from the body over each fixed dosage time interval when the biological half-life of the drug is increased.

Patients who develop severe renal impairment normally exhibit smaller apparent elimination rate constants and consequently longer biological half-lives for drugs which are eliminated substantially by renal excretion than do patients with normal renal function. For instance, the average apparent elimination rate constant for digoxin may be reduced from 0.021 h^{-1} in patients with normal renal function to 0.007 h^{-1} severe renal impairment. The average steady-state amount of drug in the body is only achieved and maintained when the overall rate of supply equals the overall rate of elimination over successive dosing time intervals. Any reduction in the overall rate of elimination of a drug as a result of renal disease, without a corresponding compensatory reduction in the overall rate of supply, will result in increased steady-state amounts of drug in the body. This effect in turn may lead to side-effects and toxic effects if the increased steady-state levels exceed the maximum safe concentration of the drug.

In order to illustrate this concept, consider that curves A and B in Figure 19.9 correspond to the plasma concentration–time curves obtained for a given drug in patients having normal renal function and severe renal impairment, respectively, and that the upper and lower dashed lines represent the maximum safe and minimum effective plasma concentrations, respectively. It is thus evident that the administration of a drug according to a multiple-dosage regimen which produces therapeutic steady-state plasma levels in patients with normal renal function, will give plasma concentrations that exceed the maximum safe plasma concentration of the drug in patients with severe renal impairment. Hence the adjustment of multiple-dosage regimens in terms or dose size, frequency of administration or both is necessary if patients suffering with renal disease are to avoid the possibility of overmedication.

Influence of the 'overnight no-dose period'

So far we have considered that multiple-dosage regimens comprise of doses being administered at uniform time intervals around the clock, but in practice this is unusual. If a multiple-dosage regimen requires a dose to be administered 'four times a day' it is unlikely that a dose will be administered at 6-hourly intervals around the clock. Instead, the four doses are likely to be administered during 'waking' hours, e.g. 10 am–2 pm –6 pm–10 pm or 9 am–1 pm–5 pm–9 pm. The significant feature of both these schedules is that the patient will experience an overnight no-dose period of 12 hours. Although this will undoubtedly give the patient periods of undisturbed sleep, it may also cause problems in maintaining therapeutic steady-state plasma concentrations of drug in the body.

It is conceivable that overnight no-dose periods of 8–12 hours could result in substantial decreases in the amount of a drug in the plasma and body, particularly for drugs having biological half-lives which are relatively short compared to the overnight no-dose period. For instance, in the case of a drug having a biological half-life of 4 hours, an overnight no-dose period of 12 hours would correspond to the elapse of three biological half-lives and consequently a large reduction in the amount of drug in the body.

The potential problems of overnight no-dose periods with respect to maintaining therapeutic steady-state drug levels is illustrated in Figure 19.10. This shows that for a drug having a biological half-life of 4 hours, a multiple-dosage regimen comprising one 60 mg dose administered perorally four times each day according to the timetable 9 am–1 pm–5 pm–9 pm does not permit a true steady state to be attained. Thus the concentration of drug in the plasma does not fluctuate between constant maximum and minimum values over successive dosage time intervals, as would occur if the doses were administered every 4 hours around the clock.

Furthermore, Figure 19.11 shows that even if a loading dose of 120 mg were included in the dosage regimen to ensure that a true steady state was obtained before the first overnight no-dose period, the steady state would not be re-established after the first overnight no-dose period. If the upper and lower dashed lines in Figures 19.10 and 19.11 represent the therapeutic range of the drug, then the patient would experience periods during which the level of drug in the plasma and body would fall below that necessary to elicit the therapeutic effect. Hence, unless the therapeutic range of the drug is sufficiently large to accommodate the fluctuations in concentration associated with overnight no-dose periods, problems could arise with regard to maintaining therapeutic drug levels in patients. The potential problems associated with overnight no-dose periods are even further complicated by patients who forget to take one of their daytime doses.

Concluding comments

This chapter explains the interrelationship between the rate at which drug enters the body and the rate at which it leaves. It also discusses how, in turn, this balance influences the concentration of drug in the plasma at any given time. It is clearly important for pharmaceutical scientists to come to terms with this problem and then overcome it by finding ways of

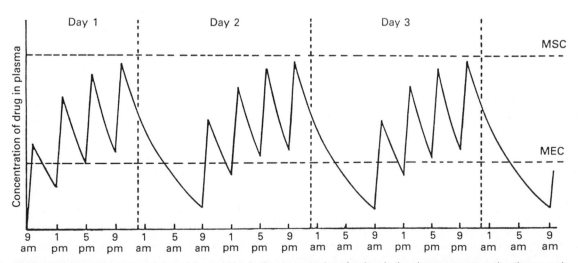

Fig. 19.10 Diagrammatic representation of the variation in the concentration of a drug in the plasma accompanying the peroral administration of a single dose of 60 mg four times a day according to the time schedule 9 am–1 pm–5 pm–9 pm. The biological half-life of the drug is 4 hours.

Fig. 19.11 Diagrammatic representation of the variation in the concentration of drug in the plasma accompanying the peroral administration of a loading dose of 120 mg followed by single maintenance doses of 60 mg four times a day according to the time schedule 9 am–1 pm–5 pm–9 pm. The biological half-life of the drug is 4 hours.

maintaining therapeutic drug levels appropriate to a particular disease state. This can be achieved by the careful design of the appropriate drug delivery system. This aspect of the design and formulation of modified-release drug delivery systems is discussed fully in Chapter 20.

BIBLIOGRAPHY

Gibaldi, M. (1991) *Biopharmaceutics and Clinical Pharmacokinetics*, 4th edn. Lea & Febiger.

Rowland, M. and Tozer, T.N. (1995) *Clinical Pharmacokinetics: Concepts and Applications*, 3rd edn. Lea & Febiger.

20

Modified-release peroral dosage forms

John Collett, Chris Moreton

MAINTENANCE OF THERAPEUTIC DRUG CONCENTRATIONS BY MODIFIED-RELEASE PERORAL DOSAGE FORMS

For many disease states the ideal dosage regimen is that by which an acceptable therapeutic concentration of drug at the site(s) of action is attained immediately and is then maintained constant for the desired duration of the treatment. It is evident from the preceding chapter that, provided dose size and frequency of administration are correct, therapeutic 'steady-state' plasma concentrations of a drug can be achieved promptly and maintained by the repetitive administration of conventional peroral dosage forms. However, there are a number of potential limitations associated with this. In the context of this section a 'conventional' peroral oral dosage form is assumed to be one that is designed to release rapidly the complete dose of drug contained therein immediately following administration. In addition, the released drug is assumed to be in a form which is therapeutically active and immediately available for absorption into the systemic circulation.

These limitations are:

1. The concentration of drug in the plasma and hence at the site(s) of action of the drug fluctuates over successive dosing intervals, even when the so-called 'steady-state' condition is achieved. Hence it is not possible to maintain a therapeutic concentration of drug **which remains constant** at the site(s) of action for the duration of treatment. At best, the mean value of the maximum and minimum plasma concentrations associated with each successive dose remains constant for the period of drug treatment.
2. The inevitable fluctuations of steady-state concentrations of drug in the plasma, and hence at the site(s) of action, can lead to a patient being over- or undermedicated for periods of time if the values of C_{max}^{ss} and C_{min}^{ss} (Chapter 19) rise or fall, respectively, beyond the therapeutic range of the drug.
3. For drugs with short biological half-lives frequent doses are required to maintain steady-state plasma concentrations within the therapeutic range. For such drugs the maintenance of therapeutic plasma concentrations is particularly susceptible to the consequence of forgotten doses and the overnight no-dose period. Lack of patient compliance, which is more likely in the case of

regimens requiring frequent administration of conventional dosage forms, is often an important reason for therapeutic inefficiency or failure. Clearly, not even a peroral dosage regimen which has been designed to perfection can achieve and maintain clinically efficacious concentrations of a drug at its site(s) of action if the patient does not comply with it.

These limitations and requirements led pharmaceutical scientists to consider presenting therapeutically active molecules in 'extended-release' preparations. In reality the scientists were attempting to take the control of medication away from the patient, and to some extent the physician, and to place it in the drug delivery system.

Over the years there has been an enormous amount of work put into designing drug delivery systems that can eliminate or reduce the cyclical plasma concentrations seen after conventional drug delivery systems are administered to a patient according to a specified dosage regimen.

One of the first commercially available products to provide sustained release of a drug was Dexedrine Spansules®, made by Smith Kline & French. After this many more sustained-release products came to the market, some successful, others potentially lethal. Each delivery system was aimed at eliminating the cyclical changes in plasma drug concentration seen after the administration of a conventional delivery system. A variety of terms was used to describe these systems:

- *Delayed release* indicates that the drug is not being released immediately following administration but at a later time, e.g. enteric-coated tablets, pulsatile-release capsules.
- *Repeat action* indicates that an individual dose is released fairly soon after administration, and second or third doses are subsequently released at intermittent intervals.
- *Prolonged release* indicates that the drug is provided for absorption over a longer period of time than from a conventional dosage form. However, there is an implication that onset is delayed because of an overall slower release rate from the dosage form.
- *Sustained release* indicates an initial release of drug sufficient to provide a therapeutic dose soon after administration, and then a gradual release over an extended period.
- *Extended release* (ER) dosage forms release drug slowly, so that plasma concentrations are maintained at a therapeutic level for a prolonged period of time (usually between 8 and 12 hours).

- *Controlled release* (CR) dosage forms release drug at a constant rate and provide plasma concentrations that remain invariant with time.
- *Modified release* (MR) dosage forms are defined by the USP as those whose drug release characteristics of time course and/or location are chosen to accomplish therapeutic or convenience objectives not offered by conventional forms, whereas an extended-release (ER) dosage form allows a twofold reduction in dosing frequency or increase in patient compliance or therapeutic performance. It is interesting to note that the USP considers that the terms controlled release, prolonged release and sustained release are interchangeable with extended release. From a biopharmaceutical perspective this is not strictly a concern.

Time following peroral administration of ONE dosage form

Fig. 20.1 Plasma concentration–time curves obtained following peroral administration of (a) one repeat-action dosage form containing two doses, and (b) one MR dosage form containing the same drug. MSC = maximum safe concentration, MEC = minimum effective concentration (see Chapter 19).

Repeat-action versus sustained-action drug therapy

A repeat-action tablet or hard gelatin capsule may be distinguished from its sustained-released counterpart by the fact that the repeat-action product does not release the drug in a slow controlled manner, and consequently does not give a plasma concentration–time curve which resembles that of a sustained-release product. A repeat-action tablet usually contains two doses of drug, the first being released immediately following peroral administration in order to provide a rapid onset of the therapeutic response. The release of the second dose is delayed, usually by means of an enteric coat. Consequently, when the enteric coat surrounding the second dose is breached by the intestinal fluids, the second dose is released immediately. Figure 20.1 shows that the plasma concentration–time curve obtained following the administration of one repeat-action preparation exhibits the 'peak and valley' profile associated with the intermittent administration of conventional dosage forms. The primary advantage provided by a repeat-action tablet over a conventional one is that two (or occasionally three) doses are administered without the need to take more than one tablet.

Modified release

The term modified release (MR) will be used in this chapter to describe peroral dosage forms that continuously release drugs at rates which are sufficiently controlled to provide periods of prolonged therapeutic action following each adminis-

tration of a 'single dose'. Although all MR products could be described literally as controlled-release systems, the term 'controlled release' will only be used in this chapter to describe a peroral sustained-release product which is able to maintain a constant therapeutic steady-state concentration of drug in the plasma, the tissues, or at the site of action. This use of the term is in accordance with the proposals of Chien (1995).

The degree of precision of control over the rate of drug release from an MR dosage form varies according to the particular formulation technique employed. Consequently, depending on the degree of control over release (and consequently over drug absorption) that is achieved, peroral MR products are generally designed to provide either:

1. the prompt achievement of a plasma concentration of drug that remains essentially constant at a value within the therapeutic range of the drug for a satisfactorily prolonged period of time, or
2. the prompt achievement of a plasma concentration of drug which, although not remaining constant, declines at such a slow rate that the plasma concentration remains within the therapeutic range for a satisfactorily prolonged period of time.

Typical drug plasma concentration–time profiles corresponding to the above criteria for modified-release products are shown in Figure 20.2.

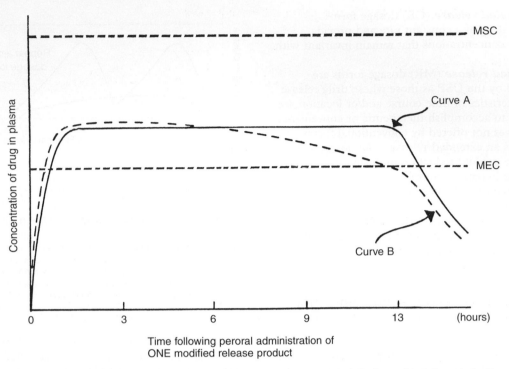

Fig. 20.2 Typical plasma concentration – time profiles for MR peroral products which, following rapid attainment of a therapeutic plasma concentration of drug, provide a period of prolonged therapeutic action by either (a) maintaining a *constant* therapeutic plasma concentration (curve A) or, (b) ensuring that the plasma concentration of drug remains within the therapeutic range for a satisfactorily prolonged period of time (curve B).

Kinetic pattern of drug release required for the ideal modified controlled-release peroral dosage form

If it is assumed that the drug which is to be incorporated into the ideal MR dosage form confers upon the body the characteristics of a one-compartment open model, then the basic kinetic design of such a product may be represented diagrammatically as shown in Figure 20.3.

To achieve a therapeutic concentration promptly in the body and then to maintain that concentration for a given period of time requires that the total drug in the dosage form consists of two portions, one that provides the **initial** priming/loading dose, D_i, and one that provides the **maintenance** or sustained dose, D_m.

The initial priming dose of drug D_i is released rapidly into the gastrointestinal fluids immediately following administration of the MR dosage form (see step 1 in Fig. 20.3). The released dose is required to be absorbed into the body compartment rapidly following a first-order kinetic process that is characterized by the apparent absorption rate constant, k_a^1 (see step 2 in Fig. 20.3). The aim of this initial rapid

release and subsequent absorption of the initial priming dose is the rapid attainment of a therapeutic concentration of drug in the body. This priming dose provides a rapid onset of the desired therapeutic response in the patient.

Following this period of rapid drug release, the portion D_m of drug remaining in the dosage form is released at a slow but defined rate (see step 3 in Fig. 20.3). In order to maintain a constant plasma level of drug, the maintenance dose, D_m, must be released by the dosage form according to zero-order kinetics. It thus follows that the rate of release of drug will remain constant and be independent of the amount of the maintenance dose remaining in the dosage form at any given time. The rate of release of the maintenance dose may be characterized by the zero-order rate constant k_m^o.

Two further conditions must be fulfilled in order to ensure that the therapeutic concentration of drug in the body remains constant.

1. The zero-order rate of release of drug from the maintenance dose must be rate determining with respect to the rate at which the released drug is subsequently absorbed into the body.

RELEASE AND ABSORPTION OF INITIAL PRIMING DOSE

RELEASE AND ABSORPTION OF MAINTENANCE DOSE

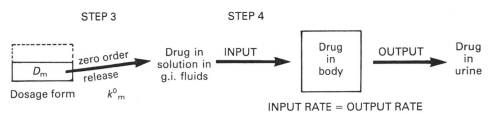

Fig. 20.3 A one-compartment open model of drug disposition in which the source of drug input is an *ideal* MR peroral drug product. D_i is the initial priming dose of drug in dosage form; D_m is the maintenance dose of drug in the dosage form; k^1_a is the first-order apparent absorption rate constant of drug from the priming dose; k^o_m is the zero-order release rate constant of drug from the maintenance dose.

The kinetics of absorption of the maintenance dose will thus be characterized by the same zero-order release rate constant, k^o_m (step 3 in Fig. 20.3).

2. The rate at which the maintenance dose is released from the dosage form, and hence the rate of absorption (input) of drug into the body, must be equal to the rate of drug output from the body when the concentration of drug in the body is at the required therapeutic value (see step 4 in Fig. 20.3).

In practice, the design of an ideal modified- or controlled-release product, which is capable of releasing the maintenance dose at a precise controlled rate which is in mass balance with the rate of drug elimination corresponding to the required therapeutic concentration of drug in the plasma, is difficult to achieve. There are problems in achieving and maintaining zero-order release and absorption of the maintenance dose of drug in the presence of all the variable physiological conditions associated with the gastrointestinal tract (see Chapter 16). In addition, the apparent elimination rate constant of a given drug varies from patient to patient, depending on such factors as genetic differences, age differences and differences in the severity of disease. Consequently it is likely that most peroral MR products in current use will not fall into the category of ideal MR/controlled-release peroral dosage forms. However, such products may be referred to

simply as MR products and may be differentiated from their ideal counterparts by the following definition. A modified-release product/dosage form is a system in which a portion (the initial priming dose) of the drug is released immediately in order to achieve the desired therapeutic response promptly. The remaining dose of drug (the 'maintenance' dose) is then released slowly, thereby resulting in a therapeutic drug/tissue drug concentration which is prolonged but not maintained constant.

Formulation methods of achieving modified drug release

It is evident from the preceding discussion that formulation techniques that permit rapid release of the priming dose, followed by slow release of the maintenance dose, are required in order to design peroral MR products. All MR formulations use a chemical or physical 'barrier' to provide slow release of the maintenance dose. Many formulation techniques have been used to 'build' the barrier into the peroral dosage form. These include the use of coatings, embedding of the drug in a wax or plastic matrix, microencapsulation, chemical binding to ion-exchange resins, and incorporation in an osmotic pump. The initial rapidly releasing priming dose may be provided by incorporating that portion of the drug in a separate, rapidly releasing form in the dosage form, for instance as uncoated, rapidly releasing granules or pellets in a tablet or hard gelatin capsule. Alternatively, immediate and rapid release of the priming dose has been achieved by that portion of the drug being positioned at the surface of a porous wax or plastic matrix.

Potential advantages of modified-release dosage forms over conventional dosage forms

1. Improved control over the maintenance of therapeutic plasma drug concentration of drugs permits:
    (a) improved treatment of many chronic illnesses where symptom breakthrough occurs if the plasma concentration of drug drops below the minimum effective concentration, e.g. asthma, depressive illnesses;
    (b) maintenance of the therapeutic action of a drug during overnight no-dose periods, e.g. overnight management of pain in terminally ill patients permits improved sleep;
    (c) a reduction in the incidence and severity of untoward systemic side-effects related to high peak plasma drug concentrations;
    (d) a reduction in the total amount of drug administered over the period of treatment. This contributes to the reduced incidence of systemic and local side-effects observed in the cases of many drugs administered in MR formulations.

2. Improved patient compliance, resulting from the reduction in the number and frequency of doses required to maintain the desired therapeutic response, e.g. one peroral MR product every 12 hours contributes to the improved control of therapeutic drug concentration achieved with such products.

3. There is a reduction in the incidence and severity of localized gastrointestinal side-effects produced by 'dose dumping' of irritant drugs from conventional dosage forms, e.g. potassium chloride. The more controlled, slower release of potassium chloride from its peroral MR formulations minimizes the build-up of localized irritant concentrations in the gastrointestinal tract. Consequently, potassium chloride is now administered perorally almost exclusively in MR form.

4. It is claimed that cost savings are made from the better disease management that can be achieved with MR products.

Potential limitations of peroral modified-release dosage forms

1. Variable physiological factors, such as gastrointestinal pH, enzyme activities, gastric and intestinal transit rates, food and severity of disease, which often influence drug bioavailability from conventional peroral dosage forms, may also interfere with the precision of control of release and absorption of drugs from peroral MR dosage forms. The achievement and maintenance of prolonged drug action depends on such control.

2. The rate of transit of MR peroral products along the gastrointestinal tract limits the maximum period for which a therapeutic response can be maintained following administration of a 'single dose' to approximately 12 hours, plus the length of time that absorbed drug continues to exert its therapeutic activity.

3. MR products, which tend to remain intact, may become lodged at some site along the gastrointestinal tract. If this occurs, slow release of the drug may produce a high localized concentration that causes local irritation to the gastrointestinal mucosa. MR products which are formulated to disperse in the gastrointestinal fluids are less likely to cause such problems.

4. There are constraints on the types of drugs that are suitable candidates for incorporation into peroral MR formulations. For instance, drugs having biological half-lives of 1 hour or less are difficult to formulate for modified release. The high rates of elimination of such drugs from the body mean that an extremely large maintenance dose would be required to provide 8–12 hours of continuous therapy following a single administration. Apart from the potential hazards of administering such a large dose, the physical size of the MR dosage form could make it difficult to swallow. Drugs having biological half-lives between 4 and 6 hours make good candidates for inclusion in MR formulations. Factors other than the biological half-life can also preclude a drug from being formulated as an MR product. Drugs that have specific requirements for their absorption from the gastrointestinal tract are poor candidates. In order to provide a satisfactory period of prolonged drug therapy, a drug is required to be well absorbed from all regions as the dosage form passes along the gastrointestinal tract.

5. MR products normally contain a larger total amount of drug than the single dose normally

administered in a conventional dosage form. There is the possibility of unsafe overdosage if an MR product is improperly made and the total drug contained therein is released at one time or over too short a time interval. Consequently, it may be unwise to include very potent drugs in such formulations.

6. As a general rule, MR formulations cost more per unit dose than conventional dosage forms containing the same drug. However, fewer 'unit doses' of an MR formulation should be required.

DESIGN OF PERORAL MODIFIED-RELEASE DRUG DELIVERY SYSTEMS

Factors influencing design strategy

Having made the decision that a drug is to be included in a modified-release delivery system intended for oral administration, it is necessary to take account of the physiology of the gastrointestinal tract; the physicochemical properties of the drug; the design of the dosage form; the drug release mechanism; the particular disease factors; and the biological properties of the drug. All of these can influence or interact with one another.

The physiology of the gastrointestinal tract and drug absorption

The influence of gastrointestinal physiology on drug delivery is discussed in detail in Chapter 16. It should also be noted that the residence time of a dosage form in the gastrointestinal tract is influenced by both stomach emptying time and intestinal transit time. It has been reported that:

- solution and pellets (<2 mm) leave the stomach rapidly;
- single dose units (>7 mm) can stay in the stomach for up to 10 hours if the delivery system is taken with a heavy meal;
- the transit time through the small intestine is approximately 3 hours.

Physicochemical properties of the drug

Several physicochemical properties of the active drug can influence the choice of dosage form. This is discussed fully in Chapter 17; these properties include aqueous solubility and stability; pK_a; partition coefficient (or, more appropriately, permeability values) and salt form.

The aqueous solubility and intestinal permeability of drug compounds are of paramount importance. A classification has been made (Amidon et al 1995) whereby drugs can be considered to belong to one of four categories:

- high solubility and high permeability (best case);
- high solubility and low permeability;
- low solubility and high permeability;
- low solubility and low permeability (worst case).

This is now codified as the Biopharmaceutical Classification System (see Chapter 18 for further details).

Consider first the influence of solubility. A drug that is highly soluble at intestinal pH and absorbed by passive diffusion (i.e. not site-specific absorption) would probably present the ideal properties for inclusion in an MR dosage form. However, there may be some problems associated with the choice of actual formulation. At the other end of the scale, compounds that have a low aqueous solubility (<1 mg mL^{-1}) may already posses inherent sustained-release potential as a result of their low solubility. The innate advantages of low aqueous solubility in relation to modified release would be negated if the drug also had low membrane permeability.

Having achieved dissolution of the drug in the gastrointestinal tract then permeability considerations become important. An indication of drug permeability values can be obtained using Caco-2 tissue culture models (see Chapter 18). More than 90% absorption in vivo may be expected for compounds with permeability, P, values $> 4 \times 10^{-6}$ mm s^{-1}, whereas less than 20% absorption is expected when P is $<0.5 \times 10^{-6}$ mm s^{-1} (Bailey et al 1996). Drug candidates with a permeability $<0.5 \times 10^{-6}$ mm s^{-1} are likely to be unsuitable for presentation as MR preparations.

Drug compounds that satisfy the solubility and permeability requirements should also ideally have:

- a biological half-life of between two and six hours so that accumulation in the body does not occur
- a lack of capability to form pharmacologically active metabolites by, for example, first-pass metabolism. Modified release is actually used for drugs which undergo first-pass metabolism but this should not be to such an extent that only inactive metabolites are left after absorption
- a dosage not exceeding 125–325 mg in order to limit the size of the delivery system. There are a few examples where this dose is exceeded, e.g. Brufen Retard.

Choice of the dosage form

The first decision to be made is whether to formulate the active ingredient as a single or a multiple unit system. Single-unit dosage forms include tablets, coated tablets, matrix tablets and some capsules. A multiple-unit dosage form includes granules, beads, capsules and microcapsules.

Modified-release dosage forms include inert insoluble matrices, hydrophilic matrices, ion-exchange resins, osmotically controlled formulations and reservoir systems.

The selection of the appropriate dosage form will need to take account of an acceptable level of variability of performance, the influence of GI tract structure and function on the delivery system, and the release mechanism and release profile of the dosage form.

Drug-release mechanisms

The two basic mechanisms controlling drug release are dissolution of the active drug component and the diffusion of dissolved or solubilized species. Within the context of these mechanisms there are four processes operating:

- Hydrating of the device (swelling of the hydrocolloid or dissolution of the channelling agent)
- Diffusion of water into the device
- Dissolution of the drug
- Diffusion of the dissolved (or solubilized) drug out of the device.

These mechanisms may operate independently, together or consecutively.

Drug delivery systems can be designed to have either continuous release, a delayed gastrointestinal transit while continuously releasing, or delayed release. Drug release may be constant, declining or bimodal.

Constant release The general belief has been that the ideal MR system should provide and maintain constant drug plasma concentrations. This led to considerable effort being put into developing systems that release drugs at a constant rate. (Although with the advent of chronotherapy, i.e. drug delivered at both the appropriate time *and* rate, zero-order release may not be such a desirable goal in the future.) In general these systems rely on diffusion of the drug or, occasionally, osmosis.

Declining release Drug release from these systems is commonly a function of the square root of time or follows first-order kinetics. These systems cannot maintain a constant plasma drug concentration but can provide sustained release.

Bimodal release Although constant drug release may be ideal, this may not always be the case. If the gastrointestinal tract behaves as a one-compartment model (Chapter 19), i.e. the different segments are homogeneous, then the situation is ideal. However, we know from Chapter 16 that absorption rate is not invariant along the gastrointestinal tract. So, whatever happens, the rate of release from the dosage form must regulate drug absorption – in other words, release rate must always be slower than absorption rate. This situation may not be easy to achieve: a release rate suited to absorption from the intestine may be far too great for that required in the stomach or colon. One possible solution to this problem is to prepare a dosage form that provides a rapid initial delivery of drug followed by a slower rate of delivery and then an increased rate at a later time.

FORMULATION OF MODIFIED-RELEASE DOSAGE FORMS

For convenience of description oral modified release delivery systems can be considered under the following headings:

- Monolithic or matrix systems
- Reservoir or membrane-controlled systems
- Osmotic pump systems.

These are the main classes of delivery system and they are considered in turn below. However, there are other systems and the above is not an exhaustive list.

There is a basic principle that governs all these systems. In a solution, drug diffusion will occur from a region of high concentration to a region of low concentration. This concentration difference is the driving force for drug diffusion out of a system. Water diffuses into the system in an analogous manner. There is an abundance of water in the surrounding medium and the system should allow water penetration. The inside of the system normally has a lower water content initially than the surrounding medium.

Components of a modified-release delivery system

These include:

- active drug;
- release-controlling agent(s): matrix formers, membrane formers;

Table 20.1 Suitable excipients for modified-release dosage forms categorized as inert, lipid or hydrophilic

Inert excipients
Dibasic calcium phosphate
Ethyl cellulose
Methacrylate copolymer
Polyamide
Polyethylene
Polyvinyl acetate

Lipid excipients
Carnauba wax
Cetyl alcohol
Hydrogenated vegetable oils
Microcrystalline waxes
Mono- and triglycerides
PEG monostearate
PEG

Hydrophilic excipients
Alginates
Carbopol
Gelatin
Hydroxypropylcellulose
Hydroxypropyl methylcellulose
Methylcellulose

- matrix or membrane modifier, such as channelling agents for wax matrices and solubilizers, and wicking agents for hydrophilic matrices;
- solubilizer, pH modifier and/or density modifiers;
- lubricant and flow aid, such as magnesium stearate, stearic acid, hydrogenated vegetable oil, sodium stearyl fumarate, talc, colloidal silicon dioxide;
- supplementary coatings to extend lag time, further reduce drug release, etc.;
- density modifiers (if required).

These types of components are virtually the same for all oral solid MR dosage forms. The differences are in the excipients, how they are incorporated into the formulation and what role they play.

The delivery systems may also be classified as inert, lipid or hydrophilic, depending on the nature of the excipients used. Suitable excipients for modified-release dosage systems are listed in Table 20.1.

Monolithic matrix delivery systems

These systems can be considered as two groups:

- Those with drug particles dispersed in a soluble matrix, with drug becoming available as the matrix dissolves or swells and dissolves (**hydrophilic colloid matrices**);
- Those with drug particles dispersed in an insoluble matrix, with drug becoming available as

a solvent enters the matrix and dissolves the particles (**lipid matrices** and **insoluble polymer matrices**).

Drugs dispersed in a soluble matrix rely on a slow dissolution of the matrix to provide sustained release. Excipients used to provide a soluble matrix often are those used to make soluble film coatings. Alternatively, slowly dissolving fats and waxes can be used. Synthetic polymers, such as polyorthoesters and polyanhydrides, have been used. These undergo surface erosion with little or no bulk erosion. If the matrix is presented with a conventional tablet geometry, then on contact with dissolution media the surface area of the matrix decreases with time, with a concomitant decrease of drug release.

Drug particles may be incorporated into an insoluble matrix. Drug release from these matrices follows penetration of fluid, followed by dissolution of the drug particles and diffusion through fluid-filled pores. This type of delivery system would not be suitable for the release of compounds that are insoluble or which have a low aqueous solubility.

Excipients used in the preparation of insoluble matrices include hydrophobic polymers, such as polyvinyl acetate, ethylcellulose and some waxes.

It is useful to consider each of the matrix systems mentioned above separately.

Lipid matrix systems

Principle of design Wax matrices are a simple concept. They are easy to manufacture using standard direct compression, roller compaction or hot-melt granulation.

The matrix compacts are prepared from blends of powdered components. The active compound is contained in a hydrophobic matrix that remains intact during drug release. Release depends on an aqueous medium dissolving the channelling agent, which leaches out of the compact so forming a porous matrix of tortuous capillaries. The active agent dissolves in the aqueous medium and, by way of the water-filled capillaries, diffuses out of the matrix.

Wax matrices are a simple unsophisticated delivery system with a fairly coarse control of rate and extent of drug release. The release is generally not zero order and there are few opportunities to modify it.

These matrices are not now in common usage, but the concept is worth considering. A typical formulation consists of:

- active drug
- wax matrix former

- channelling agent
- solubilizer and pH modifier
- antiadherent/glidant
- lubricant.

Matrix formers Hydrophobic materials that are solid at room temperature and do not melt at body temperature are used as matrix formers. These include hydrogenated vegetable oils, cottonseed, oil, soya oil, microcrystalline wax and carnauba wax. In general such waxes form 20–40% of the formulation.

Channelling agents Channelling agents are chosen to be soluble in the gastrointestinal tract and to leach from the formulation, so leaving tortuous capillaries through which the dissolved drug may diffuse in order to be released. The drug itself can be a channelling agent, but a water-soluble pharmaceutically acceptable solid material is more likely to be used. Typical examples include sodium chloride, sugars and polyols. The choice will depend on the drug and the desired release characteristics. These agents can be 20–30% of the formulation.

Solubilizers and pH modifiers It is often necessary to enhance the dissolution of the drug. This may be achieved by the inclusion of solubilizing agents, such as PEGs, polyols or surfactants. If the drug is ionizable then the inclusion of buffers or counter-ions may be appropriate. On occasions the dissolution enhancer may also be the channelling agent.

Antiadherent/glidant Heat generated during compaction of the matrix can cause melting of the wax matrix-forming compound and sticking to the punches. Something is needed to cope with the sticking; suitable antiadherents include talc and colloidal silicon dioxide.

These materials also act as glidants and improve the flow of formulations on the tablet machine. The typical amounts used will depend on the antiadherent used, for example 0.5–1% for colloidal silicon dioxide and 4–6% for talc.

This type of formulation usually does not need a lubricant per se, as the fats are themselves liquid-film lubricants (i.e. they melt during compaction). Magnesium stearate, if added, can also act as an antiadherent.

Insoluble polymer matrix systems

An inert matrix system is one in which a drug is embedded in an inert polymer which is not soluble in the gastrointestinal fluids. Drug release from inert matrices has been compared to the leaching from a sponge. The release rate depends on drug molecules in aqueous solution diffusing through a network of capillaries formed between compacted polymer par-

ticles. The concept of using inert matrices as drug delivery systems was considered in the late 1950s and led to the development of Duretter (Astra Hassle) and Gradumet (Abbott) technologies, and products such as Ferro-Gradumet (Abbott). There have been concerns that residual catalysts and initiators used in the preparation of the polymer(s) of the matrix could be leached along with active drug. The matrices remain intact during gastrointestinal transit, and there have also been concerns that impaction may occur in the large intestine and that patients may be concerned to see the matrix 'ghosts' in stools. More recently there has been renewed interest in this type of matrix, and polymers such as ethylcellulose are finding favour.

The release rate of a drug from an inert matrix can be modified by changes in the porosity and tortuosity of the matrix, i.e. its pore structure. The addition of pore-forming hydrophilic salts or solutes will have a major influence, as can the manipulation of processing variables. Compression force controls the porosity of the matrix, which in turn controls drug release. Generally a more rigid and less porous matrix will release drug more slowly than a less consolidated matrix.

The addition of excipients, such as lubricants, fillers etc., is a necessary part of the formulation process. However, the presence of excipients is likely to influence drug release. It may be anticipated that water-soluble excipients will enhance the wetting of the matrix, or increase its tortuosity and porosity on dissolution. Insoluble excipients will tend to decrease the wettability of the matrix and reduce the penetration of the dissolving medium.

The particle size of the insoluble matrix components influences release rate, larger particles leading to an increase in release rate. This is attributed to these coarser particles producing matrices with a more open pore structure.

An increase in drug loading tends to enhance release rate, but the relationship between the two is not clearly defined. One possible explanation may be a decrease in the tortuosity of the matrix. As may be expected, release rate can be related to drug solubility.

Drug release from insoluble matrices The release of drugs from insoluble matrices has been investigated and four types of drug matrix system can be considered:

- Drug molecularly dissolved in the matrix and drug diffusion occurs by a solution–diffusion mechanism;
- Drug dispersed in the matrix and then, after dissolution of the drug, diffusion occurs via a solution–diffusion mechanism;

- Drug dissolved in the matrix and diffusion occurs through water-filled pores in the matrix;
- Drug dispersed in the matrix and then, after dissolution, diffusion occurs through water-filled pores.

The amount of drug released from matrix dosage forms is normally proportional to the square root of the time of exposure to the dissolution medium:

$$M_t = Kt^{0.5} \qquad (20.1)$$

where M_t is the amount of drug released with time t, and K is a constant.

The amount of drug released decreases with time of exposure to the dissolution medium. The reason for this is that the drug is released initially from the surface region, and there is then only a short diffusion pathway. As the period of dissolution progresses, the area of drug exposed to dissolution medium decreases. Also, an ever-increasing 'zone of depletion' is formed within the matrix as the drug dissolves, and so the diffusion pathway increases in length.

A simple exponential relationship has been used to characterize drug release from non-swelling delivery systems:

$$\frac{M_t}{M_\alpha} = Kt^n \qquad (20.2)$$

where M_t/M_α is the fractional solute release, K is a constant and n is the diffusional exponent.

The numerical value of the diffusional exponent is indicative of the release mechanism and is influenced by the matrix aspect ratio (i.e. diameter:length ratio). If the matrix is presented as a thin film a value of $n = 0.5$ would be indicative of Fickian diffusion, whereas values of n not equal to 0.5 are indicative of anomalous or non-Fickian process. Zero-order release is considered to be happening if $n = 1.0$. In other words, the rate of surface erosion is controlling the rate of drug release and not its rate of diffusion within the matrix.

Hydrophilic colloid matrix systems

These delivery systems are also called swellable–soluble matrices. In general they comprise a compressed mixture of drug and water-swellable hydrophilic polymer. The systems are capable of swelling, followed by gel formation erosion and dissolution in aqueous media. Their behaviour is in contrast to a true hydrogel, which swells on hydration but does not dissolve.

Principle of design of hydrophilic matrices The system comprises a mixture of drug, hydrophilic colloid, any release modifiers and lubricant/glidant.

On contact with water the hydrophilic colloid components swell to form a hydrated matrix layer. This then controls the further diffusion of water into the matrix. Diffusion of the drug through the hydrated matrix layer controls its rate of release. The outer hydrated matrix layer will erode as it becomes more dilute; the rate of erosion depends on the nature of the colloid.

Hydrophilic colloid gels can be regarded as a network of polymer fibrils that interlink in some way. There is also a continuous phase in the interstices between the fibrils through which the drug diffuses. These interstices connect together and are analogous to the tortuous capillaries seen in wax matrices.

The tortuosity of the diffusion path and the 'microviscosity' and interactions within the interstitial continuum govern the diffusion of the drug through the hydrated gel layer, and hence the release of the drug.

Types of hydrophilic matrix

True gels These systems interact in the presence of water to form a crosslinked polymeric structure with a continuous phase trapped in the interstices of the gel network. The crosslinks are more than just random hydrogen bonds between adjacent polymer chains (e.g. alginic acid in the presence of di or trivalent cations, gelatin): here they limit the mobility of the polymer chains and give a structure to the gel (Fig. 20.4). The crosslinks can be chemical bonds or physical bonds, e.g. triple-helix formations in gelatin gels which are based on hydrogen bonds. The portions of the polymer chains between crosslinks can move, but the crosslinks restrict the overall movement of the chains.

Viscous or 'Viscolized' matrices Not all matrix systems form 'true' gels: in reality some are more

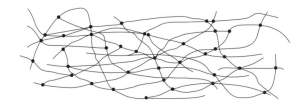

Fig. 20.4 Representation of a 'true' gel matrix.

Fig. 20.5 Representation of a 'viscolized' matrix.

Table 20.2 Comparison of different types of hydrocolloid matrix

True gels	Viscous matrices
The diffusion pathway is via the continuous phase in the interstices of the gel	The diffusion pathway is via the continuous phase trapped between the adjacent polymeric chains
The crosslinks are more or less 'fixed' after the gel has formed	There are no 'fixed' cross-links
The bulk viscosity of the gel is derived from the structure of the crosslinked polymeric chains with a contribution from the continuous phase	The bulk viscosity is related to the entanglement of adjacent polymer chains which are free to move within the continuous phase
Bulk viscosity generally does not correlate well with diffusion	Bulk viscosity may correlate with diffussion
Diffusion in the gel correlates with 'microviscosity'	

properly described as very viscous solutions. In the presence of water these systems form a matrix in which the increased viscosity occurs as a result of simple entanglement of adjacent polymer chains, but without proper crosslinking (Fig. 20.5). It is a dynamic structure. The chains are able to move relative to one another and the drug diffuses through the interstitial continuum, but the pathway is not fixed. Examples are hydroxypropyl methylcellulose and sodium alginate in water.

Comparison of different types of hydrocolloid matrix
The differences between the various different types of hydrocolloid matrix are summarized in Table 20.2. It should be appreciated that these are simplifications. In general bulk viscosity is not a good test for the functionality of either system. It may be satisfactory as a quality control test for the matrix-forming materials.

Advantages of hydrophilic matrix systems
- Comparatively simple concept;
- Excipients are generally cheap and are usually GRAS (generally regarded as safe);
- Capable of sustaining high drug loadings;
- Erodible, so reducing the possibility of 'ghost' matrices;
- Easy to manufacture using commonly available equipment, by direct compression, wet granulation or roller compaction;
- Well established technology;

- Uses readily available pharmaceutical manufacturing equipment;
- Possible to obtain different types of release profile: zero order, first order, biomodal etc.

Disadvantages of hydrophilic matrix delivery systems
- Release of the drug is dependent on two diffusion processes, penetration of the water through the hydrated matrix into the non-hydrated core, and diffusion of the dissolved drug through the hydrated matrix.
- If the outer layer of the hydrated matrix erodes, this can complicate the release profile.
- Requires batch-to-batch consistency in the matrix-forming materials, other components and process parameters.
- Scale-up of manufacture can be a problem.
- Need optimal rate-controlling polymers for different actives.

These matrices are comparatively simple in concept. However, the events following hydration can be quite complex.

The key is that there are two diffusion processes (water in and then drug out). The drug will only diffuse through a hydrated gel layer. This really only applies to drugs that are solid at room temperature. Liquid drugs may diffuse in the non-hydrated state and would not be suitable for some types of system.

Components of hydrophilic matrix delivery systems
- Active drug
- Hydrophilic colloid(s)
- (Matrix modifier)
- (Solubilizer and/or pH modifier)
- Compression aid
- Lubricant
- (Glidant).

Those components listed in parentheses are optional and not always necessary.

Matrix-forming agents for hydrophilic matrices
Hydrophilic colloids which, on contact with water, form a hydrated gel that remains 'sufficiently intact' during passage through the gastrointestinal tract are suitable matrix-forming agents for hydrophilic matrices. Examples of hydrophilic colloids include:
- Hydroxypropyl methylcellulose (high-viscosity grades)
- Sodium carboxymethyl cellulose
- Alginates
- Xanthan gum
- Xanthan gun/locust bean gum combinations
- Carbopol.

These agents generally occupy 20–80% of the mass; the actual amount will depend on the drug and the desired release characteristics.

Hydration and swelling are the key factors in the functioning of a hydrophilic matrix, as has already been stated.

Gel modifiers for hydrophilic matrix delivery systems
These are materials that are incorporated into the matrix to modify the diffusional characteristics of the gel layer, very often to enhance drug diffusion and hence release of the drug. Examples include sugars, polyols and soluble salts.

The type of modifier will depend very much on the chemical nature of the hydrocolloid(s) used. They may also modify the rate and extent of hydration of the hydrophilic matrix material.

Gel modifiers can have a number of other functions. For example, they may act:

• to allow more complete, more uniform hydration of the gel matrix;
• to allow more rapid hydration of the gel matrix;
• to associate with the matrix molecules and thus to influence the interactions at a molecular level, e.g. crosslinking;
• to modify the environment in the interstices of the gel, either to speed up or slow down diffusion;
• to suppress or promote the ionization of ionizable polymers.

Few materials will have only a single action. It is more likely that they will work in several ways.

Solubilizers and pH modifiers for drugs in hydrophilic matrices Many drugs will not dissolve sufficiently in gastrointestinal fluids to allow them to be released from a hydrophilic colloid matrix. Dissolution can be improved by the inclusion of solubilizing agents (e.g. PEGs, polyols, surfactants etc.). The only restriction is that the formulation can be formed into a tablet and that the material is acceptable. Many drugs are ionizable. The inclusion of appropriate counter-ions can facilitate release from the system. Some materials can act as both dissolution enhancer and matrix modifier: the amount of excipient needed will be determined by the amount of drug.

The above relates to the drug molecule, rather than the matrix material. It is necessary for any drug to be in solution for diffusion to occur. For insoluble drugs, solubilization is therefore an important consideration.

With some gel materials the use of certain ions causes changes in the nature of the gel matrix.

The solubilizers and pH modifiers might also influence the release process through a direct effect on the matrix. Different materials could augment crosslinking, whereas others might perhaps weaken the crosslinks.

Lubricants for hydrophilic delivery systems As with any tablet compacted on a tablet machine, a lubricant is necessary. Lubricants can have four functions:

• Reduce interparticulate friction during compression and compaction;
• Reduce die-wall friction;
• Prevent sticking to the punches;
• Improve flow of the formulation on to the machine and into the die.

The requirement for lubricants for hydrophilic matrix tablets are no different from those for any other tablet, and are thus analogous to those for conventional immediate-release tablets and capsules. Generally the choice is not governed by the same constraints as in immediate release. For example, overblending or excess magnesium stearate may not be a major problem here.

It is not essential that the lubricant is soluble. Such lubricants are available but are generally not very effective and tend to be reserved for effervescent products.

Suitable lubricants and recommended concentrations to be included in the formulation are listed in Table 20.3.

Drug release from hydrophilic colloid matrices The classic description of the events following immersion of a matrix in aqueous media are as follows:

• Surface drug (if water soluble) dissolves and gives a 'burst effect'.
• The hydrophilic polymer hydrates and an outer gel layer forms.
• The gel layer becomes a barrier to uptake of further water and to the transfer of drug.

Table 20.3 Concentration of lubricants used in hydrophilic matrix systems

Lubricants	%
Hydrophobic lubricants	
Magnesium stearate	0.25–2
Calcium stearate	0.25–2
Stearic acid	1–4
Hydrogenated vegetable oil	1–4
Hydrophilic lubricants (the latter two examples are only partially soluble in water)	
Glyceryl palmitostearate	0.5–5
Glyceryl behenate	2–5
Sodium stearyl fumarate	0.25–2
Inorganic lubricants	
Colloidal silicon dioxide	0.05–0.25 as glidant
	0.2–0.5 as antiadherent
Talc	1–4 as antiadherent

- Drug (if soluble) release occurs by diffusion through the gel layer; insoluble drug is released by erosion followed by dissolution.
- Following erosion the new surface becomes hydrated and forms a new gel layer.

It may be anticipated that the relative importance of each release mechanism will depend on the physico-chemical properties of the gel layer; the aqueous solubility of the drug; and the mechanical attrition of the matrix in the aqueous environment.

When a drug/glassy polymer matrix is placed in an aqueous environment, the water penetrates the polymer network. As the amount of water increases a transition from a glassy to a rubbery state occurs as the glass transition temperature is decreased by the presence of water to the temperature of the medium. The intake of solvent (water) induces stresses within the matrix polymer. Eventually the matrix polymer relaxes, and this manifests itself as swelling. It is possible to differentiate three 'fronts' during hydration: eroding, diffusing and swelling.

The actual drug release mechanism depends on the relative contributions of swelling and dissolution. Drug release from swellable, soluble matrices is constant when swelling and eroding fronts synchronize, but is non-linear when this is not the case. The release of sodium diclofenac from PVA and from HPMC matrices has been investigated. It was noted that if the fronts synchronized then the gel layer thickness was constant and zero-order release was observed. When synchronization did not take place the gel layer tended to increase in thickness and there was a decrease in the amount released, providing non-linear kinetics.

Membrane-controlled drug delivery systems

Membrane-controlled delivery systems function as follows. The rate-controlling part of the system is a membrane through which the drug must diffuse. To allow the drug to diffuse out, the membrane has to become permeable, e.g. through hydration by water normally present in the gastrointestinal tract, or by the drug being soluble in a membrane component, such as the plasticizer. Unlike hydrophilic matrix systems, the membrane polymer does not swell on hydration to form a hydrocolloid matrix, and does not erode.

A drug reservoir, e.g. a tablet or multiparticulate pellet, is coated with a membrane. The drug should not diffuse in the solid state, although loading of the membrane might be an advantage if an initial release on contact with dissolution medium is desired.

Aqueous medium diffusing into the system and forming a continuous phase through the membrane initiates drug diffusion and release.

The essential difference between a membrane and a matrix system is that in the former the polymer membrane is only at the surface of the system, whereas in the latter the polymer is throughout the whole system. In both cases the hydration of the polymer is the step that allows the drug to diffuse. With the classic membrane system there are the two diffusion processes: 'water in' followed by 'drug out'.

The delivery systems may be presented either as single or as multiple unit.

Components of a membrane-controlled system

Core
- Active drug
- Filler or substrate
- (Solubilizer)
- Lubricant/glidant.

The exact composition of the core formulation will depend on the formulation approach adopted.

Coating
- Membrane polymer
- Plasticizer
- (Membrane modifier)
- (Colour/opacifier).

Single-unit systems

This is essentially a tablet formulation, but with differences from conventional dosage forms in that modified-release tablet cores should not disintegrate but dissolve; and a formulation is required that allows water to penetrate and the drug to dissolve so that diffusion can occur.

Core formulation for single-unit systems   Generally, water-insoluble materials that compact by brittle fracture are not suitable if used alone. Suitable fillers include lactose, microcrystalline cellulose, dextrose, sucrose and polyols (mannitol, sorbitol, xylitol etc.).

Care is needed in the choice of soluble fillers to minimize osmotic effects. An inappropriate choice will result in increased internal osmotic pressure followed by rupture of the release-controlling membrane. The choice of solubilizer (if required) will be governed by the solubility characteristics of the drug. Materials that have been used include buffers, surfactants, polyols and PEGs.

Because single-unit cores are most often compressed tablets, a satisfactory lubricant system will also be required. Again, this is the same as for any tablet except that soluble lubricants may not be necessary. Suitable lubricants are listed in Table 20.3.

Multiple-unit systems

As the name implies, this type of dosage unit comprises more than one discrete unit. Typically, such systems comprise coated spheroids (pellets approximately 1 mm in diameter) filled into a hard gelatin capsule shell or, less commonly, compressed into a tablet.

There are two main approaches that can be adapted to the manufacture of drug-containing multiple units:

- The use of inert sugar spheres ('nonpareils') coated first with drug and then with the release-controlling membrane;
- The formulation of small spheroids containing the drug using an extrusion/spheronization process (see Chapter 25). This approach is better if a high drug loading is required.

Typical formulations comprise drug with combinations of lactose and microcrystalline cellulose. Other materials can be used. A typical formulation for a wet mass for extrusion/spheronization might comprise:

	Parts by weight
Active drug	1–20
Lactose	60
Microcrystalline cellulose	40
Binder	2–4
Water	40

After spheronization the material is dried prior to coating.

Release-controlling membrane The membrane is a critical part of the formulation as it controls the release of the drug. The requirement is that the polymer remain intact for the period of release, i.e. there should be no swelling or subsequent erosion, as seen in hydrophilic matrices. Typical polymers used include ethyl cellulose, acrylic copolymers, e.g. Eudragit RL and RS grades, shellac and zein. Shellac and zein are natural products and their quality can vary.

The release-controlling polymer is film-coated on to the system. For the coating to be successful the coating droplets must coalesce. The plasticizer is used to lower the glass transition temperature (T_g) of the film (see Chapter 28). The choice of plasticizer will depend on the polymer used, the active drug and the desired release characteristics. In addition, the plasticizer may modify the diffusional characteristics of the membrane with respect to the drug. The final choice of plasticizer will probably be a compromise of all these different requirements.

Examples of suitable plasticizers for ethyl cellulose films include dibutyl phthalate, diethyl phthalate, dibutyl sebecate and citric acid esters. These are water-insoluble materials; a water-soluble plasticizer might increase the permeability of the membrane excessively. The amount of plasticizer required will depend on the several factors mentioned above, but is typically 10–25% of the polymer dry weight.

The smallest amount of plasticizer is used that will produce the most consistent result, i.e. complete coalescence of the droplets to form the film without making it too elastic, plastic, soft or permeable. The plasticizer is not present only for processing but is added to have an effect on the mechanical properties of the film, i.e. film flexibility should be induced and maintained. Plasticizers should be permanent to avoid stability problems.

It may be necessary to add components to the coating formulation to modify the release characteristics of the film, particularly to increase the rate of release. Typically this will be a less hydrophobic, water-soluble component. Examples of such materials include polyethylene glycols, propylene glycol, glycerol or other polyols, and water-soluble polymers. Some of these may also act as plasticizers. It is important to recognize that many materials can have different functions in a formulation, and also to understand what the implications of these different functionalities are for the finished product.

Advantages of membrane-controlled systems
- For multiple-unit systems the gastrointestinal transit of small particulates is more consistent than that of a larger single-unit system.
- Multiple-unit systems are also less likely to suffer from the problems associated with total dose dumping due to overall catastrophic failure of a film around a monolith (tablet), which would then release the whole dosage.
- In addition, multiple-unit systems allow the release mechanism to be optimized for individual drugs in a system delivering two or more active components.

Disadvantages of membrane-controlled systems
- Dose dumping can occur from single-unit system as a result of film failure.
- Multiple-unit systems can be difficult to retain in the higher gastrointestinal tract.
- The control of the membrane characteristics in film-coated membranes can be difficult.
- Filling of the multiunit spheroids into capsules can be a problem owing to build-up of static charge.

Osmotic pump systems

In one sense osmotic pump systems are another form of membrane-controlled release drug delivery system and work in the following way. A drug is included in a tablet core which is water soluble, and which will solubilize (or suspend) the drug in the presence of water. The tablet core is coated with a semipermeable membrane which will allow water to pass through into the core, which then dissolves. As the core dissolves, a hydrostatic pressure builds up and forces (pumps) drug solution (or suspension) through a hole drilled in the coating. The rate at which water is able to pass in through the membrane, and how quickly the drug solution (or suspension) can pass out of the hole, govern the rate of release.

The rate at which the drug solution/suspension is forced out can be modified by changes in the viscosity of the solution formed inside the system. The essential difference between an osmotic pump system and a 'classic' membrane-controlled system is that for the osmotic pump only one diffusion process is required (in this case, 'water in'). As mentioned above, in the 'classic' system two processes are key: water in, drug out.

Components of osmotic pump systems

Core This consists of the active drug, a filler or substrate, a (viscosity modifier), (solubilizer) and, lubricant/glidant.

Coating Coatings contain a membrane polymer, a plasticizer, a (membrane modifier) and (colour/opacifier).

This is the same list of components as for matrix-controlled systems, and the types of excipient used are essentially similar. However, it is important to remember that the diffusing species is only water; an agent must be included in the core which is soluble enough to generate the osmotic pressure; and there must be a hole through which the drug solution/suspension can be pumped out. Otherwise, the same considerations apply for the formulation of the core as with other membrane-controlled systems. The coating must also be fully coalesced and be free from unintentional pinholes, and it should act as a semipermeable membrane.

Advantages of osmotic pump systems
- They are well characterized and understood.
- The diffusing species is water.
- Modification of the rate of water diffusion is more straightforward than for many drugs.
- The release mechanism is not dependent on the drug.

- They are suitable for a wide range of drugs.
- The coating technology is straightforward.
- They typically give a zero-order release profile after an initial lag.

Disadvantages of osmotic pump systems
- Size of hole is critical.
- Laser drilling is capital intensive.
- Integrity and consistency of the coating is essential:
  - If the coating process is not well controlled there is a risk of film defects, which could result in dose dumping.
  - The film droplets or particles must be induced to coalesce into a film with consistent properties.

Delivery systems for targeting to specific sites in the gastrointestinal tract

Systems that target specific sites in the gastrointestinal tract are a form of modified-release delivery system and are considered briefly here. Targeting of drugs in the gastrointestinal tract is considered useful as a means of taking advantage of and/or overcoming efflux systems (Chapter 16) and intestinal cell metabolism; specific carrier mechanisms; and cell recognition sites. It can be achieved by gastric retentive delivery systems and by colonic drug delivery systems.

Gastric retentive systems

The advantages of using these drug delivery systems include reduced variability of drug release, local drug delivery and action, and enhanced bioavailability for those drugs with a restricted absorption window in the gastrointestinal tract.

Methods to achieve gastric retention are:

- the addition of passage-delaying agents, such as food material, for example triethanolamine myristate, or drugs, for example propantheline;
- the use of high-density materials: high-density particles ($>2.5 \text{g/cm}^3$) have prolonged gastric residence times. This can be achieved by the addition of materials such as barium sulphate;
- modification of the size/shape of delivery system by the use of unfolding polymer sheets, swelling hydrogel balloons, or polymer units that are too large to pass through the pyloric sphincter.
- bioadhesive systems. Systems have been used which will adhere to surfaces such as the mucosa. The problems when these systems are used for gastrointestinal delivery are that first, high local

concentrations of drug may result, and second, there is a turnover of mucosa, leading to detachment of the delivery system;

- the use of floating dosage forms. These systems resist gastric emptying by floating on the stomach contents. They should not alter the intrinsic emptying rate of the stomach and their specific gravity should be less than that of the stomach contents. Systems used are (a) hydrodynamically balanced systems; (b) carbon dioxide-generating systems; (c) freeze-dried systems.

Colonic delivery systems

Applications for these systems include local delivery for the treatment of inflammatory diseases, infections, and diarrhoea; and systemic delivery.

Design principles for these delivery systems make use of:

- the specific pH of the colon: pH-sensitive polymers are used in their manufacture, e.g. combinations of Eudragit 100-55 (pH 5.5) with Eudragit S (pH 7.0). The principle is that drug is released at a specific pH environment;
- small-intestine transit time. These depend on timed release of the active drug;

- colonic bacteria. The principle here is to coat the drug/delivery system with a polymer that is sensitive to bacteria in the colon. Degradation of the polymer permits release of the active drug. Polymers used include glassy amylase (mixed with ethylcellulose); or pectin as a thick compression coat, crosslinked with calcium, with different degrees of methoxylation or amidation, or mixed with ethylcellulose.

REFERENCES

Amidon, G.L., Lenneras, H, Shah, V.P. and Crison, J.R. (1995) *Pharm. Res.*, **10**, 413.

Bailey, C.A., Bryla, P. and Malick, A.W. (1996) *Adv. Drug Dev. Rev.*, **22**, 85.

Chien Y.W. (1995) Novel drug delivery systems. Marcel Dekker, New York.

ACKNOWLEDGEMENT

The authors wish to thank, Dr L.G. Martini and Dr P.B. Geraghty (Glaxo SmithKline Pharmaceuticals, Harlow, UK) for their assistance and advice in the preparation of this chapter.

DOSAGE FORM DESIGN AND MANUFACTURE

PART FOUR

DOSAGE FORM DESIGN AND MANUFACTURE

21

Solutions

Michael Billany

INTRODUCTION

An understanding of the properties of solutions, the factors that affect solubility and the process of dissolution is essential because of the importance of solutions in so many areas of pharmaceutical formulation. These basic topics are covered in Chapters 2 and 3 and it is recommended that they be read in conjunction with this chapter for a full understanding of principles involved in the formulation of solutions.

Ways of expressing solubility and definitions of terms are also explained in these earlier chapters, but it is worth reiterating that a solution is a homogenous one-phase system consisting of two or more components. The solvent, or mixture of solvents, is the phase in which the dispersion occurs, and the solute is the component which is dispersed as molecules or ions in the solvent.

In general the solvent is present in the greater amount, but there are several exceptions. For example, Syrup BP contains 66.7% w/w of sucrose as the solute in 33.3% w/w of water as the solvent.

For most pharmaceutical solutions the solvent system is likely to be liquid, and the solute will be either a liquid or a solid. Solid dispersions, in which both solute and solvent are solids, are used for the improvement of the bioavailability of poorly soluble drugs. The solute is present as a molecular dispersion and will therefore exhibit a fast rate of dissolution, owing to its very high specific surface area. In addition, the particles are already in a deaggregated and wetted state, and so there is little air adsorbed on the particle surfaces to inhibit dissolution. There may even be a slight increase in actual solubility.

Solutions of gases in liquids are characteristic of aerosols, in which the propellant gas is dispersed or dissolved in the solvent under pressure. On actuation of the valve mechanism the propellant ejects the product from the container. The propellant immediately evaporates, leaving the active agent in the form of tiny droplets or particles or within a foam structure.

ADVANTAGES AND DISADVANTAGES OF SOLUTIONS AS AN ORAL DOSAGE FORM

Although tablets and capsules are more widely used than liquid preparations for oral administration, the latter possess several advantages:

- Liquids are easier to swallow than solids and are therefore particularly acceptable for paediatric and geriatric use.
- A drug must usually be in solution before it can be absorbed. If it is administered in the form of a solution, the drug is immediately available for absorption. Therefore, the therapeutic response is faster than if using a solid dosage form, which must first disintegrate in order to allow the drug to dissolve in the gastrointestinal fluid before absorption can begin. Even if the drug should precipitate from solution in the acid conditions of the stomach, it will be in a sufficiently wetted and finely divided state to allow rapid absorption to occur.
- A solution is a homogenous system and therefore the drug will be uniformly distributed throughout the preparation. In suspension or emulsion formulations uneven dosage can occur as a result of phase separation on storage.
- Some drugs, including aspirin and potassium chloride, can irritate and damage the gastric mucosa, particularly if localized in one area, as often occurs after the ingestion of a solid dosage form. Irritation is reduced by the administration of a solution of a drug because of the immediate dilution by the gastric contents.

There are, however, several problems associated with the manufacture, transport, stability and administration of solutions:

- Liquids are bulky and therefore inconvenient to transport and store. If the container should break the whole of the product is immediately and irretrievably lost.
- The stability of ingredients in aqueous solution is often poorer than if formulated as a tablet or capsule, particularly if they are susceptible to hydrolysis. The shelf-life of a liquid dosage form is often much shorter than that of the corresponding solid preparation. Not only is the stability of the drug important, but also that of other excipients, such as surfactants, preservatives, flavours and colours. The chemical stability of some ingredients can, however, be improved by the use of a mixed solvent system. The inclusion of a surfactant above its critical micelle concentration can also improve chemical stability because the hydrolytic degradation of a material may be reduced by its solubilization within the micelles.
- Solutions often provide suitable media for the growth of microorganisms and may therefore require the incorporation of a preservative.

- Most liquid preparations are designed so that the normal dosage of the drug is present in 5 mL, or a multiple of 5 mL, of product. Accurate dosage depends on the ability of the patient to use a 5 mL spoon or a volumetric dropper.
- The taste of a drug, which is usually unpleasant, is always more pronounced when in solution than in a solid form. Solutions can, however, easily be sweetened and flavoured to make them more palatable.

CHOICE OF SOLVENT

Aqueous solutions

Water is the solvent most widely used as a vehicle for pharmaceutical products, because of its physiological compatibility and lack of toxicity. It possesses a high dielectric constant, which is essential for ensuring the dissolution of a wide range of ionizable materials. In some cases this property may be an advantage, but the lack of selectivity can be responsible for aqueous solutions containing unwanted substances such as inorganic salts and organic impurities. This is one reason why water is rarely used for the extraction of active constituents from vegetable sources.

Types of pharmaceutical water

For many preparations potable water can be used. This is water freshly drawn from the mains system and which is suitable for drinking. If this type is unobtainable, then a suitable, though more expensive, alternative is pharmacopoeial Purified Water BP, which has been freshly boiled and cooled immediately before use to destroy any vegetative microorganisms that might be present. Purified Water must, however, be used on all occasions where the presence of salts – often dissolved in potable water – is undesirable. Purified Water is normally prepared by the distillation or deionization of potable water, or by the process of reverse osmosis.

Water for Injections must be used for the formulation of parenteral solutions and is obtained by sterilizing pyrogen-free distilled water immediately after its collection. For the formulation of aqueous solutions of drugs, such as phenobarbitone sodium or aminophylline, which are sensitive to the presence of carbon dioxide, Water for Injections free from carbon dioxide must be used. Similarly, drugs which are liable to oxidation, such as apomorphine and ergotamine maleate, require Water for Injections BP free from dissolved air to be used.

These are both obtained from apyrogenic distilled water in the same way as before, but are then boiled for at least 10 minutes, cooled, sealed in their containers while excluding air, and then sterilized by autoclaving. For further details on parenteral solutions see Chapter 35.

Approaches to the improvement of aqueous solubility

Although water is very widely used for inclusion in pharmaceutical preparations, it may not be possible to ensure complete solution of all ingredients at all normal storage temperatures. Strongly ionized materials are likely to be freely soluble in water over a wide pH range. Similarly, weak acids and bases should be adequately soluble at favourable pHs. Even if in solution, it is still important to ensure that the concentration of any material is not close to its limit of solubility, as precipitation may occur if the product is cooled or if any evaporation of the vehicle should occur. For unionized drugs or for weak electrolytes at a pH that is unfavourable for extensive ionization, one or more of the following methods should be used to improve aqueous solubility.

Cosolvency The solubility of a weak electrolyte or non-polar compound in water can often be improved by altering the polarity of the solvent. This can be achieved by the addition of another solvent that is both miscible with water and in which the compound is also soluble. Vehicles used in combination to increase the solubility of a drug are called cosolvents, and often the solubility in this mixed system is greater than can be predicted from the material's solubility in each individual solvent.

Because it has been shown that the solubility of a given drug is maximal at a particular dielectric constant of any solvent system, it is possible to eliminate those solvent blends possessing other dielectric constants. In some cases, however, it has been shown that the chemical nature of the solvent system used may be of greater importance. A more detailed explanation of the effects of the molecular structure of the solute and the physicochemical properties of the solvent can be found in Chapter 2.

The choice of suitable cosolvents is somewhat limited for pharmaceutical use because of possible toxicity and irritancy, particularly if required for oral or parenteral use. Ideally, suitable blends should possess values of dielectric constant between 25 and 80. The most widely used system that will cover this range is a water/ethanol blend. Other suitable solvents for use with water include sorbitol, glycerol, propylene glycol and syrup. For example, a blend of propylene glycol and water is used to improve the solubility of co-trimoxazole, and paracetamol is formulated as an elixir by the use of alcohol, propylene glycol and syrup. For external application to the scalp, betamethasone valerate is available dissolved in a water/isopropyl alcohol mixture.

For further details covering the suitability of different cosolvents see under their individual headings in this chapter.

pH control A large number of drugs are either weak acids or weak bases, and therefore their solubilities in water can be influenced by the pH of the system. A quantitative application of the Henderson–Hasselbalch equation will enable the solubility of such a drug in water at a given pH to be determined, provided its pK_a and the solubility of its unionized species are known (see Chapter 3). The solubility of a weak base can be increased by lowering the pH of its solution, whereas the solubility of a weak acid is improved by an increase in pH. Some compounds will accept or donate more than one hydrogen ion per molecule, and will therefore possess more than one pK_a value and so will exhibit a more complex solubility profile.

In controlling the solubility of a drug in this way, it must be ensured that the chosen pH does not conflict with other product requirements. For example, the chemical stability of a drug may also depend on pH, and in many cases the pH of optimum solubility does not coincide with the pH of optimum stability. This may also be true for other ingredients, especially colours, preservatives and flavours.

The pH of solutions for parenteral and ophthalmic use, for application to mucous membranes or for use on abraded skin must also be controlled, as extremes can cause pain, irritation and even tissue damage. This is particularly true for subcutaneous, intramuscular and intraspinal injections because the solutions will not be rapidly diluted after administration.

In some instances the bioavailability of drugs may be influenced by the pH of their solutions (Chapter 17), and changes in pH can also affect a preservative's activity by altering the extent to which it is ionized. Often a compromise must be reached during formulation to ensure that the stability and solubility of all ingredients, physiological compatibility and bioavailability are all adequate for the product's intended purpose.

The values of molar solubilities and dissociation constants of drugs that are reported in the literature, or determined during preformulation studies, are usually for the drug alone in distilled water. These values may differ in the final formulation owing to the presence of other ingredients. For example, the inclusion of cosolvents such as alcohol or propylene glycol with water will lower the dielectric constant of the vehicle and therefore increase the solubility of the unionized form of the drug. This lowering of the polarity of the solvent system will also reduce the degree of dissociation of the drug and increase its pK_a. As this effect will increase the concentration of the unionized (less soluble) species, an increase in the pH of the system may be necessary in order to maintain solubility.

It must be appreciated that maximum solubility may best be achieved by a judicious balance between pH control and concentration of cosolvent, and can be determined, as before, by the Henderson–Hasselbalch equation, substituting the new values both for pK_a and for the molar solubilities of the unionized species.

Suitable buffer systems for the control of pH are discussed later in this chapter, but care must be taken because the solubilities of sparingly soluble electrolytes can be decreased still further by the addition of a soluble electrolyte, should they contain a common ion. The opposite can be true if they do not possess common ions.

As solutions of non-electrolytes are not significantly affected by pH, other methods of improving their solubilities must be found.

Solubilization The solubility of a drug that is normally insoluble or poorly soluble in water can often be improved by the addition of a surface-active agent. These molecules form different types of micelles, ranging from simple spherical structures to more complex liposomes and liquid crystals. Details of their formation can be found in Chapter 6. This phenomenon of micellar solubilization has been widely used for the formulation of solutions of poorly soluble drugs. In aqueous systems, non-polar molecules will dissolve in the interior of the micelle, which consists of the lipophilic hydrocarbon moiety.

The amount of surfactant to be used for this purpose must be carefully controlled. A large excess is undesirable because of cost, possible toxicity and its effect on product aeration during manufacture. Excessive amounts may also reduce the bioavailability of a drug if it is strongly adsorbed within the micelle. An insufficient amount of surfactant, however, may not solubilize all the drug, or may lead to precipitation either on storage or on dilution of the product.

Reference to Fig. 6.15 will show that hydrophilic surfactants possessing HLB values above 15 will be particularly valuable as solubilizing agents.

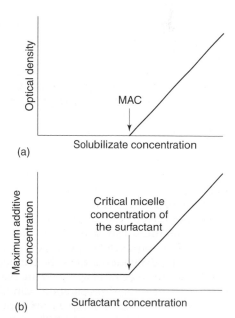

The surfactant chosen must be non-toxic and non-irritant, bearing in mind its intended route of administration. It must also be miscible with the solvent system, compatible with the other ingredients, free from disagreeable odour and taste and be non-volatile.

Examples include the solubilization of fat-soluble vitamins such as phytomenadione using polysorbates. This enables their inclusion with water-soluble vitamins in the same aqueous-based formulation. For parenteral administration of these vitamins, a mixture of glycocholic acid and lecithin provides a mixed micelle system.

The solubility of amiodarone hydrochloride can similarly be improved, although this drug can exhibit autosolubilization at high concentrations.

The solubilization of iodine to produce iodophores is achieved by the use of macrogol ethers. These products exhibit several advantages over simple iodine solutions, including an improved chemical stability, reduced loss of active agent due to sublimation, less corrosion of surgical instruments and, in some cases, enhanced activity.

Polyoxyethylated castor oil is used as a solubilizing agent for a number of intravenous injections, including the immunosuppressant cyclosporin as an intravenous infusion. Care must be taken with this surfactant, as anaphylactic reactions are known to occur when it is injected.

Other drugs that have been solubilized include antibiotics such as griseofulvin, which has been formulated with cetomacrogol. Poloxamers (polyoxyethylene/polyoxypropylene copolymers), some of which are also suitable for parenteral administration, are used to maintain the clarity of solutions for oral use (Garcia Sagredo et al 1994). Lanolin derivatives have also been used for the solubilization of volatile and essential oils.

The solubility of phenolic compounds such as cresol and chloroxylenol, which are normally soluble in water up to 2% and 0.03% respectively, can be improved by solubilization with soaps. Lysol contains 50% cresol in an aqueous system by the use of the potassium soaps of oleic, linoleic and linolenic acids.

It may also be possible to combine the beneficial effects of solubilization and cosolvency in one formulation. A 5% chloroxylenol solution can be formulated by the inclusion of potassium ricinoleate. This soap is formed in situ by the reaction between potassium hydroxide and castor oil. Ethanol and terpineol are included as cosolvents.

To ensure that the optimum concentration of surfactant is chosen, a known weight or volume is added to each of a series of vials containing the solvent. Ensuring adequate temperature control, varying amounts of solubilizate (the material to be solubilized) are added to each vial in ascending order of concentration. The maximum concentration of drug that will form a clear solution with a given concentration of surfactant can be determined visually or by optical density measurement (Fig. 21.1(a)), and is known as the maximum additive concentration (MAC). This method can be repeated for different amounts of surfactant to enable a graph to be constructed of MAC against surfactant concentration, from which the optimum amount of solubilizing agent can be chosen for any required amount of drug (Fig. 21.1(b)).

Alternatively, a ternary-phase diagram can be constructed (Fig. 21.2) that will present a more comprehensive picture of the effects of solubilizate, surfactant and solvent concentrations on the physical characteristics of the system.

The three axes form the three sides of an equilateral triangle, each axis representing 0–100% of one of the components. Point A thus represents a formulation consisting of 50% solubilizate, 20% surfactant and 30% water. By plotting at each point a number

Fig. 21.1 (a) Graph of optical density of a solubilizate/surfactant/solvent system against solubilizate concentration showing the maximum additive concentration (MAC). (b) Determination of the MAC for a range of concentrations of a given surfactant will provide the data for this graph, enabling the optimum concentration of the surfactant to be chosen for the solubilization of a given concentration of active agent.

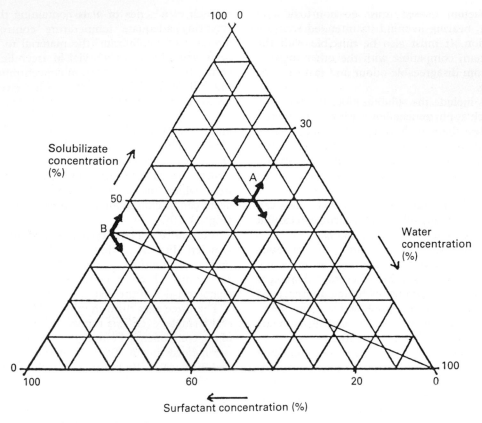

Fig. 21.2 Construction of a ternary-phase diagram.

representing one particular system (e.g. 1 = clear solution, 2 = emulsion, 3 = transparent gel etc.) and enclosing each system within a boundary, a phase diagram can be constructed. Suitable formulations, which will be clear solutions, become immediately apparent and the best can then be chosen, bearing in mind the properties required for this type of product.

It is also important to ensure that the formulation chosen does not lie too close to a phase boundary, as the positions of these can depend on the storage temperature of the product. In general the degree of solubilization of a drug increases as the temperature increases. From this type of phase diagram the physical composition of diluted preparations can also be shown. Point B, for example, represents a product consisting of 40% solubilizate and 60% surfactant. The construction of a straight line from here to point C represents the dilution of the product with increasing concentrations of water.

Should the concentration of drug to be included in the product be fixed, then the third axis can be used to represent varying concentrations of a third excipient such as a cosolvent. These values must, however, be plotted as percentage drug plus excipient to ensure a maximum value of 100%.

Alternatives to the use of surface-active agents as solubilizing agents include the cyclodextrins (Szejtli 1994). This range of compounds is based on a series of glucopyranose units that form cyclical structures resembling hollow cylinders (Fig. 21.3). As the inside surface of the ring is hydrophobic, owing to the presence of -CH$_2$ groups, drugs that are poorly soluble in water can be accommodated here. The outer part of the structure is hydrophilic and therefore freely soluble in water (Stella and Rajewski 1997).

Fig. 21.3 Representation of the structure of cyclodextrins.

There are three natural cyclodextrins, the α, β and γ forms, the ring structures of which are composed of 6, 7 and 8 glucopyranose units, respectively, as well as an expanding series of derivatives.

Poorly soluble drugs of appropriate size slot into the interior of these structures, forming soluble inclusion complexes, usually with one 'host' molecule per cyclodextrin molecule (Pagington 1987). Examples of marketed drugs formulated with cyclodextrins include a range of prostaglandins for intra-arterial infusion, an antiseptic gargle based on iodine, and an oral liquid containing the antifungal drug itraconazole.

Complexation In some cases it may be possible to interact a poorly soluble drug with a soluble material to form a soluble intermolecular complex. As most complexes are macromolecular, however, they tend to be inactive, being unable to cross lipid membranes. It is therefore essential that complex formation is easily reversible, so that the free drug is released during or before contact with biological fluids.

It is not easy to predict whether a given drug will complex with a particular compound to improve solubility. Many complexes are not water soluble and may, in fact, be better suited for the prolonged release of the drug. Several well known examples are in general use, however, and include the complexation of iodine with a 10–15% solution of polyvinylpyrrolidone to improve the aqueous solubility of the active agent. Similarly, the interaction of salicylates and benzoates with xanthines, such as theophylline or caffeine, or with carbazochrome is carried out for the same effect.

Chemical modification As a last resort, chemical modification of a drug may be necessary in order to produce a water-soluble derivative. Examples include the synthesis of the sodium phosphate salts of hydrocortisone, prednisolone and betamethasone. The water-soluble chloramphenicol sodium succinate has no antibacterial activity of its own but is suitable for parenteral administration as a solution in order to obtain high blood levels, after which it is converted back to the less soluble active base. There are many examples of poorly soluble acids and bases being converted to a salt form to increase water solubility.

Particle size control The size and shape of very small particles, if less than 1 μm diameter, can affect their solubilities. As particle size decreases solubility will increase, and molecular dispersions of drugs in solid/solid solutions can exhibit improved bioavailability owing to the increase in solubility of the dispersed drug. In practice, however, this phenomenon has little application in the formulation of solutions, but is of particular relevance in suspension formulation.

Non-aqueous solutions

If it is not possible to ensure complete solution of the ingredients at all storage temperatures, or if the drug is unstable in aqueous systems it may be necessary to use an alternative, non-aqueous solvent. The use of non-aqueous systems may also have other advantages. For example, the intramuscular injection of solutions of drugs in oils is often used for depot therapy, and some drugs are specifically synthesized to improve their oil solubilities. The propionate and benzoate esters of testosterone and estradiol, respectively, are good examples of this. The oily solution remains as a discrete entity within the muscle tissue, releasing the drug slowly into the surrounding tissue by partitioning. A similar aqueous solution would diffuse readily and, being miscible with tissue fluid, would cause the drug to be released quickly.

It is essential that, in choosing a suitable solvent, its toxicity, irritancy and sensitizing potential are taken into account, as well as its flammability, cost, stability and compatibility with other excipients. It will be obvious that there is a greater choice of solvents available for inclusion into products for external application than those for internal use, and that for parenteral products the choice is limited even further.

A far wider range of solvents, however, is available for use as part of the manufacture of pharmaceutical products. In these instances the solvent is removed before packaging and is therefore not present in the final product. Examples include acetone, light petroleum and chloroform, although the latter is also used as a flavour and preservative in some extemporaneously prepared formulations. The following is a classification of some of the more widely used non-aqueous solvents in pharmaceutical preparations.

Fixed oils of vegetable origin

These are non-volatile oils that consist mainly of fatty acid esters of glycerol. Almond oil, for example, which consists of glycerides mainly of oleic acid, is used as a solvent for oily phenol injections, water being unsuitable because of the caustic nature of aqueous phenol solutions. Of similar chemical composition is arachis oil, which is used as the solvent in Dimercaprol Injection. Olive oil, sesame oil, maize oil, cottonseed oil, soya oil and castor oil are all suitable for parenteral use, the latter also being used as the solvent in miconazole eye drops (Lee 1985) and in some formulations of triamcinolone ear drops.

Ethyl oleate, which is a useful solvent for both Ergocalciferol Injection and Testosterone Propionate

Injection, is less viscous than the oils described above and therefore more easily injected intramuscularly. Of similar viscosity is benzyl benzoate, which can be used as an alternative solvent for dimercaprol.

Some fixed oils are sufficiently tasteless and odourless to be suitable for oral use as solvents for such materials as vitamins A and D. Fractionated coconut oil is occasionally used as the solvent for some antibiotics, which would otherwise hydrolyse rapidly if formulated as aqueous systems.

Veterinary formulations may also contain these solvents, arachis oil, for example, being used for hexachlorophene in the treatment of fascioliasis in ruminants.

Oils tend to be unpleasant to use externally, however, unless presented as an emulsion. Arachis oil is one of the few examples and is used as the solvent in Methyl Salicylate Liniment.

Alcohols

Ethyl alcohol is the most widely used solvent in this class, particularly for external application, where its rapid evaporation after application to the skin imparts a cooling effect to such products as salicylic acid lotion. It is also particularly useful for the extraction of crude drugs, being more selective than water. At concentrations greater than 15% ethanol exhibits antimicrobial activity, but because of its toxicity it is used orally or parenterally only at low concentrations, usually as a cosolvent with water.

If required for external use then industrial methylated spirit (IMS), which is free from excise duty, is usually included rather than the more expensive ethanol. Because industrial methylated spirit contains 5% methyl alcohol as a denaturant it is rendered too toxic for internal use.

An alcohol possessing similar properties is isopropyl alcohol, which is used externally as a solvent for dicophane. Its main advantage is that it is less likely to be abused than ethanol and that denaturation is not necessary.

Polyhydric alcohols

Alcohols containing two hydroxyl groups per molecule are known as glycols, but because of their toxicity they are rarely used internally. One important exception to this is propylene glycol.

$$CH_3.CH(OH)CH_2OH$$

which is often used in conjunction with water or glycerol as a cosolvent. It is used, for example, in the formulation of Digoxin Injection, Phenobarbital Injection, and some formulations of Diazepam Injection, Co-trimoxazole Intravenous Infusion and as the diluent for both Chloramphenicol Ear Drops and some brands of hydrocortisone ear drops, and in many preparations for oral use.

The lower molecular weight polyethylene glycols (PEG) or macrogols have the general formula:

$$HOCH_2(CH_2CH_2O)_nCH_2OH$$

and are available in a range of viscosity grades. PEG 400, for example, is used as a solvent in clotrimazole topical solution. They are also widely used as cosolvents with alcohol or water, although their main use is in the formulation of water-miscible ointment bases. There are also other glycols available which, although rarely included in products for human use, can be used for extraction processes or as solvents in the formulation of veterinary and horticultural solutions. Examples include dipropylene glycol, diethylene glycol, ethylene glycol and their monoethyl ethers. Glycerol, an alcohol possessing three hydroxyl groups per molecule, is also widely used, particularly as a cosolvent with water for oral use. At higher concentrations it is used in, for example, Phenol and Glycerol Injection.

Dimethylsulphoxide

This is a highly polar compound and is thought to aid the penetration of drugs through the skin. Although used mainly as a solvent for veterinary drugs, it is used as a carrier for idoxuridine, an antiviral agent, for application to human skin.

Ethyl ether

This material is widely used for the extraction of crude drugs, but because of its own therapeutic activity it is not used for the preparation of formulations for internal use. It is, however, used as a cosolvent with alcohol in some collodions.

Liquid paraffin

The oily nature of this material makes it unpleasant to use externally, although it is often used as a solvent for the topical application of drugs in emulsion formulations. At one time light liquid paraffin was widely used as the base for oily nasal drops. (These are now rarely used because of the possibility of causing lipoidal pneumonia if they are inhaled into the lungs.) It has a minor use in veterinary formulation as a solvent in, for example, anthelminthic drenches containing carbon tetrachloride.

Miscellaneous solvents

Isopropyl myristate and isopropyl palmitate are used as solvents for external use, particularly in cosmetics, where their low viscosity and lack of greasiness make them pleasant to use. Dimethylformamide and dimethylacetamide have both been used as solvents in veterinary formulation, but their toxicities render them unsuitable for human use. Kerosene too is also limited in its application, being used mainly as a solvent for insecticides such as pyrethrum and piperonyl butoxide.

Xylene is present in some ear drops for human use to dissolve ear wax, and glycofurol is a useful solvent for parenteral products.

As with aqueous systems, it may be possible to improve the solubility of a drug in a particular vehicle by the addition of a cosolvent. For example, nitrocellulose is poorly soluble in both alcohol and ether but adequately soluble in a mixture of both. The formulation of Digoxin Injection, too, is best achieved by the inclusion of both ethyl alcohol and propylene glycol.

OTHER FORMULATION ADDITIVES

Buffers

These are materials which, when dissolved in a solvent, will enable the solution to resist any change in pH should an acid or an alkali be added. The choice of suitable buffer depends on the pH and buffering capacity required. It must be compatible with other excipients and have a low toxicity. Most pharmaceutically acceptable buffering systems are based on carbonates, citrates, gluconates, lactates, phosphates or tartrates. Borates can be used for external application, but not to mucous membranes or to abraded skin.

Although solutions of drugs that are themselves weak electrolytes will act as buffers, their buffering capacities are not usually sufficiently robust and should be enhanced by one of the systems described above.

As the pH of most body fluids is 7.4, products such as injections, eye drops and nasal drops should, in theory, be buffered at this value to avoid irritation. Many body fluids themselves, however, have a buffering capacity and, when formulating low-volume intravenous injections or eye drops, a wider pH range can be tolerated. This is potentially useful should a compromise be necessary when choosing a pH that is physiologically acceptable for a drug whose optimum stability, solubility and/or bioavail-

ability may depend on different pHs. For further details on the use of buffers see Chapters 3 and 35.

Density modifiers

It is rarely necessary to control the density of solutions except when formulating spinal anaesthetics. Solutions of lower density than cerebrospinal fluid will tend to rise after injection and those of higher density will fall. Careful control both of the density of such injections and of the position of the patient on the operating table will enable precise control of the area to be anaesthetized. The terms used to describe the density of injections in relation to that of spinal fluid are isobaric, hypobaric and hyperbaric, meaning of equal, lower and higher density, respectively. The most widely used material for density modification is dextrose.

Isotonicity modifiers

Solutions for injection, for application to mucous membranes, and large-volume solutions for ophthalmic use must be made iso-osmotic with tissue fluid to avoid pain and irritation.

The most widely used isotonicity modifiers are dextrose and sodium chloride. Isotonicity adjustments can only be made after the addition of all other ingredients, because each ingredient will contribute to the overall osmotic pressure of a solution.

Viscosity enhancement

It may be difficult for aqueous-based topical solutions to remain in place on the skin or in the eyes for any significant time because of their low viscosities. To counteract this effect, low concentrations of gelling agents can be used to increase the apparent viscosity of the product. Examples include povidone, hydroxyethylcellulose and carbomer.

Preservatives

When choosing a suitable preservative it must be ensured that:

- adsorption of the preservative onto the container from the product does not occur, and
- its efficiency is not impaired by the pH of the solution or by interactions with other ingredients.

For example, many of the widely used parahydroxybenzoic acid esters can be adsorbed into the micelles of some non-ionic surfactants and, although their presence can be detected by chemical analysis, they are in fact unable to exert their antimicrobial activities. It is only by full micro-biological challenge testing that the efficiency of a preservative system can be properly assessed.

A more comprehensive discussion on the preservation of pharmaceuticals can be found in Chapter 42.

Reducing agents and antioxidants

The decomposition of pharmaceutical products by oxidation can be controlled by the addition of reducing agents such as sodium metabisulphite, or antioxidants such as butylated hydroxyanisole or butylated hydroxytoluene. For unit-dose parenteral products, such as injections of nicotinamide and ascorbic acid, it is possible to use Water for Injections free from dissolved air and to replace the air in the headspace by nitrogen or another inert gas.

Sweetening agents

Low molecular weight carbohydrates, and in particular sucrose, are traditionally the most widely used sweetening agents. Sucrose has the advantage of being colourless, very soluble in water, stable over a pH range of about 4–8 and, by increasing the viscosity of fluid preparations, will impart to them a pleasant texture in the mouth. It will mask the tastes of both salty and bitter drugs and has a soothing effect on the membranes of the throat. For this reason, despite its cariogenic properties, sucrose is particularly useful as a vehicle for antitussive preparations.

Polyhydric alcohols such as sorbitol, mannitol and, to a lesser extent glycerol, also possess sweetening power and can be included in preparations for diabetic use, where sucrose is undesirable. Other less widely used bulk sweeteners include maltilol, lactilol, isomalt, fructose and xylitol. Treacle, honey and liquorice are now very rarely used, having only a minor application in some extemporaneously prepared formulations.

Artificial sweeteners can be used in conjunction with sugars and alcohols to enhance the degree of sweetness, or on their own in formulations for patients who must restrict their sugar intake. They are also termed intense sweeteners because, weight for weight, they are hundreds and even thousands of times sweeter than sucrose and are therefore rarely required at a concentration greater than about 0.2%.

Only about six artificial sweeteners are permitted for oral use within the European Union, the most widely used being the sodium or calcium salts of saccharin (E954). Both exhibit high water solubility and are chemically and physically stable over a wide pH range. Less widely used are aspartame (E951), which is a compound of L-aspartic acid and L-phenylalanine, acesulfame potassium (E950), thaumatin (E957), sodium cyclamate (E952) and neohesperidine DC (E959). The main disadvantage of all artificial sweeteners is their tendency to impart a bitter or metallic aftertaste, and they are therefore often formulated with sugars to mask this.

Flavours and perfumes

The simple use of sweetening agents may not be sufficient to render palatable a product containing a drug with a particularly unpleasant taste. In many cases, therefore, a flavouring agent can be included. This is particularly useful in paediatric formulation to ensure patient compliance. The inclusion of flavours has the additional advantage of enabling the easy identification of liquid products.

Flavouring and perfuming agents can be obtained from either natural or synthetic sources. Natural products include fruit juices, aromatic oils such as peppermint and lemon, herbs and spices, and distilled fractions of these. They are available as concentrated extracts, alcoholic or aqueous solutions, syrups or spirits, and are particularly widely used in the manufacture of products for extemporaneous use. Artificial perfumes and flavours are of purely synthetic origin, often having no natural counterpart. They tend to be cheaper, more readily available, less variable in chemical composition and more stable than natural products. They are usually available as alcoholic or aqueous solutions or as powders.

The choice of a suitable flavour can only be made as a result of subjective assessment and, as consumer preferences vary considerably, this is not easy. Some guidance can, however, be given by reference to Table 21.1, which shows that certain flavours are particularly useful for the masking of one or more of the basic taste sensations of saltiness, bitterness, sweetness and sourness. These tastes are detected by sensory receptors on various areas of the tongue,

Table 21.1 Suitable masking flavours for various product tastes	
Taste of product	Suitable masking flavour
Salty	Apricot, butterscotch, liquorice, peach, vanilla
Bitter	Anise, chocolate, mint, passion fruit, wild cherry
Sweet	Vanilla, fruits, berries
Sour	Citrus fruits, liquorice, raspberry

whereas the more subtle flavours are detected by the olfactory receptors.

In some cases there is a strong association between the use of a product and its flavour or perfume content. For example, products intended for the relief of indigestion are often mint flavoured. This is because for many years mint has been used in such products for its carminative effect, but even in products containing other active agents the odour and taste of mint are now firmly associated with antacid activity. Similarly, the odour of terpineol is often associated with antiseptic activity and, in a competitive market, it may therefore be unwise to alter these flavours or perfumes to any appreciable extent.

The fact that personal preferences for flavours and perfumes often vary with age can also aid the formulator. Children, in general, prefer fruity tastes and smells, whereas adults choose flowery odours and acid flavours. Other suitable materials for the masking of unpleasant tastes include menthol, peppermint oil and chloroform. In addition to having their own particular tastes and odours they also act as desensitizing agents by exerting a mild anaesthetic effect on the sensory taste receptors.

Flavour-enhancing agents such as citric acid for citrus fruits and glycine or monosodium glutamate for general use are now becoming more widely used.

Colours

Once a suitable flavour has been chosen, it is often useful to include a colour associated with that flavour in order to improve the attractiveness of the product. Another reason for the inclusion of colours is to enable easy product identification, particularly of poisonous materials, including weedkillers and mineralized methylated spirit, and, for example, to differentiate between the many types of antiseptic solution used in hospitals for the disinfection of skin, instruments, syringes etc.

The presence of a strongly coloured degradation product, which does not affect the use of the product, may occasionally be masked by the use of a suitable colour. It is however, essential to ensure that any colour chosen is acceptable in the country in which the product is to be sold. A colour that is acceptable in one country may not be acceptable in another, and as aspects of colour legislation can change quite frequently it is necessary to ensure that only the latest regulations are consulted. The legal departments of most dye manufacturers are usually willing to supply up-to-date information.

The proliferation of nomenclature that exists for most colours can also cause confusion. For example,

the water-soluble dye amaranth is also known as Bordeaux S, Cl Food Red 9 and Cl Acid Red 27. It has been allocated the Colour Index Number 16185 by the Society of Dyers and Colourists and the American Association of Textile Chemists and Colorists. Under the USA Food, Drug and Cosmetics Act it is known as FD and C Red Number 2, and a directive of the Council of European Communities has allocated it the reference number E 123.

As with flavours and perfumes, there is a range of both natural and synthetic colours. The former, which tend to be more widely acceptable, can be classified into carotenoids, chlorophyll, anthocyanins, and a miscellaneous group which includes riboflavines, caramel and extracts of beetroot. They can, however, exhibit the usual problems associated with natural products, namely variations in availability and chemical composition, both of which may cause formulation difficulties.

Synthetic or 'coal tar' dyes tend to give bright colours and are generally more stable than natural materials. Most of those that are suitable for pharmaceutical use are the sodium salts of sulphonic acids, and therefore they may be incompatible with cationic drugs. Care must also be taken to ensure that any dye used is not adversely affected by pH or by ultraviolet radiation, or by the inclusion of oxidizing or reducing agents or surfactants.

TYPES OF PREPARATION

The terminology used for the titles of different forms of liquid preparation for both oral and topical use can sometimes be confusing, with overlap between definitions and more than one definition being appropriate for one particular product. Furthermore, definitions can vary between different official compendia and may be at variance with definitions used within the pharmaceutical industry. This section attempts to give an overview of the types of pharmaceutical solution available.

Liquids for cutaneous application

Lotions, liniments, paints and collodions

Lotions can be formulated as solutions, and are designed to be applied to the skin without friction. They may contain humectants, so that moisture is retained on the skin after application of the product, or alcohol, which evaporates quickly, imparting a cooling effect and leaving the skin dry.

Liniments, however, are intended for massage into the skin and can contain such ingredients as methyl salicylate or camphor as counterirritants.

Liquids for application to the skin or mucous membranes in small amounts are often termed paints, and are usually applied with a small brush. The solvent is normally alcohol, acetone or ether, which evaporates quickly leaving a film on the skin that contains the active agent. A viscosity modifier such as glycerol is often added to ensure prolonged contact with the skin.

Collodions are similar preparations which, after evaporation of the solvent, leave a tough, flexible film that will seal small cuts or hold a drug in intimate contact with the skin. The film former is usually pyroxylin (nitrocellulose) in an alcohol/ether or alcohol/acetone solvent blend. Often a plasticizer such as castor oil and an adherent such as colophony resin are included.

Ear preparations

Also known as otic or aural products, these are simple solutions of drugs in either water, glycerol, propylene glycol or alcohol/water mixtures for local use, and include antibiotics, antiseptics, cleansing solutions and wax softeners. They are applied to the external auditory canal as drops, sprays or washes.

Eye preparations

These are small-volume sterile liquids designed to be instilled on to the eyeball or within the conjunctival sac for a local effect.

Irrigations

Irrigations are sterile, large-volume aqueous-based solutions for the cleansing of body cavities and wounds. They should be made isotonic with tissue fluid.

Mouthwashes and gargles

Aqueous solutions for the prevention and treatment of mouth and throat infections can contain antiseptics, analgesics and/or astringents. They are usually diluted with warm water before use.

Nasal products

These are formulated as small-volume solutions in an aqueous vehicle, oils being no longer used for nasal administration. Because the buffering capacity of nasal mucus is low, formulation at a pH of 6.8 is necessary. Nasal drops should also be made isotonic with nasal secretions using sodium chloride, and viscosity can also be modified using cellulose derivatives if necessary. Active agents for administration by this route for local use include antibiotics, anti-inflammatories and decongestants. The nasal route is also of major importance for specific types of drugs, and a full description of this method of drug delivery can be found in Chapter 32.

Oral liquids

This is a general term used to describe a solution, suspension or emulsion in which the active ingredient is dissolved or dispersed in a suitable liquid vehicle.

Elixirs

The terms mixture and elixir are often confused, although an elixir is strictly a solution of a potent or nauseous drug. If the active agent is sensitive to moisture, it may be formulated as a flavoured powder or granulation by the pharmaceutical industry and then simply dissolved in water immediately prior to administration. The dosage is usually taken using a 5 mL medicine spoon, although smaller volumes can be given using a volumetric dropper.

Linctuses

A linctus is a viscous preparation, usually prescribed for the relief of cough. It normally consists of a simple solution of the active agent in a high concentration of sucrose, often with other sweetening agents. This type of product, which is also designed to be administered in multiples of 5 mL, should be sipped slowly and not be diluted beforehand. The syrup content has a demulcent action on the mucous membranes of the throat. For diabetic use the sucrose is usually replaced by sorbitol and/or synthetic sweeteners.

Mixtures and draughts

Mixtures are usually aqueous preparations that can be in the form of either a solution or a suspension. Most preparations of this type are manufactured on a small scale as required, and are allocated a shelf-life of a few weeks before dispensing. Doses are usually given in multiples of 5 mL using a metric medicine spoon. A draught is a mixture of which only one or two large doses of about 50 mL are given, although smaller doses are often necessary for children.

Parenteral products

Sterile solutions for injection or infusion into the body are also available.

Rectal preparations

Aqueous or oily solutions, as well as emulsions and suspensions, are available for the rectal administration of medicaments for cleansing, diagnostic or therapeutic reasons, and are termed enemas.

Intermediate products

Aromatic waters and spirits

There are many pharmaceutical solutions that are designed for use during the manufacture of other preparations and which are rarely administered themselves. Aromatic waters, for example, are aqueous solutions of volatile materials and are used mainly for their flavouring properties. Examples include peppermint water and anise water, which also have carminative properties, and chloroform water, which also acts as a preservative.

They are usually manufactured as concentrated waters and are then diluted, traditionally 1:40 in the final preparation.

Spirits are also alcoholic solutions but of volatile materials, which are mainly used as flavouring agents.

Extracts, infusions and tinctures

Infusions, extracts and tinctures are terms used for concentrated solutions of active principles from animal or vegetable sources. Infusions are prepared by extracting the drug using 25% alcohol, but without the application of heat. Traditionally these preparations are then diluted 1:10 in the final product. Extracts are similar products that are then concentrated by evaporation. Tinctures are alcoholic extracts of drugs but are relatively weak compared with extracts.

Syrups

Syrups are concentrated solutions of sucrose or other sugars to which medicaments or flavourings are often added. For example, Codeine Phosphate Syrup is used as a cough suppressant and Orange Syrup contains dried bitter orange peel as a flavouring agent. Although syrups are used in the manufacture of other preparations, such as mixtures or elixirs, they can also be administered as products in

their own right, the high concentrations of sugars imparting a sweetening effect.

As syrups can contain up to 85% of sugars, they are capable of resisting bacterial growth by virtue of their osmotic effect. Syrups can contain lower concentrations of sugars but will often include sufficient of a polyhydric alcohol such as sorbitol, glycerol or propylene glycol in order to maintain a high osmotic gradient. In addition, by acting as cosolvents they will help to prevent crystallization and to maintain solubility of all ingredients.

It is possible, however, in a closed container, for surface dilution of a syrup to take place. This occurs as a result of solvent evaporation that condenses on the upper internal surfaces of the container and then flows back on to the surface of the product, thereby producing a diluted layer which provides an ideal medium for the growth of certain microorganisms. For this reason syrups often contain additional preservatives.

A further problem with the storage and use of syrups involves the crystallization of the sugar within the screw cap used to seal the containers, thereby preventing its release. This can be avoided by the addition of the polyhydric alcohols previously mentioned, or by the inclusion of invert syrup, which is a mixture of glucose and fructose.

STABILITY OF SOLUTIONS

Both the chemical and the physical stability of solutions in their intended containers are important. A solution must retain its initial clarity, colour, odour, taste and viscosity over its allocated shelf-life. Clarity can easily be assessed by visual examination or by a measurement of its optical density after agitation. Colour too may be assessed both visually and spectrophotometrically, and equipment suitable for the measurement of rheological properties of solutions has been covered earlier.

The stability of flavours and perfumes is perhaps more difficult to assess. Although chromatographic methods are used with varying success to quantify these properties, considerable reliance must be placed on the organoleptic powers of a panel of assessors, who must be screened to ensure that their powers of olfaction and gustation are sufficiently sensitive. If a suitable majority of the panel members is unable to detect a difference between a stored sample and a freshly prepared reference material, it may be assumed that the taste or odour of the sample has not changed significantly.

MANUFACTURE OF SOLUTIONS

For both small- and large-scale manufacture of solutions the only equipment necessary is suitable mixing vessels, a means of agitation and a filtration system to ensure clarity of the final solution. During manufacture, the solute is simply added to the solvent in a mixing vessel and stirring is continued until dissolution is complete. If the solute is more soluble at elevated temperatures it may be advantageous to apply heat to the vessel, particularly if the dissolution rate is normally slow. Care must be taken, however, should any volatile or thermolabile materials be present. Size reduction of solid materials to increase their surface areas should also speed up the process of solution.

Solutes present in low concentrations, particularly dyes, are often predissolved in a small volume of the solvent and then added to the bulk. Volatile materials such as flavours and perfumes are, where possible, added at the end of a process and after any cooling, to reduce loss by evaporation. Finally, it must be ensured that significant amounts of any of the materials are not irreversibly adsorbed on to the filtration medium used for final clarification. For a discussion of suitable packaging materials and containers for solutions see Chapter 36.

REFERENCES

Garcia Sagredo, F., Guzman, M., Molpereces, J., Aberturas, M.R. (1994) Pluronic copolymers – characteristics, properties and pharmaceutical applications. *Pharm. Tech. Europe*, **1**, 46–56, **2**, 38–44.

Lee, R.L.H. (1985) *Aust. J. of Hosp. Pharm.*, **15**, 233

Pagington, I.S. (1987) β-cyclodextrin: the success of molecular inclusion. *Chemistry in Britain*, **23**, 455.

Stella, V.J. and Rajewski, R.A. (1997) Cyclodextrins: their future in drug formulation and delivery. *Pharm. Res.*, **14**, 556–567.

Szejtli, J. (1994) Medicinal applications of cyclodextrins. *Med. Res. Rev.*, **14**, 353–386.

BIBLIOGRAPHY

Martindale, W. (1999) *The Extra Pharmacopoeia* Pharmaceutical Press, London.

22

Clarification

Andrew Twitchell

Clarification is a term used to describe processes that involve the removal or separation of a solid from a fluid, or a fluid from another fluid. The term 'fluid' encompasses both liquids and gases. Clarification can be achieved using either filtration or centrifugation techniques, both of which are described in this chapter.

In pharmaceutical processing there are two main reasons for such processes:

1. To remove unwanted solid particles from either a liquid product or from air;
2. To collect the solid as the product itself (e.g. following crystallization).

FILTRATION

Types of filtration

Solid/fluid filtration

Solid/fluid filtration can be defined as the separation of an insoluble solid from a fluid by means of a porous medium that retains the solid but allows the fluid to pass. It is the most common type of filtration encountered during the manufacture of pharmaceutical products. Solid/fluid filtration may be further subdivided into two types, namely solid/liquid filtration and solid/gas filtration.

Solid/liquid filtration   There are numerous applications of solid/liquid filtration in pharmaceutical processing, some of which are listed below:

• Improvement of the appearance of solutions, mouthwashes etc. to give them a 'sparkle' or 'brightness'; this is often referred to as 'clarifying' a product;
• Removal of potential irritants, e.g. from eye-drop preparations or solutions applied to mucous membranes;

- Recovery of desired solid material from a suspension or slurry, e.g. to obtain a drug or excipient after a crystallization process;
- Certain operations, such as the extraction of vegetable drugs with a solvent, may yield a turbid product with a small quantity of fine suspended colloidal matter; this can be removed by filtration;
- Sterilization of liquid or semisolid products where processes involving heat (such as auto-claving) are not appropriate;
- Detection of microorganisms present in liquids. This can be achieved by analysing a suitable filter on which the bacteria are retained. This method can also be used to assess the efficiency of preservatives.

Solid/gas filtration   There are two main applications of solid/gas filtration in pharmaceutical processing. One of particular importance in manufacturing is the removal of suspended solid material from air in order to supply air of the required standard for either processing equipment or manufacturing areas. This includes the provision of air for equipment such as fluidized-bed processors (see Chapters 25 and 26), film-coating machinery (Chapter 28) and bottle-cleaning equipment, so that product appearance and quality are maintained. The use of suitable filters also enables the particulate contamination of air in manufacturing areas to be at an appropriate level for the product being manufactured; for example, air free from microorganisms can be supplied to areas where sterile products are being manufactured.

It is also often necessary to remove particulate matter generated during a manufacturing operation from the process air in order to prevent the material being vented to the atmosphere. Examples of this include filtering of exhaust air from fluidized-bed and coating processes.

Fluid/fluid filtration

Flavouring oils are sometimes added to liquid preparations in the form of a spirit, i.e. dissolved in alcohol. When these spirits are added to aqueous-based formulations some of the oil may come out of solution, giving the product a degree of turbidity. Removal of the oil droplets by passing them through an appropriate filter (a liquid/liquid filtration process) is used to produce the desired product appearance.

Compressed air is used in a number of pharmaceutical processes (e.g. film-coating spray guns, bottle-cleaning equipment and fluid energy mills; see Chapter 11). Before use the compressed air needs to

be filtered to ensure that any entrained oil or water droplets are removed. This is an example of a liquid/gas filtration process.

Mechanisms of filtration

The mechanisms by which material may be retained by a filter medium (i.e. the surface on or in which material is deposited) are discussed below.

Straining/sieving

If the pores in the filter medium through which the fluid is flowing are smaller than the material that is required to be removed, the material will be retained. Filtration occurs on the surface of the filter in this case, and therefore the filter can be very thin. Filter media of this type are referred to as **membrane filters**. Because filtration occurs on the surface there is a tendency for them to become blocked unless the filter is carefully designed (see later). On a small scale, filters using the straining mechanism are used where the contaminant level is low or small volumes need to be filtered.

Examples of the use of membrane filters include the removal of bacteria and fibres from parenteral preparations.

Impingement

As a flowing fluid approaches and passes an object, for example a filter fibre, the fluid flow pattern is disturbed, as shown in Figure 22.1. Suspended solids may, however, have sufficient momentum that they do not follow the fluid path but impinge on the filter fibre and are retained, owing to attractive forces between the particle and the fibre. Where the pores between filter fibres are larger than the material being removed some particles may follow the fluid

Collected solids

A

B

―――― Streamlines
― ― ― ― Particle paths

Fig. 22.1 Mechanisms of filtration by impingement.

streamlines and miss the fibre, this being more likely if the particles are small (owing to their lower momentum) and as the distance from the centre of the fibre towards which they approach increases. To ensure the removal of all unwanted material, filter media using the impingement mechanism must be sufficiently thick that material not trapped by the first fibre in its path is removed by a subsequent one. These types of filter are therefore referred to as depth filters. The fluid should flow through the filter medium in a streamlined manner to ensure the filter works effectively, as turbulent flow may carry the particles past the fibres. Depth filters are the main type of filter used for removing material from gases.

Attractive forces

Electrostatic and other surface forces may exert sufficient hold on the particles to attract and retain them on the filter medium (as occurs during the impingement mechanism).

Air can be freed from dust particles in an electrostatic precipitator by passing the air between highly charged surfaces, which attract the dust particles.

Autofiltration

Autofiltration is the term used to describe the situation when filtered material (termed the *filter cake*) acts as its own filter medium. This mechanism is used by the metafilter which is covered later in this chapter.

Factors affecting the rate of filtration

The filtration process chosen must remove the required 'contaminants' or product but must also do so at an acceptably fast rate to ensure that the manufacturing process can be carried out economically. The laboratory Buchner funnel and flask (Fig. 22.2) is a convenient filter that can be used to illustrate the factors that influence the rate at which a product can be filtered. This filter is used for solid/liquid filtration processes, but the same basic principles are valid whatever filtration process is being evaluated.

The rate of filtration (volume of filtered material (V, m^3) obtained in unit time (t, s)) depends on the following factors:

1. The area available for filtration (A, m^2), which in this case is the cross-sectional area of the funnel;
2. The pressure difference (ΔP, Pa) across the filter bed (filter medium and any cake formed). With

Fig. 22.2 Buchner funnel and vacuum flask.

the Buchner funnel apparatus this difference is due to the 'head' of unfiltered product (slurry) and decreases as filtration proceeds and the level drops. Note that it is the pressure *difference* that is important, and this can be increased by drawing a vacuum in the collection flask. The difference between atmospheric pressure and the lower pressure in the flask is added to the pressure due to the unfiltered product to give the total pressure difference;

3. The viscosity of the fluid passing through the filter, i.e. the filtrate (μ Pa s). A viscous fluid will filter more slowly than a mobile one owing to the greater resistance to movement offered by more viscous fluids (see Chapter 4).

4. The thickness of the filter medium and any deposited cake (L, m). The cake will **increase** in thickness as filtration proceeds, so if this is not removed the rate of filtration will fall.

The above factors are combined in the Darcy equation:

$$\frac{V}{t} = \frac{KA\Delta P}{\mu L} \qquad (22.1)$$

In this equation the driving force for this particular 'rate process' is the pressure difference across the filter, and the resistance to the process is a function of the properties of the filter bed, its thickness, and the viscosity of the filtrate. The contribution to resistance to filtration from the filter medium is usually small compared to that of the filter cake, and can often be neglected in calculations.

The proportionality constant K (m^2) expresses the **permeability** of the filter medium and cake and will increase as the porosity of the bed increases. It is clearly desirable that the K value should be large in order to maximize the filtration rate. If K is taken to represent the permeability of the cake it can be shown that K is given by:

$$K = \frac{e^3}{5(1-e)^2 S^2} \qquad (22.2)$$

where e is the porosity of the cake and S is the surface area of the particles comprising the cake. If the solid material is one that forms an impermeable cake the filtration rate may be improved by adding a **filter aid** (see later), which aids the formation of open porous cakes.

Methods used to increase filtration rate

Darcy's equation can be used to determine ways in which the filtration rate can be increased or controlled in practice. These are discussed below.

Increase the area available for filtration   The total volume of filtrate flowing through the filter will be directly proportional to the area of the filter, and hence the rate of filtration can be increased by using either larger filters or a number of small units in parallel. Both of these approaches will also distribute the cake over a larger area and thus decrease the value of L, thereby further increasing the rate.

Increase the pressure difference across the filter cake   The simplest filters, e.g. the laboratory filter funnel, use the gravitational force of the liquid 'head' to provide the driving force for filtration. Often this driving force is too low for a sufficiently quick filtration and there is a requirement to increase it. If a vacuum is 'pulled' on the far side of the filter medium (see Fig. 22.1) then the pressure difference can be increased up to atmospheric pressure, i.e. approximately 1×10^5 Pa, or 1 bar. In practice, however, it will be less, as the liquids will boil in the collecting vessel if the pressure is reduced to too low a value (see Chapter 39). Despite the limited pressure difference generated, vacuum filtration is used in the laboratory where there are safety advantages when using glassware, because if the glassware is damaged it will implode rather than explode. One important industrial filter – the rotary vacuum filter – also utilizes a vacuum; this is described later in this chapter.

With industrial-scale liquid filtration, commonly used means of obtaining a high-pressure difference are either pumping the material to be filtered into the filter using a suitable pump, or using a pressurized vessel to drive the liquid through the filter. Most industrial filters have positive-pressure feed, the pressure used being limited only by the pump and the ability of the filter to withstand the high-pressure stress. Pressures up to 15×10^5 Pa (15 bar) are commonly used.

Although increasing the ΔP value in the absence of any other changes will cause a proportional increase in filtration rate, care needs to be taken to ensure that a phenomenon known as **cake compression** does not occur. Too high an applied pressure may cause the particles making up the cake to deform and therefore decrease the voidage (bed porosity). It can be seen from Eqn 22.2 that small decreases in the value of the porosity (e) lead to large decreases in cake permeability (K), and therefore in the filtration rate. The effect on decreasing K greatly outweighs any increase in filtration rate arising from a thinner cake. There is also a danger of 'blinding' the filter medium at high pressures by forcing particles into it. This is most likely in the early stages before a continuous layer of cake has formed. As a general rule filtration should start at moderate pressure, which can be increased as filtration proceeds and the cake thickness builds up.

Decrease the filtrate viscosity   The flow through a filter cake can be considered as the total flow through a large number of capillaries formed by the voids between the particles of the cake. The rate of flow through each capillary is governed by Poiseuille's law, which is a mathematical relationship that includes viscosity as a factor contributing to the resistance to flow. To increase the filtration rate the viscosity of the filtrate can be reduced in most cases by heating the formulation to be filtered. Many industrial filters, e.g. the metafilter, can be fitted with a steam jacket which can control temperature and hence viscosity. Care needs to be taken with this approach, however, when filtering formulations containing volatile components, or if components are thermolabile. In such cases dilution of the formulation with water may be an alternative means of reducing the viscosity providing that the increase in filtration rate exceeds the effect of increasing the total volume to be filtered.

Decrease the thickness of filter cake Darcy's equation (Eqn 22.1) shows that the filtration rate falls off as the cake increases in thickness. This effect is commonly observed when filtering in the laboratory using filter paper in a funnel. In some cases if the cake is allowed to build up the process slows to an unacceptable rate, or may almost stop altogether. In these situations it may be necessary to remove the cake periodically or maintain it at a constant thickness, as occurs for example with the rotary drum filter. As previously mentioned, the cake thickness can be kept lower by using a large filter area.

Increase the permeability of the cake One way of increasing the permeability of the cake is to include filter aids. A filter aid is a material that, when included in the formulation to be filtered, forms a cake of a more open porous nature and thus increases the K value in Darcy's equation. In addition, it may reduce the compressibility of the cake and/or prevent the filtered material blocking the filter medium. Filter aids that are used include diatomite (a form of diatomaceous earth) and perlite, which is a type of volcanic glass. The use of filter aids is obviously not appropriate if the filtered material is the intended end product.

FILTRATION EQUIPMENT

The filtration equipment described in this chapter is that used for filtering liquids. Equipment for filtering gases (mainly air) are also available.

Equipment selection

Ideally the equipment chosen should allow a fast filtration rate to minimize production costs, be cheap to buy and run, be easily cleaned and resistant to corrosion, and be capable of filtering large volumes of product before the filter needs stripping down for cleaning or replacing.

There are a number of product-related factors that should be considered when selecting a filter for a particular process. These include:

- the chemical nature of the product. Interactions with the filter medium may lead to leaching of the filter components, degradation or swelling of the filter medium or adsorption of components of the filtered product on the filter. All of these may influence the efficiency of the filtration process or the quality of the filtered product;
- the volume to be filtered and the filtration rate required. These dictate the size and type of equipment and the amount of time needed for the filtration process;
- the operating pressure needed. This is important in governing the filtration rate (Eqn 22.1) and influences whether a vacuum filter (where the pressure difference is limited to 1×10^5 Pa) is appropriate. High operating pressures require that the equipment be of sufficient strength and that appropriate safe operating procedures be adopted;
- the amount of material to be removed. This will influence the choice of filter, as a large 'load' may necessitate the use of prefilters or may require a filter where the cake can be continuously removed;
- the degree of filtration required. This will dictate the pore size of membrane filters or the filter grade to be used. If sterility is required then the equipment should itself be capable of being sterilized, and must ensure that contamination does not occur after the product has passed the filter;
- the product viscosity and filtration temperature. A high product viscosity may require elevated pressures to be used. The incoming formulation can be heated, or steam-heated jackets be fitted to the equipment. Care should be taken to ensure the equipment seals etc. can operate at elevated temperatures.

Industrial filtration equipment

Filters for liquid products may be classified by the method used to drive the filtrate through the filter medium. Filters can be organized into three classes, namely gravity, vacuum and pressure filters.

Gravity filters

Filters that rely solely on gravity only generate low operating pressures, and therefore use on a large scale is limited. Gravity filters are, however, simple and cheap, and are frequently used in laboratory filtration, where volumes are small and a low filtration rate is relatively unimportant.

Vacuum filters

The rotary vacuum filter In large-scale filtration continuous operation is often desirable, and this may be difficult when it is necessary to filter slurries containing a high proportion of solids. The rotary vacuum filter is continuous in operation and has a system for removing the cake so that it can be run for long periods handling concentrated slurries. A rotary drum filter is shown in section in Figure 22.3. It can be visualized as two concentric cylinders with the annular space between them divided into a number of septa by radial partitions. The outer cylinder is perforated and covered with a filter cloth. Each septum has a radial connection to a complicated rotating valve, whose function is to perform the sequence of operations listed in Table 22.1.

The cylinder rotates slowly in the slurry, which is kept agitated, and a vacuum applied to the segments draws filtrate into the septa, depositing cake on the filter cloth. When the deposited cake leaves the slurry bath vacuum is maintained to draw air through the cake, thus aiding drainage. This is followed by washing and then further drainage in the drying zone. The cake is removed by the scraper blade, aided by compressed air forced into the septa. It is the function of the rotary valve to direct these services into the septa where they are required.

Fig. 22.3 Rotary drum filter.

Table 22.1	Rotary vacuum filter operation		
Zone	Position	Service	Connected to
Pick-up	Slurry trough	Vacuum	Filtrate receiver
Drainage	–	Vacuum	Filtrate receiver
Washing	Wash sprays	Vacuum	Wash water receiver
Drying	–	Vacuum	Wash receiver
Cake removal	Scraper knife	Compressed air	Filter cake conveyor
In some cases, for example when the solid is the required product, the same receiver may he used for filtrate and for wash water.			

Rotary filters can be up to 2 m in diameter and 3.5 m in length, with a filtration area of around 20 m². Cake compression rollers are often fitted to improve the efficiency of washing and draining if the cake on the drum becomes cracked. Difficult solids, which tend to block the filter cloth, necessitate a preliminary precoat of a thickness of filter aid to be deposited on the cloth prior to filtration of the slurry. During the actual filtration the scraper knife is set to move slowly inwards, removing the blocked outer layer of the filter aid and exposing fresh surface.

If removal of the cake presents problems, a string discharge filter may be employed. This is useful for filtration of the fermentation liquor in the manufacture of antibiotics, when a felt-like cake of mould mycelia must be removed. The filter cloth in this case has a number of loops of string passing round the drum and over two additional small rollers, as shown in Figure 22.4. In operation the strings lift the cake off the filter medium. The cake is broken by the sharp bend over the rollers and collected, and the strings return to the drum.

The advantages of the rotary vacuum filter can be summarized as follows:

1. It is automatic and continuous in operation, so that labour costs are very low.
2. The filter has a large capacity.
3. Variation of the speed of rotation enables the cake thickness to be controlled, and for solids that form an impenetrable cake the thickness may be limited to less than 5 mm. On the other hand, if the solids are coarse, forming a porous cake, the thickness may be 100 mm or more.

Fig. 22.4 String discharge rotary drum filter.

Disadvantages include:

1. The rotary filter is a complex piece of equipment with many moving parts and is very expensive. In addition to the filter itself, ancillary equipment such as vacuum pumps, vacuum receivers and traps, slurry pumps and agitators are required.
2. The cake tends to crack because of the air drawn through by the vacuum system, so that washing and drying are not efficient.
3. Being a vacuum filter, the pressure difference is limited to 1 bar and hot filtrates may boil.
4. The rotary filter is suitable only for straightforward slurries, being less satisfactory if the solids form an impermeable cake or will not separate cleanly from the cloth.

Uses of the rotary filter The rotary filter is most suitable for continuous operation on large quantities of slurry, especially if the slurry contains considerable amounts of solids, that is, in the range 15–30%.

Examples of pharmaceutical applications include the collection of calcium carbonate, magnesium carbonate and starch, and the separation of the mycelia from the fermentation liquor in the manufacture of antibiotics.

Pressure filters

Pressure filters feed the product to the filter at a pressure greater than that which would arise from gravity alone. This is the most common type of filter used in the processing of pharmaceutical products.

The metafilter In its simplest form, the metafilter consists of a grooved drainage rod on which is packed a series of metal rings. These rings, usually of stainless steel, are about 15 mm inside diameter, 22 mm outside diameter and 0.8 mm in thickness, with a number of semicircular projections on one surface (Fig. 22.5). The height of the projections and the shape of the section of the ring are such that when the rings are packed together, all the same way up, and tightened on the drainage rod with a nut, channels are formed that taper from about 250 μm down to 25 μm. One or more of these packs is mounted in a vessel, and the filter operated by pumping in the slurry under pressure.

In this form the metafilter can be used as a strainer for coarse particles, but for finer particles a bed of a suitable material (such as a filter aid) is first built up over the rings. The pack of rings, therefore, serves essentially as a base on which the true filter medium is supported.

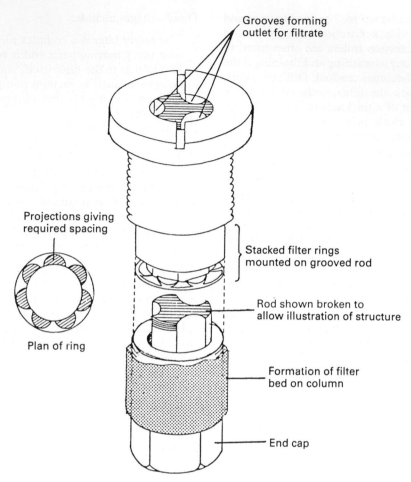

Fig. 22.5 Metafilter. Construction of the filter element (courtesy of Metafiltration Co. Ltd.).

The advantages of the metafilter can be summarized as follows:

1. It possesses considerable strength and high pressures can be used with no danger of bursting the filter medium.
2. As there is no filter medium as such, the running costs are low and it is very economical.
3. The metafilter can be made from materials (such as stainless steel) that can provide excellent resistance to corrosion and avoid contamination of the product.
4. By selecting of a suitable grade of material to form the filter bed it is possible to remove very fine particles; in fact, it is possible to sterilize a liquid using this filter

Uses of the metafilter The small surface area of the metafilter restricts the amount of solid that can be collected. This, together with the ability to separate

very fine particles, means that the metafilter is used almost exclusively for clarifying liquids where the contaminant level is low.

Furthermore, the strength of the metafilter permits the use of high pressures (up to 15 bar), making the method suitable for viscous liquids.

Specific examples of pharmaceutical uses include the clarification of syrups, injection solutions, and products such as insulin liquors.

Cartridge filters Cartridge filters are now commonly used in the preparation of pharmaceutical products, as they possess a very large filtration area in a small unit and are easy and relatively cheap to operate. In simple form they consist of a cylindrical cartridge containing highly pleated material (e.g. PTFE or nylon) or 'string-wound' material (i.e. wound like a ball of string). This cartridge then fits in a metal supporting cylinder and the product is pumped under pressure into one end of the cylinder surrounding the filter cartridge. The filtrate is forced through the filter cartridge from the periphery to the inner hollow core, from where it exits through the other end of the support cylinder. The filter cartridges are often disposable and are good for applications where there is a low contaminant level, e.g. during the filtration of liquid products as they are filled into bottles.

Cross-flow microfiltration It is possible to form membrane filters within 'hollow fibres'. The membrane, which may consist of polysulphone, acrylonitrile or polyamide, is laid down within a fibre which forms a rigid porous outer support (Fig. 22.6). The lumen of each fibre is small – typically 1–2 μm – but a large number of them can be contained in a surrounding shell to form a cartridge which may have an effective filtration area of over 2 m².

In use the liquid to be treated is pumped through the cartridge in a circulatory system, so that it passes through many times. The filtrate, which in this technique is often called the 'permeate', flows **radially** through the membrane and porous support. The great advantage of this mode of operation is that the high fluid velocity and turbulence minimize blocking of the membranes. Fresh liquid enters the system from a reservoir as filtration proceeds. Because the fluid flows **across** the surface, rather than at rightangles, this technique is known as **cross-flow** microfiltration.

Uses The method has been used for fractionation of biological products by first using a filter of pore size sufficient to let all the wanted molecules through, and then passing the permeate through a filter which will retain the required molecules while passing smaller unwanted molecules. It is claimed that blood plasma can be processed to remove alcohol and water and prepare concentrated purified albumin. The process has been suggested for the recovery of antibiotics from fermentation media.

CENTRIFUGATION

Centrifugal force can be used either to provide the driving force (ΔP) for the filtration process (refer to Darcy's law above, Eqn 22.1) or to replace the gravitational force in sedimentation processes (refer to Stokes' law, Chapter 4). Centrifuges are often used in the laboratory to separate solid material from a liquid, the solid typically forming a 'plug' at the bottom of the test tube at the end of the process.

Principles of centrifugation

If a particle (mass = m kg) spins in a centrifuge (radius r m) at a velocity (v m s⁻¹) then the centrifugal force (F N) acting on the particle equals $m\,v^2/r$.

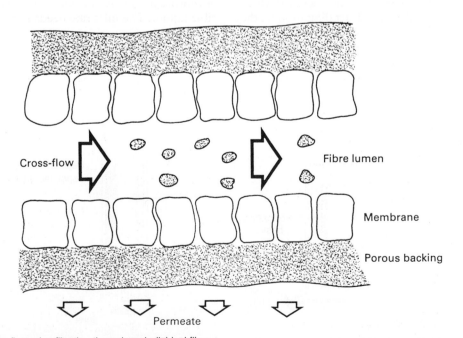

Fig. 22.6 Cross-flow microfiltration through an individual fibre

The same particle experiences gravitational force $(G, \mathrm{N}) = m\,g$ (where g = gravitational constant).

The **centrifugal effect** (C) is the ratio of these two forces, so $C = F/G$, i.e. C indicates how much greater F is than G. Therefore, $C = v^2/g\,r$. If the velocity is taken to be $\pi\,d\,n$, where n is rotation speed (s^{-1}) and d is diameter of rotation (m), then $C = 2.01\,d\,n^2$.

In order to increase the centrifugal effect it is therefore more efficient to increase the centrifuge speed than to use a larger diameter at the same speed.

Larger centrifuges also generate greater pressures on the centrifuge wall for the same value of C, and are therefore more costly to make.

Industrial centrifuges

There are two main types of centrifuge used to achieve separation on an industrial scale, those using perforated baskets, which perform a filtration-type operation (work like a spin-dryer) and those with a solid walled vessel, where particles sediment towards the wall under the influence of the centrifugal force.

Perforated-basket centrifuges (centrifugal filters)

A diagram of a perforated basket centrifuge is shown in Figure 22.7. It consists of a stainless steel perforated basket (typically 1–2 m in diameter) lined with a filter cloth. The basket rotates at a speed which is typically <25 s^{-1}, higher speeds tending to stress the basket excessively. The product enters centrally and is thrown outwards by centrifugal force and held against the filter cloth. The filtrate is forced through the cloth and removed via the liquid outlet; the solid material is retained on the cloth. The cake can be washed if required by spraying water into the centrifuge.

The centrifugal filter has been used for separating crystalline materials from the preparation liquor, e.g. in the preparation of aspirin, and for removing precipitated proteins from insulin. It has the advantages of being compact and efficient, a 1 m centrifuge being able to process about 200 kg in 10 minutes. It can also handle concentrated slurries which might block other filters, and gives a product with a very low moisture content (typically around 2% w/w), which saves energy during drying.

The centrifuge described above is operated batchwise but continuous centrifuges are available for large-scale work. These have means for automatic discharge of the cake from a basket, which rotates around a horizontal axis in contrast to the vertical axis. Most of the energy required to run a centrifuge is used to bring it up to operating speed and little more is needed to maintain that speed. Continuous centrifuges are therefore cheaper to run, but the initial cost is considerably more.

Tubular-bowl centrifuges (centrifugal sedimenters)

These consist of a cylindrical 'bowl', typically around 100 mm in diameter and 1 m long, which rotates at 300–1000 s^{-1}. The product enters at the bottom and centrifugal force causes solids to be deposited on the wall as it passes up the bowl, the liquid overflowing from the top (Fig. 22.8). This type of centrifuge can also be adapted to separate immiscible liquids. The inlet rate needs to be controlled so

Fig. 22.7   Centrifugal dewatering filter.

Fig. 22.8   Tubular-bowl centrifuge.

that there is sufficient time for sedimentation to occur before the product leaves the bowl.

The uses of centrifugal sedimenters include liquid/liquid separation, e.g. during antibiotic manufacture and purification of fish oils, the removal of very small particles, the removal of solids that are compressible or 'slimy' and which easily block the filter medium, the separation of blood plasma from whole blood (need $C \approx 3000$), the separation of different particle size fractions, and examining the stability of emulsions.

These centrifuges are compact, have a high separating efficiency and are good for separating 'difficult' solids, but have a limited capacity and are complicated to construct to achieve the required speed and minimize vibration.

Bibliography

Meltser, T.H. (1987) *Filtration in the Pharmaceutical Industry*, Marcel Dekker.

23

Suspensions and emulsions

Michael Billany

CHAPTER CONTENTS

INTRODUCTION

A coarse suspension is a dispersion of finely divided, insoluble solid particles (the disperse phase) in a fluid (the dispersion medium or continuous phase). Most pharmaceutical suspensions consist of an aqueous dispersion medium, although in some instances it may be an organic or oily liquid. A disperse phase with a mean particle diameter of up to 1 μm is usually termed a colloidal dispersion, and includes such examples as aluminium hydroxide and magnesium hydroxide suspensions. A solid in liquid dispersion, in which the particles are above colloidal size, is termed a coarse suspension.

An emulsion may be defined as two immiscible liquids, one of which is finely subdivided and uniformly distributed as droplets throughout the other. The system is stabilized by the presence of an emulsifying agent. The dispersed liquid or internal phase usually consists of globules of diameters down to 0.1 μm which are distributed within the external or continuous phase.

The physical properties of both colloidal and coarse suspensions and of emulsions are discussed in Chapter 6.

PHYSICAL PROPERTIES OF WELL-FORMULATED SUSPENSIONS AND EMULSIONS

- The product must remain sufficiently homogenous for at least the period between shaking the container and removing the required amount.
- The sediment or creaming produced on storage, if any, must be easily resuspended by moderate agitation of the container.
- The product may be required to be thickened in order to reduce the rate of settling of the particles or the rate of creaming of oil globules. The resulting viscosity must not be so high that removal of the product from the container and transfer to the site of application are difficult.
- Any suspended particles should be small and uniformly sized in order to give a smooth, elegant product, free from a gritty texture.

PHARMACEUTICAL APPLICATIONS OF SUSPENSIONS

Suspensions can be used as oral dosage forms, applied topically to the skin or mucous membrane surfaces, or given parenterally by injection.

Suspensions as oral drug delivery systems

Many people have difficulty in swallowing solid dosage forms and therefore require the drug to be dispersed in a liquid.

Some materials are required to be present in the gastrointestinal tract in a finely divided form, and their formulation as suspensions will provide the desired high surface area. Solids such as kaolin, magnesium carbonate and magnesium trisilicate, for example, are used for the adsorption of toxins, or to neutralize excess acidity. A dispersion of finely divided silica in dimethicone 1000 is used in veterinary practice for the treatment of 'frothy bloat'.

The taste of most drugs is more noticeable if it is in solution rather than in an insoluble form. Paracetamol is available both in solution as Paediatric Paracetamol Oral Solution and also as a suspension. The latter is more palatable, and therefore particularly suitable for children. For the same reason chloramphenicol mixtures can be formulated as suspensions containing the insoluble chloramphenicol palmitate.

Suspensions for topical administration

Suspensions of drugs can also be formulated for topical application (Chapter 33). They can be fluid preparations, such as Calamine Lotion, which are designed to leave a light deposit of the active agent on the skin after quick evaporation of the dispersion medium. Some suspensions, such as pastes, are semisolid in consistency and contain high concentrations of powders dispersed – usually – in a paraffin base. It may also be possible to suspend a powdered drug in an emulsion base, as in Zinc Cream.

Suspensions for parenteral use and inhalation therapy

Suspensions can also be formulated for parenteral administration in order to control the rate of absorption of the drug. By varying the size of the dispersed particles of active agent, the duration of activity can be controlled. The absorption rate of the drug into the bloodstream will then depend simply on its rate of dissolution. If the drug is suspended in a fixed oil such as arachis or sesame, the product will remain after injection in the form of an oil globule, thereby presenting to the tissue fluid a small surface area from which the partitioning of drug can occur. The release of drug suspended in an aqueous vehicle will be faster, as some diffusion of the product will occur along muscle fibres and become miscible with tissue fluid. This will present a larger surface area from which the drug can be released.

Vaccines for the induction of immunity are often formulated as dispersions of killed microorganisms, as in Cholera Vaccine, or of the constituent toxoids adsorbed on to a substrate of aluminium hydroxide or phosphate, as in Adsorbed Diphtheria and Tetanus Vaccine. Thus a prolonged antigenic stimulus is provided, resulting in a high antibody titre.

Some X-ray contrast media are also formulated in this way. Barium sulphate, for the examination of the alimentary tract, is available as a suspension for either oral or rectal administration, and propyliodone is dispersed in either water or arachis oil for examination of the bronchial tract.

The adsorptive properties of fine powders are also used in the formulation of some inhalations. The volatile components of menthol and eucalyptus oil would be lost from solution very rapidly during use, whereas a more prolonged release is obtained if the two active agents are adsorbed on to light magnesium carbonate prior to the preparation of a suspension.

Chapter 31 describes some aspects of the formulation of aerosols, many of which are also available as suspensions of the active agent in a mixture of propellants.

Solubility and stability considerations

If the drug is insoluble or poorly soluble in a suitable solvent, then formulation as a suspension is usually required. Some eye drops, notably Hydrocortisone Acetate and Neomycin Eye Drops, are formulated as suspensions because of the poor solubility of hydrocortisone in a suitable solvent.

The degradation of a drug in the presence of water may also preclude its use as an aqueous solution. In this case it may be possible to synthesize an insoluble derivative that can then be formulated as a suspension. For example, oxytetracycline hydrochloride is used in solid dosage forms, but in aqueous solution would rapidly hydrolyse. A stable liquid dosage form has been made by suspending the insoluble calcium salt in a suitable aqueous vehicle.

Prolonged contact between the solid drug particles and the dispersion medium can be considerably reduced by preparing the suspension immediately prior to issue to the patient. Amoxicillin, for example, is provided by the manufacturer as the trihydrate salt mixed with the other powdered or granulated ingredients. The pharmacist then makes the product up to volume with water immediately before issue to the patient, allocating a shelf-life of 14 days at a temperature at or below 25°C.

A drug that degrades in the presence of water may alternatively be suspended in a non-aqueous vehicle. Fractionated coconut oil is used as the vehicle for some formulations of antibiotics for oral use, and in some countries tetracycline hydrochloride is dispersed in a similar base for ophthalmic use.

FORMULATION OF SUSPENSIONS

Particle size control

It is first necessary to ensure that the drug to be suspended is of a fine particle size prior to formulation. This is to ensure a slow rate of sedimentation of the suspended particles. Large particles, if greater than about 5 μm diameter, will also impart a gritty texture to the product, and may cause irritation if injected or instilled into the eyes. The ease of administration of a parenteral suspension may depend upon particle size and shape, and it is quite possible to block a hypodermic needle with particles over about 25 μm diameter, particularly if they are acicular in shape rather than isodiametric. A particular particle size range may also be chosen in order to control the rate of dissolution of the drug and hence its bioavailability.

Even though the particle size of a drug may be small when the suspension is first manufactured, there is always a degree of crystal growth that occurs on storage, particularly if temperature fluctuations occur. This is because the solubility of the drug may increase as the temperature rises, but on cooling, the drug will crystallize out. This is a particular problem with slightly soluble drugs such as paracetamol.

If the drug is polydispersed, then the very small crystals of less than 1 μm diameter will exhibit a greater solubility than the larger ones. Over a period of time the small crystals will become even smaller, whereas the diameters of the larger particles will increase. It is therefore advantageous to use a suspended drug of a narrow size range. The inclusion of surface-active agents or polymeric colloids, which

adsorb on to the surface of each particle, may also help to prevent crystal growth.

Different polymorphic forms of a drug may exhibit different solubilities, the metastable state being the most soluble. Conversion of the metastable form, in solution, to the less soluble stable state, and its subsequent precipitation, will lead to changes in particle size.

The use of wetting agents

Some insoluble solids may be easily wetted by water and will disperse readily throughout the aqueous phase with only minimal agitation. Most, however, will exhibit varying degrees of hydrophobicity and will not be easily wetted. Some particles will form large porous clumps within the liquid, whereas others remain on the surface and become attached to the upper part of the container. The foam produced on shaking will be slow to subside because of the stabilizing effect of the small particles at the liquid/air interface.

To ensure adequate wetting, the interfacial tension between the solid and the liquid must be reduced so that the adsorbed air is displaced from the solid surfaces by the liquid. The particles will then disperse readily throughout the liquid, particularly if an intense shearing action is used during mixing. If a series of suspensions is prepared, each containing one of a range of concentrations of wetting agent, then the concentration to choose will be the lowest that provides adequate wetting.

The following is a discussion of the most widely used wetting agents for pharmaceutical products.

Surface-active agents

Figure 6.15 shows that surfactants possessing an HLB value between about 7 and 9 would be suitable for use as wetting agents. The hydrocarbon chains would be adsorbed by the hydrophobic particle surfaces, whereas the polar groups project into the aqueous medium and become hydrated. Wetting of the solid occurs as a result of a fall both in interfacial tension between the solid and the liquid and, to a lesser extent, between the liquid and air.

Most surfactants are used at concentrations of up to about 0.1% as wetting agents and include, for oral use, the polysorbates (Tweens) and sorbitan esters (Spans). For external application, sodium lauryl sulphate, sodium dioctylsulphosuccinate and quillaia extract can also be used.

The choice of surfactant for parenteral administration is obviously more limited, the main ones used being the polysorbates, some of the poloxamers (polyoxyethylene/polyoxypropylene copolymers) and lecithin.

Disadvantages in the use of this type of wetting agent include excessive foaming and the possible formation of a deflocculated system, which may not be required.

Hydrophilic colloids

These materials include acacia, bentonite, tragacanth, alginates, xanthan gum and cellulose derivatives, and will behave as protective colloids by coating the solid hydrophobic particles with a multimolecular layer. This will impart a hydrophilic character to the solid and so promote wetting. These materials are also used as suspending agents and may, like surfactants, produce a deflocculated system, particularly if used at low concentrations.

Solvents

Materials such as alcohol, glycerol and glycols, which are water miscible, will reduce the liquid/air interfacial tension. The solvent will penetrate the loose agglomerates of powder displacing the air from the pores of the individual particles, so enabling wetting to occur by the dispersion medium.

Flocculated and deflocculated systems

Having incorporated a suitable wetting agent, it is then necessary to determine whether the suspension is flocculated or deflocculated and to decide which state is preferable. Whether or not a suspension is flocculated or deflocculated depends on the relative magnitudes of the forces of repulsion and attraction between the particles. The effects of these particle–particle interactions have been adequately covered in Chapter 6.

In a deflocculated system the dispersed particles remain as discrete units and, because the rate of sedimentation depends on the size of each unit, settling will be slow. The supernatant of a deflocculated system will continue to remain cloudy for an appreciable time after shaking, due to the very slow settling rate of the smallest particles in the product, even after the larger ones have sedimented. The repulsive forces between individual particles allow them to slip past each other as they sediment. The slow rate of settling prevents the entrapment of liquid within the sediment, which thus becomes compacted and can be very difficult to redisperse. This phenomenon is also called caking or claying,

and is the most serious of all the physical stability problems encountered in suspension formulation.

The aggregation of particles in a flocculated system will lead to a much more rapid rate of sedimentation or subsidence because each unit is composed of many individual particles and is therefore larger. The rate of settling will also depend on the porosity of the aggregate, because if it is porous the dispersion medium can flow through, as well as around, each aggregate or floccule as it sediments.

The nature of the sediment of a flocculated system is also quite different from that of a deflocculated one. The structure of each aggregate is retained after sedimentation, thus entrapping a large amount of the liquid phase. As explained in Chapter 6, aggregation in the primary minimum will produce compact floccules, whereas a secondary minimum effect will produce loose floccules of higher porosity. Whichever occurs, the volume of the final sediment will still be large and will easily be redispersed by moderate agitation.

In a flocculated system the supernatant quickly becomes clear, as the large flocs that settle rapidly are composed of particles of all sizes. Figure 23.1 illus-

Flocculated system

Deflocculated system

(a)   (b)   (c)

Fig. 23.1 The sedimentation behaviour of flocculated and deflocculated suspensions. Within a few minutes of manufacture (a) there is no apparent change within the deflocculated system compared to its initial appearance. Even after several hours (b) there is still little obvious change, except that the concentration of solids in the lower layers has increased at the expense of the upper layers owing to slow particle sedimentation. There is a small amount of a compact sediment. After prolonged storage (c), depending on the physical stability of the system, the supernatant has cleared, leaving a compact sediment. In the flocculated system at (a) there is some clear supernatant with a distinct boundary between it and the sediment. At (b) there is a larger volume of clear supernatant with a relatively large volume of a porous sediment, which does not change further even after prolonged storage (c).

trates the appearance of both flocculated and deflocculated suspensions at given times after shaking.

In summary, deflocculated systems have the advantage of a slow sedimentation rate, thereby enabling a uniform dose to be taken from the container, but when settling does occur the sediment is compacted and difficult to redisperse. Flocculated systems form loose sediments which are easily redispersible, but the sedimentation rate is fast and there is a danger of an inaccurate dose being administered; also, the product will look inelegant.

Controlled flocculation

A deflocculated system with a sufficiently high viscosity to prevent sedimentation would be an ideal formulation. It cannot be guaranteed, however, that the system would remain homogenous during the entire shelf-life of the product. Usually a compromise is reached in which the suspension is partially flocculated to enable adequate redispersion if necessary, and viscosity is controlled so that the sedimentation rate is at a minimum.

The next stage of the formulation process, after the addition of the wetting agent, is to ensure that the product exhibits the correct degree of flocculation. Underflocculation will give those undesirable properties that are associated with deflocculated systems. An overflocculated product will look inelegant and, to minimize settling, the viscosity of the product may have to be so high that any necessary redispersion would be difficult.

Controlled flocculation is usually achieved by a combination of particle size control, the use of electrolytes to control zeta potential, and the addition of polymers to enable crosslinking to occur between particles. Some polymers have the advantage of becoming ionized in an aqueous solution, and can therefore act both electrostatically and sterically. These materials are also termed polyelectrolytes.

Flocculating agents

In many cases, after the incorporation of a non-ionic wetting agent a suspension will be found to be deflocculated, either because of the reduction in solid/liquid interfacial tension, or because of the hydrated hydrophilic layer around each particle forming a mechanical barrier to aggregation. The use of an ionic surfactant to wet the solid could produce either a flocculated or a deflocculated system, depending on any charge already present on the particles. If particles are of opposite charge to that of the surfactant then neutralization will occur. If a high charge density is imparted to the suspended particles then deflocculation will be the result.

If it is necessary for the suspension to be converted from a deflocculated to a partially flocculated state, this may be achieved by the addition of electrolytes, surfactants and/or hydrophilic polymers.

Electrolytes The addition of an inorganic electrolyte to an aqueous suspension will alter the zeta potential of the dispersed particles and, if this value is lowered sufficiently, flocculation may occur.

The Schultz–Hardy rule shows that the ability of an electrolyte to flocculate hydrophobic particles depends on the valency of its counter-ions. Although they are more efficient, trivalent ions are less widely used than mono- or divalent electrolytes because they are generally more toxic. If hydrophilic polymers, which are usually negatively charged, are included in the formulation they may be precipitated by the presence of trivalent ions.

The most widely used electrolytes include the sodium salts of acetates, phosphates and citrates, and the concentration chosen will be that which produces the desired degree of flocculation. Care must be taken not to add excessive electrolyte or charge reversal may occur on each particle, so forming, once again, a deflocculated system.

Surfactants Ionic surface-active agents may also cause flocculation by neutralizing the charge on each particle, thus resulting in a deflocculated system. Non-ionic surfactants will, of course, have a negligible effect on the charge density of a particle but may, because of their linear configurations, adsorb on to more than one particle, thereby forming a loose flocculated structure.

Polymeric flocculating agents Starch, alginates, cellulose derivatives, tragacanth, carbomers and silicates are examples of polymers that can be used to control flocculation. Their linear branched-chain molecules form a gel-like network within the system and become adsorbed on to the surfaces of the dispersed particles, thus holding them in a flocculated state. Although some settling can occur, the sedimentation volume is large, and usually remains so for a considerable period.

Care must be taken to ensure that, during manufacture, blending is not excessive as this may inhibit the crosslinking between adjacent particles and result in the adsorption of each molecule of polymer on to one particle only. If this should occur then a deflocculated system may result, because the formation of the hydrophilic barrier around each particle will inhibit aggregation. A high concentration of polymer may have a similar effect if the whole surface of each particle is coated. It is essential that areas on each suspended particle remain free from adsorbate, so that crosslinking can recur after the product is sheared. Further details of the use of polymers can be found in the next section.

Rheology of suspensions

An ideal pharmaceutical suspension would exhibit a high apparent viscosity at low rates of shear so that, on storage, the suspended particles would either settle very slowly or, preferably, remain permanently suspended. At higher rates of shear, such as those caused by moderate shaking of the product, the apparent viscosity should fall sufficiently for the product to be poured easily from its container. The product, if for external use, should then spread easily without excessive dragging, but should not be so fluid that it runs off the skin surface. If intended for injection, the product should pass easily through a hypodermic needle with only moderate pressure applied to the syringe plunger. It would then be important for the initial high apparent viscosity to be reformed after a short time to maintain adequate physical stability.

A flocculated system partly fulfils these criteria. In such a system pseudoplastic or plastic behaviour (see Chapter 4) is exhibited as the structure progressively breaks down under shear. The product then shows the time-dependent reversibility of this loss of structure, which is termed thixotropy.

A deflocculated system, however, would exhibit newtonian behaviour owing to the absence of such structures and may even, if high concentrations of disperse phase are present, exhibit dilatancy.

Although a flocculated system may exhibit some thixotropy and plasticity, unless a high concentration of disperse phase is present it may not be sufficient to prevent rapid settling, particularly if a surfactant or an electrolyte is present as a flocculating agent. In these cases suspending agents may be used to increase the apparent viscosity of the system.

Suitable materials are the hydrophilic polymers discussed above. These exert their effect by entrapping the solid dispersed particles within their gel-like network, so preventing sedimentation. At low concentrations many suspending agents can be used to control flocculation, and it must be realized that if large quantities are to be used to enhance viscosity the degree of flocculation may also be altered.

Viscosity modifiers

The following materials are those most widely used for the modification of suspension viscosity.

Polysaccharides

Acacia This natural material is often used as a suspending agent for extemporaneously prepared suspensions. Acacia is not a good thickening agent and its value as a suspending agent is largely due to its action as a protective colloid. It is therefore useful for preparations containing tinctures of resinous materials that precipitate on addition to water. It is essential to ensure that any precipitated resin is well coated by the protective colloid before any electrolyte (which should be well diluted) is added. Acacia is not very effective for dense powders, and for these it is often combined with other thickeners such as tragacanth, starch and sucrose in compound tragacanth powder.

Unfortunately, acacia mucilage becomes acidic on storage as a result of enzyme activity, and it also contains an oxidase enzyme which may cause deterioration of active agents that are susceptible to oxidation. This enzyme can, however, be inactivated by heat.

Because of the stickiness of acacia it is rarely used in preparations for external use.

Tragacanth This product will form viscous aqueous solutions. Its thixotropic and pseudoplastic properties make it a better thickening agent than acacia and it can be used both for internal and external products. Like acacia it is mainly, though not exclusively, used for the extemporaneous preparation of suspensions with a short shelf-life.

Tragacanth is stable over a pH range of 4–7.5 but takes several days to hydrate fully after dispersion in water. The maximum viscosity of its dispersions is not, therefore, achieved until after this time, and can also be affected by heating. There are several grades of this material and only the best quality is suitable for use as a pharmaceutical suspending agent.

Alginates Alginic acid, a polymer of D-mannuronic acid, is prepared from kelp, and its salts have suspending properties similar to those of tragacanth. Alginate mucilages must not be heated above 60°C as depolymerization occurs, with a consequent loss in viscosity. They are most viscous immediately after preparation, after which there is a fall to a fairly constant value after about 24 hours. Alginates exhibit a maximum viscosity over a pH range of 5–9, and at low pH the acid is precipitated. Sodium alginate (Manucol) is the most widely used material in this class but it is, of course, anionic and will be incompatible with cationic materials and with heavy metals. The addition of calcium chloride to a sodium alginate dispersion will produce calcium alginate, which has a much higher viscosity. Several different viscosity grades are commercially available.

Starch Starch is rarely used on its own as a suspending agent but is one of the constituents of compound tragacanth powder, and it can also be used with carmellose sodium. Sodium starch glycollate (Explotab, Primojel), a derivative of potato starch, has also been evaluated for its use in the extemporaneous preparation of suspensions.

Xanthan gum (Keltrol) This is an anionic heteropolysaccharide produced by the action of *Xanthomonas campestris* on corn sugars. It is very soluble in cold water and is one of the most widely used thickening agents for the extemporaneous preparation of suspensions for oral use. It is used in concentrations up to about 2% and is stable over a wide pH range.

Water-soluble celluloses

Several cellulose derivatives are available that will disperse in water to produce viscous colloidal solutions suitable for use as suspending agents.

Methylcellulose (Celacol, Methocel) This is a semi-synthetic polysaccharide of the general formula:

$$[C_6H_7O_2(OH_2)OCH_3]_n$$

and is produced by the methylation of cellulose. Several grades are available, depending on their degree of methylation and on the chain length. The longer the chain, the more viscous is its solution. For example, a 2% solution of methylcellulose 20 exhibits an apparent viscosity of 20 millipascal seconds (mPa s) and methylcellulose 4500 has value of 4500 mPa s at 2% concentration. Because these products are more soluble in cold water than in hot, they are often dispersed in warm water and then, on cooling with constant stirring, a clear or opalescent viscous solution is produced. Methylcelluloses are non-ionic and therefore stable over a pH range of 3–11, and are compatible with many ionic additives. When these dispersions are heated, the methylcellulose molecules become progressively dehydrated and eventually gel at about 50°C; on cooling the original form is regained.

Hydroxyethylcellulose (Natrosol) This compound has hydroxyethyl instead of methyl groups attached to the cellulose chain and is also available in different viscosity grades. It has the advantage of being soluble in both hot and cold water and will not gel on heating. Otherwise it exhibits the same properties as methylcellulose.

Carmellose sodium (sodium carboxymethylcellulose) This material can be represented by:

$$[C_6H_{10-x}O_5(CH_2COONa)_x]_n$$

where x represents the degree of substitution, usually about 0.7, which in turn affects its solubility. The viscosity of its solution depends on the value of n, which represents the degree of polymerization. The numerical suffix gives an indication of the viscosity of a 2% solution. For example sodium carboxymethylcellulose 50 at a concentration of 2% will have a viscosity of 50 mPa s. This material produces clear solutions in both hot and cold water, which are stable over a pH range of about 5–10. Being anionic, this material is incompatible with polyvalent cations and the acid will be precipitated at low pHs. Heat sterilization of either the powder or its mucilage will reduce the viscosity, and this must be taken into account during formulation. It is widely used at concentrations of up to 1% in products for oral, parenteral or external use.

Microcrystalline cellulose This material consists of crystals of colloidal dimensions which disperse readily in water (but are not soluble) to produce thixotropic gels. It is a widely used suspending agent and the rheological properties of its dispersions can often be improved by the incorporation of additional hydrocolloid, in particular carboxymethylcellulose, methylcellulose and hydroxypropylmethylcellulose. These will aid dispersion and also stabilize the product against the flocculating effects of added electrolyte.

Hydrated silicates

There are three important materials within this classification, namely bentonite, magnesium aluminium silicate and hectorite, and they belong to a group called the montmorillonite clays. They hydrate readily, absorbing up to 12 times their weight of water, particularly at elevated temperatures. The gels formed are thixotropic and therefore have useful suspending properties. As with most naturally occurring materials they may be contaminated with spores, and this must be borne in mind when considering a sterilization process and choosing a preservative system.

Bentonite This has the general formula:

$$Al_2O_3.4SiO_2.H_2O$$

It is used at concentrations of up to 2 or 3% in preparations for external use, such as calamine lotion. As this product may contain pathogenic spores it should be sterilized before use.

Magnesium aluminium silicate (Veegum) Also known as attapulgite, this is available as insoluble flakes that disperse and swell readily in water by absorbing the aqueous phase into its crystal lattice. Several grades are available, differing in their particle size, their acid demand and the viscosity of their dispersions. They can be used both internally and externally at concentrations of up to about 5%, and are stable over a pH range of 3.5–11. Veegum/water dispersions will exhibit thixotropy and plasticity with a high yield value, but the presence of salts can alter these rheological properties because of the flocculating effect of their positively charged counter-ions. Some grades, however, have a higher resistance to flocculation than others.

This material is often combined with organic thickening agents such as sodium carboxymethylcellulose or xanthan gum to improve yield values and degree of thixotropy, and to control flocculation (Ciullo 1981).

Hectorite This material is similar to bentonite and can be used at concentrations of 1–2% for external use. It is also possible to obtain synthetic hectorites (Laponite) that do not exhibit the batch variability or level of microbial contamination associated with natural products, and which can also be used internally.

As with other clays it is often advantageous to include an organic gum to modify its rheological properties.

Carbomers (carboxypolymethylene)

This material is a totally synthetic copolymer of acrylic acid and allyl sucrose. It is used at concentrations of up to 0.5%, mainly for external application, although some grades can be taken internally. When dispersed in water it forms acidic, low-viscosity solutions which, when adjusted to a pH of between 6 and 11, become highly viscous.

Colloidal silicon dioxide (Aerosil)

When dispersed in water this finely divided product will aggregate, forming a three-dimensional network. It can be used at concentrations of up to 4% for external use, but has also been used for thickening non-aqueous suspensions.

TYPES OF EMULSION

Pharmaceutical emulsions usually consist of a mixture of an aqueous phase with various oils and/or waxes. If the oil droplets are dispersed throughout the aqueous phase the emulsion is termed oil-in-water (o/w). A system in which the water is dispersed throughout the oil is a water-in-oil (w/o) emulsion. It is also possible to form multiple emulsions. For example, many small water droplets can be enclosed within larger oil droplets, which are themselves then dispersed in water. This gives a water-in-oil-in-water (w/o/w) emulsion. The alternative o/w/o emulsion is also possible.

If the dispersed globules are of colloidal dimensions (1 nm to 1 μm diameter) the preparation, which is quite often transparent or translucent, is called a microemulsion. This type has similar properties to a micellar system and will therefore exhibit the properties of hydrophobic colloids. As the size of the dispersed droplets increases more of the characteristics of coarse dispersions will be exhibited (see Chapter 6).

Tests for identification of emulsion type

Several simple methods are available for distinguishing between o/w and w/o emulsions (Table 23.1). The most common of these involve:

- miscibility tests with oil or water. The emulsion will only be miscible with liquids that are miscible with its continuous phase;
- conductivity measurements. Systems with aqueous continuous phases will readily conduct electricity, whereas systems with oily continuous phases will not;
- staining tests. Water-soluble and oil-soluble dyes are used, one of which will dissolve in, and colour the continuous phase.

FORMULATION OF EMULSIONS

Because of the very wide range of emulsifying agents available, considerable experience is required to choose the best emulgent system for a particular product. The final choice will depend to a large extent on the properties and use of the final product and the other materials required to be present.

Choice of emulsion type

The decision as to whether an o/w or a w/o emulsion is to be formulated will eliminate many unsuitable emulsifying systems.

Fats or oils for oral administration, either as medicaments in their own right or as vehicles for oil-soluble drugs, are invariably formulated as oil-in-water emulsions. In this form they are pleasant to take, and the inclusion of a suitable flavour in the aqueous phase will mask any unpleasant taste.

Table 23.1 Tests for identification of emulsion type

Oil-in-water emulsions	Water-in-oil emulsions
Miscibility tests	
Are miscible with water but immiscible with oil	Are miscible with oil but not with water
Staining tests by incorporation of an oil-soluble dye	
Macroscopic examination	
Paler colour than a w/o emulsion	More intense colouration than with an o/w emulsion
Microscopic examination	
Coloured globules on a colourless background	Colourless globules against a coloured background
Conductivity tests	
Water, being the continuous phase, will conduct electricity throughout the system. Two electrodes, when placed in such a preparation with a battery and suitable light source connected in series, will cause the lamp to glow	A preparation in which oil is the continuous phase will not conduct electricity. The lamp will not glow, or will only flicker spasmodically

Emulsions for intravenous administration must also be of the o/w type, although intramuscular injections can also be formulated as w/o products if a water-soluble drug is required for depot therapy.

Emulsions are most widely used for external application. Semisolid emulsions are termed creams and more fluid preparations are called either lotions or, if intended for massage into the skin, liniments. Both o/w and w/o types are available. The former is used for the topical application of water-soluble drugs, mainly for local effect. They do not have the greasy texture associated with oily bases and are therefore pleasant to use and easily washed from skin surfaces.

Water-in-oil emulsions will have an occlusive effect by hydration of the upper layers of the stratum corneum and the inhibition of evaporation of eccrine secretions. This, in turn, may influence the absorption rates of drugs from these preparations.

This type of emulsion is also useful for cleansing the skin of oil-soluble dirt, although its greasy texture is not always cosmetically acceptable. Oil-in-water emulsions are less efficient as cleansers but are usually more acceptable to the consumer, particularly for use on the hands. Similarly, moisturising creams, designed to prevent moisture loss from the skin and thus inhibit drying of the stratum corneum, are more efficient if formulated as w/o emulsions, which produce a coherent, water-repellent film.

Choice of oil phase

In many instances the oil phase of an emulsion is the active agent, and therefore its concentration in the product is predetermined. Liquid paraffin, castor oil, cod liver oil and arachis oil are all examples of medicaments which are formulated as emulsions for oral administration. Cottonseed oil, soya bean oil and safflower oil are used for their high calorific value in emulsions for intravenous feeding, and examples of externally applied oils that are formulated as emulsions include turpentine oil and benzyl benzoate.

Many emulsions for external use contain oils that are present as carriers for the active agent. It must be realized that the type of oil used may also have an effect both on the viscosity of the product and on the transport of the drug into the skin (see Chapter 33). One of the most widely used oils for this type of preparation is liquid paraffin. This is one of a series of hydrocarbons, which also includes hard paraffin, soft paraffin and light liquid paraffin. They can be used individually or in combination with each other to control emulsion consistency. This will ensure that the product can be spread easily but will be sufficiently viscous to form a coherent film over the skin. The film-forming capabilities of the emulsion can be further modified by the inclusion of various waxes, such as beeswax, carnauba wax or higher fatty alcohols. Continuous films can therefore be formed that are sufficiently tough and flexible to prevent contact between the skin and aqueous-based irritants. These preparations are called barrier creams, and many are of the w/o variety. The inclusion of silicone oils, such as dimethicone at 10–20%, which have exceptional water-repellent properties, may also permit the formulation of o/w products that are equally effective.

A variety of fixed oils of vegetable origin are also available, the most widely used being arachis, sesame, cottonseed and maize. Those expressed from seeds or fruits are often protein rich and contain useful vitamins and minerals. They are often, therefore, formulated for oral use as emulsions. Because of their lack of toxicity they can be used both internally and externally as vehicles for other materials.

Emulsion consistency

The texture or feel of a product intended for external use must also be considered. A w/o preparation will have a greasy texture and often exhibits a higher apparent viscosity than o/w emulsions. This fact is often used to convey a feeling of richness to many cosmetic formulations. Oil-in-water emulsions will, however, feel less greasy or sticky on application to the skin, will be absorbed more readily because of their lower oil content, and can be more easily washed from the skin surface.

Ideally emulsions should exhibit the rheological properties of plasticity/pseudoplasticity and thixotropy (see Chapter 4). A high apparent viscosity at the very low rates of shear caused by movement of dispersed phase globules is necessary in order to retard this movement and maintain a physically stable emulsion. It is important, however, that these products should flow freely when shaken, poured from the container or injected through a hypodermic needle. Therefore, at these high rates of shear, a lower apparent viscosity is required. This change in apparent viscosity must be reversible after a suitable time delay so as to retard creaming and coalescence.

For an externally applied product a wide range of emulsion consistencies can be tolerated. Low-viscosity lotions and liniments can be formulated that are dispensed from a flexible plastic container via a nozzle on to the skin. Only light shearing is then required to spread this type of product over the skin surface. This is particularly advantageous for painful or inflamed skin conditions.

The main disadvantage with low-viscosity emulsions is their tendency to cream easily, especially if formulated with a low oil concentration. It is rarely possible to formulate low-viscosity w/o products because of the consistency of the oil phase.

Emulsions of high apparent viscosity for external use are termed creams and are of a semisolid consistency. They are usually packed into collapsible plastic or aluminium tubes, although large volumes or very high-viscosity products are often packed into glass or plastic jars.

It is important not to ignore the patient/consumer acceptability of topically applied preparations, particularly in a competitive market.

There are several methods by which the rheological properties of an emulsion can be controlled.

Volume concentration of the dispersed phase

As discussed in Chapters 4 and 6, Einstein developed an equation relating the viscosity of a suspension to the volume fraction of the particles in that suspension. A qualitative application of this equation to the behaviour of emulsions shows that the viscosity of the product as a whole would be higher than the viscosity of the continuous phase on its own. So, as the concentration of dispersed phase increases, so does the apparent viscosity of the product.

Care must be taken to ensure that the dispersed phase concentration does not increase above about 60% of the total, as phase inversion may occur.

Particle size of the dispersed phase

It is possible, under certain conditions, to increase the apparent viscosity of an emulsion by a reduction in mean globule diameter. This can be achieved by homogenization. There are two postulated mechanisms for this occurrence:

1. A smaller mean globule size can cause increased flocculation. In a flocculated system a significant part of the continuous phase is trapped within aggregates of droplets, thus effectively increasing the apparent disperse phase concentration. Emulsions consisting of polydispersed droplets will tend to exhibit a lower viscosity than a monodispersed system, due to differences in electrical double-layer size and thus in the energy of interaction curves. These variations in interaction between globules during shear may be reflected in their flow behaviour,
2. If a hydrophilic colloid is used to stabilize the emulsion it will form a multimolecular film round the dispersed globules. A reduction in mean globule size will increase the total surface area, and therefore more colloid will be adsorbed on to the droplet surface. This will effectively increase the volume concentration of the dispersed phase.

The particle size of the dispersed phase is therefore controlled mainly by the method and conditions of manufacture of the emulsion, and by the type of emulgent used and its concentration.

Viscosity of the continuous phase

It has been well documented that a direct relationship exists between the viscosity of an emulsion and the viscosity of its continuous phase. Syrup and glycerol, which are used in oral emulsions as sweetening agents, will increase the viscosity of the continuous phase. Their main disadvantage is in increasing the density difference between the two phases, and thus possibly accelerating creaming.

Hydrocolloids, when used as emulsifying agents in o/w emulsions, will stabilize them not only by the formation of multimolecular layers around the dispersed globules, but also by increasing the continuous phase viscosity. They do not have the disadvantage of altering the density of this phase. If oil is the continuous phase, then the inclusion of soft or hard paraffin or certain waxes will increase its viscosity.

Viscosity of the dispersed phase

For most practical applications it is doubtful whether this factor would have any significant effect on total emulsion viscosity. It is possible, however, that a less viscous dispersed phase would, during shear, be deformed to a greater extent than a more viscous phase, and thus the total interfacial area would increase slightly. This may affect double-layer interactions and hence the viscosity of the emulsion.

Nature and concentration of the emulsifying system

It has already been shown that hydrophilic colloids, as well as forming multimolecular films at the oil/water interface, will also increase the viscosity of the continuous phase of an o/w emulsion. Obviously, as the concentration of this type of emulgent increases so will the viscosity of the product.

Surface-active agents forming condensed monomolecular films will, by the nature of their chemical structure, influence the degree of flocculation in a similar way, by forming linkages between adjacent globules and creating a gel-like structure. A flocculated system will exhibit a greater apparent viscosity than its deflocculated counterpart and will depend on surfactant concentration.

Choice of emulsifying agent

Toxicity and irritancy considerations

The choice of emulgent to be used will depend not only on its emulsifying ability, but also on its route of administration and, consequently, on its toxicity. Although there is no approved list of emulsifying agents for use in pharmaceutical products there is an approved list of emulsifiers as food additives for use in the European Union. It can be assumed that emulsifiers contained in this list would be suitable for internally used pharmaceutical emulsions. The regulations mainly include naturally occurring materials and their semisynthetic derivatives, such as the

polysaccharides, as well as glycerol esters, cellulose ethers, sorbitan esters and polysorbates.

It will be noted that most of these are non-ionic, having a tendency to be less irritant and less toxic than their anionic, and particularly their cationic counterparts. The concentrations of ionic emulsifying agents necessary for emulsification will be irritant to the gastrointestinal tract and have a laxative effect, and should not be used for oral emulsions. Cationic surfactants in general are toxic even at lower concentrations. The emulgent cetrimide is limited to externally used preparations, where its antiseptic properties are of use.

Some emulgents, such as the anionic alkali soaps, often have a high pH and are thus unsuitable for application to broken skin. Even on normal intact skin with a pH of 5.5, the application of such alkaline materials can cause irritation. Some emulsifiers, in particular, wool fat can cause sensitization reactions in susceptible people.

When choosing an emulgent for parenteral use it must be realized that only certain types of non-ionic material are suitable. These include lecithin, polysorbate 80, methylcellulose, gelatin and serum albumin.

Formulation by the HLB method

It has already been shown that physically stable emulsions are best achieved by the presence of a condensed layer of emulgent at the oil/water interface, and that the complex interfacial films formed by a blend of an oil-soluble emulsifying agent with a water-soluble one produces the most satisfactory emulsions.

A useful method has been devised for calculating the relative quantities of these emulgents necessary to produce the most physically stable emulsion for a particular oil/water combination. This is called the hydrophile–lipophile balance (HLB) method. Although originally applied to non-ionic surface-active agents, its use has been extended to ionic emulgents. Each surfactant is allocated an HLB number representing the relative proportions of the lipophilic and hydrophilic parts of the molecule. High numbers (up to a theoretical maximum of 20) therefore indicate a surfactant exhibiting mainly hydrophilic or polar properties, whereas low numbers represent lipophilic or non-polar characteristics. Table 23.2 gives HLB values for some commonly used emulsifying agents. The concept of HLB values is discussed more fully in Chapter 6.

Each type of oil used will require an emulgent of a particular HLB number in order to ensure a stable

Table 23.2 HLB values for some pharmaceutical surfactants	
Sorbitan trioleate (Span 85)	1.8
Oleic acid	4.3
Sorbitan mono-oleate (Span 80)	4.3
Sorbitan monostearate (Span 60)	4.7
Sorbitan monolaurate (Span 20)	8.6
Polysorbate 60 (polyoxyethylene sorbitan monostearate)	14.9
Polysorbate 80 (polyoxyethylene sorbitan mono-oleate) (Tween 80)	15.0
Polysorbate 20 (polyoxyethylene sorbitan mono-laurate) (Tween 20)	16.7
Potassium oleate	20.0
Sodium dodecyl (lauryl) sulphate	40.0

product. For an o/w emulsion, for example, the more polar the oil phase the more polar must be the emulgent system.

Table 23.3 gives the required emulgent HLB value for particular oil phases for both types of emulsion. If a formulation contains a mixture of oils, fats or waxes the total HLB required can be calculated. The following example of an o/w emulsion will show this.

Liquid paraffin	35%
Wool fat	1%
Cetyl alcohol	1%
Emulsifier system	5%
Water	to 100%

The total percentage of oil phase is 37 and the proportion of each is:

Liquid paraffin	$35/37 \times 100$	=	94.6%
Wool fat	$1/37 \times 100$	=	2.7%
Cetyl alcohol	$1/37 \times 100$	=	2.7%

The total required HLB number is obtained as follows:

Table 23.3 Required HLB values for a range of oils and waxes		
	For a w/o emulsion	For an o/w emulsion
Beeswax	5	12
Cetyl alcohol	–	15
Liquid paraffin	4	12
Soft paraffin	4	12
Wool fat	8	10

Liquid paraffin (HLB 12)	$94.6/100 \times 12 =$	11.4
Wool fat (HLB 10)	$2.7/100 \times 10 =$	0.3
Cetyl alcohol (HLB 15)	$2.7/100 \times 15 =$	0.4
Total required HLB		**= 12.1**

From theoretical considerations, this particular formulation requires an emulgent blend of HLB 12.1 in order to produce the most stable emulsion. It must be realized, however, that the presence of other ingredients, particularly those that may partition into the oil phase, can also affect the required HLB value. It is therefore often necessary to prepare a series of emulsions using blends of a given pair of non-ionic emulsifying agents covering a wide range of HLB values. This is also important if the required HLB for an oil phase is not available. The HLB value of the emulgent blend giving the most stable emulsion is the required value for that oil phase.

Assuming that a blend of sorbitan mono-oleate (HLB 4.3) and polyoxyethylene sorbitan mono-oleate (HLB 15) is to be used as the emulsifying system, the proportions of each to be added to the emulsion to provide an HLB of 12.1 are calculated as follows.

Let A be the percentage concentration of the hydrophilic and B the percentage of the hydrophobic surfactants required to give a blend having an HLB value of x. Then:

$$A = \frac{100(x - \text{HLB of } B)}{(\text{HLB of } A - \text{HLB of } B)} \quad \text{and} \quad B = 100 - A$$

In our example, therefore:

$$A = \frac{100(12.1 - 4.3)}{(15 - 4.3)} = 72.9$$

$B = 100 - 72.9 = 27.1$

Because the total percentage of emulgent blend in the formulation is 5, the percentage of each emulsifier will be:

Sorbitan mono-oleate	$5 \times 27.1/100 = 1.36$
Polyoxyethylene sorbitan mono-oleate	$5 - 1.36 = 3.64$

The series of trial emulsions can then be assessed for stability, based on the fact that the degree of creaming or separation is at a minimum at the optimal HLB value. Should several of the series show equally poor or equally good stability, resulting in an inability to choose a suitable HLB value, then the total emulgent concentration may be increased or reduced, respectively, and the manufacture of the series repeated.

Having determined the best HLB value for a given pair of emulgents, that value can now be used to assess the suitability of other emulgent blends that may give a better emulsion than the one containing the emulgent used for the initial trials.

It must be remembered that, in choosing an emulsifier blend, the effect of chemical structure on the type of interfacial film must be taken into account. Condensed films are produced by emulgents having long, saturated hydrocarbon groups, thus providing maximum cohesion between adjacent molecules. In most cases it has been found that the most stable emulsions are formed when both emulsifying agents are of the same hydrocarbon chain length.

The use of phase inversion temperature

The use of the HLB system has several disadvantages, including the inability to take into account the effects of temperature, the presence of additives and the concentration of the emulsifier. It is possible to overcome some of these problems.

An o/w emulsion stabilized by non-ionic emulgents will, on heating, invert to form a w/o product. This is because, as the temperature increases, the HLB value of a non-ionic surfactant will decrease as it becomes more hydrophobic. At the temperature at which the emulgent has equal hydrophilic and hydrophobic tendencies (the phase inversion temperature) the emulsion will invert.

The stability of an emulsion has been related to the phase inversion temperature (PIT) of its emulsifying agent (see Chapter 6).

CLASSIFICATION OF EMULSIFYING AGENTS

The inclusion of an emulsifying agent or agents is necessary to facilitate actual emulsification during manufacture, and also to ensure emulsion stability during the shelf-life of the product.

The different methods by which emulsifying agents (also called emulsifiers or emulgents) exert their effects have been detailed in Chapter 6, but the one factor common to all of them is their ability to form an adsorbed film around the dispersed droplets between the two phases. There are many types of emulgent available, but for convenience they can be divided into two main classifications: synthetic or semisynthetic surface-active agents, and naturally occurring materials and their derivatives.

These divisions are quite arbitrary and some materials may justifiably be placed in more than one category.

Synthetic and semisynthetic surface-active agents

There are four main categories of these materials, depending on their ionization in aqueous solutions: anionic, cationic, non-ionic and amphoteric.

Anionic surfactants

In aqueous solutions these compounds dissociate to form negatively charged anions that are responsible for their emulsifying ability. They are widely used because of their cheapness, but because of their toxicity are only used for externally applied preparations.

Alkali metal and ammonium soaps Emulgents in this group consist mainly of the sodium, potassium or ammonium salts of long-chain fatty acids, such as:

$$\text{sodium stearate } C_{17}H_{35}COO^- \, Na^+$$

They produce stable o/w emulsions but may in some instances require the presence of an auxiliary non-ionic emulsifying agent in order to form a complex monomolecular film at the oil/water interface. Because in acidic conditions, these materials will precipitate out as the free fatty acids, they are most efficient in an alkaline medium.

This type of emulgent can also be formed in situ during the manufacture of the product by reacting an alkali such as potassium, sodium or ammonium hydroxide with a fatty acid. The latter may be a constituent of a vegetable oil. Oleic acid and ammonia, for example, are reacted together to form the soap responsible for stabilizing White Liniment.

These emulgents are incompatible with polyvalent cations, often causing phase reversal, and it is therefore essential that deionized water is used in their preparation.

Soaps of divalent and trivalent metals Although many different divalent and trivalent salts of fatty acids exist, and would produce satisfactory emulsions, only the calcium salts are commonly used. They are often formed in situ during preparation of the product by interacting the appropriate fatty acid with calcium hydroxide. For example, oleic acid is reacted with calcium hydroxide to produce calcium oleate, which is the emulsifying agent for both Zinc Cream BP and some formulations of oily calamine lotion.

These emulgents will only produce w/o emulsions.

Amine soaps A number of amines form salts with fatty acids. One of the most important of those used is based on triethanolamine $N(CH_2CH_2OH)_3$ and is widely used in both pharmaceutical and cosmetic products. For example, triethanolamine stearate forms stable o/w emulsions and is usually made in situ by a reaction between triethanolamine and the appropriate fatty acid. Although these emulgents are usually pH neutral they are still restricted to externally used preparations. They are also incompatible with acids and high concentrations of electrolytes.

Sulphated and sulphonated compounds The alkyl sulphates have the general formula $ROSO_3^-M^+$, where R represents a hydrocarbon chain and M^+ is usually sodium or triethanolamine. An example is sodium lauryl sulphate, which is widely used to produce o/w emulsions. Because of its high water solubility and its inability to form condensed films at the oil/water interface, it is always used in conjunction with a non-ionic oil-soluble emulsifying agent in order to produce a complex condensed film. It is used with cetostearyl alcohol to produce Emulsifying Wax, which stabilizes such preparations as Aqueous Cream and Benzyl Benzoate Application.

Sulphonated compounds are much less widely used as emulgents. Materials of this class include sodium dioctylsulphosuccinate, and are more often used as wetting agents or for their detergency.

Cationic surfactants

In aqueous solutions these materials dissociate to form positively charged cations that provide the emulsifying properties. The most important group of cationic emulgents consists of the quaternary ammonium compounds. Although these materials are widely used for their disinfectant and preservative properties, they are also useful o/w emulsifiers. Like many anionic emulgents, if used on their own they will produce only poor emulsions, but if used with non-ionic oil-soluble auxiliary emulgents they will form stable preparations.

Because of the toxicity of cationic surfactants they tend to be used only for the formulation of antiseptic creams, where the cationic nature of the emulgent is also responsible for the product's antiseptic properties.

Cationic emulsifying agents are incompatible with anionic surface-active agents and polyvalent anions, and are unstable at high pH.

Cetrimide The most useful of these cationic emulgents is cetrimide (cetyl trimethylammonium bromide) $CH_3(CH_2)_{15}N^+(CH_3)_3Br^-$. Cetrimide is used at a concentration of 0.5% with 5% cetostearyl alcohol for the formulation of Cetrimide Cream BP.

Non-ionic surfactants

These products range from oil-soluble compounds stabilizing w/o emulsions to water-soluble materials giving o/w products. It is usual for a combination of a water-soluble with an oil-soluble emulgent to be used in order to obtain the complex interfacial film necessary for optimum emulsion stability. Non-ionic emulgents are particularly useful because of their low toxicity and irritancy; some can therefore be used for orally and parenterally administered preparations. They also have a greater degree of compatibility with other materials than do anionic or cationic emulgents, and are less sensitive to changes in pH or to the addition of electrolytes. They do, however, tend to be more expensive.

Being non-ionic, the dispersed globules may not possess a significant charge density. To reduce the tendency for coalescence to occur in an oil-in-water emulsion, it is necessary that the polar groups be well hydrated and/or sufficiently large to prevent close approach of the dispersed droplets in order to compensate for the lack of charge.

Most non-ionic surfactants are based on:

- a fatty acid or alcohol (usually with 12–18 carbon atoms), the hydrocarbon chain of which provides the hydrophobic moiety;
- an alcohol (-OH) and/or ethylene oxide grouping ($-OCH_2CH_2-$), which provide the hydrophilic part of the molecule.

By varying the relative proportions of the hydrophilic and hydrophobic groupings many different products can be obtained.

If the hydrophobic part of the molecule predominates, then the surfactant will be oil-soluble. It will not concentrate at the oil/water interface but rather tend to migrate into the oil phase. Similarly, a water-soluble surfactant will migrate into the aqueous phase and away from the oil/water interface. The best type of non-ionic surfactant to use is one with an equal balance of hydrophobic and hydrophilic groupings. An alternative would be to use two emulgents, one hydrophilic and one hydrophobic. The cohesion between their hydrocarbon chains will then hold both types at the oil/water interface.

Glycol and glycerol esters Glyceryl monostearate (a polyhydric alcohol fatty acid ester) is a strongly hydrophobic material that produces weak w/o emulsions. The addition of small amounts of sodium, potassium or triethanolamine salts of suitable fatty acids will produce a 'self-emulsifying' glyceryl monostearate, which is a useful o/w emulsifier. Self-emulsifying monostearin is glyceryl monostearate to which anionic soaps (usually oleate or stearate) have been added. This combination is used to stabilize Hydrocortisone Lotion.

Other polyhydric alcohol fatty acid esters are also available either in the pure form or in the 'self-emulsifying' form containing small proportions of a primary emulsifier, and include glyceryl mono-oleate, diethylene glycol monostearate and propylene glycol mono-oleate.

Sorbitan esters These are produced by the esterification of one or more of the hydroxyl groups of sorbitan with either lauric, oleic, palmitic or stearic acids. The structure of sorbitan monostearate is shown below.

This range of surfactants exhibits lipophilic properties and tends to form w/o emulsions. They are, however, much more widely used with polysorbates to produce either o/w or w/o emulsions.

Polysorbates Polyethylene glycol derivatives of the sorbitan esters give us polysorbates. These have the general formula:

where R represents a fatty acid chain. Variations in the type of fatty acid used and in the number of oxyethylene groups in the polyethylene glycol chains produce a range of products of differing oil and water solubilities. Polyoxyethylene 20 sorbitan mono-oleate, for example, contains 20 oxyethylene groups in the molecule. This number must not be confused with the one given as part of the official name (Polysorbate 80) or in the trade name (Tween 80), which is included in order to identify the type of fatty acid in the molecule.

Polysorbates are generally used in conjunction with the corresponding sorbitan ester to form a complex condensed film at the oil/water interface (see Formulation by the HLB method, earlier).

Other non-ionic oil-soluble materials, such as glyceryl monostearate, cetyl or stearyl alcohol or

propylene glycol monostearate, can be incorporated with polysorbates to produce 'self-emulsifying' preparations. For example, Polawax contains cetyl alcohol with a polyoxyethylene sorbitan ester.

Polysorbates are compatible with most anionic, cationic and non-ionic materials. They are pH neutral and are stable to the effects of heat, pH change and high concentrations of electrolyte. Their low toxicity renders them suitable for oral use and some are also used in parenteral preparations. They have the disadvantage, however, of an unpleasant taste, and care must be taken when selecting a suitable preservative as many are inactivated by complexation with polysorbates.

Fatty alcohol polyglycol ethers These are condensation products of polyethylene glycol and fatty alcohols, usually cetyl or cetostearyl:

$$ROH + (CH_2CH_2O)_n \rightarrow RO(CH_2CH_2O)_nH$$

where R is a fatty alcohol chain.

Perhaps the most widely used is macrogol cetostearyl ether (22) or cetomacrogol 1000, which is polyethylene glycol monocetyl ether. This is a very useful water-soluble o/w emulgent, but because of its high water solubility it is necessary to include an oil-soluble auxiliary emulsifier when formulating emulsions. Cetomacrogol Emulsifying Ointment includes cetomacrogol 1000 and cetostearyl alcohol and is used to stabilize cetomacrogol creams.

They can also be produced with shorter polyoxyethylene groups as lipophilic w/o emulsifiers. Combinations of lipophilic and hydrophilic ethers can be used together to produce stable emulsions.

These materials can be salted out by the addition of high concentrations of electrolyte, but are stable over a wide pH range.

Fatty acid polyglycol esters The stearate esters or polyoxyl stearates are the most widely used of this type of emulgent. Polyoxyethylene 40 stearate (in which 40 represents the number of oxyethylene units) is a water-soluble material often used with stearyl alcohol to give o/w emulsions.

Poloxalkols Poloxalkols are polyoxyethylene/polyoxypropylene copolymers with the general formula:

$$OH(C_2H_4O)_a(C_3H_6O)_b(C_2H_4O)_a$$

and comprise a very large group of compounds, some of which are used as emulsifying agents for intravenous fat emulsions.

Higher fatty alcohols The hexadecyl (cetyl) and octadecyl (stearyl) members of this series of saturated aliphatic monohydric alcohols are useful auxiliary emulsifying agents. Part of their stabilizing effect comes from their ability to increase the viscosity of the preparation, thereby retarding creaming. Cetostearyl alcohol will also form complex interfacial films with hydrophilic surface-active agents such as sodium lauryl sulphate, cetrimide or cetomacrogol 1000, and so stabilize o/w emulsions.

Amphoteric surfactants

This type possesses both positively and negatively charged groups, depending on the pH of the system. They are cationic at low pH and anionic at high pH. Although they are not widely used as emulsifying agents, one example, lecithin, is used to stabilize intravenous fat emulsions.

Naturally occurring materials and their derivatives

Naturally occurring materials often suffer from two main disadvantages: they show considerable batch-to-batch variation in composition and hence in emulsifying properties, and many are susceptible to bacterial or mould growth. For these reasons they are not widely used in manufactured products requiring a long shelf-life, but rather for extemporaneously prepared emulsions designed for use within a few days of manufacture.

Polysaccharides

The most important emulsifying agent in this group is acacia. This stabilizes o/w emulsions by forming a strong multimolecular film round each oil globule, and so coalescence is retarded by the presence of a hydrophilic barrier between the oil and water phases.

Because of its low viscosity, creaming will occur readily, and therefore a suspending agent such as tragacanth or sodium alginate can also be included. Because of its sticky nature the use of acacia is limited to products for internal use.

Semisynthetic polysaccharides

In order to reduce the problems associated with batch-to-batch variation, semisynthetic derivatives are available as o/w emulgents or stabilizers.

Several grades of methylcellulose and carmellose sodium are available and exert their action in a similar way to that of acacia.

Methylcellulose 20, for example, is used at a concentration of 2% to stabilize Liquid Paraffin Oral Emulsion.

Sterol-containing substances

Beeswax, wool fat and wool alcohols are all used in the formulation of emulsions. Beeswax is used mainly in cosmetic creams of both o/w and w/o type, in conjunction with borax. Because of the systemic toxicity of boric acid and its salts, however, the use of beeswax/borax preparations is limited, although beeswax is used as a stabilizer for w/o creams.

Wool fat (anhydrous lanolin) consists chiefly of normal fatty alcohols with fatty acid esters of cholesterol and other sterols. It will form w/o emulsions of low dispersed phase concentration, and it can also be incorporated for its emollient properties. Some individuals exhibit sensitization to this material and, because of its characteristic odour and the need to incorporate antioxidants, it is not widely used. It is, however, to be found in low concentrations in many ointments, where its water-absorbing properties are of great value. It can be employed as an emulsion stabilizer with a primary emulsifying agent, for example with calcium oleate in oily calamine lotion, with beeswax in Proflavine Cream, and with cetostearyl alcohol in Zinc Cream and ichthammol cream.

Because wool fat has some ideal properties, attempts have been made to improve its other, less desirable, characteristics by physical and chemical modification. Processes including hydrogenation and fractionation have been carried out with some success. It has also been converted, by a reaction with ethylene oxide, to give a range of polyoxyethylene lanolin derivatives. These non-ionic products are mainly water soluble and are used as o/w emulgents possessing the properties of emollience.

The principal emulsifying agent in wool fat is wool alcohols, which consists mainly of cholesterol together with other alcohols. It is an effective w/o emulgent, being more powerful than wool fat, and is used in the formulation of Hydrous Ointment. It is also incorporated as Wool Alcohols Ointment into other ointment bases which, although not emulsions, will readily mix with aqueous skin secretions and easily wash off the skin. Wool alcohols does not have the same strong odour as wool fat but does require the presence of an antioxidant.

Finely divided solids

Certain finely divided solids can be adsorbed at the oil/water interface, forming a coherent film that physically prevents coalescence of the dispersed globules. If the particles are preferentially wetted by the aqueous phase then o/w products will result, whereas preferential wetting by the oil will produce w/o emulsions.

Montmorillonite clays (such as bentonite and aluminium magnesium silicate) and colloidal silicon dioxide are used mainly for external use. Aluminium and magnesium hydroxides are also used internally. For example, Liquid Paraffin and Magnesium Hydroxide Oral Emulsion BP is stabilized by the incorporation of the magnesium hydroxide.

Other formulation additives

Buffers

The inclusion of buffers (see Chapters 3, 21 and 35) may be necessary to maintain chemical stability, control tonicity or ensure physiological compatibility. It must be remembered, however, that the addition of electrolytes may have profound effects on the physical stability of suspensions and emulsions.

Density modifiers

From a qualitative examination of Stokes' law (Chapter 6) it can be seen that if the disperse and continuous phases both have the same densities then sedimentation or creaming will not occur. Minor modifications to the aqueous phase of a suspension or emulsion by incorporating sucrose, dextrose, glycerol or propylene glycol can be achieved, but because of the differing coefficients of expansion this can only be possible over a small temperature range.

Humectants

Glycerol, polyethylene glycol and propylene glycol are examples of suitable humectants that can be incorporated at concentrations of about 5% into aqueous suspensions for external application. They are used to prevent the product from drying out after application to the skin.

They can also be added to an emulsion formulation in order to reduce the evaporation of the water, either from the packaged product when the closure is removed or from the surface of the skin after application. High concentrations, if used topically, may actually remove moisture from the skin, thereby dehydrating it.

Antioxidants

Before including an antioxidant in emulsion formulations, it is essential to ensure that its use is not restricted in whichever country it is desired to sell the product. In Britain, butylated hydroxyanisole (BHA) is widely used for the protection of fixed oils and fats at concentrations of up to 0.02% and for some essential oils up to 0.1%. A similar antioxidant

is butylated hydroxytoluene (BHT), which is recommended as an alternative to tocopherol at a concentration of 10 ppm to stabilize liquid paraffin. Other antioxidants widely used for emulsion formulation include the propyl, octyl and dodecyl esters of gallic acid, recommended for use at concentrations up to 0.001% for fixed oils and fats and up to 0.1% for essential oils.

The efficiency of an antioxidant in a product will depend on many factors, including its compatibility with other ingredients, its oil/water partition coefficient, the extent of its solubilization within micelles of the emulgent, and its sorption on to the container and its closure. It must be realized, therefore, that the choice of antioxidant and the concentration at which it is to be used can only be determined by testing its effectiveness in the final product and in the package in which the product is to be sold.

Flavours, colours and perfumes

The use of these ingredients is discussed in Chapter 21 and the information there will be directly applicable to suspension and emulsion formulation.

Adsorption of these materials on to the surfaces of the dispersed phase of a suspension may occur, and because of the high surface area of the dispersed powders in this type of formulation, their effective concentrations in solution may be significantly reduced. The finer the degree of subdivision of the disperse phase, the paler may appear the colour of the product for a given concentration of dye.

It must also be realized that the inclusion of these adjuvants may alter the physical characteristics of both suspensions and emulsions. Either the presence of electrolytes or their effect on pH can influence the degree of flocculation.

Sweetening agents

Suitable sweeteners are discussed in Chapter 21. High concentrations of sucrose, sorbitol or glycerol, which will exhibit Newtonian properties, may adversely affect the rheological properties of the suspension. Synthetic sweeteners may be salts and can affect the degree of flocculation.

Preservation of suspensions and emulsions

Preservation of suspensions

The section covering the preservation of emulsions is applicable also to suspension formulation. It is essential that a suitable preservative be included, particularly if naturally occurring materials are to be used. This is to prevent the growth of microorganisms that may be present in the raw material and/or introduced into the product during use. Some of the natural products, particularly if they are to be applied to broken skin, should be sterilized before use. Bentonite, for example, may contain *Clostridium tetani* but can be sterilized by heating the dry powder at 160°C for 1 hour or by autoclaving aqueous dispersions.

As with emulsion formulation, care must be taken to ascertain the extent of inactivation, if any, of the preservative system caused by interaction with other excipients. Solubilization by wetting agents, interaction with polymers or adsorption on to suspended solids, particularly kaolin or magnesium trisilicate, may reduce the availability of preservatives.

Preservation of emulsions

Problems associated with the growth of microorganisms in pharmaceutical products are discussed in Chapter 43. Those microbiological factors of specific importance to the stability of emulsions are discussed later in this chapter. The necessity of including a preservative in an emulsion formulation is discussed below.

Unfortunately there is no theoretical way of choosing a suitable preservative system, the only reliable methods being based on the results of suitable challenge tests. These methods of testing preservative activity are given in official compendia, but essentially involve the addition to the test products of a mixture of Gram-positive and Gram-negative bacteria, yeasts and moulds, and comparing their survival with a control sample containing no preservative.

The desirable features of a preservative suitable for use in an emulsion include:

- a wide spectrum of activity against all bacteria, yeasts and moulds;
- bactericidal rather than bacteristatic activity. A preservative having a minimal bacteristatic activity may lose it if any physical or chemical changes occur in the system;
- freedom from toxic, irritant or sensitizing activity;
- high water solubility. Because the growth of microorganisms occurs in the aqueous phase, it is important that the preservative has a low oil/water partition coefficient. The more polar the oil phase, the more difficult it is to preserve the product adequately, owing to the solubility of the preservative in both phases. If the preservative is

more soluble in oil than in water, then increasing the proportion of oil will decrease the aqueous phase concentration. Allowance must be made for this when choosing the phase–volume ratios;
- compatibility with the other ingredients and with the container. Certain preservatives are incompatible with particular groups of emulsifying agent. Phenols and the esters of *p*-hydroxybenzoic acid, for example, will complex with some non-ionic emulgents, owing to either a reaction with oxyethylene groups or solubilization within micelles of excess surfactant. In many cases it is possible, by chemical assay, to detect the correct concentration of preservative in the product even though some of it may not be available for antimicrobial activity. If some of the added preservative has been inactivated it may be possible to overcome this problem by increasing the amount of preservative in the product to give a satisfactory concentration of free preservative in the aqueous phase. It is important to ensure that, during manufacture, the preservative is added after the emulgent has concentrated at the oil/water interface;
- stability and effectiveness over a wide range of pH and temperatures;
- freedom from colour and odour;
- retention of activity in the presence of large numbers of microorganisms. Uptake of preservative by bacterial cells may deplete the concentration of preservative in solution, thereby rendering it insufficient to maintain adequate bactericidal activity.

Because of the complex systems involved and the many factors to be taken into consideration, it is necessary to test the efficiency of a new preservative in the finished product and container by suitable challenge testing procedures.

The most widely used preservatives in emulsions include benzoic and sorbic acid and their salts, *p*-hydroxybenzoic acid esters, chlorocresol, phenoxyethanol, bronopol, quaternary ammonium compounds and, to a lesser extent, organic mercurials. Because of the irritancy and toxicity of certain preservatives, the initial choice will depend on the route of administration of the product. Further details of the use of preservatives in emulsions can be found in Chapter 42.

It must be realized that no single preservative exhibits all of the desirable properties outlined earlier. In many cases a combination is required, the most widely used being a mixture of methyl and propyl *p*-hydroxybenzoates at a ratio usually of 10:1.

PHYSICAL STABILITY OF SUSPENSIONS

The physical stability of a suspension is normally assessed by the measurement of its rate of sedimentation, the final volume or height of the sediment, and the ease of redispersion of the product.

The first two parameters can be assessed easily by a measurement of the total initial volume or height of the suspension (V_0) and the volume or height of the sediment (V_t), as shown in Figure 23.1. By plotting the value of V_t/V_0 against time for a series of trial formulations (all initial values will equal unity), it can be seen, by an assessment of the slope of each line, which suspension shows the slowest rate of sedimentation. When the value of V_t/V_0 becomes constant this indicates that sedimentation has ceased.

Alternatively, the term flocculation value can be used, which is a ratio of the final volume or height of the sediment and the volume or height of the fully sedimented cake of the same system which has been deflocculated.

Attempts have also been made to equate the zeta potential of the suspended particles with the physical stability – particularly the degree of flocculation – of the system using electrophoresis.

The ease of redispersion of the product can be assessed qualitatively by simply agitating the product in its container. The use of a mechanical shaker will eliminate variations in shaking ability.

PHYSICAL STABILITY OF EMULSIONS

A stable emulsion is one in which the dispersed globules retain their initial character and remain uniformly distributed throughout the continuous phase. Various types of deviation from this ideal behaviour can occur. Explanations for emulsion stability have been given in Chapter 6. This section will concentrate on methods of improving emulsion stability in practice.

Creaming and its avoidance

This is the separation of an emulsion into two regions, one of which is richer in the disperse phase than the other. A simple example is the creaming of milk, when fat globules slowly rise to the top of the product. This is not a serious instability problem as a uniform dispersion can be reobtained simply by shaking the emulsion. It is, however, undesirable because of the increased likelihood of coalescence of the droplets, owing to their close proximity to each other. A creamed emulsion is also inelegant and, if the emulsion is not shaken adequately, there is a risk of the patient obtaining an incorrect dosage.

Consideration of the qualitative application of Stokes' law will show that the rate of creaming can be reduced by the following methods.

Production of an emulsion of small droplet size

This factor usually depends on the method of manufacture. An efficient emulsifying agent will not only stabilize the emulsion but also facilitate the actual emulsification process to give a product of fine globule size.

Increase in the viscosity of the continuous phase

Many auxiliary emulsifying agents, in particular the hydrophilic colloids, are viscosity enhancers and this property is part of their emulsifying capability. For example, the inclusion of methylcellulose will reduce the mobility of the dispersed droplets in an o/w emulsion. The addition of soft paraffin will have the same effect on water droplets in a w/o emulsion.

Storage of the product at a low temperature (but above freezing point) will increase the viscosity of the continuous phase and also reduce the kinetic energy of the system. This will decrease the rate of migration of the globules of the disperse phase. It is unwise, however, to rely solely on this method of controlling creaming, as storage conditions after the product is sold are outside the control of the manufacturer.

Reduction in the density difference between the two phases

Creaming could be prevented altogether if the densities of the two phases were identical. In practice this method is never used, as it could only be achieved over a very narrow temperature range owing to differences in the coefficients of expansion between different ingredients.

Control of disperse phase concentration

It is not easy to stabilize an emulsion containing less than 20% disperse phase, as creaming will readily occur. A higher disperse phase concentration would result in a hindrance of movement of the droplets and hence in a reduction in rate of creaming.

Although it is theoretically possible to include as much as 74% of an internal phase, it is usually found that at about 60% concentration phase inversion occurs.

Finally, it must be realized that some of the factors above are interrelated. For example, homogenization of the emulsion would decrease globule size and, by thus increasing their number, increase the viscosity of the product.

Flocculation prevention

Flocculation involves the aggregation of the dispersed globules into loose clusters within the emulsion. The individual droplets retain their identities but each cluster behaves physically as a single unit. This, as we have already seen, would increase the rate of creaming. As flocculation must precede coalescence, any factor preventing or retarding flocculation would therefore maintain the stability of the emulsion.

Flocculation in the secondary minimum (see Fig. 6.3) occurs readily and cannot be avoided. Redispersion can easily be achieved by shaking. Primary minimum flocculation, however, is more serious and redispersion is not so easy.

The presence of a high charge density on the dispersed droplets will ensure the presence of a high energy barrier, and thus reduce the incidence of flocculation in the primary minimum. Care must be taken to ensure that the effects of any ions in the product are taken into consideration very early in the formulation process. This is particularly important when formulating emulsions for parenteral nutrition which contain high levels of electrolytes (Washington 1990).

Coalescence (breaking, cracking)

The coalescence of oil globules in an o/w emulsion is resisted by the presence of a mechanically strong adsorbed layer of emulsifier around each globule. This is achieved by the presence of either a condensed mixed monolayer of lipophilic and hydrophilic emulgents, or a multimolecular film of a hydrophilic material. Hydration of either of these types of film will hinder the drainage of water from between adjacent globules which is necessary prior to coalescence. As two globules, approach each other their close proximity causes their adjacent surfaces to flatten. As a change from a sphere to any other shape results in an increase in surface area and hence in total surface free energy, this globule distortion will be resisted and drainage of the film of continuous phase from between the two globules will be delayed.

The presence of long, cohesive hydrocarbon chains projecting into the oil phase will prevent coalescence in a w/o emulsion.

CHEMICAL INSTABILITY OF EMULSIONS

Although it is not possible to list every incompatibility, the following general points will illustrate the more common chemical problems that can cause the coalescence of an emulsion.

It is necessary to ensure that any emulgent system used is not only physically but also chemically compatible with the active agent and with the other emulsion ingredients. Ionic emulsifying agents, for example, are usually incompatible with materials of opposite charge. Anionic and cationic emulgents are thus mutually incompatible.

It has already been demonstrated that the presence of electrolyte can influence the stability of an emulsion either by:

- reducing the energy of interaction between adjacent globules, or
- a salting-out effect, by which high concentrations of electrolytes can strip emulsifying agents of their hydrated layers and so cause their precipitation.

In some cases phase inversion may occur rather than demulsification. If, for example, a sodium soap is used to stabilize an o/w emulsion, then the addition of a divalent electrolyte such as calcium chloride may form the calcium soap, which will stabilize a w/o emulsion.

Emulgents may also be precipitated by the addition of materials in which they are insoluble. It may be possible to precipitate hydrophilic colloids by the addition of alcohol. For this reason care must therefore be taken if tinctures are to be included in emulsion formulations.

Changes in pH may also lead to the breaking of emulsions. Sodium soaps may react with acids to produce the free fatty acid and the sodium salt of the acid. Soap-stabilized emulsions are therefore usually formulated at an alkaline pH.

Oxidation

Many of the oils and fats used in emulsion formulation are of animal or vegetable origin and can be susceptible to oxidation by atmospheric oxygen or by the action of microorganisms. The resulting rancidity is manifested by the formation of degradation products of unpleasant odour and taste. These problems can also occur with certain emulsifying agents, such as wool fat or wool alcohols. Oxidation of microbiological origin is controlled by the use of antimicrobial preservatives, and atmospheric oxidation by the use of reducing agents or, more usually, antioxidants. Some examples are mentioned earlier in this chapter.

Microbiological contamination

The contamination of emulsions by microorganisms can adversely affect the physicochemical properties of the product, causing such problems as gas production, colour and odour changes, hydrolysis of fats and oils, pH changes in the aqueous phase, and breaking of the emulsion. Even without visible signs of contamination an emulsion can contain many bacteria and, if these include pathogens, may constitute a serious health hazard. Most fungi and many bacteria will multiply readily in the aqueous phase of an emulsion at room temperature, and many moulds will also tolerate a wide pH range. Some of the hydrophilic colloids, which are widely used as emulsifying agents, may provide a suitable nutritive medium for use by bacteria and moulds. Species of the genus *Pseudomonas* can utilize polysorbates, aliphatic hydrocarbons and compounds. Some fixed oils, including arachis oil, can be used by some *Aspergillus* and *Rhizopus* species, and liquid paraffin by some species of *Penicillium*.

A few emulgents, particularly those from natural sources, may introduce heavy contamination into products in which they are used. Because bacteria can reproduce in resin beds, deionized water may be unsatisfactory and even distilled water, if incorrectly stored after collection, can be another source of contamination. Oil-in-water emulsions tend to be more susceptible to microbial spoilage than water-in-oil products as, in the latter case the continuous oil phase acts as a barrier to the spread of microorganisms throughout the product, and the less water there is present the less growth there is likely to be.

It is therefore, necessary to include an antimicrobial agent to prevent the growth of any microorganisms that might contaminate the product. Suitable candidates are discussed in Chapter 42.

Adverse storage conditions

Adverse storage conditions may also cause emulsion instability. It has already been explained that an increase in temperature will cause an increase in the rate of creaming, owing to a fall in apparent viscosity of the continuous phase. The temperature increase will also cause an increased kinetic motion, both of the dispersed droplets and of the emulsifying agent at the oil/water interface. This effect on the disperse phase will enable the energy barrier to be easily surmounted and thus the number of collisions between globules will increase. Increased motion of the emulgent will result in a more expanded monolayer, and so coalescence is more likely. Certain macromolecular emulsifying agents may also be coagulated by an increase in temperature.

At the other extreme, freezing of the aqueous phase will produce ice crystals that may exert unusual pressures on the dispersed globules and their adsorbed layer of emulgent. In addition, dissolved electrolyte may concentrate in the unfrozen water, thus affecting the charge density on the globules. Certain emulgents may also precipitate at low temperatures.

The growth of microorganisms within the emulsion can cause deterioration and it is therefore essential that these products are protected as far as possible from the ingress of microorganisms during manufacture, storage and use, and that they contain adequate preservatives.

STABILITY TESTING OF EMULSIONS

Methods of assessing stability

Macroscopic examination

The physical stability of an emulsion can be assessed by an examination of the degree of creaming or coalescence occurring over a period of time. This is carried out by calculating the ratio of the volume of the creamed or separated part of the emulsion and the total volume. These values can be compared for different products.

Globule size analysis

If the mean globule size increases with time (coupled with a decrease in globule numbers), it can be assumed that coalescence is the cause. It is therefore possible to compare the rates of coalescence for a variety of emulsion formulations by this method. Microscopic examination or electronic particle counting devices, such as the Coulter counter, or laser diffraction sizing are most widely used.

Viscosity changes

It has already been shown that many factors influence the viscosity of emulsions. Any variation in globule size or number, or in the orientation or migration of emulsifier over a period of time, may be detected by a change in apparent viscosity. Suitable methods and equipment are detailed in Chapter 4.

In order to compare the relative stabilities of a range of similar products it is often necessary to speed up the processes of creaming and coalescence. This can be achieved in one of the following ways.

Accelerated stability tests

To assess the physical stability of suspensions and emulsions macroscopic examination and measurement of apparent viscosity are of value. In addition, for emulsions, microscopic evaluation of globule size distribution and numbers will provide further evidence of changes in physical stability.

Storage at adverse temperatures

An assessment of these parameters at elevated temperatures for emulsions and coarse suspensions would give a speedier indication of a rank order of degree of instability, but it is essential to correlate these results with those taken from suspensions stored at ambient temperatures.

Temperature cycling By exaggerating the temperature fluctuations to which any product is subjected under normal storage conditions, it may be possible to compare the physical stabilities of a series of suspensions or emulsions. Temperature cycles consisting of storage for several hours at about 40°C, followed by refrigeration or freezing until instability becomes evident, have been used successfully. The continual formation and melting of small ice crystals will disrupt the adsorbed layer of emulgent at the oil/water interface, and any weakness in the structure of the film will quickly become apparent. Similarly, normal temperature fluctuations can be used, but at increased frequencies of only a few minutes at each extreme. This method of accelerated stability testing is particularly useful for the assessment of crystal growth in suspensions. Measurement of particle size is usually carried out microscopically, by laser diffraction or by use of a Coulter counter. It is of course important to ensure that the suspension is deflocculated to ensure that each individual particle is measured, rather than each floccule.

Centrifugation

A qualitative examination of Stokes' law (Chapters 4 and 10) would indicate centrifugation to be a suitable method for artificially increasing the rate of sedimentation of a suspension. Again, it is not always possible to predict accurately the behaviour of such a system when stored under normal conditions from data obtained after this type of accelerated testing. The process of centrifugation may destroy the structure of a flocculated system that would remain intact under normal storage conditions. The sediment formed would become tightly packed and difficult to redisperse, whether or not the initial suspension was flocculated or deflocculated. This method may, however, give a useful indication of the relative stabilities of a series of trial products, particularly if used at speeds no faster than 200–300 rpm.

Rheological assessment

Although apparent viscosity measurements are also used as a tool to assess physical stability, the high shear rates involved may also destroy the structure of a suspension or emulsion. Very low rates of shear, using for example the Brookfield viscometer with Helipath stand, can give an indication of the change in the structure of the system after various storage times. For suspensions it may be possible to combine the results from sedimentation techniques with those from rheological assessments.

A measurement of the residual apparent viscosity, after breaking down the structure of the suspension, can be used as a routine quality control procedure after manufacture.

MANUFACTURE OF SUSPENSIONS

It is important to ensure initially that the powder to be suspended is in a suitably fine degree of subdivision in order to ensure adequate bioavailability, minimum sedimentation rate and impalpability. Suitable size reduction equipment and the relative merits of wet and dry milling are detailed in Chapter 11.

For the extemporaneous preparation of suspensions on a small scale, the powdered drug can be mixed with the suspending agent and some of the vehicle using a pestle and mortar. It may also be necessary, at this stage, to include a wetting agent to aid dispersion. Other soluble ingredients should then be dissolved in another portion of the vehicle, mixed with the concentrated suspension and then made up to volume.

It is often preferable, particularly on a larger scale, to make a concentrated dispersion of the suspending agent first. This is best accomplished by adding the material slowly to the vehicle while mixing. Suitable mixers are described under Manufacture of emulsions, but can include either an impeller type of blender or a turbine mixer. This stage is important, as it is necessary to ensure that agglomerates of the suspending agent are fully broken up. If they are not, then the surface of each agglomerate may gel and cause the powder inside to remain non-wetted. Very intense shearing, however, can destroy the polymeric structure of the suspending agent, and it may be better to use milder shearing and then allow the dispersion to stand until full hydration has been achieved. This may be instantaneous or may, as with tragacanth, take several hours. If the suspending agent is blended with one of the water-soluble ingredients, such as sucrose, this will also aid dispersion.

The drug to be suspended is then added in the same way, along with the wetting agent. For very hydrophobic drugs, wetting may be facilitated by mixing under reduced pressure. This has the additional advantage of de-aerating the product and thus improving its appearance. Other ingredients should now be added, preferably dissolved in a portion of the vehicle, and the whole made up to volume if necessary. Finally, homogenization (see under Manufacture of emulsions) would ensure complete dispersion of the drug and the production of a smooth and elegant preparation.

It is also possible, though much less widely used, to suspend an insoluble drug by precipitating it from a solution. This can be accomplished either by double decomposition or, if it is a weak acid or a weak base, by altering the pH of its solution or by precipitating the drug from a water-miscible solvent on the addition of water. This method may be of use if the drug is required to be sterile but is degraded by heat or irradiation. A soluble form of the drug is dissolved in a suitable vehicle, sterilized by filtration and then precipitated to form a suspension.

In normal circumstances aqueous suspensions can be autoclaved, as long as the process does not adversely affect either physical or chemical stability.

MANUFACTURE OF EMULSIONS

It has already been explained that the smaller the globules of the disperse phase, the slower will be the rate of creaming in an emulsion. The size of these globules can also affect the viscosity of the product, and in general it has been found that the best emulsions with respect to physical stability and texture exhibit a mean globule diameter of between 0.5 and 2.5 μm. The choice of suitable equipment for the emulsification process depends mainly on the intensity of shearing required to produce this optimum particle size. Other considerations, however, include the volume and viscosity of the emulsion and the interfacial tension between the oil and the water. The presence of surfactants, which will reduce interfacial tension, will aid the process of emulsification as well as promoting emulsion stability.

In many cases simple blending of the oil and water phases with a suitable emulgent system may be sufficient to produce satisfactory emulsions. Further processing using a homogenizer can also be carried out to reduce globule size still further. The initial blending may be accomplished on a small scale by the use of a pestle and mortar or by using a mixer fitted with an impeller type of agitator, the size and type of which will depend primarily on the volume and viscosity of the emulsified product.

A more intense rate of shearing can be achieved using a turbine mixer such as the Silverson mixer–homogenizer. In this type of machine the short, vertical or angled rotor blades are enclosed within a stationary perforated ring and connected by a central rod to a motor. The liquids are therefore subjected to intense shearing, caused initially by the rotating blades, and then by the forced discharge through the perforated ring. Different models are available for a variety of batch sizes up to several thousand litres, and can include inline models.

The mixing vessel may also be fitted with baffles in order to modify the circulation of the liquid, and may be jacketed so that heating or cooling can be applied.

Homogenizers are often used after initial mixing to enable smaller globule sizes to be produced. They all work on the principle of forced discharge of the emulsion under pressure through fine interstices, formed by closely packed metal surfaces, in order to provide an intense shearing action.

If two immiscible liquids are subjected to ultrasonic vibrations, alternate regions of compression and rarefaction are produced. Cavities are then formed in the regions of rarefaction, which then collapse with considerable force causing emulsification. The required frequency of vibration is usually produced electrically, but mechanical methods are also available. Unfortunately this method of emulsification is limited to small-scale production.

Colloid mills are also suitable for the preparation of emulsions on a continuous basis. The intense shearing of the product between the rotor and the stator, which can be variably separated, will produce emulsions of very small globule size.

It is important to ensure that methods of manufacture developed on a laboratory scale can be easily extended to large-scale production, and without any change in the quality of the product.

During manufacture it is usual to add the disperse phase to the continuous phase during the initial mixing. The other ingredients are dissolved, prior to mixing, in the phase in which they are soluble. This is particularly important when making w/o emulsions. Oil-in-water emulsions, however, are sometimes made by the phase-inversion technique, in which the aqueous phase is slowly added to the oil phase during mixing. Initially a w/o emulsion is formed but, as further aqueous phase is added the emulsion inverts to form the intended product. This method often produces emulsions of very low mean droplet size.

Should any of the oily ingredients be of solid or semisolid consistency they must be melted before mixing. It is also essential that the aqueous phase be heated to the same temperature, to avoid premature solidification of the oil phase by the colder water on mixing but before emulsification has taken place. This also has the advantage of reducing the viscosity of the system, so enabling shear forces to be transmitted through the product more easily. Because of the increased kinetic motion of the emulgent molecules at the oil/water interface, however, it is necessary to continue stirring during the cooling process to avoid demulsification.

Volatile ingredients, including flavours and perfumes, are usually added after the emulsion has cooled. It must, however, be sufficiently fluid to enable adequate blending. Ingredients that may influence the physical stability of the emulsion, such as alcoholic solutions or electrolytes, require to be diluted as much as possible before adding slowly and with constant mixing.

RELEASE OF DRUGS FROM SUSPENSION AND EMULSION FORMULATIONS

Drug release from suspensions

After the oral administration of a suspension the drug, which is already in a wetted state, is presented to the gastrointestinal fluids in a finely divided form.

Dissolution therefore occurs immediately. The rate of absorption of the drug into the bloodstream is therefore usually faster than for the same drug in a solid dosage form, but not as fast as that from a solution. The rate of release of a drug from a suspension is also dependent upon the viscosity of the product. The more viscous the preparation, the slower is likely to be the release of the drug. Care must therefore be taken to ensure that the physical characteristics of the suspension do not change on addition to an acid medium, if this should affect the rate of release of the drug.

Because the rate of release of an active agent from a suspension is usually slower than the release from solution, drugs are often formulated as suspensions for intramuscular, intraarticular or subcutaneous injection in order to prolong drug release. This is often termed depot therapy. Methylprednisolone, for example, which is available as the water-soluble sodium succinate salt, can be synthesized as the insoluble acetate ester. After intramuscular injection as a suspension, the rate of release is sufficiently slowed to maintain adequate blood levels for up to 14 days.

Release will occur even more slowly if the drug is suspended in an oil, which after injection will remain as a globule, so providing a minimal area of contact with tissue fluid.

Sustained release preparations formulated as suspensions for oral use are less common, but one example is the use of the Pennkinetic system. This involves the complexation of drugs such as hydrocortone and dextromethorphan with tiny ion exchange resin particles, which are then coated with ethylcellulose (Chang 1992). After ingestion the drug is slowly released by exchanging with ions present in the gastrointestinal tract. One of the main difficulties in the formulation of this type of product is to ensure that ions are not present in any of its ingredients.

Drug release from emulsions

The main commercial use of emulsions is for the oral, rectal and topical administration of oils and oil-soluble drugs. Lipid emulsions are also widely used for intravenous feeding, although the choice of emulgent is very limited and globule size must be kept below 4 μm diameter to avoid the formation of emboli. Quite often, however, the high surface area of dispersed oil globules will enhance the rate of absorption of lipophilic drugs.

The emulsion can also be used as a sustained-release dosage form. The intramuscular injection of certain water-soluble vaccines formulated as w/o emulsions can provide a slow release of the antigen and result in a greater antibody response and hence a longer-lasting immunity. Other drugs have also been shown to have this effect, the rate of release being dependent mainly upon the oil/water partition coefficient of the drug and its rate of diffusion across the oil phase.

It is also possible to formulate multiple emulsion systems in which an aqueous phase is dispersed in oil droplets, which in turn are dispersed throughout another aqueous external phase, producing a water-in-oil-in-water (w/o/w) emulsion. These products can also be used for the prolonged release of drugs that are incorporated into the internal aqueous phase. These products have the advantage of exhibiting a lower viscosity than their w/o counterparts and hence are easier to inject.

Similarly, o/w/o emulsions can be formulated and are also under investigation as potential sustained-release bases.

Multiple emulsions, however, tend to be stable only for a relatively short time, although the use of polymers as alternatives to the traditional emulsifying agents may improve their physical stability (Florence and Whitehill 1982).

REFERENCES

Chang, R.K. (1992) Formulation approaches for sustained release oral suspensions. *Pharm. Tech.* **16**, 134–136.

Ciullo, P.A. (1981) Rheological properties of magnesium aluminium silicate/xanthan gum dispersions. *J. Soc. Cosmetic Chemists*, Sep/Oct, 32.

Florence, A.T. and Whitehill, D. (1982) Stabilisation of water/oil/water multiple emulsions by polymerisation of the aqueous phase. *J. Pharm. Pharmacol.*, **34**, 687–691.

Washington, C. (1990) The stability of intravenous fat emulsions in parenteral nutrition mixtures. *Int. J. Pharmaceutics*, **66**, 1–21.

BIBLIOGRAPHY

Florence, A.T. and Attwood, D. (1998) *Physicochemical Principles of Pharmacy*, 3rd Edn. Macmillan, Basingstoke, Chapter 7: Emulsions, suspensions and other dispersions, pp. 252–307; Chapter 8: Polymers and macromolecules, pp. 308–371.

24

Powders and granules

Malcolm Summers

POWDERED AND GRANULATED PRODUCTS AS DOSAGE FORMS

The term 'powder' when used to describe a dosage form describes a formulation in which a drug powder has been mixed with other powdered excipients to produce the final product. The function of the added excipients depends upon the intended use of the product. Colouring, flavouring and sweetening agents, for example, may be added to powders for oral use.

Conventionally, the title 'powder' should be restricted to powder mixes for internal use, and alternative titles are used for other powdered formulations, e.g. dusting powders, which are for external use. The more descriptive title 'oral powder' to differentiate powders for internal use is recommended.

Granules which are used as a dosage form consist of powder particles that have been aggregated to form a larger particle, which is usually 2–4 mm in diameter. This is much larger than granules prepared as an intermediate for tablet manufacture. The processes involved in forming granules from powders are discussed in Chapter 25.

Powdered and granulated products are traditionally dispensed as:

- bulk powders or granules for internal use
- divided powders or granules (i.e. single preparations) for internal use
- dusting powders for external use.

Other preparations which are presented as powders or granules include:

- insufflations for administration to ear, nose or throat
- antibiotic syrups to be reconstituted before use
- powders for reconstitution into injections
- dry powder inhalers.

Advantages and disadvantages of powdered and granulated products

The advantages of this type of preparation are as follows.

1. Solid preparations are more chemically stable than liquid ones. The shelf-life of powders for antibiotic syrups, for example, is 2–3 years, but once they are reconstituted with water it is 1–2 weeks. The instability observed in liquid preparations is usually the primary reason for presenting some injections as powders to be reconstituted just prior to use.
2. Powders and granules are a convenient form in which to dispense drugs with a large dose. The dose of Compound Magnesium Trisilicate Oral Powder is 1–5 g, and although it is feasible to manufacture tablets to supply this dose it is often more acceptable to the patient to disperse a powder in water and swallow it as a draught.
3. Orally administered powders and granules of soluble medicaments have a faster dissolution rate than tablets or capsules, as these must first disintegrate before the drug dissolves. Drug absorption from such powdered or granulated preparations will therefore be faster than from the corresponding tablet or capsule, if the dissolution rate limits the rate of drug absorption.

The disadvantages of powders and granules are as follows.

1. Bulk powders or granules are far less convenient for the patient to carry than a small container of tablets or capsules, and are as inconvenient as liquid preparations, such as mixtures. Modern packaging methods for divided preparations, such as heat-sealable laminated sachets, mean that individual doses can be conveniently carried.
2. The masking of unpleasant tastes may be a problem with this type of preparation. A method of attempting this is by formulating the powder into a pleasantly tasting or taste-masked effervescent product, whereas tablets and capsules are a more common alternative for low-dose products.
3. Bulk powders or granules are not suitable for administering potent drugs with a low dose. This is because individual doses are extracted from the bulk using a 5 mL spoon. This method is subject to such variables as variation in spoon fill (e.g. 'level' or 'heaped' spoonfuls) and variation in the bulk density of different batches of a powder. It is therefore not an accurate method

of measurement. Divided preparations have been used for more potent drugs, but tablets and capsules have largely replaced them for this purpose.

4. Powders and granules are not a suitable method for the administration of drugs which are inactivated in, or cause damage to, the stomach; these should be presented as enteric-coated tablets, for example.

DISPENSED PREPARATIONS

Bulk powders

The mixed ingredients are packed into a suitable bulk container, such as a wide-mouthed glass jar. Because of the disadvantages of this type of preparation the constituents are usually relatively non-toxic medicaments with a large dose, e.g. magnesium trisilicate and chalk, as present in Compound Magnesium Trisilicate Oral Powder. Relatively few proprietary examples exist, although many dietary/food supplements are packed in this way.

Divided powders

Divided powders are similar formulations to bulk powders but individual doses are separately wrapped.

Traditionally, single doses were wrapped in paper. This was unsatisfactory for most products, particularly if the ingredients were hygroscopic, volatile or deliquescent. Modern packaging materials of foil and plastic laminates have replaced such paper wrappings because they offer superior protective qualities and are amenable to use on high-speed packing machines.

Effervescent powders can now be packed in individual dose units because of the protective qualities of laminates. Such powders contain, for example, sodium bicarbonate and citric acid, which react and effervesce when the patient adds the powder to water to produce a draught. It is important to protect the powder from the ingress of moisture during manufacture and on subsequent storage to prevent the reaction occurring prematurely.

All powders and granules should be stored in a dry place to prevent deterioration due to ingress of moisture. Even if hydrolytic decomposition of susceptible ingredients does not occur, the particles will adhere and cake, producing an inelegant, often unusable product.

Bulk granules

One disadvantage of bulk powders is that, because of particle size differences, the ingredients may segregate (see Chapter 13), either on storage in the final container or in the hoppers of packaging machines. If this happens the product will be non-uniform and the patient will not receive the same dose of the ingredients on each occasion. This can be prevented by granulating the mixed powders.

Bulk granules therefore contain similar medicaments to powders, i.e. those with low-toxicity, high-dose drugs. Methylcellulose Granules, for example, are used as a bulk-forming laxative and have a dose of 1–4 g daily. Many proprietary preparations contain similar bulk-forming laxatives.

Divided granules

These are granulated products in which sufficient for one dose is individually wrapped. Effervescent granules can be formulated and presented in this manner. The comments on packaging materials discussed under Divided powders above are also equally pertinent to divided granules.

Dusting powders

Dusting powders contain ingredients used for therapeutic, prophylactic or lubricant purposes and are intended for external use.

Only sterile dusting powders should be applied to open wounds. Such preparations should be prepared using materials and methods designed to ensure sterility and to avoid the introduction of contaminants and the growth of micro-organisms.

Dusting powders for lubricant purposes or superficial skin conditions need not be sterile but they should be free from pathogenic organisms. As minerals such as talc and kaolin may be contaminated at source with spores of organisms causing tetanus and gangrene, these should be sterilized before they are incorporated into the product. Talc dusting powder is a sterile cutaneous powder containing starch and purified talc in which the talc is sterilized before incorporation with the starch, or the final product is subject to a suitable terminal sterilization procedure.

Dusting powders are normally dispensed in glass or metal containers with a perforated lid. The powder must flow well from such a container, so that they can be dusted over the affected area. The active ingredients must therefore be diluted with materials having reasonably good flow properties, e.g. purified talc or maize starch.

Hexachlorophane Dusting Powder contains an antibacterial agent and Talc Dusting Powder is used as a lubricant to prevent chafing. Proprietary products are available, usually for the treatment of bacterial or fungal infections, e.g. Canesten Powder (clotrimazole) is used as an antifungal agent and CX Powder (containing chlorhexidine acetate) is used as a general skin disinfectant.

Insufflations

Insufflations are medicated powders which are blown into regions such as the ear, nose and throat using an insufflator. The use of traditional insufflations declined because they were not very acceptable, being more inelegant and less convenient to apply than other topical preparations. A second problem was that if the powder contained a drug that had systemic activity it was difficult, with the conventional insulator, to ensure that the same dose was delivered on each occasion.

Some potent drugs are now presented in this way because they are rapidly absorbed when administered as a fine powder via the nose (see Chapter 32 for a detailed discussion of the nasal route of administration). To enhance convenience and ensure that a uniform dose is delivered on each occasion, devices have been developed to replace the traditional insufflator. Sufficient drug for one dose may be presented in a hard gelatin capsule diluted with an inert, soluble diluent such as lactose. The capsule is placed in the body of the insufflator and is broken when the device is assembled. The drug is inhaled by the patient as a fine powder.

Dry-powder inhalers

The use of dry-powder systems for pulmonary drug delivery is now extensive. This dosage form has developed into one of the most effective methods of delivering active ingredients to the lung for the treatment of asthma and chronic obstructive pulmonary disease. Its popularity is reflected in the number of commercial preparations available in a number of sophisticated and increasingly precise devices. Pulmonary delivery is discussed fully in Chapter 31, and the reader is referred there for further information.

PREPARATIONS REQUIRING FURTHER TREATMENT AT TIME OF DISPENSING

Oral antibiotic syrups

For patients who have difficulty taking capsules and tablets, e.g. young children, a liquid preparation of a drug offers a suitable alternative. However, many drugs, e.g. antibiotics, are physically or chemically unstable when formulated as a solution or suspension. The method used to overcome this instability problem is to manufacture the dry ingredients of the intended liquid preparation in a suitable container in the form of a powder or granules. When the pharmacist dispenses the product, a given quantity of water is added to reconstitute the solution or suspension. This enables sufficient time for warehouseing and distribution of the product and storage at the pharmacy without degradation. Once it is reconstituted, the patient is warned of the short shelf-life. A shelf-life of 1–2 weeks for the reconstituted syrup should not be a serious problem for the patient. Examples are Erythroped Suspension and Amoxicillin Oral Suspension.

Powders for injection

Injections of medicaments that are unstable in solution must be made immediately prior to use and are presented as sterile powders in ampoules. Sufficient diluent, e.g. sterile Water for Injections, is added from a second ampoule to produce the required drug concentration and the injection is used immediately. The powder may contain suitable excipients in addition to the drug, e.g. sufficient additive to produce an isotonic solution when the injection is reconstituted.

BIBLIOGRAPHY

British Pharmacopoeia (2000), HMSO, London.
Further information on proprietary products can be found in:
The Data Sheet Compendium, Datapharm Publications Ltd (published annually).
The Monthly Index of Medical Specialities (MIMS), Medical Publications Ltd.

25

Granulation

Malcolm Summers, Michael Aulton

INTRODUCTION TO GRANULATION

Granulation is the process in which **primary powder particles** are made to adhere to form larger, multiparticle entities called **granules**. Pharmaceutical granules typically have a size range between 0.2 and 4.0 mm, depending on their subsequent use. In the majority of cases this will be in the production of tablets or capsules, when granules will be made as an intermediate product and have a typical size range between 0.2 and 0.5 mm, but larger granules are used as a dosage form in their own right (see Chapter 24).

Granulation normally commences after initial dry mixing of the necessary powdered ingredients so that a uniform distribution of each ingredient through the mix is achieved. After granulation the granules will either be packed (when used as a dosage form), or they may be mixed with other excipients prior to tablet compaction or capsule filling.

Reasons for granulation

The reasons why granulation is often necessary are as follows.

To prevent segregation of the constituents of the powder mix

Segregation (or demixing, see Chapter 13) is due primarily to differences in the size or density of the components of the mix, the smaller and/or denser particles concentrating at the base of a container with the larger and/or less dense ones above them. An ideal granulation will contain all the constituents of the mix in the correct proportion in each granule, and segregation of the ingredients will not occur (Fig. 25.1).

It is also important to control the particle size distribution of the granules because, although the individual components may not segregate, if there is a wide size distribution the granules themselves may segregate. If this occurs in the hoppers of sachet-filling machines, capsule-filling machines or tablet machines, products with large weight variations will result. This is because these machines fill by volume rather than weight, and if different regions in the hopper contain granules of different sizes (and hence bulk density), a given volume in each region will contain a different weight of granules. This will lead to an unacceptable distribution of the drug content within the batch of finished product, even though the drug is evenly distributed, weight per weight, through the granules.

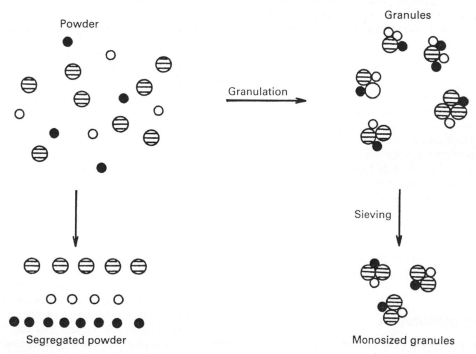

Fig. 25.1 Granulation to prevent powder segregation.

To improve the flow properties of the mix

Many powders, because of their small size, irregular shape or surface characteristics, are cohesive and do not flow well. Poor flow will often result in a wide weight variation within the final product owing to variable fill of tablet dies etc. Granules produced from such a cohesive system will be larger and more isodiametric, both factors contributing to improved flow properties.

To improve the compaction characteristics of the mix

Some powders are difficult to compact even if a readily compactable adhesive is included in the mix, but granules of the same formulation are often more easily compacted and produce stronger tablets. This is associated with the distribution of the adhesive within the granule and is a function of the method employed to produce the granule. Often solute migration (see Chapter 26) occurring during the postgranulation drying stage results in a binder-rich outer layer to the granules. This in turn leads to direct binder–binder bonding, which assists the consolidation of weakly bonding materials.

Other reasons

The above are the primary reasons for the granulation of pharmaceutical products, but there are other reasons that may necessitate the granulation of powdered material:

1. The granulation of toxic materials will reduce the hazard associated with the generation of toxic dust that may arise when handling powders. Suitable precautions must be taken to ensure that such dust is not a hazard during the granulation process. Thus granules should be non-friable and have a suitable mechanical strength.
2. Materials which are slightly hygroscopic may adhere and form a cake if stored as a powder. Granulation may reduce this hazard, as the granules will be able to absorb some moisture and yet retain their flowability because of their size.
3. Granules, being denser than the parent powder mix, occupy less volume per unit weight. They are therefore more convenient for storage or shipment.

Methods of granulation

Granulation methods can be divided into two types: **wet** methods, which use a liquid in the process, and **dry** methods in which no liquid is used.

In a suitable formulation a number of different excipients will be needed in addition to the drug. The common types used are diluents, to produce a unit dose weight of suitable size, and disintegrating agents, which are added to aid the break-up of the granule when it reaches a liquid medium, e.g. on ingestion by the patient. Adhesives in the form of a dry powder may also be added, particularly if dry granulation is employed. These ingredients will be mixed before granulation.

Dry granulation

In the dry methods of granulation the primary powder particles are aggregated under high pressure. There are two main processes. Either a large tablet (known as a '**slug**') is produced in a heavy-duty tabletting press (a process known as '**slugging**') or the powder is squeezed between two rollers to produce a sheet of material ('**roller compaction**'). In both cases these intermediate products are broken using a suitable milling technique to produce granular material, which is usually sieved to separate the desired size fraction. The unused fine material may be reworked to avoid waste. This dry method may be used for drugs that do not compress well after wet granulation, or those which are sensitive to moisture.

Wet granulation (involving wet massing)

Wet granulation involves the massing of a mix of dry **primary powder particles** using a **granulating fluid**. The fluid contains a solvent which must be volatile so that it can be removed by drying, and be non-toxic. Typical liquids include water, ethanol and isopropanol, either alone or in combination. The granulation liquid may be used alone or, more usually, as a solvent containing a dissolved **adhesive** (also referred to as a **binder** or **binding agent**) which is used to ensure particle adhesion once the granule is dry.

Water is commonly used for economical and ecological reasons. Its disadvantages as a solvent are that it may adversely affect drug stability, causing hydrolysis of susceptible products, and it needs a longer drying time than do organic solvents. This increases the length of the process and again may affect stability because of the extended exposure to heat. The primary advantage of water is that it is non-flammable, which means that expensive safety precautions such as the use of flameproof equipment need not be taken. Organic solvents are used when water-sensitive drugs are processed, as an alternative to dry granulation, or when a rapid drying time is required.

In the traditional wet granulation method the wet mass is forced through a sieve to produce wet granules which are then dried. A subsequent screening stage breaks agglomerates of granules and removes the fine material, which can than be recycled. Variations of this traditional method depend on the equipment used, but the general principle of initial particle aggregation using a liquid remains in all of the processes.

Effect of granulation method on granule structure

The type and capacity of granulating mixers significantly influences the work input and time necessary to produce a cohesive mass, adequate liquid distribution and intragranular porosity of the granular mass. The method and conditions of granulation affect intergranular and intragranular pore structure by changing the degree of packing within the granules. It has been shown that precompressed granules, consisting of compressed drug and binder particles, are held together by simple bonding during compaction. Granules prepared by wet massing consist of intact drug particles held together in a sponge-like matrix of binder. Fluidized-bed granules are similar to those prepared by the wet massing process, but possess greater porosity and the granule surface is covered by a film of binding agent. With spray-dried systems the granules consist of spherical particles composed of an outer shell and an inner core of particles. Thus the properties of the granule are influenced by the manufacturing process.

GRANULATION MECHANISMS

Particle-bonding mechanisms

To form granules, bonds must be formed between powder particles so that they adhere and these bonds must be sufficiently strong to prevent breakdown of the granule to powder in subsequent handling operations.

There are five primary bonding mechanisms between particles:

1. Adhesion and cohesion forces in the immobile liquid films between individual primary powder particles;

2. Interfacial forces in mobile liquid films within the granules;
3. The formation of solid bridges after solvent evaporation;
4. Attractive forces between solid particles;
5. Mechanical interlocking.

Different types of mechanism were identified in each group and the ones discussed below are those that are relevant to pharmaceutical granulations.

Adhesion and cohesion forces in immobile films

If sufficient liquid is present in a powder to form a very thin, immobile layer, there will be an effective decrease in interparticulate distance and an increase in contact area between the particles. The bond strength between the particles will be increased because of this, as the van der Waals forces of attraction are proportional to the particle diameter and inversely proportional to the square of the distance of separation.

This situation will arise with adsorbed moisture and accounts for the cohesion of slightly damp powders. Although such films may be present as residual liquid after granules prepared by wet granulation have been dried, it is unlikely that they contribute significantly to the final granule strength. In dry granulation, however, the pressures used will increase the contact area between the adsorption layers and decrease the interparticulate distance, and this will contribute to the final granule strength.

Thin, immobile layers may also be formed by highly viscous solutions of adhesives, and so the bond strength will be greater than that produced by the mobile films discussed below. The use of starch mucilage in pharmaceutical granulations may produce this type of film.

Interfacial forces in mobile liquid films

During wet granulation liquid is added to the powder mix and will be distributed as films around and between the particles. Sufficient liquid is usually added to exceed that necessary for an immobile layer and to produce a mobile film. There are three states of water distribution between particles, which are illustrated in Figure 25.2.

At low moisture levels, termed the *pendular state*, the particles are held together by lens-shaped rings of liquid. These cause adhesion because of the surface tension forces of the liquid/air interface and the hydrostatic suction pressure in the liquid bridge. When all the air has been displaced from between

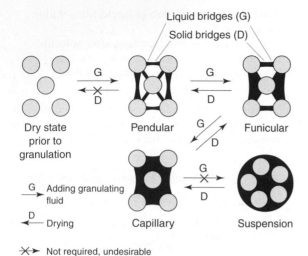

Fig. 25.2 Water distribution between particles of a granule during formation and drying.

the particles the **capillary state** is reached, and the particles are held by capillary suction at the liquid/air interface, which is now only at the granule surface. The **funicular state** represents an intermediate stage between the pendular and capillary states. Moist granule tensile strength increases about three times between the pendular and the capillary state.

It may appear that the state of the powder bed is dependent upon the total moisture content of the wetted powders, but the capillary state may also be reached by decreasing the separation of the particles. In the massing process during wet granulation, continued kneading/mixing of material originally in the pendular state will densify the wet mass, decreasing the pore volume occupied by air and eventually producing the funicular or capillary state without further liquid addition.

In addition to these three states, a further state, the droplet, is illustrated in Figure 25.2. This will be important in the process of granulation by spray-drying of a suspension. In this state, the strength of the droplet is dependent upon the surface tension of the liquid used.

These wet bridges are only temporary structures in wet granulation because the moist granules will be dried. They are, however, a prerequisite for the formation of solid bridges formed by adhesives present in the liquid, or by materials that dissolve in the granulating liquid.

Solid bridges

These can be formed by:

1. partial melting
2. hardening binders
3. crystallization of dissolved substances.

Partial melting   Although not considered to be a predominant mechanism in pharmaceutical materials, it is possible that the pressures used in dry granulation methods may cause melting of low melting-point materials where the particles touch and high pressures are developed. When the pressure is relieved, crystallization will take place and bind the particles together.

Hardening binders   This is the common mechanism in pharmaceutical wet granulations when an adhesive is included in the granulating solvent. The liquid will form liquid bridges, as discussed above, and the adhesive will harden or crystallize on drying to form solid bridges to bind the particles. Adhesives such as polyvinylpyrrolidone, the cellulose derivatives (such as carboxymethylcellulose) and pregelatinized starch function in this way.

Crystallization of dissolved substances   The solvent used to mass the powder during wet granulation may partially dissolve one of the powdered ingredients. When the granules are dried, crystallization of this material will take place and the dissolved substance then acts as a hardening binder. Any material soluble in the granulating liquid will function in this manner, e.g. lactose incorporated into dry powders granulated with water.

The size of the crystals produced in the bridge will be influenced by the rate of drying of the granules: the slower the drying time, the larger the particle size. It is therefore important that the drug does not dissolve in the granulating liquid and recrystallize, because it may adversely affect the dissolution rate of the drug if crystals larger than that of the starting material are produced.

Attractive forces between solid particles

In the absence of liquids and solid bridges formed by binding agents, there are two types of attractive force that can operate between particles in pharmaceutical systems.

Electrostatic forces may be important in causing powder cohesion and the initial formation of agglomerates, e.g. during mixing. In general they do not contribute significantly to the final strength of the granule.

Van der Waals forces, however, are about four orders of magnitude greater than electrostatic forces and contribute significantly to the strength of granules produced by dry granulation. The magnitude of these forces will increase as the distance between adjacent surfaces decreases, and in dry granulation this is achieved by using pressure to force the particles together.

Mechanisms of granule formation

In the dry methods, particle adhesion takes place because of applied pressure. A compact or sheet is produced which is larger than the granule size required, and therefore the required size can be attained by milling and sieving.

In wet granulation methods, liquid added to dry powders has to be distributed through the powder by the mechanical agitation created in the granulator. The particles adhere to each other because of liquid films, and further agitation and/or liquid addition causes more particles to adhere. The precise mechanism by which a dry powder is transformed into a bed of granules varies for each type of granulation equipment, but the mechanism discussed below serves as a useful broad generalization of the process.

The proposed granulation mechanism can be divided into three stages.

Nucleation

Granulation starts with particle–particle contact and adhesion due to liquid bridges. A number of particles will join to form the pendular state illustrated in Figure 25.2. Further agitation densifies the pendular bodies to form the capillary state, and these bodies act as nuclei for further granule growth.

Transition

Nuclei can grow in two possible ways: either single particles can be added to the nuclei by pendular bridges, or two or more nuclei may combine. The combined nuclei will be reshaped by the agitation of the bed.

This stage is characterized by the presence of a large number of small granules with a fairly wide size distribution. Providing that this distribution is not excessively large, this is a suitable end-point for granules used in capsule and tablet manufacture, as relatively small granules will produce a uniform tablet die or capsule fill. Larger granules may give rise to problems in small-diameter dies owing to bridging across the die and uneven fill.

Ball growth

Further granule growth produces large, spherical granules and the mean particle size of the granulating system will increase with time. If agitation is con-tinued, granule coalescence will continue and produce an unusable, overmassed system, although this is dependent upon the amount of liquid added and the properties of the material being granulated.

Although ball growth produces granules that may be too large for pharmaceutical purposes, some degree of ball growth will occur in planetary mixers and it is an essential feature of some spheronizing equipment.

The four possible mechanisms of ball growth are illustrated in Figure 25.3.

Coalescence Two or more granules join to form a larger granule.

Breakage Granules break into fragments which adhere to other granules, forming a layer of material over the surviving granule.

Abrasion transfer Agitation of the granule bed leads to the attrition of material from granules. This abraded material adheres to other granules, increasing their size.

Layering When a second batch of powder mix is added to a bed of granules the powder will adhere to the granules, forming a layer over the surface and increasing the granule size. This mechanism is only relevant to the production of layered granules using spheronizing equipment.

There will be some degree of overlap between these stages and it will be very difficult to identify a given stage by inspection of the granulating system. For end-product uniformity it is desirable to finish every batch of a formulation at the same stage, and this may be a major problem in pharmaceutical production.

Using the slower processes, such as the planetary mixer, there is usually sufficient time to stop the process before overmassing occurs. With faster granulation equipment the duration of granulation can only be used as a control parameter when the formulation is such that granule growth is slow and takes place at a fairly uniform rate. In many cases, however, the transition from a non-granulated to an overmassed system is very rapid, and monitoring equipment is necessary to stop the granulation at a predetermined point, known as granulation end-point control.

PHARMACEUTICAL GRANULATION EQUIPMENT

Wet granulators

There are three main types of granulator used in the pharmaceutical industry for wet granulation.

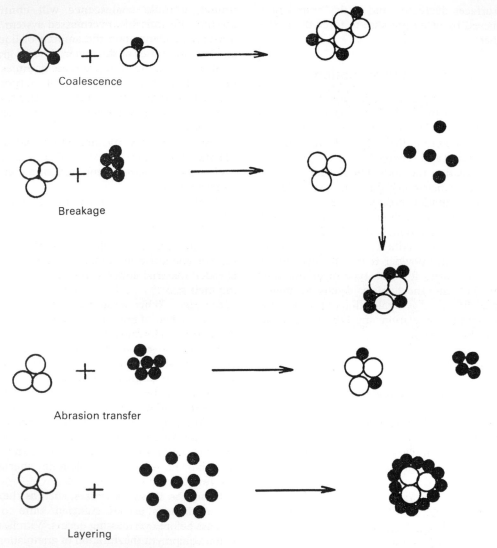

Fig. 25.3 Mechanisms of ball growth during granulation.

Shear granulators

In the traditional granulation process a planetary mixer is often used for wet massing of the powders, e.g. Hobart, Collette, Beken (Fig. 25.4). Powder mixing usually has to be performed as a separate operation using suitable mixing equipment. With some formulations, such as those containing two or three ingredients in approximately equal quantities, however, it may be possible to achieve a suitable mix in the planetary mixer without a separate stage.

The mixed powders are fed into the bowl of the planetary mixer and granulating liquid is added as the paddle of the mixer agitates the powders. The planetary action of the blade when mixing is similar to that of a household mixer.

The moist mass has then to be transferred to a granulator, such as an oscillating granulator (Fig. 25.5). The rotor bars of the granulator oscillate and force the moist mass through the sieve screen, the size of which determines the granule size. The mass should be sufficiently moist to form discrete granules when sieved. If excess liquid is added, strings of material will be formed and if the mix is too dry the mass will be sieved to powder and granules will not be formed.

The granules can be collected on trays and transferred to a drying oven, although tray drying suffers from three major disadvantages:

drying, it reduces the problems of aggregation and intergranular solute migration, thereby reducing the need for a sieving stage after drying.

The disadvantages of this traditional granulation process are its long duration, the need for several pieces of equipment, and the high material losses that can be incurred because of the transfer stages. Advantages are that the process is not very sensitive to changes in the characteristics of the granule ingredients (e.g. surface area variations in different batches of an excipient), and the end-point of the massing process can often be determined by inspection.

High-speed mixer/granulators

This type of granulator (e.g. Diosna, Fielder) is used extensively in pharmaceutics. The machines have a stainless steel mixing bowl containing a three-bladed main impeller, which revolves in the horizontal plane, and a three-bladed auxiliary chopper (breaker blade) which revolves either in the vertical or the horizontal plane (Fig. 25.6).

The unmixed dry powders are placed in the bowl and mixed by the rotating impeller for a few minutes. Granulating liquid is then added via a port in the lid of the granulator while the impeller is turning. The granulating fluid is mixed into the powders by the impeller. The chopper is usually switched on when the moist mass is formed, as its function is to break up the wet mass to produce a bed of granular material. Once a satisfactory granule has been produced, the granular product is discharged, passing through a wire mesh which breaks up any large aggregates, into the bowl of a fluidized-bed drier.

The advantage of the process is that mixing, massing and granulation are all performed within a few minutes in the same piece of equipment. The process needs to be controlled with care as the granulation progresses so rapidly that a usable granule can be transformed very quickly into an unusable, overmassed system. Thus it is often necessary to use a suitable monitoring system to indicate the end of the granulation process, i.e. when a granule of the desired properties has been attained. The process is also sensitive to variations in raw materials, but this may be minimized by using a suitable end-point monitor.

A variation of the Diosna/Fielder type of design is the Collette–Gral mixer (Fig. 25.7). This is based on the bowl and overhead drive of the planetary mixer, but the single paddle is replaced by two mixing shafts. One of these carries three blades, which rotate in the horizontal plane at the base of the bowl, and the

Fig. 25.4 Planetary mixer for wet massing.

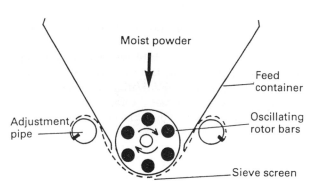

Fig. 25.5 Oscillating granulator.

1. The drying time is long.
2. Dissolved material can migrate to the upper surface of the bed of granules, as the solvent is only removed from the upper surface of the bed on the tray.
3. Granules may aggregate owing to bridge formation at the points of contact of the granules.

To deaggregate the granules and remix them, a sieving stage is necessary after drying.

An alternative method is to dry the granules using a fluidized-bed drier. This is quicker and, as it keeps the individual granules separated during

Fig. 25.6   High-speed mixer/granulator.

Fig. 25.7   Collette–Gral granulator: mixing shafts and bowl.

second carries smaller blades which act as the chopper and rotate in the horizontal plane in the upper regions of the granulating mass. Thus the operation principle is similar.

Fluidized-bed granulators

Fluidized-bed granulators (e.g. Aeromatic, Glatt) have a similar design and operation to fluidized-bed driers, i.e. the powder particles are fluidized in a stream of air, but in addition granulation fluid is sprayed from a nozzle on to the bed of powders (Fig. 25.8).

Heated and filtered air is blown or sucked through the bed of unmixed powders to fluidize the particles and mix the powders; fluidization is actually a very efficient mixing process. Granulating fluid is pumped from a reservoir through a spray nozzle positioned over the bed of particles. The fluid causes the primary powder particles to adhere when the droplets and powders collide. Escape of material from the granulation chamber is prevented by exhaust filters, which are periodically agitated to reintroduce the collected material into the fluidized bed. Sufficient liquid is sprayed to produce granules of the required size, at which point the spray is turned off but the fluidizing air continued. The wet granules are then dried in the heated fluidizing airstream.

Advantages of fluidized-bed granulation Fluidized-bed granulation has many advantages over conventional wet massing. All the granulation processes, which require separate equipment in the conventional method, are performed in one unit, saving labour costs, transfer losses and time. Another advantage is that the process can be automated once the conditions affecting the granulation have been optimized.

Fig. 25.8 Fluidized-bed granulator.

Disadvantages of fluidized-bed granulation On the downside, the equipment is initially expensive and optimization of process (and product) parameters affecting granulation needs extensive development work, not only during initial formulation work but also during scale-up from development to production. Similar development work for the traditional process and that using high-speed granulators is not as extensive.

This long and very product-specific development process has proved to be a serious problem with fluidized-bed granulation in the pharmaceutical industry. There are numerous apparatus, process and product parameters that affect the quality of the final granule. These are listed in Table 25.1. The extent of this list, coupled with the fact that each formulation presents its own individual development problems,

Table 25.1   Apparatus, process and product variables influencing fluidized-bed granulation

Apparatus parameters	Process parameters	Product parameters
Air distribution plate	Bed load	Type of binder
Shape of granulator body	Fluidizing air flow rate	Quantity of binder
Nozzle height	Fluidizing air temperature	Binder solvent
Positive or negative pressure operation	Fluidizing air humidity	Concentration of granulating solution
Scale-up	Atomization	Temperature of granulation solution
	Nozzle type	
	Spray angle	Starting Materials
	Spraying regime	Fluidization
	Liquid flow rate	Powder hydrophobicity
	Atomizing air flow rate	
	Atomizing air pressure	
	Droplet size	

has led to fluidized-bed granulation not reaching its full potential in pharmaceutical production. This is exacerbated by the reality that most pharmaceutical companies have a wide range of products made at relatively small batch sizes, unlike other industries (fertilizers, herbicides, foodstuffs) where fluidized-bed granulation is used successfully and extensively.

Spray-driers

These differ from the method discussed above in that a dry, granular product is made from a solution or a suspension rather than initially dry primary powder particles. The solution or suspension may be of drug alone, a single excipient or a complete formulation.

The process of spray-drying is discussed fully in Chapter 26. The resultant granules are free-flowing hollow spheres and the distribution of the binder in such granules (at the periphery following solute migration during drying) results in good compaction properties.

This process can be used to make tablet granules, although it is probably economically justified for this purpose only when suitable granules cannot be produced by the other methods. Spray-drying can convert hard elastic materials into more ductile ones. Spray-dried lactose is the classic example, and its advantages over α-lactose monohydrate crystals when compacted are discussed in Chapter 27.

The primary advantages of the process are the short drying time and the minimal exposure of the product to heat owing to the short residence time in the drying chamber. This means that little deterioration of heat-sensitive materials takes place, and it may be the only process suitable for this type of product.

Spheronizers/pelletizers

For some applications it may be desirable to have a dense, spherical pellet of the type difficult to produce with the equipment above. Such pellets are used for controlled drug release products following coating with a suitable polymer coat and filling into hard gelatin capsules. Capsule filling with a mixture of coated and non-coated drug-containing pellets would give some degree of programmed drug release after the capsule shell dissolves.

A commonly used process involves the separate processes of wet massing, followed by extrusion of this wet mass into rod-shaped granules and subsequent spheronization of these granules. Because this process is used so frequently to produce modified-release multiparticulates, it will be discussed in some detail.

Extrusion/spheronization

Extrusion/spheronization is a multistep process used to make uniformly sized spherical particles. It is used primarily to produce multiparticulates for controlled drug release applications. The major advantage over other methods of producing drug-loaded spheres or pellets is the ability to incorporate high levels of active ingredients without producing excessively large particles (i.e. minimal excipients are necessary).

The main steps of the process are:

1. **Dry mixing of ingredients** to achieve a homogenous powder dispersion;
2. **Wet massing** to produce a sufficiently plastic wet mass;
3. **Extrusion** to form rod-shaped particles of uniform diameter;
4. **Spheronization** to round off these rods into spherical particles;
5. **Drying** to achieve the desired final moisture content;
6. **Screening** (optional) to achieve the desired narrow size distribution.

Applications of extrusion/spheronization

Potential applications are many, but relate mainly to controlled drug release and improved processing.

Controlled drug release Both immediate-release and controlled-release pellets can be formed. In turn, these pellets can either be filled into hard gelatin capsule shells or compacted into tablets to form unit dosage forms. Pellets can contain two or more ingredients in the same individual unit, or incompatible ingredients can be manufactured in separate pellets.

Pellets can be coated in sub-batches to give, say, rapid-, intermediate- and slow-release pellets in the same capsule shell. Dense multiparticulates disperse evenly within the GI tract and have less variable gastric emptying and intestinal transit times than do single units, such as coated monolithic tablets.

Processing The process of extrusion/spheronization can be used to increase the bulk density, improve flow properties and reduce the problems of dust usually encountered with low-density, finely divided active and excipient powders.

Extrusion/spheronization is a more labour-intensive process than other forms of granulation and should therefore only be considered when other methods are either not satisfactory for that particular formulation or are inappropriate (i.e. when spheres are required).

Desirable properties of pellets

Uncoated pellets:

- Uniform spherical shape
- Uniform size
- Good flow properties
- Reproducible packing (into hard gelatin capsules)
- High strength
- Low friability
- Low dust
- Smooth surface
- Ease of coating.

Once coated:

- Maintain all of the above properties
- Have desired drug-release characteristics.

The process

Dry mixing of ingredients This uses normal powder-mixing equipment.

Wet massing This stage also employs normal equipment and processes as used in wet granulation. There are two major differences in the granulation step compared with granulation for compaction:

1. The amount of granulation fluid
2. The importance of achieving a uniform dispersion of fluid.

The amount of fluid needed to achieve spheres of uniform size and sphericity is likely to be greater than that for a similar tablet granulation. Poor liquid dispersion will produce a poor-quality product.

Extrusion Extrusion produces rod-shaped particles of uniform diameter from the wet mass. The wet mass is forced through dies and shaped into small cylindrical particles with uniform diameter. The extrudate particles break at similar lengths under their own weight. Thus the extrudate must have enough plasticity to deform, but not so much that the extruded particles adhere to other particles when collected or rolled in the spheronizer.

There are many designs of extruder, but generally they can be divided into three classes, based on their feed mechanism:

- Screw-feed extruders (axial or end-plate, dome and radial)
- Gravity-feed extruders (cylinder roll, gear roll, radial)
- Piston-feed extruders (ram).

The first two categories (Fig. 25.9) are used for both development and production, but the latter is only

Screw-feed extruders

axial   radial

Gravity-feed extruders

cylinder   gear

Fig. 25.9 Schematic representation of production extruders.

used for experimental development work as it is easy to add instrumentation.

The primary extrusion process variables are:

- the feed rate of the wet mass
- the diameter of the die
- the length of the die
- the water content of the wet mass.

The properties of the extrudate, and hence the resulting spheres, are very dependent on the plasticity and cohesiveness of the wet mass. In general, an extrudable wet mass needs to be wetter than that appropriate for conventional granulation by wet massing.

Spheronization The function of the fourth step in the process (i.e. spheronization) is to round off the rods produced by extrusion into spherical particles.

This is carried out in a relatively simple piece of apparatus (Fig. 25.10). The working part consists of a bowl with fixed side walls and a rapidly rotating bottom plate or disc. The rounding of the extrudate into spheres is dependent on frictional forces generated by particle–particle and particle–equipment collisions. The bottom disc has a grooved surface to increase these forces. Two geometric patterns are generally used:

- A cross-hatched pattern with grooves running at right-angles to one another
- A radial pattern with grooves running radially from the centre of the disc.

Wet product spheronizing during toroidal motion

Spinning friction wheel

Fig. 25.10 A spheronizer showing the characteristic toroidal (rope-like) movement of the forming pellets in the spheronizer bowl during operation.

(a)	(b)	(c)	(d)	(e)
Cylinder	Cylinder with rounded ends	Dumbbell	Ellipsoid	Sphere

Spheronization time ⟶

Fig. 25.11 Representation of a mechanism of spheronization. The diagram shows a transition from cylindrical particles (a) into cylindrical particles with rounded edges (b), then dumbbells (c), to ellipsoids (d) and finally spheres (e).

The transition from rods to spheres during spheronization occurs in various stages. These are best described by examining the following diagrams (Fig. 25.11).

If the mass is too dry spheres will not be formed: the rods will only transform as far as dumbbells.

Drying A drying stage is required in order to achieve the desired moisture content. This is often the final step in the process. The pellets can be dried in any drier that can be used for conventional wet granulations, including tray dryers and fluidized-bed driers. Both are used successfully for extrusion/spheronization. If solute migration (Chapter 26) occurs during drying of the wet spheres, this may result in:

• an increased initial rate of dissolution
• stronger pellets
• modified surfaces which might reduce the adhesion of any added film coats.

Screening Screening may be necessary to achieve the desired narrow size distribution. Normal sieves are used. If all the previous stages are performed efficiently and with careful development of process and formulation conditions, this step may not be necessary.

Formulation variables

The composition of the wet mass is critical in determining the properties of the particles produced. During the granulation step a wet mass is produced which must be plastic, deform when extruded, and break off to form uniformly sized cylindrical particles which are easily deformed into spherical particles. Thus the process has a complex set of requirements that are strongly influenced by the ingredients of the pellet formulation.

Summary

Extrusion/spheronization is a versatile process capable of producing spherical granules with very useful properties. Because it is more labour-intensive than more common wet massing techniques its use should be limited to those applications where a sphere is required and other granulation techniques are unsuitable.

The most common application of the process is to produce spherical pellets for controlled drug release.

Care must be taken to understand the required properties of the pellets and the manner in which the process and formulation influence the ability to achieve these aims.

Rotor granulation

This process allows the direct manufacture of spheres from dry powder. In the Freund granulator, the powder mix is added to the bowl and wetted with granulating liquid from a spray (Fig. 25.12). The baseplate rotates at high speed and centrifugal force keeps the moist mass at the edges of the rotor. Here, the velocity difference between the rotor and the static walls, combined with the upward flow of air around the rotor plate, causes the mass to move in a toroidal motion, resulting in the formation of discrete spherical pellets. These spheres (actually, of course, wet granules) are dried by the heated inlet air

Fig. 25.12 Freund granulator.

from the air chamber, which also acts as a positive-pressure seal during granulation.

Using this technique it is possible to continue the process and coat the pellets by subsequently spraying coating solution on to the rotating dried pellets. In addition, layered pellets can be produced by using uncoated pellets as nuclei in a second granulation with a powder mix of a second ingredient or ingredients.

Fig. 25.13 Roller compaction: (a) Alexanderwerk and (b) Hutt types.

Dry granulators

Dry granulation converts primary powder particles into granules using the application of pressure without the intermediate use of a liquid. It therefore avoids heat–temperature combinations that might cause degradation of the product.

Two pieces of equipment are necessary for dry granulation: first, a machine for compressing the dry powders into compacts or flakes, and secondly a mill for breaking up these intermediate products into granules.

Sluggers

The dry powders can be compressed using a conventional tablet machine or, more usually, a large heavy-duty rotary press can be used. This process is often known as 'slugging', the compact made in the process (typically 25 mm diameter by about 10–15 mm thick) being termed a 'slug'. A hammer mill is suitable for breaking the compacts.

Roller compactors

Roller compaction is an alternative gentler method, the powder mix being squeezed between two rollers to form a compressed sheet (Fig. 25.13). The sheet normally is weak and brittle and breaks immediately into flakes. These flakes need gentler treatment to break them into granules, and this can usually be achieved by screening alone.

BIBLIOGRAPHY

There are a large number of published papers in the field of pharmaceutical granulation and only a limited number are listed below.

Baert, L. (1992) Correlation of extrusion forces, raw materials and sphere characteristics. *J. Pharm. Pharmacol.*, **44**, 676–678.

Das, S. and Jarowski, C.I. (1979) Effect of granulating method on particle size distribution of granules and disintegrated tablets. *Drug Dev. Ind. Pharm.*, **5**, 479.

Faure, A., Grimsey, I.M., Rowe, R.C. York, P. and Cliff, M.J. (1999) Applicability of a scale-up methodology for the wet granulation process in Collette Gral high shear mixer granulators. *Eur. J. Pharm. Sci.*, **8**, 85–93.

Gandhi, R., Kaul, C.L. and Panchagnula, R. (1999). Extrusion and spheronization in the development of oral controlled-release dosage forms. *Pharm. Sci. Tech. Today*, **2(4)**, 160–81.

Gergely, G. (1981) Granulation – a new approach. *Mfg Chem. Aerosol News*, **52**, 43.

Landin, M., York, P., Cliff, M.J. and Rowe, R.C. (1999) Scale up of a pharmaceutical granulation in planetary mixers. *Pharm. Dev. Tech.*, **4(2)**, 145–150.

Law, M.F.L. et al (1997). Comparison of two commercial brands of microcrystalline cellulose for extrusion–spheronization. *J. Microencap.*, **14(6)**, 713–723.

Lindberg, N.-O. and Leander, L. (1982) Instrumentation of a Kenwood major domestic-type mixer for studies of granulation. *Drug Dev. Ind. Pharm.*, **8**, 775.

Maejima, T. et al (1998) Application of tumbling melt granulation (TMG) method to prepare controlled-release fine granules. *Chem. Pharm. Bull*, **46(3)**, 534–536.

Nurnberg, E. and Wunderlich, J. (1998). Manufacturing pellets by extrusion and spheronization (Part I). *Pharm. Technol. Eur.*, **11(2)**, 41–47; Part II **11(3)**.

Ogawa, S. et al (1994) A new attempt to solve the scale-up problem for granulation using response surface methodology. *J. Pharm. Sci.*, **83(3)**, 439–443.

Parikh, D.M. (1997). *Handbook of Pharmaceutical Granulation Technology*, Marcel Dekker, New York.

Rubino, O.R. (1999) Fluid-bed technology; overview and criteria for process selection. *Pharm. Tech.*, **(6)**, 104–113.

Shah, R.D. et al (1995) Physico-mechanical characterization of the extrusion-spheronization process. *Pharm. Res.*, **12(4)**, 496–507.

Thoma, K. and Ziegler, I. (1998) Investigations on the influence of the type of extruder for pelletization by extrusion–spheronization I. Extrusion behavior of formulations. *Drug Dev. Ind. Pharm.*, **24(5)**, 401–411; II Sphere characteristics. *Drug Dev. Ind. Pharm.*, **24(5)**, 413–422.

Wørts, O. (1998) Wet granulation – fluidized bed and high shear techniques compared. *Pharm. Techn. Europe*, **10(11)**, 27–30.

Zhang, F. and McGinity, J.M. (1999). Properties of sustained-release tablets prepared by hot-melt etrusion. *Pharm. Dev. and Tech.*, **4(2)**, 241–250.

26
Drying

Michael Aulton

CHAPTER CONTENTS

INTRODUCTION

Drying is an important operation in primary pharmaceutical manufacture (i.e. the synthesis of actives) as it is usually the last stage of manufacturing before packaging, and it is important that the residual moisture is rendered low enough to prevent product deterioration during storage and ensure free-flowing properties during use. It is equally important (and probably encountered more frequently) in secondary (dosage form) manufacture following the commonly performed operation of wet granulation (Chapter 25) during the preparation of granules prior to tablet compaction. Hence, stability, flow properties and compactability are all influenced by residual moisture (see Chapter 27).

This chapter is concerned with drying to the solid state, starting with either a wet solid or a solution or suspension of the materials that will form the final dry product. Formerly solutions or suspensions were first concentrated by evaporation of much of the liquid before drying of the intermediate paste so formed. Equipment such as the spray drier (see later) are now capable of producing a dry product from a solution or suspension in one operation.

Most pharmaceutical materials are not completely free from moisture ('bone dry') but contain some residual water, which may vary with the temperature and humidity of the ambient air to which they are exposed. This is discussed in more detail later.

Some wet crystallized product may be freed from much of its residual moisture by initial treatment in a 'dewatering' centrifuge, which is similar in construction to a domestic spindrier. For the purpose of this chapter, however, drying is defined as the removal of all or most of the liquid by supplying latent heat to cause thermal vaporization, i.e. a liquid is converted into a vapour. In the majority of cases the 'liquid' will be water, but volatile solvents such as isopropanol may also need to be removed in a drying process. The physical principles are similar regardless of the nature of the liquid, although volatile solvents are normally recovered by condensation (rather than being vented into the atmosphere). The toxicity and flammability of organic solvents pose safety considerations.

THE DRYING OF WET SOLIDS

An understanding of this operation requires some preliminary explanation of the following important terms. These will be defined and explained in the context of water (the most commonly used pharmaceutical solvent), but the explanations and concepts are equally applicable to other relevant liquids (e.g. ethanol, isopropanol etc).

Moisture content of wet solids

The moisture content of a wet solid is expressed as kilograms of moisture associated with 1 kg of the moisture-free or 'bone-dry' solid. Thus a moisture content of 0.4 means that 0.4 kg of removable water is present per kg of the 'bone-dry' solid which will remain after complete drying. It is sometimes calculated as a percentage moisture content.

Total moisture content

This is the total amount of liquid associated with a wet solid. In the context of drying, not all of it can be easily removed by the simple evaporative processes employed by most pharmaceutical driers. The easily removable water is known as the **free moisture content**, and the moisture which is more difficult to remove in practice is the **equilibrium moisture content** (see below). The easily removable water is known as **unbound water**.

Unbound water This water exists as a liquid and exerts its full vapour pressure; it can be removed readily by evaporation. During a drying process this water is easily lost but the resulting solid is not completely free from water molecules; this is known as **air dry**.

Equilibrium moisture content

Evaporative drying processes will not remove all the possible moisture present in a wet product because the solid equilibrates with the moisture present in the air. The moisture content present in a solid under steady-state ambient conditions is termed the equilibrium moisture content. Its value changes with temperature, humidity and the nature of the solid.

Bound water Part of the moisture present in a wet solid may be adsorbed on surfaces of the solid or be adsorbed within its structure to such an extent to prevent it from developing its full vapour pressure and from being easily removed by evaporation. Such moisture is described as 'bound' and is more difficult to remove than unbound water. The adsorbed water is attached to the surface of the solid as individual water molecules, which may form a mono- (or bi-) layer on the solid surface. Absorbed water exists as a liquid but is trapped in capillaries within the solid by surface tension. As such it cannot exert its full vapour pressure and is not easily lost by evaporation.

Relative humidity (RH) of air

Air at a given temperature is capable of taking up water vapour until it is saturated (at 100% RH). It is a simple solution of water in air that follows the rules of most solutions – such as increased solubility with increasing temperature, a maximum solubility at a particular temperature (saturation) and precipitation of the solute on cooling (condensation, rain). If the temperature is raised then the air will be able to take up more moisture and the relative humidity falls.

This is because the percentage RH may be defined as:

$$\frac{\text{Vapour pressure of water vapour in the air}}{\substack{\text{Vapour pressure of water vapour in air} \\ \text{saturated at the same temperature}}} \times 100$$

This is **approximately** equal to the **percentage saturation**, which is the ratio:

$$\frac{\text{Mass of vapour present per kg of dry air}}{\substack{\text{Mass of vapour required to saturate 1 kg} \\ \text{of air at the same temperature}}} \times 100$$

This relationship shows that the relative humidity of air is dependent not only on the amount of moisture in the air, but also on its temperature, as the amount of water required to saturate air is itself dependent on temperature.

It should be noted that in convective drying, where warm air is passed over the surface of a wet solid, the relative humidity may rise during the drying process as a result of two separate factors:

1. Uptake of evaporated water vapour from the wet solid;
2. The cooling of the supply air as it transfers heat to the wet solid (evaporative cooling).

If the cooling is excessive the temperature of the air may fall to a value known as the **dew point**, when liquid water will condense and be deposited.

Wet-bulb and dry-bulb temperature

If two similar thermometers are set up, one with its bulb kept moist by a wet cotton wick immersed in a water reservoir, the wet-bulb thermometer will register a lower temperature than its dry-bulb neighbour (Fig. 26.1). This is due to the **evaporative cooling** as the latent heat of evaporation (Chapter 38) is taken from the sensible heat of the water surrounding the

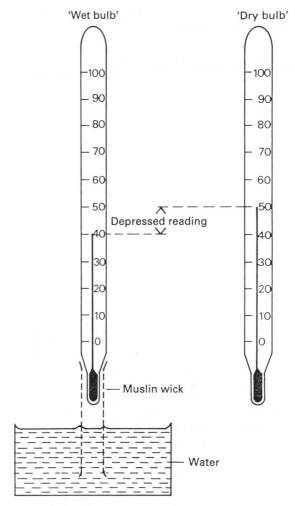

Fig. 26.1 Wet- and dry-bulb temperatures.

bulb. In a similar way, the temperature of a wet solid is kept low while free water remains, but rises towards the temperature of the drying air as drying proceeds. Fortunately, many materials can withstand higher temperatures when in the dry state.

The two temperatures will be the same only when the relative humidity is 100%, as under these conditions there will be no net evaporation of water from the sleeve. In fact, the relationship between dry-bulb temperature and the depression of the wet-bulb temperature as a result of evaporation is so precise that these readings can be used to calculate the percentage relative humidity of the air with some accuracy.

Moisture content of air

The moisture content of air, which is the moisture content expressed as kg of water per kg of 'bone-dry'

381

air, should be carefully distinguished from the relative humidity. Moisture content is not altered by change of temperature alone, only if further moisture is taken up by the air.

Relationship between equilibrium moisture content and relative humidity

The equilibrium moisture content of a solid exposed to moist air varies with the relative humidity, as shown in some typical plots (Fig. 26.2). Ordinary atmospheric conditions are of the order of 20°C and 70–75% relative humidity, so that if exposed to the atmosphere a mineral such as kaolin will contain about 1% moisture, whereas a starch-based product may have as much as 30% or more. Materials exposed to humid conditions will regain moisture, and so there is no advantage in drying to a moisture content lower than that which the material will have under the conditions of use.

Loss of water from wet solids

As explained above, unbound water is easily lost by evaporation until the equilibrium moisture content of the solid is reached. This is shown in Figure 26.3. Once the solid reaches its equilibrium moisture content, extending the time of drying will not change the moisture content as an equilibrium situation has been reached. The only way to reduce the moisture content of the solid shown in Figure 26.3 is to

Fig. 26.3   Loss of water from a drying solid. The wet solid prior to drying is at condition (1). It can lose water by evaporation to position (2), its equilibrium moisture content at that RH. The only way the solid can lose more water is to reduce the RH of the ambient or storage atmosphere, to (3) with silica gel or to (4) with phosphorus pentoxide.

reduce the relative humidity of the ambient air. This can be done mechanically on a large scale with an air-conditioning system. On a small scale, desiccators are used. Silica gel (a common laboratory desiccant) does not directly take water from a solid, instead, it acts by removing the water from the air, thereby reducing its relative humidity to around 5–10%. This in turn moves the drying curve in Figure 26.3 to the left, thus reducing the moisture content of the solids in the desiccator. Phosphorous pentoxide works in an identical manner but it has an even greater affinity for the water in the storage air.

It is worth re-emphasizing at this point that moisture may be regained very quickly from the atmosphere if a 'dry' solid is exposed to ambient air. For this reason it is unnecessary to 'overdry' a product. If a low residual moisture content is necessary because of hydrolytic instability in the material, the dried product must be efficiently sealed from the ingress of moisture. It also worthy of note that some materials (tablet granules are a classic example) have superior compaction properties with a small amount (1–2%) of residual moisture.

Fig. 26.2   Typical equilibrium moisture contents at 20°C. (1) Starch-based materials; (2) textiles and fibrous materials; (3) inorganic substances such as kaolin.

TYPES OF DRYING METHOD

When considering how to dry a material, the following points should be considered:

• Heat sensitivity of the material being dried

- Physical characteristics of the material
- The necessity for asepsis
- Nature of the liquid to be removed
- The scale of the operation
- Available sources of heat (steam, electrical).

The general principles for efficient drying can be summarized as follows:

- Large surface area for heat transfer;
- Efficient heat transfer per unit area (to supply sufficient latent heat of vaporization or heat of sublimation in the case of freeze-drying);
- Efficient mass transfer of evaporated water through any surrounding boundary layers, i.e. sufficient turbulence to minimize boundary layer thickness;
- Efficient vapour removal, i.e. low relative humidity air at adequate velocity.

It is convenient to categorize pharmaceutical driers according to the heat transfer method they use, i.e. convective, conductive or radiant.

CONVECTIVE DRYING OF WET SOLIDS

Fixed (or static) bed convective drying

The factors affecting drying in this manner can be illustrated by reference to the construction and use of a simple form of drier – the tray (shelf or compartment) drier.

Tray drier

An efficient type of tray drier is the directed circulation form shown in Figure 26.4. Air flows in the direction of the arrows over each shelf in turn. The wet material is spread on shallow trays resting on the shelves. Electrical elements or steam-heated

Fig. 26.4 Directed-circulation tray drier.

pipes are positioned as shown, so that the air is periodically reheated after it has cooled by passage over the wet material on one shelf before it passes over the material on the next.

The required latent heat of evaporation is transferred convectively from the air and the rate of heat transfer may be written as:

$$\text{Rate of heat transfer, } (dH/dt) = h_c A\, \Delta T$$

where h_c is a heat transfer coefficient (Chapter 38) for convective heat transfer. The value of h_c is commonly around only $10\text{--}20\ \text{W m}^{-2}\ \text{K}^{-1}$. Heat transfer from air is therefore relatively inefficient and so convective drying is slow and wet materials can take up to 24 hours to dry.

There is another important factor controlling the rate of drying: the water vapour must pass through the boundary layers present at the surface into the turbulent airstream. For this to occur the relative humidity of the air must be kept well below the saturation level and the boundary layers small. These conditions are achieved by having a brisk turbulent air flow over the surface and by the periodic reheating of the air as the temperature falls, so that it can pick up further moisture.

Rate of drying in fixed beds

The rate at which drying occurs has been found to show certain phases (Fig. 26.5) in which the change in moisture content is plotted against time. From A to B the relationship is linear, which is known as the **constant-rate period**, whereas from B to C the rate of loss of moisture decreases and is known as the **falling-rate period**. The end of the constant rate period, B, is referred to as the **critical moisture content**.

The **first falling-rate period** has a linear relationship, that is, the decrease in drying rate is uniform, whereas in the **second falling-rate period** there is a continuous decrease in the rate of drying until the equilibrium moisture content is reached. Each of these periods will be considered in more detail.

Constant-rate period   For given conditions of temperature and humidity, most substances dry at a similar rate in the constant-rate period. It is found that the evaporation rate from the drying bed is similar to that of the solvent alone from a free liquid surface under the same conditions, indicating that the evaporation takes place from the wet surface of the solid, and that the surface remains wet in this period as a result of the liquid being replaced from below as fast as it is vaporized.

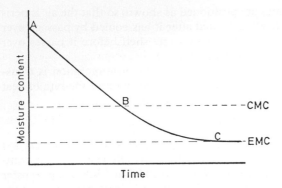

Fig. 26.5 Drying curve. CMC, critical moisture content, EMC, equilibrium moisture content.

Controlling factors in this period are the rate at which heat can be transferred and the rate of removal of the vapour, as explained earlier.

First falling-rate period As moisture is removed from the surface, a point will be reached when the rate of vaporization is insufficient to saturate the air in contact with the surface. Under these conditions, the rate of drying will be limited by the rate of capillary transfer of the liquid to the surface of the wet bed, and as this becomes increasingly difficult as the bed dries, the solvent level decreases and thus has further to travel to the point of evaporation. Consequently, the rate of drying decreases continuously.

Moisture movement may cause the 'migration' of soluble drugs or excipients. This is discussed later in this chapter.

Eventually, movement of solvent to the surface can no longer occur, for example when the water is in the pendular state (Fig. 25.2) and drying at the surface will end. As the drying rate decreases, less heat is used as latent heat of vaporization, so that the heat input should be reduced.

Second falling-rate period Any moisture that remains within the drying bed at the end of the first falling-rate period is unable to move, so that drying cannot take place on the surface. Hence, the plane of vaporization retreats from the surface into the body of the solid, and the drying rate depends on the movement of the **vapour** through the pores of the bed to the surface, in general by molecular diffusion.

Minimal atmospheric humidity above the solid will assist in maintaining the maximum vapour pressure gradient. In addition, the thermal conductivity of the solid decreases as it becomes dry; if the solid is thermostable it is safe to allow temperature gradients to increase to maintain the rate of heat transfer, but if the material is thermolabile the heating must be decreased.

In the operation of a tray drier it is usual to remove the dry material on the trays near the air inlet and replace them with the trays with partially dry material from further away. Trays with fresh wet material are placed on the empty shelves. In this way the outgoing (wetter) air contacts the wettest material.

Dynamic convective driers

Fluidized-bed drier

An excellent method of obtaining good contact between the warm drying air and wet particles is found in the **fluidized-bed drier**. The general principles of **fluidization** will be summarized before discussing its application to drying.

Consider the situation in which particulate matter is contained in a vessel, the base of which is perforated, enabling a fluid to pass through the bed of solids from below. The fluid can be liquid or gas, but for the purposes of this description air will be assumed, as it is directly relevant to the drying process.

If the air velocity through the bed is increased gradually and the pressure drop through the bed is measured, a graph of the operation shows several distinct regions, as indicated in Figure 26.6. At first, when the air velocity is low, A, flow takes place between the particles without causing disturbance, but as the velocity is increased a point, B, is reached, when the pressure drop has attained a value where the frictional drag on the particle is equal to the force of gravity on that particle. Rearrangement of the particles occurs to offer least resistance, C, and eventually they are suspended in the air and can move; pressure drop through the bed decreases slightly because of the greater porosity, D. Further increase in the air velocity causes the particles to separate and move freely and the bed is **fully fluidized**. Any additional increase in velocity separates the particles

Fig. 26.6 Effect of air velocity on pressure drop through a fluidized bed.

further, that is, the bed expands without appreciable change in the pressure drop, until E, when the air velocity is sufficient to entrain the solid particles and transport them out of the top of the bed.

In the region D–E fluidization is irregular, much of the air flowing through in bubbles, the term **boiling bed** being commonly used to describe it. The important fact is that it produces conditions of great turbulence, the particles mixing with good contact between them and the air. Hence if hot air is used the turbulent conditions lead to high heat and mass transfer rates; the fluidized-bed technique therefore offers a means of rapid drying. The arrangement of such a drier is shown in Figure 26.7. Sizes are available with capacities from 1 kg in the laboratory to 200–500 kg in production.

Advantages of fluidized-bed drying

1. Efficient heat and mass transfer give high drying rates, so that drying times are shorter than with static-bed convection driers. A batch of tablet granules, for example, can be dried in 20–30 minutes, whereas a tray drier would require many hours. Apart from obvious economic advantages, the heat challenge to thermolabile materials is minimized.
2. The fluidized state of the bed ensures that drying occurs from the surface of all the individual particles and not just from the surface of the bed. Hence, most of the drying will be at constant rate and the failing-rate period (when the danger of overheating is greatest) is very short.
3. The temperature of a fluidized bed is uniform throughout and can be controlled precisely.
4. The turbulence in a fluidized bed causes some attrition to the surface of the granule. This produces a more spherical free-flowing product.
5. The free movement of individual particles eliminates the risk of soluble materials migrating, as may occur in static beds (see later).
6. The containers can be mobile, making handling and movement around the production area simple and so reducing labour costs.
7. Short drying times mean that the unit has a high output from a small floor space.

Disadvantages of fluidized-bed drying

1. The turbulence of the fluidized state may cause excessive attrition of some materials, with damage to some granules and the production of too much dust.
2. Fine particles may become entrained in the fluidizing air and must be collected by bag filters, with care to avoid segregation and loss of fines.
3. The vigorous movement of particles in hot dry air can lead to the generation of static electricity charges, and suitable precautions must be taken. A mixture of air with a fine dust of organic materials such as starch and lactose can explode

Fig. 26.7 Fluidized-bed drier.

violently if ignited by sparking caused by static charges. The danger is increased if the fluidized material contains a volatile solvent such as isopropanol. Adequate electrical earthing is essential.

CONDUCTIVE DRYING OF WET SOLIDS

In this process the wet solid is in thermal contact with a hot surface and the bulk of heat transfer occurs by conduction.

Vacuum oven

This equipment is a good example of a conduction drier though it is not used so extensively as it was formerly. The vacuum oven (Fig. 26.8) consists of a jacketed vessel sufficiently stout in construction to withstand vacuum within the oven and steam pressure in the jacket. In addition, the supports for the shelves form part of the jacket, giving a larger area for conduction heat transfer. The oven can be closed by a door that can be locked to give an airtight seal. The oven is connected through a condenser and liquid receiver to a vacuum pump, although if the liquid to be removed is water and the pump is of the ejector type that can handle water vapour, the pump can be connected directly to the oven.

Operating pressure can be as low as 0.03–0.06 bar, at which pressures water boils at 25–35°C. Some ovens may be large (for example about 1.5 m cube and with 20 shelves), but vacuum ovens are rarely used nowadays for production, although they are frequently found in development laboratories, where they are commonly used for the drying of small development samples, particularly when the heat stability of the drug or formulation is uncertain.

The main advantage of a vacuum oven is that drying takes place at a low temperature, and as there is little air present there is minimum risk of oxidation. The temperature of the drying solid will rise to the steam or water temperature at the end of the drying, but this is not usually harmful.

Vacuum tumbling drier

Vacuum tumbling drying has found application in the pharmaceutical industry. One design of tumbler drier resembles a large Y-cone mixer (discussed in Chapter 13). The vessel is steam jacketed and is connected to a vacuum. It can be used for drying tablet granules, which tumble over the heated surface as the vessel slowly revolves. Heat transfer rates in this equipment are much higher than can be attained in a conventional vacuum oven, where the material is static.

RADIATION DRYING OF WET SOLIDS

Radiant heat transmission

Heat transmission by radiation differs from heat transfer by conduction or convection in that no transfer medium (solid, liquid or gaseous) need be present. Heat energy in the form of radiation can cross empty space or travel through the atmosphere virtually without loss. If it falls on a body capable of absorbing it then it appears as heat, although a proportion may be reflected or transmitted.

Use of infrared radiation

Infrared heating has been used in the past to dry pharmaceutical products such as wet granules, but it suffers from the disadvantage that it is absorbed very quickly and does not penetrate far into the wet mass.

Steam or water jacket

Condenser

Connection to vacuum pump

Condensate receiver

Fig. 26.8   Vacuum oven (schematic).

The surface layers dry quickly and the absorption of further energy then raises the temperature of the dry material to a high value, which is often detrimental to the product. For this reason infrared radiation is now seldom used as a heat source in pharmaceutical manufacture.

The use of microwave radiation

Although energy in the infrared region is more easily generated there are other, longer, wavelengths that can generate heat when the radiation is absorbed by a wet solid. Microwave radiation in the wavelength range 10 mm to 1 m penetrates much better than IR radiation. Microwave driers are finding some application in the pharmaceutical industry.

Generation and action of microwaves

Microwaves are produced by an electronic device known as a magnetron. Microwave energy can be reflected down a rectangular duct (termed a waveguide) or simply beamed through a transparent polypropylene window into the drying chamber. To avoid interference with radio and television it is permitted to operate only at certain frequencies, which are normally 960 and 2450 MHz.

The penetration of microwaves into the wet product is so good that heat is generated uniformly within the solid.

When microwaves fall on substances of suitable electronic structure (small polar molecules, such as water), the electrons in the molecule attempt to resonate in sympathy with the radiation and the resulting molecular 'friction' results in the generation of heat. Dry solids do not resonate as well as water, so further heating may be avoided once the water is removed. This is indicated clearly by the loss factors listed in Table 26.1. The loss factor is a measure of the ratio of the microwave energy absorbed by individual molecules; the higher the number the greater the absorption of microwave energy. Table 26.1 lists these values for some common solvents and excipients. Clearly, the absorption of the microwave energy is far greater for small polar molecules than for larger and less polar molecules.

A microwave drier for granulates

Figure 26.9 is a sketch of a microwave drier used for drying granulates. It is designed to operate under a slight vacuum. This in itself is not essential for the use of microwaves, but the air flow allows the con-

Table 26.1 Microwave energy loss factors for some pharmaceutical solvents and excipients

Material	Loss factor
Methanol	13.6
Ethanol	8.6
Water	6.1
Isopropanol	2.9
Acetone	1.25
Maize starch	0.41
Magnesium carbonate	0.08
Lactose	0.02

tinuous removal of evaporated solvent. The radiation is generated by multiple magnetrons, each producing 0.75 kW at 2450 MHz. The radiation passes through the polypropylene window into the drying chamber, where it is absorbed by the liquid in the wet granules contained on a tray. The heat generated in the mass drives off the moisture and the evolved vapour is drawn away in the air flow as it is formed. When drying is nearly complete the radiation field intensity will rise, as the dry solids do not absorb as readily as water. This rise is detected and the magnetrons are progressively turned off automatically, to give an accurate control of the final moisture content and minimize the danger of overheating.

Advantages of microwave drying The following advantages are claimed for microwave drying:

1. It provides rapid drying at fairly low temperatures.
2. The thermal efficiency is high, as the drier casing and the air remain cool. Most of the microwave energy is absorbed by the liquid in the wet material.
3. The bed is stationary, avoiding the problems of dust and attrition.
4. Solute migration is reduced as there is uniform heating of the wet mass.
5. Equipment is highly efficient and refined. All the requirements of product and operator safety have been incorporated into machines without detracting from GMP considerations.
6. Granulation end-point is possible by measuring the residual microwave energy (as this rises sharply when there is little solvent left to evaporate).

Fig. 26.9   Microwave drier (courtesy of T K Fielder).

Disadvantages of microwave drying
1. The batch size of commercial production microwave driers is smaller than those available for fluidized-bed driers.
2. Care must be taken to shield operators from the microwave radiation, which can cause damage to organs such as the eyes and testes. This is ensured by 'failsafe' devices preventing the generation of microwaves until the drying chamber is sealed.

DRIERS FOR DILUTE SOLUTIONS AND SUSPENSIONS

The objective of these driers is to spread the liquid to a large surface area for heat and mass transfer and

to provide an effective means of collecting the dry solid. Two main types are used, the first spreading the liquid to a thin film on to a drum and the second dispersing the liquid to a spray of small droplets.

Drum drier

Shown in section in Figure 26.10, the drum drier consists of a drum 0.75–1.5 m in diameter and 2–4 m in length, heated internally, usually by steam, and rotated on its longitudinal axis. The liquid is applied to the surface of the drum and spread to a film; this may be done in various ways, but the simplest method is that shown in the diagram, where the drum dips into a **feed pan**. Drying rate is controlled by manipulating the speed of rotation of the drum and its temperature. The drum can be heated by either steam or warm water. The product is scraped

Fig. 26.10 Drum drier.

from the surface of the drum by means of a *doctor knife*.

Advantages of the drum drier

1. The method gives rapid drying, the thin film spread over a large area resulting in rapid heat and mass transfer.
2. The equipment is compact, occupying much less space than the spray-drier, for example.
3. Heating time is short, being only a few seconds.
4. The drum can be enclosed in a vacuum jacket, enabling the temperature of drying to be reduced.
5. The product is obtained in flake form, which is convenient for many purposes.

The only **disadvantage** is that operating conditions are critical and it is necessary to impose careful control on feed rate, film thickness, speed of drum rotation and drum temperature.

The drum drier can handle a variety of materials, either as solutions or as suspensions; substances that are dried by this method include starch products, ferrous salts and suspensions of kaolin and zinc oxide.

Spray drier

The spray drier provides a large surface area for heat and mass transfer by atomizing the liquid to small droplets. These are sprayed into a stream of hot air, so that each droplet dries to an individual solid particle.

There are many forms of spray drier and Figure 26.11 shows a typical design, in which the drying chamber resembles a cyclone. This ensures good air circulation, facilitates heat and mass transfer and encourages the separation of dried particles from the moving air by the centrifugal action.

The character of the particles is controlled by the droplet size, and so the type of atomizer is important. Jet atomizers are easily blocked by rapid evaporation and deposition of solid on the nozzle, and the droplet size is likely to vary. This is not the case with

Fig. 26.11 Spray drier.

rotary types of atomizer, one form of which is shown in Figure 26.12. Liquid is fed on to the disc, which is rotated at high speed (up to 20 000 rpm). A film is formed and spreads from the small disc to a larger, inverted hemispherical bowl, becoming thinner and eventually being dispersed from the edge in a fine, uniform spray. In addition, the rotary atomizer has the advantage of being equally effective with either solutions or suspensions of solids, and it can operate efficiently at various feed rates.

The air enters the chamber tangentially and rotates the drying droplets around the chamber to increase their residence time and therefore time for drying. For pharmaceutical purposes it is usual to filter the air and to heat it indirectly by means of a heat exchanger. Dust carried over in the air outlet stream may be recovered by a cyclone separator or filter bag.

Fig. 26.12 Rotary atomizer.

Spray-dried products are easily recognizable, being uniform in appearance. The particles have a characteristic shape, in the form of hollow spheres sometimes with a small hole. This arises from the drying process, as the droplet enters the hot air stream and dries on the outside to form an outer crust with liquid still in the centre. This liquid then vaporizes, and the internal vapour escapes by blowing a hole in the sphere. Figure 26.13 shows the mechanism of formation of the spherical product.

Advantages of the spray drying process
1. There are millions of small droplets which give a large surface area for heat and mass transfer, so that evaporation is very rapid. The actual drying time of a droplet is only a fraction of a second, and the overall time in the drier only a few seconds.
2. Because evaporation is very rapid, the droplets do not attain a high temperature. Most of the heat is used as latent heat of vaporization and so the temperature of the particles is kept low by evaporative cooling.
3. The characteristic particle form gives the product a high bulk density and, in turn, rapid dissolution (large surface area).
4. Provided that a suitable atomizer is used the resulting powder will have a uniform and controllable particle size.
5. The product is free flowing, with almost spherical particles, and is especially convenient for tablet manufacture as it has excellent flow and compaction properties.

6. Labour costs are low, the process yielding a dry, free-flowing powder from a dilute solution in a single operation with no handling.

Disadvantages of the spray drying process
1. The equipment is very bulky, and with the ancillary equipment is expensive. In a large installation the drying chamber alone may be as much as 15 m in height and 6 m in diameter.
2. The overall thermal efficiency is rather low, as the air must still be hot enough when it leaves the drier to avoid condensation of moisture. Also, large volumes of heated air pass through the chamber without contacting a particle, thus not contributing directly to the drying process.

Uses of the spray drying process The spray drier can be used for drying almost any substance, in solution or in suspension. It is most useful for thermolabile materials, particularly if handled continuously and in large quantities; outputs of 2000 kg h^{-1} can be attained, although pharmaceutical plants are usually somewhat smaller.

Examples of both soluble and insoluble substances that are spray dried include citric acid, sodium phosphate gelatin, starch, barium sulphate, calcium phosphate, and some powdered antibiotic formulations for reconstitution into syrup.

Spray drying is also capable of producing spherical particles in the respirable range of 1–7 mm that have been used satisfactorily for the delivery of drugs from dry powder inhalers.

It is possible to operate spray driers aseptically using heated filtered air to dry products such as serum hydrolysate. Also, some spray driers operate in a closed-circuit mode with an inert gas to minimize oxidation of the product. Volatile solvents can be recovered from such systems.

Modern pharmaceutical spray drying has been reviewed by Wendel and Çelik (1997) and the reader is referred to this article if additional information is required.

FREEZE DRYING

Freeze drying is a process used to dry extremely heat-sensitive materials. It allows the drying, without excessive damage, of proteins, blood products and even microorganisms, which retain a small but significant viability.

In this process the initial liquid solution or suspension is frozen, the pressure above the frozen state

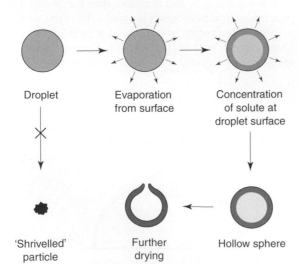

Droplet

Evaporation from surface

Concentration of solute at droplet surface

'Shrivelled' particle

Further drying

Hollow sphere

Fig. 26.13 Formation of product in spray drying.

is reduced and the water removed by sublimation. Thus a liquid-to-vapour transition takes place, as with all the previous driers discussed, but here there are three states of matter involved: liquid to solid, then solid to vapour.

The theory and practice of freeze drying is based, therefore, on an understanding and application of the phase diagram for the water system.

The phase diagram for water

The phase diagram for the water system is shown in Figure 26.14. The diagram consists of three separate areas, each representing a single phase of water, either solid, liquid or vapour. Two phases can coexist along a line under the conditions of temperature and pressure defined by any point on the line. The point O is the one unique point where all three phases can coexist, and is known as the *triple point*. Its coordinates are a pressure of 610 Pa and a temperature of 0.0075°C.

The lines on the phase diagram represent the interphase equilibrium lines, which show:

1. the boiling point of water as it is lowered by reduction of the external pressure above the water (BO in Fig. 26.14);
2. the variation of the melting point of ice on reduction of the external pressure above it. There is a very slight rise in the melting point (AO);

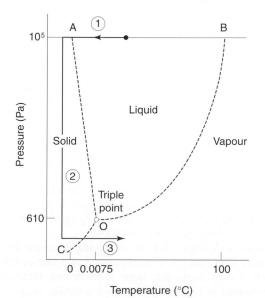

Fig. 26.14 The phase diagram for water (not to scale) with freeze drying process superimposed (see text for explanation).

3. the reduction of the vapour pressure exerted by ice as the temperature is reduced (CO).

On heating at constant **atmospheric** pressure ice will melt when the temperature rises to 0°C. At this constant temperature and pressure it will then change to water. Continued heating will raise the temperature of the water to 100°C where, if heat addition is continued, the liquid water will be converted into water vapour at 100°C.

If, however, solid ice is maintained at a pressure below the triple point then on heating the ice will sublime and pass directly to water vapour without passing through the liquid phase. This sublimation, and therefore drying, can occur at a temperature below 0°C. This will only happen if the pressure is prevented from rising above the triple point pressure and, to ensure that this is the case, the vapour evolved must be removed as fast as it is formed. It may be thought that as the process takes place at a low temperature the heat required to sublime the ice will be small. In fact, the latent heat of sublimation of ice at 2900 kJ kg^{-1} is appreciably greater than the latent heat of evaporation of water at atmospheric pressure, and this heat must be supplied for the process to take place.

Application of the phase diagram of water to freeze drying

The freeze drying of products such as blood plasma, although simple in theory, presents a number of practical problems.

1. The depression of the freezing point caused by the presence of dissolved solutes means that the solution must be cooled to well below the normal freezing temperature for pure water, and it is usual to work in the range −10 to −30°C. In part this is because it is obviously not pure water that is being dried, and thus the presence of dissolved solutes will shift the pure-water phase diagram.
2. Sublimation can only occur at the frozen surface and is a slow process (approximately 1 mm thickness of ice per hour). For all but very small volumes the surface area must therefore be increased and the liquid thickness prior to freezing be reduced in order to reduce the thickness of ice to be sublimated.
3. At low pressures large volumes of water vapour are produced which must be rapidly removed to prevent the pressure rising above the triple point pressure.

4. The dry material often needs to be sterile, and it must also be prevented from regaining moisture prior to final packing.

Stages of the freeze drying process

Freezing stage

The liquid material is frozen before the application of vacuum to avoid frothing, and several methods are used to produce a large frozen surface.

Shell freezing   This is employed for fairly large volumes such as blood products. The bottles are rotated slowly and almost horizontally in a refrigerated bath. The liquid freezes in a thin shell around the inner circumference of the bottle. Freezing is slow and large ice crystals form, which is a drawback of this method as they may damage blood cells and reduce the viability of microbial cultures.

In vertical spin freezing the bottles are spun individually in a vertical position so that centrifugal force forms a circumferential layer of solution, which is cooled by a blast of cold air. The solution supercools and freezes rapidly, with the formation of small ice crystals.

Centrifugal evaporative freezing   This is a similar method, where the solution is spun in small containers within a centrifuge. This prevents foaming when a vacuum is applied. The vacuum causes boiling at room temperature and this removes so much latent heat that the solution cools quickly and snap freezes. About 20% of the water is removed prior to freeze drying and there is no need for refrigeration. Ampoules are usually frozen in this way, a number being spun in a horizontal angled position in a special centrifuge head so that the liquid is thrown outwards and freezes as a wedge.

Vacuum application stage

The containers and the frozen material must be connected to a vacuum source sufficient to drop the pressure below the triple point and remove the large volumes of low-pressure vapour formed during drying. Again an excess vacuum is normal in practice, to ensure that the product in question is below its triple point.

Commonly a number of bottles or vials are attached to individual outlets of a manifold, which is connected to a vacuum.

Sublimation stage

Heat of sublimation must be supplied. Under these conditions the ice slowly sublimes, leaving a porous solid which still contains about 0.5% moisture after primary drying.

Primary drying   Primary drying can reduce the moisture content of a freeze-dried solid to around 0.5%. Further reduction can be effected by secondary drying. During the primary drying, the latent heat of sublimation must be provided and the vapour removed.

Heat transfer   Heat transfer is critical: insufficient heat input prolongs the process, which is already slow, and excess heat will cause melting.

Prefrozen bottles – of blood, for example – are placed in individually heated cylinders, or are connected to a manifold when heat can be taken from the atmosphere.

Shelf-frozen materials are heated from the drier shelf, whereas ampoules may be left on the centrifuge head or may be placed on a manifold, but in either case heat from the atmosphere is sufficient.

In all cases the heat transfer must be controlled, as only about 5 W m^{-2} K^{-1} is needed and overheating will lead to melting. It is important to appreciate here that although a significant amount of heat is required there should be no significant increase in temperature – the added heat should be sufficient to provide the latent heat of sublimation only and little sensible heat.

Vapour removal   The vapour formed must be continually removed to avoid a pressure rise that would stop sublimation. To reduce the pressure sufficiently it is necessary to use efficient vacuum pumps, usually two-stage rotary pumps on the small scale, and ejector pumps on the large scale. On the small scale, vapour is absorbed by a desiccant such as phosphorus pentoxide, or is cooled in a small condenser with solid carbon dioxide. Mechanically refrigerated condensers are used on the large scale.

For vapour flow to occur the vapour pressure at the condenser must be less than that at the frozen surface, and a low condenser temperature is necessary. On the large scale vapour is commonly removed by pumping, but the pumps must be of large capacity and not affected by moisture. The extent of the necessary pumping capacity will be realized from the fact that, under the pressure conditions used during primary drying, 1 g of ice will form 1000 L of water vapour. Ejector pumps are most satisfactory for this purpose.

Rate of drying   The rate of drying in freeze drying is very slow, the ice being removed at a rate of about only 1 mm depth per hour. The drying rate curve illustrated in Figure 26.15 shows a similar shape to a normal drying curve, the drying being at constant rate during most of the time.

Fig. 26.15 Sublimation drying: rate of drying curve.

Computer control enables the drying cycle to be monitored. There is an optimum vapour pressure for a maximum sublimation rate and the heat input and other variables are adjusted to maintain this value. Continuous freeze drying is possible in modern equipment, where the vacuum chamber is fitted with a belt conveyor and vacuum locks, but despite these advances the overall drying rate is still slow.

Secondary drying

The removal of residual moisture at the end of primary drying is performed by raising the temperature of the solid to as high as 50 or 60°C. A high temperature is permissible for many materials because the small amount of moisture remaining is not sufficient to cause spoilage.

Packaging

Attention must be paid to packaging freeze-dried products to ensure protection from moisture. Containers should be closed without contacting the atmosphere, if possible, and ampoules, for example, are sealed on the manifold while still under vacuum. Otherwise, the closing must be carried out under controlled atmospheric conditions.

Freeze drying in practice

Advantages

As a result of the character of the process, freeze drying has certain special advantages:

1. Drying takes place at very low temperatures, so that enzyme action is inhibited and chemical decomposition, particularly hydrolysis, is minimized.

2. The solution is frozen such that the final dry product is a network of solid occupying the same volume as the original solution. Thus, the product is light and porous.
3. The porous form of the product gives ready solubility.
4. There is no concentration of the solution prior to drying. Hence, salts do not concentrate and denature proteins, as occurs with other drying methods.
5. As the process takes place under high vacuum there is little contact with air, and oxidation is minimized.

Disadvantages

There are two main disadvantages of freeze drying:

1. The porosity, ready solubility and complete dryness yield a very hygroscopic product. Unless products are dried in their final container and sealed in situ, packaging requires special conditions.
2. The process is very slow and uses complicated plant, which is very expensive. It is not a general method of drying, therefore, but is limited to certain types of valuable products which, because of their heat sensitivity, cannot be dried by any other means.

Uses of freeze drying

The method is used for products that cannot be dried by any other heat method. These include biological products, for example some antibiotics, blood products, vaccines (such as BCG, yellow fever, smallpox), enzyme preparations (such as hyaluronidase) and microbiological cultures. The latter enables specific microbiological species and strains to be stored for long periods with a viability of about 10% on reconstitution.

SOLUTE MIGRATION DURING DRYING

Solute migration is the phenomenon that can occur during drying which results from the movement of a solution within a wet system. The solvent moves towards the surface of a solid (from where it evaporates), taking any dissolved solute with it. Many drugs and binding agents are soluble in granulating fluid, and during the convective drying of granulates these solutes can move towards the surface of the drying bed or granule and be deposited there when the solvent evaporates. Solute migration during drying can lead to localized variability in the concentration of soluble drugs and excipients within the dried product.

Migration associated with drying granules can be of two types, intergranular (between granules) and intragranular (within individual granules).

Intergranular migration

Intergranular migration, where the solutes move from granule to granule, may result in gross maldistribution of the active drug. It can occur during the drying of static beds of granules (e.g. tray drying), as the solvent and accompanying solute(s) move from granule to granule towards the top surface of the bed where evaporation takes place. When the granules are compressed the tablets may have a deficiency or an excess of drug. For example, experiments found that only 12% of tablets made from a tray-dried warfarin granulate were within the USP limits for drug content.

Intragranular migration

Drying methods based on fluidization and vacuum tumbling keep the granules separate during drying and so prevent the intergranular migration that may occur in fixed beds. However, intragranular migration, where the solutes move towards the periphery of each granule, may take place.

Consequences of solute migration

Solute migration of either type can result in a number of problems and occasional benefits.

Loss of active drug

The periphery of each granule may become enriched, with the interior suffering a depletion. This will be of no consequence unless the enriched outer layer is abraded and lost, as may happen during fluidized-bed drying, when the fine drug-rich dust can be eluted in the air and carried to the filter bag or lost. The granules suffer a net loss of drug and, as a result, will be below specification with respect to quantity of active ingredient.

Mottling of coloured tablets

Coloured tablets can be made by adding soluble colour during wet granulation. Intragranular migration of the colour may give rise to dry granules with a highly coloured outer zone and a colourless interior (Fig. 26.16). During compaction granules are fractured and the colourless interior is exposed. The eye then sees the coloured fragments against a colourless background and the tablets appear mottled.

Migration may be reduced by using the insoluble aluminium 'lake' of the colouring material (in which the soluble dye is adsorbed strongly on to insoluble alumina particles) in preference to the soluble dye itself. This is not the complete answer, as factors such as an unfavourable pH can allow dyes to detach from lakes and then migrate. They suggest that small granules, which do not fracture so readily, are preferable to larger ones if mottling is troublesome.

Migration of soluble binders

Intragranular migration may deposit a soluble binder at the periphery of the granules and so confer

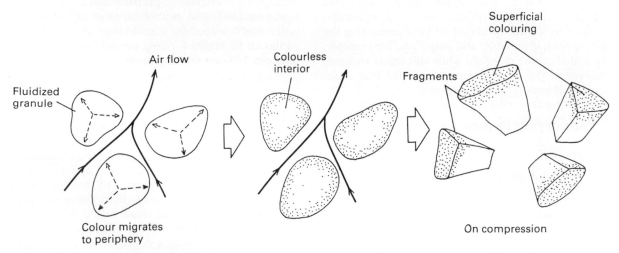

Fig. 26.16 Diagram of mottling caused by intragranular migration.

a 'hoop stress' resistance, making the granules harder and more resistant to abrasion. This migration can aid the bonding process during tablet compaction as a result of binder–binder (rather than drug–drug or drug–excipient) contact, and is therefore sometimes beneficial.

Many other factors, such as granulate formulation, drying method and moisture content, have been shown to affect solute migration.

The influence of formulation factors on solute migration

Nature of substrate

The principles governing solute migration are similar to those of thin-layer chromatography. Thus, if the granule substrate has an affinity for the solute then migration will be impeded. Luckily, many of the common tablet excipients seem to possess this affinity.

It is likely, therefore, that the presence of absorbent materials, such as starch and microcrystalline cellulose, will minimize tablet solute migration.

The use of water-insoluble aluminium lakes (pigments) rather than water-soluble dyes reduces mottling. This effect has also been seen with film-coat colours.

Viscosity of granulating fluid

The popular granulating fluids are solutions of polymers whose viscosity is appreciably greater than that of water alone. This viscosity impedes the movement of moisture by increasing the fluid friction. Increasing the concentration and therefore the viscosity of PVP solution has been shown to slow the migration of drugs in fixed beds of wet granules. Solutions of methylcellulose with comparable viscosities gave similar migration rates, showing that the effect is due to viscosity alone and not to any specific action of either of the binders.

The influence of process factors on solute migration

Drying method

Intergranular migration in fixed beds of granules will occur whenever a particular method of drying creates a temperature gradient. This results in greater evaporation from the hotter zones.

In slow convective drying (e.g. during static tray drying) the maximum concentration of migrated solute will normally occur in the surface of the drying bed, as the process of drying is slow enough to maintain a capillary flow of solvent/solute to the surface over a long period of time.

Drying by microwave radiation results in the uniform heating that is a characteristic of this technique, which in turn minimizes solute migration.

Drying methods that keep the granules in motion will abolish the problem of intergranular migration, but intragranular migration can still occur. This is marked in fluidized granules. Vacuum tumbling methods, on the other hand, greatly reduce migration.

Initial moisture content

The initial moisture content of the granulate will also influence the extent of migration. The greater the moisture content, the greater will be the moisture movement before the pendular state is reached, at which migration cannot continue as there is no longer a continuous layer of mobile liquid water within the wet solid (see Fig. 25.2).

Some practical means of minimizing solute migration

It may be useful to list the measures that can be taken to minimize migration.

1. Use the minimum quantity of granulating fluid and ensure that it is well distributed. High-speed mixer/granulators give better moisture distribution than earlier equipment, and granulates prepared in this way show less migration.
2. Prepare the smallest granules that will flow easily. These are generally satisfactory if mottling is troublesome.
3. Avoid tray drying unless there is no alternative.
4. If tray drying is unavoidable, the dry granules should be remixed before compression. This will ensure that a random mix of enriched and depleted granules will be fed to the tablet machines. This remixing will be more effective if the granule size is small, as there will be a greater number of granules per die fill.
5. If intragranular migration is likely to be troublesome, consider vacuum or microwave drying as an alternative to fluidized-bed drying.

REFERENCES

Wendel, S. and Çelik, M. (1997) An overview of spray-drying applications. *Pharm. Technol.*, **10**, 124–144

BIBLIOGRAPHY

Broadhead, J. et al (1994) The effect of process and formulation variables on the properties of spray-dried beta-galactosidase. *J. Pharm. Pharmacol.*, **46(6)**, 458–467

Masters, K. (1991) *Spray drying handbook*, 5th edn. Longman, Harlow

Nielson, F. (1983) Spray drying of pharmaceuticals. *Mfg Chem. Aerosol News*, **53(7)**, 38–41

Powell, M. (1983) Developments in freeze drying. *Mfg Chem. Aerosol News*, **53(7)**, 47–50

Travers, D.N. (1983) Problems with solute migration. *Mfg Chem. Aerosol News*, **53(3)**, 67–71

Wan, L.S., Heng, P.W., Chia, C.G. (1991) Preparation of coated particles using a spray drying process with an aqueous system. *Int. J. Pharm.*, 77, 183–191

INTRODUCTION

The oral route is the most common way of administering drugs, and among the oral dosage forms tablets of various different types are the most common. Although a variety of tablets exist, with few exceptions (primarily sugar lozenges) tablets are formed by the compression of a powder held within a confined space. The idea of forming a solid dosage form by powder compression is not new. In 1843 the first patent for a hand-operated device used to form a tablet was granted. The use of tablets as dosage form became of interest to the growing pharmaceutical industry, but within pharmacies the pill (a dosage form for oral administration formed by hand into spherical particles about 4–6 mm in diameter) remained the most popular solid dosage form for a long time.

A tablet consists of one or more drugs (active ingredients) as well as a series of other substances used in the formulation of a complete preparation. In the European Pharmacopoeia (3rd edition, 1997) tablets are defined as 'solid preparations each containing a single dose of one or more active ingredients and obtained by compressing uniform volumes of particles. They are intended for oral administration. Some are swallowed whole, some after being chewed, some are dissolved or dispersed in water before being administered and some are retained in the mouth, where the active ingredient is 'liberated'. Thus, a variety of tablets exists and the type of excipients and also the way in which they are incorporated in the tablet vary between the different types. There are also other dosage forms that can be prepared in a similar way, such as suppositories, but which are administered by other routes.

Tablets are used mainly for systemic drug delivery but also for local drug action. For systemic use the drug must be released from the tablet, i.e. normally dissolved in the fluids of the mouth, stomach or intestine, and thereafter be absorbed into the systemic circulation, by which it reaches its site of action. Alternatively, tablets can be formulated for local delivery of drugs in the mouth or gastrointestinal tract, or can be used to increase temporarily the pH of the stomach.

Tablets are popular for several reasons:

- The oral route represents a convenient and safe way of drug administration.
- Compared to liquid dosage forms tablets have general advantages in terms of the chemical and physical stability of the dosage form.
- The preparation procedure enables accurate dosing of the drug.
- Tablets are convenient to handle and can be prepared in a versatile way with respect to their use and to the delivery of the drug.
- Finally, tablets can be mass produced, with robust and quality-controlled production procedures giving an elegant preparation of consistent quality and, in relative terms, low price.

The main disadvantage of tablets as a dosage form concerns the bioavailability of poorly water-soluble or poorly absorbable drugs. In addition, some drugs may cause local irritant effects or otherwise cause harm to the gastrointestinal mucosa.

QUALITY ATTRIBUTES OF TABLETS

Like all other dosage forms, tablets should fulfil a number of specifications regarding their chemical, physical and biological properties. Quality issues relating to the final product are worth considering early in the development process (and thus early in this chapter) as they give an indication of the goal to be achieved during the development and manufacture of tablets.

Tests and specifications for some of these properties are given in pharmacopoeias. The most important of these are dose content and dose uniformity, the release of the drug in terms of tablet disintegration and drug dissolution, and the microbial quality of the preparation. In addition, the authorities and manufacturers define a set of other specifications. One such important property is the resistance of the tablet towards attrition and fracture.

The quality attributes a tablet must fulfil can be summarized as follows:

1. The tablet should include the correct dose of the drug.
2. The appearance of the tablet should be elegant and its weight, size and appearance should be consistent.
3. The drug should be released from the tablet in a controlled and reproducible way.
4. The tablet should be biocompatible, i.e. not include excipients, contaminants and microorganisms that could cause harm to patients.
5. The tablet should be of sufficient mechanical strength to withstand fracture and erosion during handling.
6. The tablet should be chemically, physically and microbiologically stable during the lifetime of the product.

7. The tablet should be formulated into a product acceptable by the patient.
8. The tablet should be packed in a safe manner.

TABLET MANUFACTURING

Stages in tablet formation

Tablets are prepared by forcing particles into close proximity to each other by powder compression, which enables the particles to cohere into a porous, solid specimen of defined geometry. The compression takes place in a die by the action of two punches, the lower and the upper, by which the compressive force is applied. Powder compression is defined as the reduction in volume of a powder owing to the application of a force. Because of the increased proximity of particle surfaces accomplished during compression, bonds are formed between particles which provides coherency to the powder, i.e. a compact is formed. Compaction is defined as the formation of a porous specimen of defined geometry by powder compression.

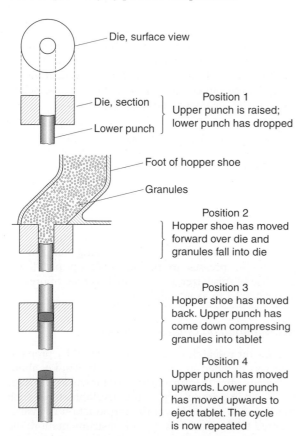

- Die, surface view

- Die, section
- Lower punch

Position 1
Upper punch is raised; lower punch has dropped

- Foot of hopper shoe
- Granules

Position 2
Hopper shoe has moved forward over die and granules fall into die

Position 3
Hopper shoe has moved back. Upper punch has come down compressing granules into tablet

Position 4
Upper punch has moved upwards. Lower punch has moved upwards to eject tablet. The cycle is now repeated

Fig. 27.1 The sequence of events involved in the formation of tablets.

The process of tabletting can be divided into three stages (sometimes known as the **compaction cycle**) (Fig. 27.1).

Die filling

This is normally accomplished by gravitational flow of the powder from a hopper via the die table into the die (although presses based on centrifugal die filling are also used). The die is closed at its lower end by the lower punch.

Tablet formation

The upper punch descends and enters the die and the powder is compressed until a tablet is formed. During the compression phase, the lower punch can be stationary or can move upwards in the die. After maximum applied force is reached, the upper punch leaves the powder, i.e. the decompression phase.

Tablet ejection

During this phase the lower punch rises until its tip reaches the level of the top of the die. The tablet is subsequently removed from the die and die table by a pushing device.

Tablet presses

There are two types of press in common use during tablet production: the single-punch press and the rotary press. In addition, in research and development work hydraulic presses are used as advanced equipment for the evaluation of the tabletting properties of powders and the prediction of scale-up on the properties of the formed tablets (scale-up refers to the change to a larger apparatus for performing a certain operation on a larger scale).

Single-punch press (eccentric press)

A single-punch press possesses one die and one pair of punches (Fig. 27.2). The powder is held in a hopper which is connected to a hopper shoe located at the die table. The hopper shoe moves to and fro over the die, by either a rotational or a translational movement. When the hopper shoe is located over the die, the powder is fed into the die by gravity. The amount of powder filled into the die is controlled by the position of the lower punch. When the hopper shoe is located beside the die, the upper punch descends and the powder is compressed. The lower punch is stationary during compression and the pressure is thus applied by the upper punch and

Fig. 27.2 A single-punch tablet press.

1 Die filling
2 Powder volume control
3 Powder compaction
4 Tablet ejection

Fig. 27.3 Schematic illustration of the events involved in the formation of tablets with a rotary press.

controlled by the upper punch displacement. After ejection the tablet is pushed away by the hopper shoe as it moves back to the die for the next tablet.

The output of tablets from a single-punch press is about 200 tablets per minute. A single-punch press thus has its primary use in the production of small batches of tablets, such as during formulation development, and during small-scale production, such as production for clinical trials.

Rotary press

The rotary press (also referred to as a multistation press) was developed to increase the output of tablets. The primary use of this machine is thus during scale-up in the latter part of the formulation work, and during large-scale production. Outputs of over 10 000 tablets per minute can be achieved by rotary presses.

A rotary press operates with a number of dies and sets of punches, which can vary considerably from three for small rotary presses up to 60 or more for large presses. The dies are mounted in a circle in the die table and both the die table and the punches rotate together during operation of the machine, so that one die is always associated with one pair of punches (Figs. 27.3 and 27.4). The vertical movement of the punches is controlled by tracks that pass over cams and rolls used to control the volume of powder fed into the die and the pressure applied during compression.

The powder is held in a hopper whose lower opening is located just above the die table. The powder flows by gravity on to the die table and is fed into the die by a feed frame. The reproducibility of the die feeding can be improved by a rotating device, referred to as a force-feeding device. During powder compression both punches operate by vertical movement. After tablet ejection, the tablet is knocked away as the die passes the feed frame.

Computerized hydraulic press

For computerized hydraulic presses the movement of the punches can be controlled and varied considerably. Thus, tablets can be prepared under controlled conditions with respect to the loading pattern and loading rate. Possible applications are the investigation of the sensitivity of a drug to such variations, or to mimic the loading pattern of production presses to predict scale-up problems. Because of this latter application, this type of press is also referred to as a 'simulator'.

Instrumentation of tablet presses

Significant research on the process of tablet preparation was initiated in the 1940s and 1950s, i.e. about 100 years after the introduction of tablets as a dosage form. An important step in the development of such fundamental research was the introduction of instrumented tablet machines. By this instrumentation, the forces involved in the compaction process, i.e. the press forces from the upper and lower punches and

Fig. 27.4   Diagram of punch tracks of a rotary tablet press. UR, upper roller; LR, lower roller; W, powder volume adjuster; F, feed frame with granules. U1 to U8, upper punches in raised position; L1, lower punch at top position, tablet ejected; L2 to L7, lower punches dropping to lowest position and filling die with granules to an overfill at L7; L8, lower punch raised to expel excess granules giving correct volume; U9 to U12, upper punches lowering to enter die at U12; L13 and U13, upper and lower punches pass between rollers and granules are compacted to a tablet; U14 to U16, upper punch rising to top position; L14 to L16, lower punch rising to eject tablet.

the force transmitted to the die, and the displacement of the upper and lower punch during the compression and decompression phases, could be recorded.

Instrumented presses are used in research, in development and in the production of tablets. In research and development, instrumented machines are used to provide fundamental information on the mechanical and compaction properties of powders that should be used in tablet formulations. With this application, the work is normally carried out by instrumented single-punch presses or with instrumented hydraulic presses (compaction simulators). The two main applications for an instrumented press in research and development are:

1. to prepare tablets under defined conditions, e.g. in terms of applied force during compaction. These tablets are thereafter characterized by different procedures, such as imaging, surface area and tensile strength analysis;
2. to describe and analyse the compression properties of materials by studying punch forces and punch displacements during the compression and decompression phases. A series of different procedures exists involving, for example, the assessment of deformation behaviour of particles during compression and friction properties during ejection. Some of these are described below.

In production, instrumented production machines, i.e. rotary presses, are used to control the tabletting operation and to ensure that tablets of consistent quality are produced. Normally, only force signals are used on production machines and the variation in force signal during compression is followed as it reflects variations in tablet weight.

Force transducers commonly used in the instrumentation of tablet machines are of two types. The most common type is called a *strain gauge*, which consists of wires through which an electric current is passed. The strain gauge is bonded to a punch or punch holder. During powder compression, a force is applied to the punches and they will temporarily deform. The magnitude of this deformation is dependent on the elastic modulus of the punches and the force applied. When the punch is deformed the wire of the strain gauge is also deformed, and the electrical resistance of the strain gauge will change. This change in electrical resistance can be recorded and calibrated in terms of a force signal. Another, less common, type of force transducer, employs piezoelectric crystals. These are devices which emit an electrical charge when loaded, the magnitude of which is proportional to the applied force.

Displacement transducers measure the distance which the punches travel during the compression and decompression processes. The most common type of displacement transducer delivers an analogue signal. It consists of a rod and some inductive elements mounted in a tube. When the rod moves within the tube, a signal is obtained which directly reflects the position of the rod. The movable rod is connected to the punch so that they move in parallel, i.e. the signal from the displacement transducer reflects the position of the punch. Digital displacement transducers are also used in instrumented tablet machines. Such transducers are based on differences in signal level depending on the position of an indicator. One advantage of a digital displacement transducer is that it is insensitive to electrical noise.

Displacement transducers are necessarily mounted some distance from the punch tip. There is therefore a difference in the position given by the transducer and the real position of the punch tip owing to deformation of the punch along the distance between its tip and the connection point of the transducer. This deviation must be determined by a calibration procedure, e.g. by compressing the punch tips against each other, and a correction for this error must be made before the displacement data can be used.

The signals from the force and displacement transducers are normally amplified and sampled into a computer. After conversion into digital form, the signals are transformed into physically relevant units, i.e. N, Pa, μm etc., and organized as a function of time. To obtain reliable data the calibration of the signals, the resolution of the measuring systems and the reproducibility of the values must be carefully considered.

Technical problems during tabletting

A number of technical problems can arise during the tabletting procedure, among which the most important are:

- high weight and dose variation of the tablets
- low mechanical strength of the tablets
- capping and lamination of the tablets
- adhesion or sticking of powder material to punch tips
- high friction during tablet ejection.

Such problems are related to the properties of the powder intended to be formed into tablets, and also to the design and conditions of the press. They should therefore be avoided by ensuring that the powder possesses adequate technical properties and also that a suitable, well conditioned tablet press is used, e.g. in terms of the use of forced-feed devices and polished and smooth dies and punches.

Important technical properties of a powder which must be controlled to ensure the success of a tabletting operation are:

- homogeneity and segregation tendency
- flowability
- compression properties and compactability
- friction and adhesion properties.

The technical properties of the powder are controlled by the ingredients of the formulation (i.e. the drug and excipients) and by the way by which the ingredients are combined into a powder during precompaction processing. The precompaction processing often consists of a series of unit operations in sequence. The starting point is normally the drug in a pure, most often crystalline form; the subsequent treatment of the drug particles is sometimes referred to as *downstream processing*. The unit operations used during this precompaction treatment are mainly particle size reduction, powder mixing, particle size enlargement and powder drying. For further details see Chapters 11,13, 25 and 26, respectively. Traditionally, the use of a particle size enlargement operation, normally referred to as granulation, is the dominant procedure in preparing a powder for tabletting. To save time and energy, precompaction processing without a particle size enlargement operation is chosen if possible. This procedure is called **tablet production by direct compression**, or **direct compaction**.

Tablet production via granulation

Rationale for granulating powders prior to tabletting

Because both granulation and tabletting involve the formation of aggregates, tablet production by granulation is based on the combination of two size enlargement processes in sequence. The main rationales for granulating the powder (drug and filler mixture) before tabletting are:

- to increase the bulk density of the powder mixture and thus ensure that the required volume of powder can be filled into the die;
- to improve the flowability of the powder in order to ensure that tablets with a low and acceptable tablet weight variation can be prepared;
- to improve mixing homogeneity and reduce segregation by mixing small particles which subsequently adhere to each other;
- to improve the compactability of the powder by adding a solution binder, which is effectively distributed on the particle surfaces;
- to ensure a homogenous colour in a tablet by adding the colour so it is distributed effectively over the particle surfaces;
- to affect the dissolution process for hydrophobic, poorly soluble particles by using a fine particulate drug which is thoroughly mixed with a hydrophilic filler and a hydrophilic binder.

Before granulation the drug might be processed separately in order to obtain a suitable quality in terms of solid-state and particulate properties, such as spray-drying and milling. Normally, the drug exists in dry particulate form before granulation. However, it might be suspended or dissolved in a liquid and be added to the filler as a part of the agglomeration liquid.

Different procedures may be used to prepare a granulation, among which the most important are the use of convective mixers, fluidized-bed driers, spray driers and compaction machines (see Chapter 25 for further detail).

Granulation by convective mixing

Agitation of a powder by convection in the presence of a liquid followed by drying, is the main procedure for the preparation of a pharmaceutical granulation.

This is considered to be the most effective means in terms of production time and cost to prepare good-quality granulations. The process is often referred to as *wet granulation*.

The ingredients to be granulated in a convective mixer are first dry mixed. The objective is to achieve a good homogeneity. As the components are often cohesive powders, a convective mixer operating at high intensity is normally used (a high-shear mixer). The mixture often consists of the drug and a filler. A disintegrant may also be included (i.e. an intragranular disintegrant), but it is also common to add the disintegrant to the dry granulation (i.e. an extragranular disintegrant). After wet mixing the wet mass is dried in a separate drier (a fluidized-bed dryer or a tray dryer). Because granulation in a convective mixer is not a very well controlled operation, large granules (above 1 mm) are often formed which must be broken down into smaller units. This is normally done by milling in a hammer mill or by pressing the granulation through a screen in an oscillating granulator. Granules ranging in size from about 100 to 800 μm are thus obtained.

The prepared granulation is finally dry-mixed with the other ingredients, for example in a double-cone mixer, before tabletting. Common excipients added in this final mixing operation are disintegrants, lubricants, glidants and colourants. Figure 27.5 summarizes the sequence of unit operations used in the production of tablets with precompaction treatment by granulation.

Fig. 27.5 Overview of the sequence of unit operations used in the production of tablets with precompaction treatment by granulation.

Alternative granulation procedures

A series of alternative granulation procedures can be preferable in certain situations. Granulation in a fluidized-bed apparatus is less common than the use of convective mixers as it is considered to be more time-consuming. However, granulations of high quality in terms of homogeneity, flowability and compactability can be prepared by this operation.

By spray drying a suspension of drug particles in a liquid, which can contain a dissolved binder, relatively small spherical granules with uniform size can be prepared. The process is of limited use except for the preparation of fillers or diluents for direct compaction. The granulation can show a good compactability and presents a possibility to granulate a drug suspension without a separate drying step for the drug substance.

The formation of granules by compacting the powder into large compacts which are subsequently comminuted into smaller granules (often referred to as **dry granulation**, or **slugging**) is a possible granulation procedure which, however, is not widely used in pharmaceutical production. The procedure can be employed as a means to avoid exposure of the powder to moisture and heat. In addition, for powders of very low bulk density compaction can be an effective means to increase markedly their bulk density.

Tablet production by direct compaction

An obvious way to reduce production time and hence cost is to minimize the number of operations involved in the pretreatment of the powder mixture before tabletting. Tablet production by direct compaction involves only two operations in sequence, powder mixing and tabletting (Fig. 27.6). The advantage with direct compaction is primarily a reduced production cost. However, in a direct compactable formulation specially designed fillers and dry binders are normally required, which usually are more expensive than the traditional ones. They may also require a larger number of quality tests before processing. As heat and water are not involved, product stability can be improved. Finally, drug dissolution might be faster from a tablet prepared by direct compaction owing to fast tablet disintegration into primary drug particles.

The disadvantages of direct compaction are mainly technological. In order to handle a powder of acceptable flowability and bulk density, relatively large particles must be used which, firstly, may be difficult to mix to a high homogeneity, and secondly are prone to segregate. Moreover, a powder consist-

Fig. 27.6 Overview of the sequence of unit operations used in the production of tablets by direct compaction.

ing mainly of drug will be difficult to form into tablets if the drug itself has poor compactability. Finally, an even colouring of tablets can be difficult to achieve with a colourant in dry particulate form.

Direct compaction has been used mainly for two types of drug, firstly, relatively soluble drugs which can be processed as coarse particles (to ensure good flowability) and, secondly, relatively potent drugs which are present in a few milligrams in each tablet and can be mixed with relatively coarse excipient particles (in this latter case the flow and compaction properties of the formulation are controlled mainly by the excipients).

TABLET EXCIPIENTS

In addition to the active ingredient(s), a series of excipients are normally included in a tablet; their role is to ensure that the tabletting operation can run satisfactorily and to ensure that tablets of specified quality are prepared. Depending on the intended main function, excipients to be used in tablets are subcategorized into different groups. However, one excipient can affect the properties of a powder or the tablet in a series of ways, and many substances used in tablet formulations can thus be described as multifunctional. The functions of the most common types of excipients used in tablets are described below. Examples of substances used as excipients in tablets are given in Table 27.1.

Filler (or diluent)

In order to form tablets of a size suitable for handling, a lower limit in terms of powder volume and weight is required. Tablets weigh normally at least 50 mg. Therefore, a low dose of drug per tablet requires the incorporation of a substance into the formulation to increase the bulk volume of the powder and

Table 27.1 Examples of substances used as excipients in tablet formulation

Type of excipient	Example of substances
Filler	Lactose Sucrose Glucose Mannitol Sorbitol Calcium phosphate Calcium carbonate Cellulose
Disintegrant	Starch Cellulose Crosslinked polyvinyl pyrrolidone Sodium starch glycolate Sodium carboxymethyl cellulose
Solution binder	Gelatin Polyvinyl pyrrolidone Cellulose derivatives (e.g. hydroxypropylmethyl cellulose) Polyethylene glycol Sucrose Starch
Dry binder	Cellulose Methyl cellulose Polyvinyl pyrrolidone Polyethylene glycol
Glidant	Silica Magnesium stearate Talc
Lubricant	Magnesium stearate Stearic acid Polyethylene glycol Sodium lauryl sulphate Sodium stearyl fumarate Liquid paraffin
Antiadherent	Magnesium stearate Talc Starch Cellulose

hence the size of the tablet. This excipient, known as the filler or the diluent, is not necessary if the dose of the drug per tablet is high.

The ideal filler should fulfil a series of requirements, such as:

- be chemically inert
- be non-hygroscopic
- be biocompatible
- possess good biopharmaceutical properties (e.g. water soluble or hydrophilic)
- possess good technical properties (such as compactability and dilution capacity)
- have an acceptable taste
- be cheap.

As all these requirements cannot be fulfilled by a single substance, different substances have gained use as fillers in tablets, mainly carbohydrates but also some inorganic salts.

Lactose is the most common filler in tablets. It possesses a series of good filler properties, e.g. dissolves readily in water, has a pleasant taste, is non-hygroscopic and fairly non-reactive and shows good compactability. Its main limitation is that some people have an intolerance to lactose.

Lactose exists in both crystalline and amorphous form. Crystalline lactose is formed by precipitation and, depending on the crystallization conditions, α-monohydrate or β-lactose (an anhydrous form) can be formed. By thermal treatment of the monohydrate form, crystalline α-anhydrous particles can be prepared. Depending on the crystallization conditions and the use of subsequent size reduction by milling, lactoses of different particle sizes is obtained.

Amorphous lactose can be prepared by spray-drying a lactose solution (giving nearly completely amorphous particles) or a suspension of crystalline lactose particles in a lactose solution (giving aggregates of crystalline and amorphous lactose). Amorphous lactose dissolves more rapidly than crystalline and shows better compactability. Its main use is therefore in the production of tablets by direct compaction. The amorphous lactose is, however, hygroscopic and physically unstable, i.e. it will spontaneously crystallize if crystallization conditions are met as a result of elevated temperature or high relative humidity.

Other sugars or sugar alcohols, such as glucose, sucrose, sorbitol and mannitol, have been used as alternative fillers to lactose, primarily in lozenges or chewable tablets because of their pleasant taste. Mannitol has a negative heat of solution and imparts a cooling sensation when sucked or chewed.

Apart from the sugars perhaps the most widely used fillers are celluloses in powder forms of different types. Celluloses are biocompatible, chemically inert and have good tablet-forming and disintegrating properties. They are therefore used also as dry binders and disintegrants in tablets. They are compatible with many drugs but, owing to their hygroscopicity, may be incompatible with drugs prone to hydrolyse in the solid state.

The most common type of cellulose powder used in tablet formulation is microcrystalline cellulose. The name indicates that the particles have both crystalline and amorphous regions, depending on the relative position of the cellulose chains within the solid. The crystallinity might vary depending on the source of the cellulose and the preparation procedure. The degree of crystallinity will affect the physical and technical properties of the particles, e.g. in terms of hygroscopicity and powder compactability.

Microcrystalline cellulose is prepared by hydrolysis of cellulose followed by spray drying. The particles thus formed are aggregates of smaller cellulose fibres. Depending on the preparation conditions, aggregates of different particle size can be prepared which have different flowabilities.

A final important example of a common filler is an inorganic substance, dicalcium phosphate dihydrate. This is insoluble in water and non-hygroscopic but is hydrophilic, i.e. easily wetted by water. The substance can be obtained both in a fine particulate form, mainly used in granulation, and in an aggregated form. The latter possesses good flowability and is used in tablet production by direct compaction. Calcium phosphate is slightly alkaline and may thus be incompatible with drugs sensitive to alkaline conditions.

Disintegrant

A disintegrant is included in the formulation to ensure that the tablet, when in contact with a liquid, breaks up into small fragments, which promotes rapid drug dissolution. Ideally, the tablet should break up into individual drug particles in order to obtain the largest possible effective surface area during dissolution.

The disintegration process for a tablet occurs in two steps. First, the liquid wets the solid and penetrates the pores of the tablet. Thereafter, the tablet breaks into smaller fragments. The actual fragmentation of the tablet can also occur in steps, i.e. the tablet disintegrates into aggregates of primary particles which subsequently deaggregate into their primary drug particles. A deaggregation directly into primary powder particles will set up conditions for the fastest possible dissolution of the drug. A scheme for the release of the drug from a disintegrating tablet is shown in Fig. 27.7.

Several mechanisms of action of disintegrants have been suggested, such as swelling of particles, exothermic wetting reaction, particle repulsion and particle deformation recovery. However, as two main processes are involved in the disintegration event, disintegrants to be used in plain tablets are here classified into two types:

1. *Disintegrants that facilitate water uptake.* These disintegrants act by facilitating the transport of liquids into the pores of the tablet, with the consequence that the tablet may break into fragments. One obvious type of substance that can promote liquid penetration are surface active agents. Such substances are used to make the drug particle surfaces more hydrophilic and thus promote the wetting of the solid and the penetration of the liquid into the pores of the tablet. It has also been suggested that other substances can promote the liquid penetration using capillary forces to suck water into the pores of the tablet.

2. *Disintegrants that will rupture the tablet.* Rupturing of tablets can be caused by swelling of the disintegrant particles during sorption of water. However, it has also been suggested that non-swelling disintegrants can break the tablet, and different mechanisms have been suggested. One such concerns a repulsion of particles in contact with water and another the recovery of deformed particles to their original shape in contact with water, i.e. particles which have been deformed during compaction.

The most traditionally used disintegrant in conventional tablets is starch, among which potato, maize and corn starches are the most common types used. The typical concentration range of starch in a tablet formulation is up to 10%. Starch particles swell in contact with water and this swelling can subsequently disrupt the tablet. However, it has also been suggested that starch particles may facilitate disintegration by particle–particle repulsion.

The most common and effective disintegrants act via a swelling mechanism and a series of effective swelling disintegrants have been developed which can swell dramatically during water uptake and thus quickly and effectively break the tablet. These are normally modified starch or modified cellulose. High-swelling disintegrants are included in the formulation at relatively low concentrations, typically 1–5% by weight.

Disintegrants can be mixed with other ingredients prior to granulation and thus be incorporated within the granules (intragranular addition). It is also common for the disintegrant to be mixed with the dry granules before the complete powder mix is compacted (extragranular addition). The latter procedure will contribute to an effective disintegration of the tablet into smaller fragments. Disintegrants may also be incorporated as both an intragranular and an extragranular portion.

A third group of disintegrants functions by producing gas, normally carbon dioxide, in contact with water. Such disintegrants are used in effervescent tablets and normally not in tablets that should be swallowed as a solid. The liberation of carbon dioxide is

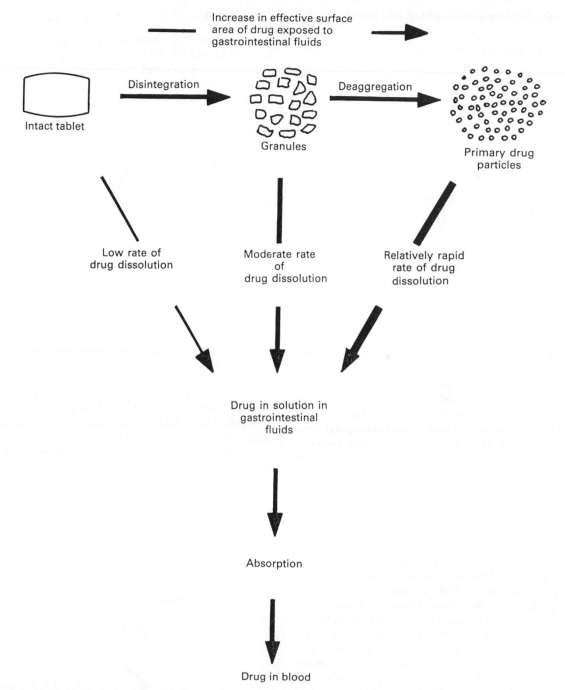

Fig. 27.7 Mechanistic representation of the drug release process from a tablet by disintegration and dissolution. From Wells, J.I. and Rubinstein, M.W. (1976) *Pharm. J.* **217**, 629.

obtained by the decomposition of bicarbonate or carbonate salts in contact with acidic water. The acidic pH is accomplished by the incorporation of a weak acid in the formulation, such as citric acid and tartaric acid.

Binder

A binder (also sometimes called adhesive) is added to a drug–filler mixture to ensure that granules and tablets can be formed with the required mechanical strength. Binders can be added to a powder in different ways:

- As a dry powder which is mixed with the other ingredients before wet agglomeration. During the agglomeration procedure the binder might thus dissolve partly or completely in the agglomeration liquid;
- As a solution which is used as agglomeration liquid during wet agglomeration. The binder is here often referred to as a **solution binder**.
- As a dry powder which is mixed with the other ingredients before compaction (slugging or tabletting). The binder is here often referred to as a **dry binder**.

Both solution binders and dry binders are included in the formulation at relatively low concentrations, typically 2–10% by weight. Common traditional solution binders are starch, sucrose and gelatin. More commonly used binders today, with improved adhesive properties, are polymers such as polyvinylpyrrolidone and cellulose derivatives (in particular hydroxypropyl methylcellulose). Important examples of dry binders are microcrystalline cellulose and crosslinked polyvinylpyrrolidone.

Solution binders are generally considered the most effective, and this is therefore the most common way of incorporating a binder into granules; the granules thus formed are often referred to as binder–substrate granules. It is not uncommon, however, for a dry binder to be added to the dry binder–substrate granules before tabletting in order to further improve the compactability of the granulation.

Glidant

The role of the glidant is to improve the flowability of the powder. This is especially important during tablet production at high production speeds and during direct compaction. However, because the requirement for adequate flow is high, a glidant is often also added to a granulation before tabletting.

Traditionally, talc has been used as a glidant in tablet formulations, in concentrations of about 1–2% by weight. Today, the most commonly used glidant is probably colloidal silica, added in very low proportions (about 0.2% by weight). Because the silica particles are very small they adhere to the particle surfaces of the other ingredients and improve flow by reducing interparticulate friction. Magnesium stearate, normally used as a lubricant, can also promote powder flow at low concentrations (< 1% by weight).

Lubricant

The function of the lubricant is to ensure that tablet formation and ejection can occur with low friction between the solid and the die wall. High friction during tabletting can cause a series of problems, including inadequate tablet quality (capping or even fragmentation of tablets during ejection, and vertical scratches on tablet edges) and may even stop production. Lubricants are thus included in almost all tablet formulations.

Lubrication is achieved by mainly two mechanisms: **fluid lubrication** and **boundary lubrication** (Fig. 27.8). In fluid lubrication a layer of fluid is located between and separates the moving surfaces of the solids from each other and thus reduces the friction. Fluid lubricants are seldom used in tablet formulations. However, liquid paraffin has been used, such as in formulations for effervescent tablets.

Boundary lubrication is considered as a surface phenomenon, as here the sliding surfaces are separated by only a very thin film of lubricant. The nature of the solid surfaces will therefore affect friction. In boundary lubrication the friction coefficient and wear of the solids are higher than with fluid lubrication. All substances that can affect interaction between sliding surfaces can be described as boundary lubricants, including adsorbed gases. The lubricants used in tablet formulations acting by boundary lubrication are fine particulate solids.

A number of mechanisms have been discussed for these boundary lubricants, including that lubricants are substances that show a low resistance towards shearing. The most effective of the boundary lubricants are stearic acid or stearic acid salts, primarily

Fig. 27.8 Schematic illustration of lubrication mechanisms by fluid and boundary lubrication.

magnesium stearate. Magnesium stearate has become the most widely used lubricant owing to its superior lubrication properties. The stearic acid salts are normally used at low concentrations (< 1% by weight).

Besides reducing friction lubricants may cause undesirable changes in the properties of the tablet. The presence of a lubricant in a powder is thought to interfere in a deleterious way with the bonding between the particles during compaction, and thus reduce tablet strength (Fig. 27.9). Because many lubricants are hydrophobic, tablet disintegration and dissolution are often retarded by the addition of a lubricant. These negative effects are strongly related to the amount of lubricant present, and a minimum amount is normally used in a formulation, i.e. concentrations of 1% or below. In addition, the way in which the lubricant is mixed with the other ingredients should also be considered. It can, for example, be important if the excipients are added sequentially to a granulation rather than simultaneously. The total mixing time and the mixing intensity are also important in this context.

The commonly observed retardation of disintegration and dissolution of tablets is related to the hydrophobic character of the most commonly used lubricants. In order to avoid these negative effects more hydrophilic substances have been suggested as alternatives to the hydrophobic lubricants. Examples are surface-active agents and polyethylene glycol. A combination of hydrophobic and hydrophilic substances might also be used.

Both the effect on friction and the effect on the changes in tablet properties of a lubricant are related to the tendency of lubricants to adhere to the surface of drugs and fillers during dry mixing. Lubricants are often fine particulate substances which thus are prone to adhere to larger particles. In addition, studies on the mixing behaviour of magnesium stearate have indicated that this substance has the ability to form a film which can cover a fraction of the surface area of the drug or filler particles (the substrate particles). This film can be described as being continuous rather than particulate. A number of factors have been suggested to affect the development of such a lubricant film during mixing, and hence also affect friction and changes in tablet properties, such as the shape and surface roughness of the substrate particles; the surface area of the lubricant particles; mixing time and intensity; and the type and size of mixer.

Concerning the tablet strength-reducing effect of a lubricant, apart from the degree of surface coverage of the lubricant film obtained during mixing, the compression behaviour of the substrate particles will also be important. Drugs and fillers can thus be evaluated in terms of their lubricant sensitivity, i.e. the reduction in tablet strength due to the addition of a lubricant compared to a tablet formed from a powder without a lubricant. An important property for this lubricant sensitivity seems to be the degree of fragmentation the substrate particles undergo during compression (see below). It is thus assumed that, during compression,

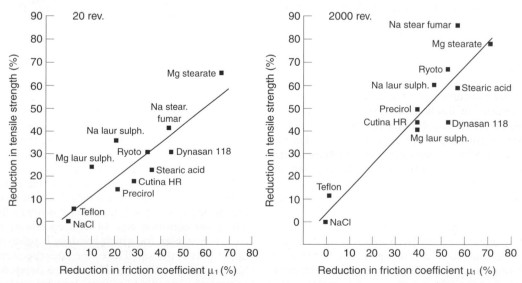

Fig. 27.9 The reduction in tablet tensile strength as a function of the reduction in friction coefficient during tabletting of a sodium chloride powder mixed with 0.1% by weight of a series of lubricants admixed at two different mixing intensities. (From Hölzer, A.H. and Sjögren, J. Acta Pharm. Suec. 18, 139, 1981, with permission).

particle surfaces which are not covered with a lubricant film are formed during particle fragmentation, and that these clean surfaces will bond differently from the lubricant-covered particle surfaces.

To explain the effect of lubricant film formation on the tensile strength of tablets, a coherent matrix model has been developed. This suggests that when a continuous matrix of lubricant-covered particle surfaces exists in a tablet, along which a fracture plane can be formed, the tablet strength is considerably lower than that of tablets formed from unlubricated powder. However, if the mixing and compression processes do not result in such a coherent lubricant matrix within the tablet, for example due to irregular substrate particles or particle fragmentation, the lubricant sensitivity appears to be lower.

Antiadherent

The function of an antiadherent is to reduce adhesion between the powder and the punch faces and thus prevent particles sticking to the punches. Many powders are prone to adhere to the punches, a phenomenon (known in the industry as *sticking* or *picking*) which is affected by the moisture content of the powder. Such adherence is especially prone to happen if the tablet punches are engraved or embossed. Adherence can lead to a build-up of a thin layer of powder on the punches, which in turn will lead to an uneven and matt tablet surface with unclear engravings.

Many lubricants, such as magnesium stearate, have also antiadherent properties. However, other substances with limited ability to reduce friction can also act as antiadherents, such as talc and starch.

Sorbent

Sorbents are substances that are capable of sorbing some quantities of fluids in an apparently dry state. Thus, oils or oil–drug solutions can be incorporated into a powder mixture which is granulated and compacted into tablets. Microcrystalline cellulose and silica are examples of sorbing substances used in tablets.

Flavour

Flavouring agents are incorporated into a formulation to give the tablet a more pleasant taste or to mask an unpleasant one. The latter can be achieved also by coating the tablet or the drug particles.

Flavouring agents are often thermolabile and so cannot be added prior to an operation involving heat. They are often mixed with the granules as an alcohol solution.

Colourant

Colourants are added to tablets to aid identification and patient compliance. Colouring is often accomplished during coating (see Chapter 28 for further information), but a colourant can also be included in the formulation prior to compaction. In the latter case the colourant can be added as an insoluble powder or dissolved in the granulation liquid. The latter procedure may lead to a colour variation in the tablet caused by migration of the soluble dye during the drying stage (see Chapter 26 for more information on the phenomenon of solute migration).

TABLET TYPES

Classification of tablets

Based on their drug-release characteristics, tablets can be classified into three types, immediate release, extended release and, delayed release. For immediate-release tablets the drug is intended to be released rapidly after administration, or the tablet is dissolved and administered as a solution. This is the most common type of tablet and includes disintegrating, chewable, effervescent, sublingual and buccal tablets.

Modified-release tablets should normally be swallowed intact. The formulation and thus also the type of excipients used in such tablets might be quite different from those of immediate-release tablets. The drug is released from an extended-release tablet slowly at a nearly constant rate. If the rate of release is constant during a substantial period of time, a zero-order type of release is obtained, i.e. $M = kt$ (where M is the cumulative amount of drug released and t is the release time). This is sometimes described as an ideal type of extended-release preparation. However, for most type of extended-release tablets a perfect zero-order release is not obtained.

For delayed-release tablets the drug is liberated from the tablet some time after administration. After this period has elapsed, the release is normally rapid. The most common type of delayed-release tablet is an enteric tablet, for which the drug is released in the upper part of the small intestine after the preparation has passed the stomach. However, a delayed-release can also be combined with a slow drug release, e.g. for local treatment in the lower part of the intestine or in the colon.

The type of release obtained from immediate-, extended- and delayed-release tablets is illustrated in Figure 27.10.

Disintegrating tablets

The most common type of tablet is intended to be swallowed and to release the drug in a relatively short time thereafter by disintegration and dissolution, i.e. the goal of the formulation is fast and complete drug release in vivo. Such tablets are often referred to as conventional or plain tablets. A disintegrating tablet includes normally at least the following type of excipients: filler (if the dose of the drug is low), disintegrant, binder, glidant, lubricant and antiadherent.

As discussed above, the drug is released from a disintegrating tablet in a sequence of processes, including tablet disintegration, drug dissolution and drug absorption (see Fig. 27.7). All these processes will affect, and can be rate-limiting steps for, the rate of drug bioavailability. The rate of the processes is affected by both formulation factors and production conditions.

The disintegration time of the tablet can be markedly affected by the choice of excipients, especially disintegrant (Fig. 27.11). The type of filler and lubricant can also be of significant importance for tablet disintegration.

Tablet disintegration may also be affected by production conditions during manufacture. Important examples are the design of the granulation procedure (which will affect the physical properties of the granules), mixing conditions during the addition of lubricants and antiadherents, and the applied punch force during tabletting and the punch

Fig. 27.11 The dissolution rate of salicylic acid, as assessed by an in vitro dissolution method based on agitated baskets, from tablets formed from mixtures of salicylic acid (325 mg) and a series of different types of starches as disintegrant. (From Underwood, T.W. and Cadwallader, D.E., J. Pharm. Sci. 61, 239, 1972.) □ potato starch, ● arrowroot starch, ▲ rice starch, ● corn starch, △ compressible starch.

force–time relationship. It has been reported that an increased compaction pressure can either increase or decrease disintegration time, or give complex relationships with maximum or minimum disintegration times.

For poorly water-soluble drugs the dissolution rate is often the rate-limiting step for bioavailability. The dissolution rate is a function of the solubility and the surface area of the drug (see Chapter 2). Thus, dissolution rate will increase if the solubility of the drug is increased, e.g. by the use of a salt of the drug. It is also possible to speed up the dissolution process by incorporating into the formulation a substance that forms a salt with the drug during dissolution. This has been a common means to increase the dissolution rate of aspirin by using magnesium oxide in the formulation.

The drug dissolution rate will also increase with an increase in the surface area of the drug. Thus,

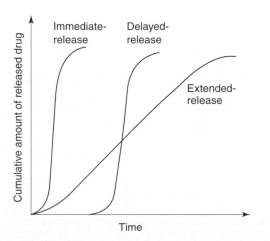

Fig. 27.10 Schematic representation of the cumulative amount of drug released from immediate-, extended- and delayed-release tablets.

control of drug particle size is important to control drug dissolution. However, a reduced particle size will make a powder more cohesive. A reduction in drug particle size might thus give aggregates of particles which are difficult to break up, with the consequence that the drug dissolution rate from the tablet will be reduced. It is thus important to ensure that the tablet is formulated in such a way that it will disintegrate, and the aggregates thus formed break up into small drug particles so that a large surface area of the drug is exposed to the dissolution medium.

For drugs with poor absorption properties the absorption can be affected (see Chapter 17) by modifying the drug lipophilicity, e.g. by esterification of the drug. The use of substances in the formulation that affect the permeability of the gastrointestinal cell membranes, often referred to as absorption enhancers, is also a possible means to increase the drug absorption rate and degree.

Single disintegrating tablets can also be prepared in the form of multilayers, i.e. the tablet consists of two or three layers cohered to each other (double- and triple-layered tablets). During the preparation of multilayer tablets the die is filled in two or three consecutive steps with different granulations from separate feed stations. Each layer is normally compressed after each fill.

Multilayer tablets are made primarily to separate incompatible drugs from each other, i.e. incompatible drugs can be incorporated into the same tablet. Although intimate contact exists at the surface between the layers, the reaction between the incompatible drugs is limited. The use of layered tablets where the layers are differently coloured represents an approach to preparing easily identifiable tablets.

Another variation of the disintegrating tablet is coated tablets which are intended to disintegrate and release the drug quickly (in contrast to coated tablets intended for modified release). The rationale for using coated tablets and detailed descriptions of the procedures used for tablet coating (sugar coating, film coating and press coating) are given in Chapter 28.

Chewable tablets

Chewable tablets are chewed and thus mechanically disintegrated in the mouth. The drug is, however, normally not dissolved in the mouth but swallowed and dissolves in the stomach or intestine. Thus, chewable tablets are used primarily to accomplish a quick and complete disintegration of the tablet – and hence obtain a rapid drug effect – or to facilitate the intake of the tablet. A common example of the former is antacid tablets. In the latter case, the elderly and children in particular have difficulty in swallowing tablets, and so chewable tablets are attractive forms of medication. Important examples are vitamin tablets. Another general advantage of a chewable tablet is that this type of medication can be taken when water is not available.

Chewable tablets are similar in composition to conventional tablets except that a disintegrant is normally not included in the composition. Flavouring and colouring agents are common, and sorbitol and mannitol are common examples of fillers.

Effervescent tablets

Effervescent tablets are dropped into a glass of water before administration, during which carbon dioxide is liberated. This facilitates tablet disintegration and drug dissolution; the dissolution of the tablet should be complete within a few minutes. As mentioned above, the effervescent carbon dioxide is created by a reaction in water between a carbonate or bicarbonate and a weak acid such as citric or tartaric.

Effervescent tablets are used to obtain rapid drug action, for example for analgesic drugs (Fig. 27.12), or to facilitate the intake of the drug, for example for vitamins.

The amount of sodium bicarbonate in an effervescent tablet is often quite high (about 1 g). After dissolution of such a tablet, a buffered water solution will be obtained which normally temporarily increases the pH of the stomach. The result is a rapid emptying of the stomach and the residence time of the drug in the stomach will thus be short. As drugs

Fig. 27.12 Concentration of salicylates in plasma after administration of acetylsalicylic acid tablets (1 g). Circles, effervescent tablet; squares, conventional tablet. (From Ekenved, G., Elofsson, R. and Sölvell, L. Acta Pharm. Suec. 12, 323, 1975.)

are absorbed more effectively in the small intestine than in the stomach, effervescent tablets can thus show a fast drug bioavailability, which can be advantageous, for example, for analgesic drugs. Another aspect of the short residence time of the drug in the stomach is that drug-induced gastric irritation can be avoided, e.g. for aspirin tablets, as the absorption of aspirin in the stomach can cause irritation.

Effervescent tablets also often include a flavour and a colourant. A water-soluble lubricant is preferable in order to avoid a film of a hydrophobic lubricant on the surface of the water after tablet dissolution. A binder is normally not included in the composition.

Effervescent tablets are prepared by both direct compaction and by compaction via granulation. In the latter case, traditional wet granulation is seldom used; instead, granules are formed by the fusion of particles as a result of their partial dissolution during wet massing of a moistened powder.

Effervescent tablets should be packaged in such a way that they are protected against moisture. This is accomplished with waterproof containers, often including a dessicant, or with blister packs or aluminium foils.

Lozenges

Lozenges are tablets that dissolve slowly in the mouth and so release the drug dissolved in the saliva. Lozenges are used for local medication in the mouth or throat, e.g. with local anaesthesia, antiseptic and antibiotic drugs. They can thus be described as slow-release tablets for local drug treatment.

Disintegrants are not used in the formulation, but otherwise such tablets are similar in composition to conventional tablets. In addition, lozenges are often coloured and include a flavour. The choice of filler and binder is of particular importance in the formulation of lozenges, as these excipients should contribute to a pleasant taste or feeling during tablet dissolution. The filler and binder should therefore be water soluble and have a good taste. Common examples of fillers are glucose, sorbitol and mannitol. A common binder in lozenges is gelatin.

Lozenges are normally prepared by compaction at high applied pressures in order to obtain a tablet of high mechanical strength and low porosity which can dissolve slowly in the mouth.

Sublingual and buccal tablets

Sublingual and buccal tablets are used for drug release in the mouth followed by systemic uptake of the drug. A rapid systemic drug effect can thus be obtained without first-pass liver metabolism. Sublingual tablets are placed under the tongue and buccal tablets are placed in the side of the cheek.

Sublingual and buccal tablets are often small and porous, the latter facilitating fast disintegration and drug release.

Extended-release tablets

Classification of extended-release tablets

In recent years there has been great interest in the development and use of tablets which should be swallowed and thereafter slowly release the drug in the gastrointestinal tract. Such tablets are denominated in various ways, such as slow release, prolonged release, sustained release and extended-release. In the European Pharmacopoeia the term extended-release has been chosen as denominator for these types of tablets and so is used here. Extended-release tablets are often referred to as controlled-release preparations. This latter term is somewhat misleading, as all tablets, irrespective of their formulation and use, should release the drug in a controlled and reproducible way. (The nomenclature for extended-release preparations is subject to some debate and no worldwide acceptable system exists. The reader is referred to Chapter 20 for further discussion on this subject.)

After the release of the drug from the tablet the drug should normally be absorbed into the systemic circulation. The aim is normally to increase the time period during which a therapeutic drug concentration level in the blood is maintained. However, the aim can also be to increase the release time for drugs that can cause local irritation in the stomach or intestine if they are released quickly. Examples of the latter are potassium chloride and iron salts. In addition, drugs for local treatment of diseases in the large intestine are sometimes formulated as extended-release tablets.

An extended-release tablet contains one dose of the drug which is released for a period of about 12–24 hours. The release pattern can vary, from being nearly continuous to two or more pulses. In the latter case the pulses can correspond to a rapid release of the drug, or can be a combination of a rapid release of one portion of drug followed by a slow release of a second portion.

An extended-release preparation can also be categorized as a single-unit or a multiple-unit dosage form. In the first case the drug dose is incorporated into a single-release unit, and in the latter is divided into a large number of small release units. A multiple-unit dosage form is often considered to give a more reproducible drug action.

There are a series of rationales behind the increased interest in administering drugs orally for systemic uptake in the form of extended-release tablets. However, the drug must fulfil certain criteria in order to render itself suitable for sustained-release medication, otherwise another type of tablet is a more feasible alternative. These rationales and criteria, as well as the pharmacokinetic aspects of extended-release drug administration, are described elsewhere in this book (Chapters 19 and 20). In Chapter 20 the formulation principles used to achieve extended drug release are described.

Extended-release tablets are often classified according to the mechanism of drug release. The following are the most common means used to achieve a slow, controlled release of the drug from tablets:

- Drug transport control by diffusion
- Dissolution control
- Erosion control
- Drug transport control by convective flow (accomplished by, for example, osmotic pumping)
- Ion-exchange control.

Diffusion-controlled release systems

In diffusion-controlled extended-release systems the transport by diffusion of dissolved drugs in pores filled with gastric or intestinal juice or in a solid (normally polymer) phase is the release-controlling process. Depending on the part of the release unit in which the drug diffusion takes place, diffusion-controlled release systems are divided into matrix systems (also referred to as monolithic systems) and reservoir systems. The release unit can be a tablet or a nearly spherical particle of about 1 mm in diameter (a granule or a millisphere). In both cases the release unit should stay more or less intact during the course of the release process. In matrix systems diffusion occurs in pores located within the bulk of the release unit, and in reservoir systems diffusion takes place in a thin water-insoluble film or membrane, often about 5–20 μm thick, which surrounds the release unit. Diffusion through the membrane can occur in pores filled with fluid, or in the solid phase that forms the membrane.

Drug is released from a diffusion-controlled release unit in two steps:

1. The liquid that surrounds the dosage form penetrates the release unit and dissolves the drug. A concentration gradient of dissolved drug

is thus established between the interior and the exterior of the release unit.
2. The dissolved drug will diffuse in the pores of the release unit or the surrounding membrane and thus be released, or, alternatively, the dissolved drug will partition into the membrane surrounding the dose unit and diffuse in the membrane.

A dissolution step is thus normally involved in the release process, but the diffusion step is the rate-controlling step. The rate at which diffusion will occur depends on four variables: the concentration gradient over the diffusion distance, the area and distance over which diffusion occurs; and the diffusion coefficient of the drug in the diffusion medium. Some of these variables are used to modulate the release rate in the formulation.

Reservoir systems   In a reservoir system the diffusion occurs in a thin film surrounding the release unit (Fig. 27.13). This film is normally formed from a high molecular weight polymer. The diffusion distance will be constant during the course of the release and, as long as a constant drug concentration gradient is maintained, the release rate will be constant, i.e. a zero-order release ($M = kt$).

One possible process for the release of the drug from a reservoir system involves partition of the drug dissolved inside the release unit to the solid membrane, followed by transport by diffusion of the drug within the membrane. Finally, the drug will partition to the solution surrounding the release unit. The driving force for the release is the concentration gradient of dissolved drug over the membrane. The release rate can be described in a simplified way by the following equation, which also summarizes the formulation factors by which the release rate can be controlled, i.e.

$$M/t = C\,A\,K\,D/h \qquad (27.1)$$

where C is the solubility of the drug in the liquid, A and h are the area and thickness of the membrane, D is the diffusion coefficient of the drug in the

Fig. 27.13   Schematic illustration of the mechanism of drug release from a diffusion-based reservoir tablet (t = time).

membrane and K the partition coefficient for the drug between the membrane and the liquid at equilibrium.

In practice, the membrane surrounding the release unit often includes a water-soluble component. This can be small particles of a soluble substance, such as sucrose, or a water-soluble polymer, such as a water-soluble cellulose derivative (e.g. hydroxypropyl methylcellulose). In the latter case the polymer is used together with a water-insoluble polymer as the film-forming materials that constitute the coating. In such a membrane the water-soluble component will dissolve and form pores filled with liquid in which the drug can thereafter diffuse. The area and length of these pores will thus constitute the diffusion area and distance. These factors can be estimated from the porosity of the membrane (E) and the tortuosity (τ) of the pores (the tortuosity refers to the ratio between the actual transport distance in the pores between two positions and the transport distance in a solution). The release rate can thus be described in a simplified way as follows:

$$M/t = C\,A\,E\,D/h\,\tau \qquad (27.2)$$

The membrane porosity and pore tortuosity can be affected by the addition of water-soluble components to the membrane.

For oral preparations the film surrounding the release units is normally based on high molecular weight, water-insoluble polymers, such as certain cellulose derivatives (e.g. ethyl cellulose) and acrylates. The film often also includes a plasticizer. In the case of drug release through liquid-filled pores a small amount of a water-soluble compound is also added, as described above. Reservoir systems today are normally designed as multiple-unit systems rather than single units.

Matrix systems In a matrix system the drug is dispersed as solid particles within a porous matrix formed of a water-insoluble polymer, such as

polyvinyl chloride (Fig. 27.14). Initially, drug particles located at the surface of the release unit will be dissolved and the drug released rapidly. Thereafter, drug particles at successively increasing distances from the surface of the release unit will be dissolved and released by diffusion in the pores to the exterior of the release unit. Thus, the diffusion distance of dissolved drug will increase as the release process proceeds. The drug release, in terms of the cumulative amount of drug (M) released from a matrix in which drug particles are suspended is proportional to the square root of time i.e. $M = kt^{1/2}$.

The main formulation factors by which the release rate from a matrix system can be controlled are the amount of drug in the matrix, the porosity of the release unit, the length of the pores in the release unit (dependent on the size of the release unit and the pore tortuosity) and the solubility of the drug (which regulates the concentration gradient). The characteristics of the pore system can be affected by, for example, the addition of soluble excipients and by the compaction pressure during tabletting.

Matrix systems are traditionally designed as single-unit systems, normally tablets, prepared by tabletting. However, alternative preparation procedures are also used, especially for release units that are smaller than tablets. Examples of such techniques are extrusion, spray-congealing and casting.

Dissolution-controlled release systems

In dissolution-controlled extended-release systems the rate of dissolution in the gastrointestinal juices of the drug or another ingredient is the release-controlling process. It is obvious that a sparingly water-soluble drug can form a preparation of a dissolution-controlled extended-release type. A reduced drug solubility can be accomplished by preparing poorly soluble salts or derivatives of the

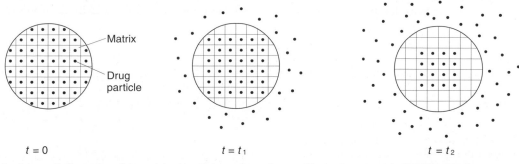

$t = 0$ $t = t_1$ $t = t_2$

Fig. 27.14 Schematic illustration of the mechanism of drug release from a diffusion-based matrix tablet (t = time).

drug. In practice, this approach is a less common way of formulating an extended-release preparation. An alternative means to achieve extended release based on dissolution is to incorporate the drug in a slowly dissolving carrier.

Dissolution-controlled extended-release systems can also be obtained by covering drug particles with a slowly dissolving coating. The release of the drug from such units occurs in two steps:

1. The liquid that surrounds the release unit dissolves the coating (rate-limiting dissolution step).
2. The solid drug is exposed to the liquid and subsequently dissolves.

In order to obtain an extended release based on dissolution of a coating, the tablet is designed to release the drug in a series of pulses. Although this type of release is not continuous it is normally referred to as extended release, as a similar bioavailability as with continuous-release systems can often be achieved. A pulsatile drug release can be accomplished by dividing the drug dose into a number of smaller release units, which are coated in such a way that the dissolution time of the coatings will vary (Fig. 27.15). The release unit is often a nearly spherical granule about 1 mm in diameter. A variation in dissolution time of the coating can be accomplished by varying its thickness or its solubility. Release units with different release times will be mixed and formed into tablets. After disintegration of the tablet, the release units will deliver the drug in a sequence of pulses.

The procedure described here is also the most common means to prepare a delayed-release system, such as enteric-coated dosage forms. In this case dissolution is inhibited until the preparation reaches the higher pH of the small intestine, where the drug is released in a relatively short time.

Erosion-controlled release systems

In erosion-controlled extended-release systems the rate of drug release is controlled by the erosion of a

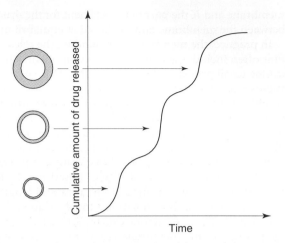

Fig. 27.15 Schematic representation of the cumulative amount of drug released from a dissolution-based (due to differences in coating thickness) pulsatile-release preparation.

matrix in which the drug is dispersed. The matrix is normally a tablet, i.e. the matrix is formed by a tabletting operation, and the system can thus be described as a single-unit system. The erosion in its simplest form can be described as a continuous liberation of matrix material (both drug and excipient) from the surface of the tablet, i.e. a surface erosion. The consequence will be a continuous reduction in tablet weight during the course of the release process (Fig. 27.16). Drug release from an erosion system can thus be described in two steps:

1. Matrix material, in which the drug is dissolved or dispersed, is liberated from the surface of the tablet.
2. The drug is subsequently exposed to the gastrointestinal fluids and mixed with (if the drug is dissolved in the matrix) or dissolved in (if the drug is suspended in the matrix) the fluid.

This release scheme is in practice a simplification, as erosion systems may combine different mechanisms for drug release. For example, the drug may be released both by erosion and by diffusion within the

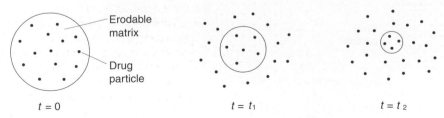

$t = 0$ $t = t_1$ $t = t_2$

Fig. 27.16 Schematic illustration of the mechanism of drug release from an erosion tablet.

matrix. Thus, a mathematical description of drug release from an erosion system is complex. However, drug release can often approximate zero-order for a significant part of the total release time.

The eroding matrix can be formed from different substances. One example is lipids or waxes, in which the drug is dispersed. Another example is polymers that gel in contact with water (e.g. hydroxyethyl cellulose). The gel will subsequently erode and release the drug dissolved or dispersed in the gel. Diffusion of the drug in the gel may occur in parallel.

Osmosis-controlled release systems

In osmosis-controlled extended-release systems the flow of liquid into the release unit, driven by a difference in osmotic pressure between the inside and the outside of the release unit, is used as the release-controlling process. Osmosis can be defined as the flow of a solvent from a compartment with a low concentration of solute to a compartment with a high concentration. The two compartments are separated by a semipermeable membrane, which allows flow of solvent but not of the solute.

In the most simple type of osmosis-controlled drug release the following sequence of steps is involved in the release process:

1. Osmotic transport of liquid into the release unit;
2. Dissolution of drug within the release unit;
3. Convective transport of a saturated drug solution by pumping of the solution through a single orifice or through pores in the semipermeable membrane.

The pumping of the drug solution can be accomplished in different ways. One example is a tablet which includes an expansion layer, i.e. a layer of a substance that swells in contact with water, the expansion of which will press out the drug solution from the release unit. Alternatively, the increased volume of fluid inside the release unit will increase the internal pressure, and the drug solution will thus be pumped out.

If the flow rate of incoming liquid to the release unit is the rate-controlling process, the drug release rate can be described as:

$$M/t = C\,V/t \qquad (27.3)$$

where V is the volume of incoming liquid. The flow rate of incoming liquid under steady-state conditions is a zero-order process, and the release rate of the drug will therefore also be a zero-order process. The water flow is not affected by the flow and pH of the dissolution medium. However, the water flow rate

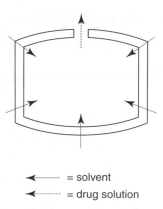

= solvent

= drug solution

Fig. 27.17 Schematic illustration of the mechanism of drug release from an osmosis-controlled release system designed as a single-unit tablet with a single release orifice.

and hence drug release rate can be affected by a number of formulation factors, such as the osmotic pressure of the drug solution within the release unit, the drug solubility and the permeability and mechanical properties of the membrane.

Osmosis-controlled release systems can be designed as single-unit or multiple-unit tablets. In the first case the drug solution can be forced out from the tablet through a single orifice (Fig. 27.17) formed in the membrane by boring with a laser beam. Alternatively, the drug solution can flow through a number of pores formed during the uptake of water. Such pores can be formed by the dissolution of water-soluble substances in the membrane, or by straining of the membrane owing to the increased internal pressure in the release unit. In the case of multiple-unit release tablets the transport occurs in formed pores.

TABLET TESTING

Uniformity of content of active ingredient

A fundamental quality attribute for all pharmaceutical preparations is the requirement for a constant dose of drug between individual tablets. In practice, small variations between individual preparations are accepted and the limits for this variation are defined as standards in pharmacopoeias. For tablets, uniformity of dose or dose variation is tested in two separate tests: uniformity of weight and uniformity of active ingredient. These either reflect indirectly or measure directly the amount of drug substance in the tablet.

The test for uniformity of weight is carried out by collecting a sample of tablets, normally 20, from a batch and determining their individual weights. The average weight of the tablets is then calculated. The sample complies with the standard if the individual weights do not deviate from the mean more than is permitted in terms of percentage.

If the drug substance forms the greater part of the tablet mass, any weight variation obviously reflects variations in the content of active ingredient. Compliance with the standard thus helps to ensure that uniformity of dosage is achieved. However, in the case of potent drugs which are administered in low doses, the excipients form the greater part of the tablet weight and the correlation between tablet weight and amount of active ingredient can be poor (Fig. 27.18). Thus, the test for weight variation must be combined with a test for variation in content of the drug substance. Nevertheless, the test for uniformity of weight is a simple way to assess variation in drug dose, which makes the test useful as a quality control procedure during tablet production.

The test for uniformity of drug content is carried out by collecting a sample of tablets, normally 10, followed by a determination of the amount of drug in each. The average drug content is calculated and the content of the individual tablets should fall within specified limits in terms of percentage deviation from the mean.

Disintegration

As discussed above, the drug release process from immediate-release tablets often includes a step at which the tablet disintegrates into smaller fragments. In order to assess this, disintegration test methods have been developed and examples are described as official standards in pharmacopoeias.

The test is carried out by agitating a given number of tablets in an aqueous medium at a defined temperature, and the time to reach the end-point of the test is recorded. The preparation complies with the test if the time to reach this end-point is below a given limit. The end-point of the test is the point at which all visible parts of the tablets have been eliminated from a set of tubes in which the tablets have been held during agitation. The tubes are closed at the lower end by a screen and the tablet fragments formed during the disintegration are eliminated from the tubes by passing the screen openings, i.e. disintegration is considered to be achieved when no tablet fragments remain on the screen (fragments of coating may remain).

A disintegration apparatus (Fig. 27.19) consists normally of six chambers, i.e. tubes open at the upper end and closed by a screen at the lower. Before disintegration testing, one tablet is placed in each tube and normally a plastic disc is placed upon it. The tubes are placed in a water bath and raised and lowered at a constant frequency in the water in such a way that at the highest position of the tubes, the screen remains below the surface of the water.

Tests for disintegration do not normally seek to establish a correlation with in vivo behaviour. Thus, compliance with the specification is no guarantee of an acceptable release and uptake of the drug in vivo and hence an acceptable clinical effect. However, it is reasonable that a preparation that fails to comply with the test is unlikely to be efficacious. Disintegration tests are, however, useful as a means to assess the potential importance of formulation and process variables on the biopharmaceutical properties of the tablet, and as

Fig. 27.18 Correlation between amount of active ingredient and tablet weight for (a) a low dose (drug content 23% of tablet weight) and (b) a high dose (drug content 90% of tablet weight) tablet. (From Airth, J.M., Bray, D.F., and Radecka, C. (1967). J. Pharm. Sci., 56, 233–235.

Fig. 27.19 Diagram of a disintegration instrument for the testing of tablet disintegration time.

a control procedure to evaluate the quality reproducibility of the tablet during production.

Dissolution

Dissolution testing is the most important way to study, under in vitro conditions, the release of a drug from a solid dosage form, and thus represents an important tool to assess factors that affect the bioavailability of a drug from a solid preparation. During a dissolution test the cumulative amount of drug that passes into solution is studied as a function of time. The test thus describes the overall rate of all the processes involved in the release of the drug into a bioavailable form.

Dissolution studies are carried out for several reasons:

- To evaluate the potential effect of formulation and process variables on the bioavailability of a drug;
- To ensure that preparations comply with product specifications;
- To indicate the performance of the preparation under in vivo conditions.

This last point requires that in vitro dissolution data correlate with the in vivo performance of the dosage form, which must be experimentally verified. The term in vitro/in vivo correlation in this context is related to the correlation between in vitro dissolution and the release or uptake of the drug in vivo. The establishment of such a correlation is one of the

most important aspects of a dissolution test for a preparation under formulation development, and is discussed further in Chapter 18.

Dissolution is accomplished by locating the tablet in a chamber containing a flowing dissolution medium. So that the method is reproducible, all factors that can affect the dissolution process must be standardized. This includes factors that affect the solubility of the substance (i.e. the composition and temperature of the dissolution medium) and others that affect the dissolution process (such as the concentration of dissolved substance in, and the flow conditions of, the fluid in the dissolution chamber). Normally, the concentration of the drug substance in the bulk of the dissolution medium shall not exceed 10% of the solubility of the drug, i.e. sink conditions. Under sink conditions, the concentration gradient between the diffusion layer surrounding the solid phase and the concentration in the bulk of the dissolution medium is often assumed to be constant.

A number of official and unofficial methods exist for dissolution testing, which can be applied to both drug substances and formulated preparations. With respect to preparations, the main test methods are based on forced convection of the dissolution medium and can be classified into two groups: stirred-vessel methods and continuous-flow methods.

Stirred-vessel methods

The most important stirred-vessel methods are the paddle method (Fig. 27.20) and the rotating-basket method (Fig. 27.21). Details of these can be found in official monographs in the European or US Pharmacopoeias. Both use the same type of vessel, which is filled with a dissolution medium of controlled volume and temperature. In the paddle method, the tablet is placed in the vessel and the dissolution medium is agitated by a rotating paddle. In the rotating-basket method, the tablet is placed in a small basket formed from a screen. This is then immersed in the dissolution medium and rotated at a given speed.

Continuous-flow methods

In the continuous-flow method the preparation is held within a flow cell, through which the dissolution medium is pumped at a controlled rate from a large reservoir. The liquid which has passed the flow cell is collected for analysis of drug content. The continuous-flow cell method may have advantages over stirred-vessel methods, e.g. it maintains sink conditions throughout the experiment and avoids floating of the preparation.

Speed (rpm) USP/NF –
Monograph ± 4%
25– 150 rpm – lower speed preferred

Shaft
USP/NF – 9.5– 10.5 mm diameter:
lower part polyfluorocarbon
coated if desired

Centring (or tilt)
USP/NF – ± 2 mm at all points

Eccentricity
USP/NF – no
significant wobble

Sampling point
USP/NF – midway
between top of blade and
top of fluid; no closer than
1 cm to side of flask

Flask
USP/NF – cylindrical with
spherical bottom; 16– 17.5 cm high,
inside diameter 10– 10.5 cm, glass
or plastic

A

Paddle

Paddle position
USP/NF – 2.5± 0.2 cm

Stainless or glass helix may be
attached to floating dosage forms

Fig. 27.20 Diagram of a dissolution instrument based on the rotating paddle method for the testing of tablet dissolution rate. (From Banakar, U.V. Pharmaceutical Dissolution Testing. Marcel Dekker, Inc., New York 1992.)

The amount of drug dissolved is normally analysed more or less continuously as the concentration in the vessel at a series of consecutive times. However, sometimes a single measurement can be performed if required in the Pharmacopoeia or product specification, i.e. the amount of drug dissolved within a certain time period is determined.

The composition of the dissolution medium might vary between different test situations. Pure water may be used, but in many cases a medium that shows a closer resemblance to some physiological fluid is used. In such media the pH and ionic strength can be controlled, and surface-active agents might be added to affect the surface tension of the liquid and the solubility of the drug. Such fluids are often referred to as simulated gastric or intestinal fluids. Also, other dissolution media might be used, such as solvent mixtures, if the solubility of the drug is very low.

Mechanical strength

The mechanical strength of a tablet is associated with the resistance of the solid specimen towards fracturing and attrition. An acceptable tablet must remain intact during handling between production and administration. Thus, an integrated part of the

Speed (rpm) as specified in monograph
25 –150 rpm (± 4% USP/NF, ± 5% BP)

Shaft
USP/NF – 6– 10.5 mm diameter;
BP – approximately 6 mm diameter;
2 mm vent in disc drive

Centring (or tilt)
± 2 mm at all points

Eccentricity
USP/NF – no significant wobble;
BP – no perceptible wobble

Sampling point
USP/NF – midway from top of
basket to top of fluid and no
closer than 1 cm to side of flask
BP – halfway between basket
and side at middle of basket

Flask
USP/NF – cylindrical with
spherical bottom; 16– 17.5 cm high,
inside diameter 10– 10.5 cm,
plastic or glass
BP – cylindrical, flat bottomed,
glass

Basket

Basket position
USP/NF – 2.5 ± 0.2 cm
BP – 2.0 ± 0.2 cm

Fig. 27.21 Diagram of a dissolution instrument based on the rotating-basket method for the testing of tablet dissolution rate. (From Banakar, U.V. Pharmaceutical Dissolution Testing. Marcel Dekker, Inc., New York 1992.)

formulation and production of tablets is the determination of their mechanical strength. Such testing is carried out for several reasons, such as:

- To assess the importance of formulation and production variables for the resistance of a tablet towards fracturing and attrition during formulation work, process design and scaling up;
- To control the quality of tablets during production (in-process and batch control);
- To characterize the fundamental mechanical properties of materials used in tablet formulation.

A number of methods are available for measuring mechanical strength and they give different results.

Especially for the use of strength data to assess material properties, a number of test methods originating from materials science are used, such as beam bending and uniaxial tensile testing. In this context also the hardness of a tablet can be measured by indentation. The hardness of a specimen is associated with its resistance to local permanent deformation, and is thus not a measure of the resistance of the tablet towards fracturing.

The most commonly used methods for strength testing can be subcategorized into two main groups: attrition-resistance methods and fracture-resistance methods.

Attrition-resistance methods

The idea behind attrition resistance methods is to mimic the kind of forces to which a tablet is subjected during handling between its production and its administration. These are also referred to as friability tests: a friable tablet is one that is prone to erode mechanically during handling. During handling, tablets are subjected to stresses from collisions and tablets sliding towards one another and other solid surfaces, which can result in the removal of small fragments and particles from the tablet surface. The result will be a progressive reduction in tablet weight and a change in its appearance. Such attrition can occur even though the stresses are not high enough to break or fracture the tablet into smaller pieces. Thus, an important property of a tablet is its ability to resist attrition so as to ensure that the correct amount of drug is administered and that the appearance of the tablet does not change during handling. Another application of a friability method is to detect incipient capping, as tablets with no visible defects can cap or laminate when stressed by an attrition method, e.g. a rotating cylinder.

The most common experimental procedure to determine attrition resistance involves the rotation of tablets in a cylinder followed by the determination of weight loss after a given number of rotations. Another approach is to shake tablets intensively in a jar of similar dimensions to a pack-jar. Normally, weight loss of less than 1% during a friability test is required. In addition, the tablets should not show capping or cracking during such testing.

Fracture-resistance methods

Analysis of the fracture resistance of tablets involves the application of a load on the tablet and the determination of the force needed to fracture or break the specimen along its diameter. In order to obtain a controlled loading, care must be taken to ensure that the load is applied under defined and reproducible conditions in terms of the type of load applied (compression, pulling, twisting etc.) and the loading rate.

For compressive loading of tablets, the test is simple and reproducible under controlled conditions, and the diametric compression test has therefore a broad use during formulation development and tablet production. In such compression testing the tablet is placed against a platen and the load is applied along its diameter by a movable platen. The tablet fails ideally along its diameter, i.e. parallel to the compression load, in a single fracture into two pieces of similar size (Fig. 27.22), and the fracture force is recorded. This mode of failure is actually a tensile failure even though it is accomplished here by compressive loading. The force needed to fracture the tablet by diametral compression is often somewhat unfortunately referred to as the crushing or breaking strength of the tablet. The term hardness is also used in the literature to denote the failure force, which is in this context incorrect as hardness is a deformation property of a solid.

The force needed to fracture a tablet depends on the tablet's dimensions. An ideal test, however, should allow comparison between tablets of different sizes or even shapes. This can be accomplished by assessing the strength of the tablet, i.e. the force needed to fracture the tablet per unit fracture area. A strength test requires that the fracture mode (i.e. the way by which the crack is formed) can be controlled and that the stress state along the fracture plane can be estimated. The simplest and most common tensile strength test is the indirect diametral compression test described above. For a cylindrical flat-faced tablet the tensile strength (σ_t) can be calculated by Eqn 27.4, provided that the tablet fails in a tensile fracture mode characterized by a single linear fracture across the diameter of the cylindrical specimen:

$$\sigma_t = 2F/\pi D\,t \qquad (27.4)$$

where F is the force needed to fracture the tablet and D and t are the diameter and the thickness of the cylindrical flat-faced tablet, respectively.

In practice, more complicated failure characteristics than tensile failure are often obtained during diametral compression (Fig. 27.23), which will prevent the strict application of the calculation procedure. It should be pointed out that the tensile strength of convex-faced tablets can also be calculated by using other equations.

An alternative procedure to measure the tensile strength of a tablet is to directly pull the tablet apart

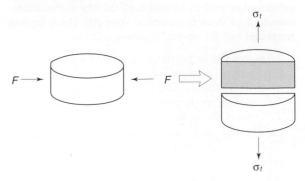

Fig. 27.22 Illustration of the tensile failure of a tablet during diametral compression.

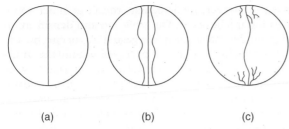

(a)   (b)   (c)

Fig. 27.23 Examples of different types of failure induced by diametral compression. (a) Simple tensile failure. (b) Triple cleft failure. (c) Failure due to shear at platen edges. (From Davies, P.N. and Newton, J.M. In: Pharmaceutical Powder Compaction Technology (Eds. Alderborn G. and Nyström, C.), Marcel Dekker Inc., New York 1996.)

by the application of stresses along its main axes until fracture occurs, i.e. a direct axial tensile test. The use of this method is primarily to detect weaknesses in the compact in the axial direction, which is an indication of capping or lamination tendencies in the tablet. Thus, the strength value obtained by this procedure indicates weak zones in the tablet rather than the mean strength of the whole tablet.

FUNDAMENTAL ASPECTS OF THE COMPRESSION OF POWDERS

Mechanisms of compression of particles

The compressibility of a powder is defined as its propensity, when held within a confined space, to reduce in volume while loaded. The compression of a powder bed is normally described as a sequence of processes. Initially, the particles in the die are rearranged, resulting in a closer packing structure and reduced porosity. At a certain load the reduced space and the increased interparticulate friction will prevent any further interparticulate movement. The subsequent reduction of the tablet volume is therefore associated with changes in the dimensions of the particles.

Particles, either whole or a part, can change their shape temporarily by elastic deformation and permanently by plastic deformation (Fig. 27.24). Particles can also fracture into a number of smaller, discrete particles, i.e. particle fragmentation. The particle fragments can then find new positions, which will further decrease the volume of the powder bed. When the applied pressure is further increased the smaller particles formed could again undergo deformation. Thus, one single particle may undergo this cycle of events several times during one compression. As a

Particles deform under compressive force

Compressive force removed

Elastic deformation.
Particles return to their former shape.
Cohesion lost.

Plastic deformation.
Particles remain deformed.
Cohesion retained.

Fig. 27.24 Schematic illustration of particle deformation, elastic and plastic, during compression. (From Armstrong, N.A. Mfg. Chem. October, 64 1982.)

consequence of compression particle surfaces are brought into close proximity to each other and particle–particle bonds can be formed.

Elastic and plastic deformation of particles are a time-independent processes, i.e. the degree of deformation is related to the applied stress and not the time of loading. However, it can also be time-dependent, i.e. the degree of deformation is related to the applied stress *and* the time of loading. This deformation behaviour is referred to as viscoelastic and viscous deformation of a material. The consequence is that the compression behaviour of a material might depend on the loading conditions during the formation of a tablet in terms of the punch displacement–time relationship. Many pharmaceutical substances seem to have a viscous character, i.e. be strain-rate sensitive, and the properties of the tablet is thus dependent on the punch displacement–time relationship for the compression process.

Elastic deformation can be described as a densification of the particle due to a small movement of the cluster of molecules or ions that forms the particle, e.g. a crystal lattice or a cluster of disordered molecules. Plastic deformation is considered to occur by the sliding of molecules along slip planes within the particles. For real crystals, such slip planes are formed at defects in the crystal lattice, especially dislocations.

The majority of powders handled in pharmaceutical production consist not of non-porous primary particles but rather of granules, i.e. porous secondary particles formed from small dense primary particles. For granules, a larger number of processes are involved in their compression. These can be classified into two groups:

- Physical changes in the granules, i.e. the secondary particles;
- Physical changes in the primary particles from which the granules are formed.

The latter concern changes in the dimensions of the primary particles due to elastic and plastic deformation and fragmentation. Such processes may be significant for the strength of tablets. It is, for example, common for a capping-prone substance, when compacted as dense particles, to also be prone to cap or laminate during compaction in the form of granules, such as substrate-binder granules. However, in terms of the evolution of the tablet structure, the physical changes in the granules that occur during compression are of primary importance.

At low compression forces the reduction in volume of the bed of granules can occur by a rearrangement within the die. However, granules are normally fairly coarse, which means that they spontaneously form a powder bed of relatively low voidage (i.e. the porosity of the intergranular spaces). Therefore, this initial rearrangement phase is probably of limited importance with respect to the total change in bed volume of the mass. With increased loading, a further reduction in bed volume therefore requires changes in the structure of the granules. The granules can deform, both elastically and permanently, but also densify, i.e. reduce their intragranular porosity. By these processes granules can still be described as coherent units, but their shape and porosity will change.

Granules can also be broken down into smaller units by different mechanisms:

1. Primary particles might be removed from the surface of granules when they slide against each other or against the die wall. This can be described as erosion or attrition, rather than fracturing. This mechanism occurs primarily for granules with a rough surface texture.
2. Granules can fracture into a number of smaller ones i.e. granule fragmentation.

Studies on the compression properties of granules formed from pharmaceutical substances have indicated that granules are not prone to fracture into smaller units during compression over a normal range of applied pressures. Thus, permanent deformation and densification dominate the compression event. However, for irregular, rough granules some attrition might occur. Deformation and densification of granules have been suggested to occur by the repositioning of primary particles within the granules, i.e. these processes involves an internal flow of primary particles. In this context, the terms **degree** and **mode** of deformation have been used to describe granule deformation. Degree of deformation refers to some quantitative change in the shape of the granules, whereas mode of deformation refers to the type of shape change, such as a flattening of the granule, or a more complicated shape change towards irregular granules.

The dominating compression mechanisms for dense particles and granules are summarized in Table 27.2. The relative occurrence of fragmentation and deformation of solid particles during compression is related to the fundamental mechanical characteristics of the substance, such as their elasticity and plasticity. For granules, both the mechanical properties of the primary particles from which the granules are formed and the physical structure of the granule, such as their porosity and shape, will affect the relative occurrence of each compression mechanism.

Evaluation of compression behaviour

Procedures

The procedures used in research and development work to evaluate the compression behaviour of particles and the mechanisms of compression involved in the volume reduction process are of two types:

- Characterization of ejected tablets;
- Characterization of the compression and decompression events.

Concerning the characterization of ejected tablets, the most important procedures used are inspection and the determination of the pore structure of the

Table 27.2 Dominating compression mechanisms for dense particles and granules (porous particles)

Dense particles	Granules
Repositioning of particles	Repositioning of granules
Particle deformation	Granule deformation
elastic	(permanent)
plastic	Granule densification
viscous/viscoelastic	Granule attrition
Particle fragmentation	Deformation of primary particles

tablet, in terms of a mean pore size, pore size distribution and specific surface area. A less common approach is to calculate ratios between the mechanical strengths of tablets measured in different directions.

Concerning characterization of the compression and decompression events, these procedures are based on relationships between parameters that can be derived from the compaction process (Table 27.3). Some of the most common approaches used in this context are described below.

Inspection of tablets

The inspection of tablets, e.g. by scanning electron microscopy, is an important means to study changes in the physical properties of particles during compression. Such changes include fragmentation into smaller particles, permanent shape changes due to deformation, and finally, the formation of cracks within the particles. Such inspection will also give information about the relative positions of particles within the tablet and hence the interparticulate pore structure. The fracture path during strength testing, i.e. failure around or across the particles, can also be estimated from inspection of the tablet fracture surface.

In addition to the inspection of intact tablets, studies of the fragmentation of particles during compression can be obtained by analysing the size and size distribution of particles obtained by deaggregation of a tablet. Such deaggregation can occur spontaneously by disintegration of the tablet in a liquid, or be created mechanically. Studies on such

---

Table 27.3 Parameters used in procedures to describe compression and decompression events

Upper punch force/pressure versus compression time*

Lower punch force/pressure versus compression time†

Upper punch force/pressure versus lower punch force/pressure

Upper punch force versus die-wall force

Punch force versus punch displacement (mainly upper punch)

Tablet volume versus upper punch pressure/force

Tablet porosity versus upper punch pressure/force

---

* Used both during ordinary compression and also as prolonged loading after maximum applied force/pressure has been reached (referred to as stress relaxation measurements).
† Used primarily to describe the ejection phase.

---

deaggregated tablets have indicated that powder compression can effectively reduce the size of particles and result in a wider particle size distribution of the cohered particles within a tablet.

Pore structure and specific surface area of tablets

One of the most important ways to study the evolution of tablet structure during compression is to measure some characteristic of the pore structure of the tablet. Information on pore size distribution can be obtained by mercury intrusion measurements and by gas adsorption–desorption. However, the most common way to evaluate the pore system of a tablet has been to measure the surface area of the tablet by air permeability or gas adsorption. The former has also been used to derive an indication of the mean pore size in a tablet.

Fragmentation is a size reduction process and so can be assessed by measuring the specific surface area of a particulate solid before and after compaction, or measuring changes in tablet surface area with compaction pressure. The surface area of tablets can be determined by several procedures, including gas adsorption and mercury intrusion. Both these methods can provide useful information on particle fragmentation. However, by these methods it is difficult to differentiate between inter- and intraparticulate pores, and the procedure might thus not reflect particle fragmentation only, but also the formation or closure of cracks or intraparticulate pores.

A method which measures the external surface area is thus advantageous in this context. Air permeametry is one such method which also has the advantage of being simple and fast. The procedure involves the formation of tablets at a series of applied pressures, followed by the measurement of the tablet's specific surface area. The slope of the relationship between tablet surface area and applied pressure represents the degree of fragmentation and can be used to classify materials with respect to their fragmentation propensity (Fig. 27.25). It should be pointed out that the calculation of tablet surface area from air permeability measurements may give erroneous values as a result of the assumptions made in the derivation of the calculation procedure. In spite of this, the method has been shown to give useful data in terms of describing the fragmentation propensity of a substance.

The relationship between tablet surface area and applied pressure is, however, strongly dependent on the original surface area of the powder, i.e. the tablet

Fig. 27.25 The tablet surface area, measured by air permeametry, as a function of compaction pressure for a series of pharmaceutical substances. (From Alderborn, G., Pasanen, K., and Nyström, C. Int. J. Pharm., 23, 79 1985. □ sodium chloride, ▲ sodium bicarbonate, ○ saccharose, ■ sodium citrate, △ ascorbic acid, ● lactose, ◇ paracetamol, ◆ Emcompress.

surface area increases more markedly with applied pressure when the original particle size was smaller. Attempts have been made in the literature to derive an expression similar to those describing the size reduction of particles during milling (see Chapter 11), by which a measure of the propensity of particles to fragment independent of the original powder surface area can be calculated.

It is generally assumed that a change in the size of a particle affects the mechanics of particle deformation, i.e. how a particle responds to an applied load. Such a size-related change in the mechanics of particles can, for example, be attributed to a reduced probability of the presence of flaws in the crystal structure at which a catastrophic failure is initiated. It seems possible, therefore, that at a limiting particle size fragmentation might cease. Examples of such transitions from a brittle to a plastic behaviour have been reported, and the particle size at which this transition takes place is referred to as the critical particle size. An example is that of α-lactose monohy-

drate crystals, where this transition takes place at about 20 μm. This critical size has been suggested to vary markedly between different substances.

The use of surface area data to estimate particle fragmentation from gas adsorption and permeability measurements can only be applied to powders consisting of solid particles, and not to those consisting of porous particles, such as granules. The problem for the latter type is related to the internal surface area and the intraparticulate porosity of the granules.

As granules are porous particles, the pore structure of a bed of granules is dualistic, i.e. there will be pores both within and between the granules. The compression process will dramatically affect the pore structure, and for tablets prepared from granules it is in practice difficult to distinguish between inter- and intragranular pores. It seems, though, that granules tend to keep their integrity during compaction, and hence the pore structure of the tablet is principally dualistic. It has been shown that the porosity of the intragranular pore space constitutes a significant portion of the total porosity of a tablet formed from granules. As granules densify during compression, measures of their porosity before compression is not sufficient compensation for the intragranular part of the pore system.

In order to avoid the problem of defining the porosity of the intergranular pore space, a simplified approach based on air permeability measurements has been used instead to characterize the compression behaviour of granules. In this case, a tablet permeability coefficient is measured and studied in relation to the applied pressure. By this procedure, the change in intergranular tablet pore structure with applied pressure can be assessed, which is suggested to reflect the deformation and densification behaviour of granules during tabletting.

Force–displacement profiles

The relationship between upper punch force and upper punch displacement during compression, often referred to as force–displacement profile, has been used as a means to derive information on the compression behaviour of a powder and to make predictions on its tablet-forming ability. The area under a force–displacement curve represents the work or energy involved in the compression process. Different procedures have been used to analyse the curves.

One suggested approach is based on the division of the force–displacement curve into different regions (denoted E1, E2 and E3 in Fig. 27.26). It has been suggested that the areas of E1 and E3 should be as small as possible if the powder will perform well in a tabletting operation and give tablets of a high

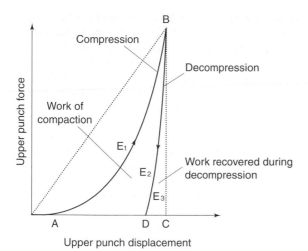

Fig. 27.26 The relationship between upper punch force and upper punch displacement during compression and decompression of a powder. (From Ragnarsson, G. In: Pharmaceutical Powder Compaction Technology (Eds. Alderborn G. and Nyström, C.), Marcel Dekker Inc., New York 1996.)

mechanical strength. An alternative proposed approach is based on mathematical analysis of the force–displacement curve from the compression phase, e.g. in terms of a hyperbolic function.

Force–displacement curves have some use in pharmaceutical development as an indicator of the tablet-forming ability of powders, including the assessment of the elastic properties of materials from the decompression curve. It can also be used as a means to monitor the compression behaviour of a substance in order to document and evaluate reproducibility between batches. However, the interpretation of the force–displacement relationship in terms of mechanisms of particle compression, or compression mechanics, is not clarified, which limits the use of force–displacement curves in fundamental compression studies.

Force–displacement measurements have also been used in fundamental studies on the energy conditions during compaction of powders, i.e. a thermodynamic analysis of the process of compact formation. The energy applied to the powder can be calculated from the area under the force–displacement curve. This compaction energy is used to overcome friction between particles, to deform particles both permanently and reversibly, and to create new particle surfaces by fragmentation. The thermal energy released during compaction can be assessed by calorimetry, i.e. the die is constructed as a calorimeter. The heat released during compression is the result of particle deformation – i.e. energy is consumed during deformation and thereafter partly

released when the deformation is completed – and the result of the formation of interparticulate bonds.

Data have been reported indicating that the net effect of a compaction process is exothermal, i.e. more thermal energy is released during compaction than is applied to the powder in terms of mechanical energy. The main explanation for this is released bonding energy in the form of heat due to the formation of bonds between particles.

Tablet volume–applied pressure profiles

In both engineering and pharmaceutical sciences, the relationship between volume and applied pressure during compression is the main approach to deriving a mathematical representation of the compression process. A large number of tablet volume–applied pressure relationships exist. In addition to tablet volume and applied pressure parameters, such expressions include some constants which often are defined in physical terms. However, only for a few equations has the physical significance of the constants been generally accepted. Among these, the most recognized expression in both engineering and pharmaceutical science is the tablet porosity–applied pressure function according to Heckel.

Heckel equation Tablet porosity can be measured either on an ejected tablet or on a powder column under load, i.e. in die. The latter approach is more common as it can be performed rapidly with a limited amount of powder. A problem might be that the compression time is different at each pressure, which could affect the profile for materials having pronounced time-dependent compression behaviour.

The compression of a powder can be described in terms of a first-order reaction where the pores are the reactant and the densification the product. Based on this assumption, the following expression was derived:

$$\ln (1/E) = KP + A$$

where E is the tablet porosity, P the applied pressure, A a constant suggested to reflect particle rearrangement and fragmentation, and K the slope of the linear part of the relationship which is suggested to reflect the deformation of particles during compression. The reciprocal of the slope value K is often calculated and considered to represent the **yield stress** or **yield pressure** (P_y) for the particles, i.e.:

$$\ln (1/E) = (P/P_y) + A$$

The yield stress is defined as the stress at which particle plastic deformation is initiated. To be able to use the Heckel yield pressure parameter to compare different substances, it is important to standardize the experimental conditions, such as tablet dimensions and speed of compaction.

Figure 27.27 shows a typical Heckel profile. This often shows an initial curvature (phase I) which has been suggested to reflect particle fragmentation and repositioning. Thereafter, the relationship is often linear over a substantial range of applied pressures (phase II), and thus obeys the expression. From the gradient of this linear part the yield pressure can be calculated, which is thus a measure of the particle plasticity. Finally, during decompression an expansion in tablet height is represented by increased tablet porosity (phase III). From this decompression phase a measure of the particle elasticity can be calculated as the relative change in tablet porosity or height.

Strain-rate sensitivity Another proposed use of yield pressure values from Heckel profiles is to assess the time-dependent deformation properties of particles during compression by comparing yield pressure values derived under compression at different punch velocities. A term denoted the **strain-rate sensitivity** (SRS) has been proposed (Roberts and Rowe 1985) as a characteristic of the time dependency of a powder:

$$SRS = (P_y' - P_y'')/P_y''$$

where P_y' is the yield pressure derived at a high punch velocity and P_y'' is that derived at a low punch velocity. P_y' is normally higher than P_y'' and the SRS is thus a positive value.

The discussion on the use of Heckel profiles to derive a measure of the compression yield pressure is applicable to the compression of powders consisting of solid particles. It should be emphasized that the interpretation of $1/K$ in terms of a mean yield stress for the particles is under debate. Nevertheless, support has been presented that such an interpretation is valid for solid (non-porous) particles. For porous particles, i.e. granules and pellets, the Heckel procedure is inadequate for the derivation of a measure of deformability or granule strength. The problem of applying the Heckel approach to the compression of porous particles is related to the need to assess the porosity of the reactant pore system. The pore space of interest in relation to the Heckel equation is intergranular, and the problem of quantifying this is discussed above.

Kawakita equation A promising means of assessing the compression mechanics of granules is to calculate a compression shear strength from the **Kawakita equation**. This was derived from the assumption that, during powder compression in a confined space, the system is in equilibrium at all stages, so that the product of a pressure term and a volume term is constant. The equation can be written in the following linear form:

$$P/C = (1/ab) + (P/a)$$

where P is applied pressure, C the degree of volume reduction and a and b are constants. The degree of volume reduction relates the initial height of the powder column (h_o) to the height of the powder column (the compact) at an applied pressure P (h_p) as follows:

$$C = (h_o - h_p)/h_o$$

The equation has been applied primarily to powders of solid particles. However, it has been suggested (Adams et al 1994) that the compression parameter $1/b$ corresponds to the strength of granules in terms of a compression strength. The procedure thus represents a possible means to characterize the mechanical property of granules from a compression experiment.

Evaluation of die-wall friction during compression

Friction is a serious problem during tabletting. A series of procedures has thus been developed with the aim of assessing the friction between the powder or tablet and the die wall during compression and ejection, which can be used during tablet formulation to evaluate lubricants. These methods are based mainly on the use of force signals during powder compression or tablet ejection. The most common type of compression situation used in this context is

Fig. 27.27 A typical example of a Heckel profile during compression and decompression of a powder. (From Duberg, M. and Nyström, C. Powder Technol. 46, 67, 1986.)

to use a single-punch press with a movable upper punch and a stationary lower punch. In such a rig the force is applied by the upper punch and transmitted axially to the lower punch, and also laterally to the die. The ejection of the tablet involves the application of an ejection force by the lower punch. Typical force profiles during compression in a single-punch press with a stationary lower punch are given in Figure 27.28.

When the descending upper punch establishes contact with the powder bed in the die, the force increases with compression time. The applied force rises to a maximum value and thereafter decreases during the decompression phase to zero. Parallel with the force trace from the upper punch, force traces from the lower punch and the die will be obtained. These can be described as transmitted forces and the force values are thus generally lower than the applied force. The force transmitted from the upper punch to the lower is considered to depend on a number of factors, including the friction between the powder and the die wall. These factors can be summarized in the following expression:

$$F_a = F_b \, e(KL/D)$$

where F_a and F_b are applied and transmitted forces, L and D are the length and diameter of the powder column within the cylindrical die (Fig. 27.29) and K is a constant. The constant K is a function of the friction coefficient between particles and the die wall. Thus, the transmission of force from the upper to the lower punch depends on the friction between the powder and the die wall. Both the difference in transmitted force, i.e. upper punch force–lower punch force, and the ratio between the upper and lower punch force, i.e. lower punch force/upper punch force (often denoted the R value), are used as measures of die-wall friction during compression. For a well lubricated powder the force transmission corresponds to $R > 0.9$.

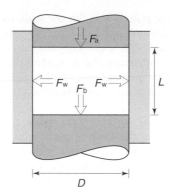

Fig. 27.29 Schematic illustration of punch and die-wall forces involved during uniaxial powder compression in a cylindrical die

In addition to studies on transmitted forces during uniaxial compression of a powder, studies have been performed with the intention of describing the distribution of the compression pressure within the powder column in a more detailed way. A complex pressure pattern will be developed during the compression, an example of which is given in Figure 27.30. This distribution in pressure will probably be associated with local variations in porosity, pore size and strength within the tablet, caused by, for example, pressure-related variations in the degree of particle deformation within the tablet.

After the upper punch has lost contact with the tablet and its force has consequently decreased to zero, the tablet will be positioned in the die in contact

Fig. 27.28 Force–time signals (from punches and die) during uniaxial powder compression.

Fig. 27.30 The distribution of compression pressure (in MPa) during uniaxial powder compression (From Train, D. Trans. Inst. Chem. Engrs. 35, 258, 1957.)

with the lower punch and the die wall. In this situation, the tablet will apply a force to both the lower punch and the die wall. The magnitude of these forces is dependent on the mechanical character of the particles formed into the tablet, but also by the friction conditions at the interface between tablet and die wall.

The ejection of the tablet will result in an increased force signal from the lower punch, referred to as the ejection force. This is a function of the lateral die-wall force, but also of the friction condition at the interface between tablet and die wall. The maximum ejection force is thus also used as a measure of friction between tablet and die wall. One approach to assess friction during ejection is to calculate the dimensionless friction coefficient (μ) as the ratio between the ejection force (F_e) and the die-wall force (F_w) at the beginning of the ejection phase, i.e.:

$$\mu = F_e/F_w$$

To summarize, the following procedures are mainly used to derive measures of friction between powder or tablet and the die wall from force signals during tabletting in a single-punch press:

- Force difference between upper and lower punch;
- Force ratio between lower and upper punch;
- Maximum ejection force;
- Friction coefficient during ejection.

FUNDAMENTAL ASPECTS OF THE COMPACTION OF POWDERS

Bonding in tablets

The transformation of a powder into a tablet is fundamentally an interparticulate bonding process, i.e. the increased strength of the assembly of particles is the result of the formation of bonds between them. The nature of these bonds is traditionally subdivided into five types – known as the Rumpf classification:

1. Solid bridges
2. Bonding by liquids (capillary and surface tension forces)
3. Binder bridges (viscous binders and adsorption layers)
4. Intermolecular and electrostatic forces
5. Mechanical interlocking.

In the case of compaction of dry powders, two of the suggested types of bond are often considered to dominate the process of interparticulate bond formation, i.e. bonding due to intermolecular forces

and bonding due to the formation of solid bridges. Mechanical interlocking between particles is also considered as a possible but less significant bond type in tablets.

Bonding by intermolecular forces is sometimes also known as **adsorption bonding**, i.e. the bonds are formed when two solid surfaces are brought into intimate contact and subsequently adsorb to each other. Among the intermolecular forces, dispersion forces are considered to represent the most important bonding mechanism. This force operates in vacuum and in a gaseous or liquid environment up to a separation distance between the surfaces of approximately 10–100 nm.

The formation of solid bridges, also referred to as the **diffusion theory of bonding**, occurs when two solids are mixed at their interface and accordingly form a continuous solid phase. Such a mixing process requires that molecules in the solid state are movable, at least temporarily, during compression. An increased molecular mobility can occur due to melting, or as a result of a glass–rubber transition of an amorphous solid phase.

Mechanical interlocking is the term used to describe a situation where strength is provided by interparticulate hooking. This phenomenon usually requires that the particles have an atypical shape, such as needle-shaped, or highly irregular and rough particles.

For tablets of a porosity in the range 5–30% it is normally assumed that bonding by adsorption is the dominant bond type between particles. In tablets formed from amorphous substances or from substances with low melting points, it is possible that solid bridges can be formed across the particle–particle interface. It is also reasonable that if tablets of a very low porosity, i.e. close to zero, are formed, particles can fuse together to a significant degree.

Often granules, i.e. secondary particles formed by the aggregation of primary particles, are handled in a tabletting operation. When granules are compacted, bonds will be formed between adjacent granule surfaces. For granules that do not include a binder the fusion of adjacent surfaces during compaction is probably not a significant bonding mechanism. Thus, intermolecular bonding forces acting between intergranular surfaces in intimate contact will probably be the dominant bond type in such tablets.

Granules often include a binder. When such binder–substrate granules are compacted it is reasonable to assume that the binder also plays an important role in the formation of intergranular bonds. The binder may fuse together locally and form binder bridges between granule surfaces which cohere the granules to each other. Such bridges may be the result of a softening or melting of binder layers during the compression phase. These bonds can be described as solid bridges according to the Rumpf classification (see above). However, different types of adsorption bonds may be active between granule surfaces. These may be subdivided into three types: binder–binder, binder–substrate and substrate–substrate bonds.

For adsorption bonds between granules in a tablet, the location of the failure during fracturing of the tablet can vary. Fractures occurring predominantly through binder bridges between substrate particles, as well as predominantly at the interface between the binder and the substrate particle, may occur. The location of the failure has been attributed to the relative strength of the cohesive (binder bridge) and adhesive (binder–substrate interface) forces acting within the granules, which can be affected by, for example, the surface geometry of the substrate particles.

The main bond types in tablets formed from dense particles (interparticulate bonds) and from granules (intergranular bonds) are summarized in Table 27.4.

The compactability of powders and the strength of tablets

The compactability of a powder refers to its propensity to form a coherent tablet and thus represents a critical powder property in successful tabletting operations. The ability of a powder to cohere is understood in this context in a broad sense, i.e. a powder with a high compactability forms tablets with a high resistance towards fracturing and without tendencies to cap or laminate (Fig. 27.31). In practice, the most common way to assess powder compactability is to study the effect of compaction pressure on the strength of the resulting tablet, as assessed by the force needed to fracture the formed tablet while loaded dia-

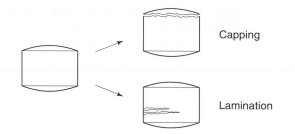

Fig. 27.31 Illustration of tablet defects referred to as capping and lamination.

metrically, or the tensile strength of the tablet. Such relationships are often nearly linear (Fig. 27.32) above a lower pressure threshold needed to form a tablet and up to a pressure corresponding to a tablet of a few percent porosity. At low porosities the relationship between tablet strength and compaction pressure will often level out. This relationship can thus be described simply in terms of a three-region relationship characterized by lower and upper tablet strength thresholds and an intermediate region in which the tablet strength is pressure dependent in an almost linear way. However, if cracks are formed in the tablet during tabletting, e.g. during the ejection phase, this will often affect the assessed strength. Cracking and capping can often be induced at relatively high compaction pressures. This can often be reflected as a drop in the tablet strength–compaction pressure profile.

By determining the tensile strength of a tablet by direct pulling in the axial direction, weaknesses in the tablet caused by small cracks can be observed as a reduction in axial tensile strength without a parallel effect on the tablet's tensile strength.

Alternatives to tablet strength–compaction pressure relationships for representing the compactability of powders are also used, such as the relationship

Table 27.4 Suggested predominant bond types in tablets formed from dense particles (interparticulate bonds) and from granules (intergranular bonds)	
Interparticulate bonds	Intergranular bonds
Adsorption bonds (intermolecular forces)	Adsorption bonds of three types: binder–binder binder–substrate substrate–substrate
Solid bridges	Solid binder bridges

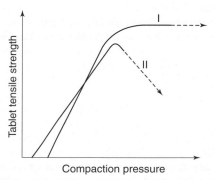

Fig. 27.32 Outline of the relationship between tablet tensile strength and compaction pressure for tablets showing no lamination (I) and for tablets showing lamination or capping (II).

between tablet strength and tablet porosity, and the relationship between tablet strength and the work done by the punches during tablet formation.

Compaction is fundamentally a bonding process, i.e. strength is provided by bonds formed at the interparticulate junctions or contact sites during the compression process. Studies on the structure of fractured tablets indicate that a tablet generally fails by the breakage of interparticulate bonds, i.e. an interparticulate fracture process. However, especially for tablets of low porosity, the tablet can also fracture by breakage of the particles that form the tablet, i.e. a combination of an inter- and an intraparticulate fracture process. In general terms it seems, though, that the interparticulate contacts in a tablet represent the preferred failure path during fracturing. This conclusion is applicable both to tablets formed from solid particles and to tablets formed from porous secondary particles (granules and pellets). Consequently, factors that affect the microstructure at the interparticulate junctions have been considered significant for the compactability of a powder.

Our understanding of the mechanical strength of a solid is based on the resistance of a solid body to fracture while loaded. It might seem reasonable that the sum of the bonding forces that cohere the molecules forming the solid will represent the strength of that solid. However, solids fail by a process of crack propagation, i.e. the fracture is initiated at a specific point within the solid and is thereafter propagated across a plane, thereby causing the solid to break. The consequence in terms of the strength of the solid is that the sum of the bonding forces acting over the fracture surface will be higher than the stress required to cause failure. It is known, for example, that for crystalline solids the theoretical strength due to the summation of intermolecular bonds is much higher than the measured strength of the solid.

In order to understand the strength of solids, the process of fracture has attracted considerable interest in different scientific areas. In this context important factors associated with the fracturing process and the strength of a specimen are the size of the flaw at which the crack is initiated and the resistance of the solid towards fracturing. The latter property can be described by the **critical stress intensity factor**, which is an indication of the stress needed to propagate a crack. Another fracture mechanics parameter, which is related to the critical stress intensity factor, is the strain energy release rate, which is a measure of the energy that is released during crack propagation. By using the critical stress intensity

factor, the tensile strength of the solid is considered to relate to the flaw size (c) and the critical stress intensity factor (K_{IC}) in the following way:

$$\sigma_t = f(K_{IC}/c^{1/2})$$

The critical stress intensity factor varies with tablet porosity. It has therefore been suggested that for compacts, such as tablets, factors such as the size of the particles within the tablet and the surface energy of the material will affect the critical stress intensity factor (Kendall 1988). These factors are also considered to control the interparticulate bond structure in a tablet.

Procedures to determine the critical stress intensity factor for a particulate solid have been described. Such a procedure involves normally the formation of a beam-shaped compact in which a notch is formed. When the compact is loaded, the fracture is initiated at the notch. The force needed to fracture the compact is determined and the critical stress intensity factor thereafter calculated. In order to assess a material characteristic, compacts of a series of porosities are formed and the series of values for the critical stress intensity factor subsequently determined is plotted as a function of the compact porosity (Fig. 27.33). The relationship is thereafter sometimes extrapolated to zero porosity, and the value thus derived is sometimes considered a fundamental material characteristic.

In addition to the fundamental studies on the strength of solids, indices and expressions have been derived within pharmaceutical science which can be described as indicators of the compactability

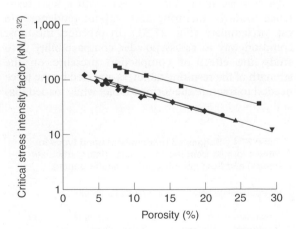

Fig. 27.33 A log-linear relationship between the critical stress intensity factor and the compact porosity for beams formed from polyethylene glycols of different molecular weight (From Al-Nasassrah, M.A., Podczeck, F., Newton, J.M. Eur. J. Pharm. Biopharm. 46, 31, 1998.)

of a powder. There are several applications of such indicators during pharmaceutical development, such as:

- the evaluation of the compactability of small amounts of particles;
- the selection of drug candidates during preformulation based on technical performance;
- the detection of batch variations of drugs and excipients;
- the selection of excipients and the evaluation of the compactability of formulations.

Examples of such indicators which have found industrial use are the indices of tabletting performance derived by Hiestand and co-workers (1996). Hiestand derived three indices of tabletting performance, among which the **bonding index** (BI) and the **brittle fracture index** (BFI) are suggested to reflect the compactability of the powder. These indices are dimensionless ratios between mechanical properties of compacts formed at some porosity. The bonding index is proposed to reflect the ability of particles to form a tablet of high tensile strength, whereas the brittle fracture index is proposed to reflect the ability of a tablet to resist fracturing and lamination during handling. These indices are defined as follows:

$$BI = T/H$$

and

$$BFI = (T/T_o - 1)/2$$

where T is the tensile strength of a normal compact, T_o is the tensile strength of a compact with a small hole and H is the hardness of the compact.

Other approaches to derive an indicator of the compactability of a powder aim to describe the microstructure of a tablet in terms of an interparticulate bond structure. They are based on the view that bond formation during compaction is significant for the development of coherence, i.e. it is postulated that the tensile strength of a tablet has some proportionality to the interparticulate bonds that act over the fracture area. The latter can be modelled in terms of, for example, the effective number of bonds and the effective contact area of the bonds. Such models can thus be described as bond summation approaches, and it is implicit that all bonds are separated simultaneously. This is not consistent with the real mode of failure of a solid and the models are thus not fundamental approaches to understanding the strength of a tablet. They can, however, be described as pragmatic models, with the aim of describing the importance of the compression

behaviour of particles for the evolution of bond structure and tablet strength.

Examples of such equations have been given by Leuenberger (1982) and Alderborn and co-workers (Eriksson and Alderborn 1995, Sebhatu and Alderborn 1999). In both cases the bond structure is modelled and related to an end-point representing the maximum tensile strength (σ_t^{max}) that can be obtained for tablets of a specific powder. This maximum tensile strength can thus be described as reflecting the bond strength. Leuenberger's approach is based on the concept of effective number of interparticulate bonds in a cross-section of the tablet. It is assumed that over a cross-section of a tablet a number of bonding and non-bonding sites exist. This number depends on the applied pressure during compression (P) and the tablet relative density (ρ, which is equivalent to 1 minus the tablet porosity). In the derivation of the expression the term **compression susceptibility** (γ) was introduced, which described the compressibility of the powder and has the unit 1/pressure. The equation takes the following form:

$$\sigma_t = \sigma_t^{max} (1 - e [\gamma P \rho])$$

Alderborn's approach is based on the concept of effective contact area between particles in a cross-section of the tablet. In the derivation it was assumed that both particle fragmentation and particle permanent deformation are bond-forming processes, and that the former controlled the number of bonds in a tablet cross-section and the latter the area of contact between a pair of particles in that section. The expression indicates that the propensity of particles to deform irreversibly during compression is a dominant factor for the microstructure of the formed tablet, which thus is considered to be of significant importance for the resistance of a tablet towards fracturing (Fig. 27.34).

Post-compaction tablet strength changes

The compactability of a powder is normally understood in terms of the ability of particles to cohere during the compression process and hence to form a porous specimen of defined shape. However, the mechanical strength of tablets can change, increase or decrease, during storage without the application of any external mechanical force. The underlying mechanisms for such changes are often a complex function of the combination of ingredients in the tablet and the storage conditions, such as relative humidity and temperature. In order to describe

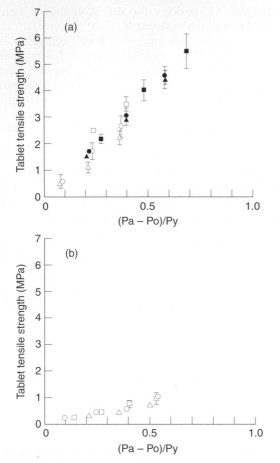

Table 27.5 Proposed mechanisms for post-compaction changes (increase or decrease) in the mechanical strength of tablets

Decreased tablet strength

Reduced bonding (intermolecular forces) due to condensation of water in tablet pores

Change in tablet microstructure due to dissolution of material in condensed water

Softening of amorphous material due to water absorption

Increased tablet strength

Formation of bonds due to crystallization of material dissolved in condensed water

Formation of bonds due to crystallization of amorphous material in rubbery state

Change in tablet microstructure due to viscous particle deformation

Change in tablet microstructure due to rearrangement of solid material in the amorphous state

Change in tablet microstructure due to polymorphic transformations

Fig. 27.34 The tensile strength of lactose tablets as a function of their microstructure, as calculated in terms of an effective contact area between the particles in the tablet by using the yield pressure from Heckel profiles (P_y). Upper graph represents tablets formed from amorphous lactose of three different particle sizes and lower graph represents tablets formed from crystalline lactose of three different particle sizes. (From Sebhatu, T. and Alderborn, G. Eur. J. Pharm. Sci. 8, 235, 1999.)

water can drastically decrease tablet strength and eventually lead to the collapse of the whole tablet. However, the dissolution of a freely soluble substance in condensed pore water can also give an increase in tablet strength if the water is allowed to evaporate owing to a change in temperature or relative humidity. The result of this evaporation can be a crystallization of solid material, with the subsequent formation of solid bridges between particles in the tablet and increased tablet strength.

In addition to the mechanisms involving the presence of condensed pore water, several other mechanisms causing an increase in tablet strength during storage at a relative humidity at which condensation of water is unlikely to occur, have been proposed. One such mechanism is a continuing viscous deformation of particles after the compaction process is completed. This phenomenon is referred to as ***stress relaxation*** of tablets. The increase in tablet strength can be significant with no or minor detectable changes in its physical structure. However, viscous deformation of small parts of particles might change the microstructure of the tablet in terms of the relative orientation of particle surfaces, and the geometry of the interparticle voids, and thus affect the resistance to fracturing of a tablet. A characteristic feature for stress relaxation changes is that the tablet strength changes occur for a limited time in connection with the compaction phase.

mechanisms responsible for post-compaction changes in tablet strength, studies on simple, one-component powders have been conducted (Table 27.5). The suggested mechanisms are probably active also in tablets formed from complete formulations of several components.

During storage at a fairly high relative humidity, tablets can be softer and their tensile strength reduced. With increased relative humidity, the state of water adsorbed at the solid surface can change from an adsorbed gas to a liquid, i.e. water condenses in the tablet pores. Furthermore, if the solid material is freely soluble in water, it can dissolve. Both the presence of condensed water in the pores and the dissolution of a substance in the condensed

Explanations for observed changes in tablet strength due to the presence of amorphous material in tablets have been presented. If the amorphous substance absorbs or desorbs moisture, the mechanical strength of the tablet can change. This is probably related to an effect of absorbed moisture on the mechanical properties of the amorphous material. If the uptake of moisture allows the amorphous material to change from a glassy to a rubbery state, the amorphous phase may crystallize. Such crystallization can subsequently affect – normally increase – tablet strength.

Another mechanistic explanation for a storage-related increase in tablet strength which involves amorphous material is a process described as a restructuring of parts of the pore system due to a rearrangement of solid material. It has been reported, for example, that a marked increase in tablet strength during storage occurred in parallel with a change to a more open pore structure. Moreover, these changes do not necessarily occur immediately after compaction, but can be initiated by exposure of the tablet to humid air for a certain period after compaction (Fig. 27.35). The restructuring of the pore system might be due to a diffusion-like transport of molecules or ions at the surface of particles, followed by a localization of material in zones where particle surfaces are close to each other. Such a mobility of molecules in the solid state has been shown by an amorphous phase.

Finally, an increase in tablet strength during storage has also been explained by a change in the crystal structure of particles, from a less to a more stable crystal form, i.e. a polymorphic transformation.

RELATIONSHIPS BETWEEN MATERIAL PROPERTIES AND TABLET STRENGTH

Factors of importance for powder compactability

A number of empirical studies exists in the pharmaceutical literature with the aim of mapping factors that affect the structure of a tablet and its mechanical strength, i.e. tensile strength, resistance towards attrition and capping tendencies. These factors can be classified into three group: material and formulation factors; processing factors (choice of tablet machine and operation conditions); and environmental factors (relative humidity etc.).

Of special importance from a formulation perspective are the physical and mechanical properties of the particles used in the formulation and how these particles are combined in granulation and mixing steps. Relationships for powders consisting both of one component and of two components, such as a filler and a lubricant or a dry binder, have been discussed in this context.

The compaction of solid particles

It is often assumed that the evolution of the interparticulate structure of a tablet, in terms of bonds between particles and the pores between the particles, will be significant for the mechanical strength of the tablet. Thus, the material-related factors that control the evolution of the microstructure of the tablet have been discussed as important factors for the compactability of a powder. In this context, the compression behaviour and the original dimensions of the particles have received special interest.

As discussed above, the degree of fragmentation and permanent deformation that particles undergo during compression are significant for tablet structure and strength. It has been suggested that both fragmentation and deformation are strength-producing compression mechanisms. The significance of particle fragmentation has been considered to be related to the formation of small particles which constitute the tablet, with the consequence that a large number of contact sites between particles at which bonds can be formed will be developed. The significance of permanent deformation has been explained in terms of an effect on the area of contact of the interparticulate contact sites, with a subse-

Fig. 27.35 The tensile strength of sodium chloride tablets as a function of storage time for tablets stored at different relative humidities. Open symbols: tablets stored 4 days at low, 4 days at high and 3 days at low relative humidity. Closed symbols: tablets stored 4 days at high, 4 days at low and 3 days at high relative humidity. (From Eriksson, M. and Alderborn, G. Int. J. Pharm. 109, 59, 1994.)

quent increased bonding force. The relative importance of these mechanisms for the bonding between particles in a tablet and the resistance of a tablet towards fracturing has, not however, been fully clarified. Concerning elastic deformation, which is recoverable, this is considered as a disruptive rather than a bond-forming mechanism. Poor compactability, in terms of low tablet strength and capping/lamination, has been attributed to elastic properties of the solid. A summary of proposed advantages and disadvantages of the different particle compression mechanisms for the ability of the particles to form tablets is given in Table 27.6.

It is sometimes considered that one of the most important properties of particles for the mechanical strength of a tablet is their size before compaction. A number of empirical relationships between particle dimensions before compaction and the mechanical strength of the resultant tablet can thus be found in the literature. As a rule, it is normally assumed that a smaller original particle size increases tablet strength. However, it is also suggested that the effect of original particle size is in relative terms limited for powder compactability, with the possible exception of very small (i.e. micronized) particles. Reported data show, however, that different and sometimes complex relationships between particle size and tablet strength can be obtained, with maximum or minimum tablet strength values. Complex relationships might be associated with a change in the shape, structure (such as the formation of aggregates) or degree of disorder of the particles with particle size. It seems also that increased compaction pressure stresses the relationship between original particle size and tablet strength in absolute terms.

Expressions quantifying the relationship between tablet strength and original particle size have been presented in the literature, such as the following:

$$F = K\, d^{-a}$$

where F is the force (N) needed to break the compact, d is the diameter (m) of the particle, and, K and a are constants. The expression thus describes the general assumption that tablet strength increases with a reduced original particle size. The compactability of sodium chloride and hexamine is described by this equation (Fig. 27.36).

Some studies have specifically reported on the effect of original particle shape on tablet strength. The results indicate that, for particles that fragment to a limited degree during compression, an increased particle irregularity improved their compactability. However, for particles that fragmented markedly during compression the original shape of the particles did not affect tablet strength. Moreover, an increased compaction pressure increased the absolute difference in strength of compacts of different original particle shape. Thus, the shape characteristics of particles that fragment markedly during compression seem not to affect the microstructure and the tensile strength of tablets, but the converse applies for particles that showed limited fragmentation.

Table 27.6 Proposed advantages and disadvantages of the different compression mechanisms in relation to the tablet-forming ability of the powder

Compression mechanism	Advantages	Disadvantages	Others
Fragmentation	No effect of particle shape Low sensitivity to additives Strain-rate insensitive	May cause fracturing of tablets (capping etc.)	Bond-forming ability (and tablet strength) dependent on degree of particle fragmentation
Plastic deformation	Resistant towards fracturing of tablets (capping etc.) Strain-rate insensitive	Sensitive to additives and variations in original particle shape	Bond-forming ability (and tablet strength) dependent on degree of particle deformation
Elastic deformation	–	May cause fracturing of tablets (capping etc.)	–
Time-dependent deformation	–	Strain rate sensitive Prone to change tablet strength after compaction due to stress relaxation	–

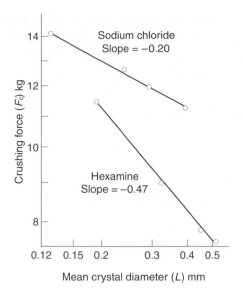

Fig. 27.36 The relationship (log-log scales) between the force needed to break the tablet and the original diameter of the particles of sodium chloride and hexamine. (From Shotton, E. and Ganderton, D. J. Pharm. Pharmacol. Suppl. 13, 144T, 1961.

The compaction of granules

The rationale for granulating a powder mixture before tabletting has been discussed above, one reason being to ensure good compactability. When granules are compacted, the mechanical characteristics of the primary particles will probably affect the compactability of the mass. For example, it is a common experience that capping-prone material will show capping tendencies in the granulated form of the substance also. However, the design of the granulation process, such as the method of granulation, will also affect the compactability of the granules. Such process conditions will control the physical properties of the aggregates formed, e.g. in terms of intragranular binder distribution and granule porosity.

Tablets formed from granules can in physical terms be described as granules bonded together by intergranular bonds. When subjected to a load, tablets formed from granules often fail because of breakage of these bonds. Hence, the bonding force of the intergranular bonds and the structure of the intergranular pores will be significant for the tensile strength of the tablets. The evolution of the intergranular tablet microstructure during compression is affected by the physical properties of the granules before compression, as well as their composition.

Thus, in order to engineer granules in terms of their compactability, two main factors can be controlled:

- The composition of the granules (e.g. choice of filler and binder);
- The physical properties of the granules (e.g. porosity and mechanical strength).

In terms of the physical properties of granules, porosity, compression shear strength and shape are significant properties that influence compactability. In general terms, increased porosity, decreased compression shear strength and increased irregularity (Fig. 27.37) will increase the compactability of the granules. As discussed above, pharmaceutical granules seem to fragment to only a limited degree during compression. The importance of these granule properties for compactability has thus been discussed in terms of a sequential relationship between the original physical character of the granules, the degree of deformation they undergo during compression, and the area of contact and the geometry of the intergranular pores of the formed tablet. The formation of large intergranular areas of contact and a closed pore system promotes a high tablet strength.

Traditionally, the most important means to control the compactability of granules has been to add a binder to the powder to be granulated. This is normally done by adding the binder in a dissolved form, thereby creating binder–substrate granules. An increased amount of binder can correspond to an increased compactability, but this is not a general rule. The importance of the presence of a binder for the compactability of such granules can be explained in two ways. First, it has been suggested that intergranular bonds that involve binder-coated granule surfaces can be described as comparatively strong,

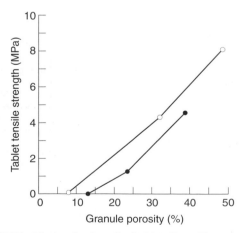

Fig. 27.37 The tensile strength of tablets formed from granules of a series of porosities and of two different shapes. Open symbol: irregular granules. Closed symbol: nearly spherical granules. (From Johansson, B. and Alderborn, G. Unpublished data.)

i.e. difficult to break. Secondly, binders are often comparatively deformable substances, which can reduce the compression shear strength of the whole granule and thus facilitate the deformation of the granules during compression. An increased degree of granule deformation is sometimes proposed to increase the compactability of the granules. Thus, the binder might have a double role in the compactability of granules, i.e. increase granule deformation and increase bond strength. Except for the presence of a binder in the granules, the combination of fillers in terms of the hardness and dimensions of the particles can affect the compression shear strength and hence the deformation properties of the granules during compression.

In the preparation of binder–substrate granules the intention is normally to spread out the binder homogenously within the granules, i.e. all substrate particles are more or less covered with a layer of binder. However, it is possible that the binder will be concentrated at different regions within the granules, e.g. due to solute migration during drying. The question of the importance of a relatively homogenous distribution versus a peripheral localization of the binder, i.e. concentration at the granule surface, has been addressed in the literature. It has been argued that a peripheral localization of the binder in the granules before compression should be advantageous, as the binder can thereby be used most effectively for the formation of intergranular bonds. However, the opposite has also been suggested, i.e. a homogenous binder distribution is advantageous for the compactability of granules. This observation was explained by assuming that, owing to extensive deformation and some attrition of granules during compression, new extragranular surfaces will be formed originating from the interior of the granule. When the binder is distributed homogenously, such compression-formed surfaces will show a high capacity for bonding.

Figure 27.38 gives an overview of the physical granule properties that affect the compactability of granules.

The compaction of binary mixtures

Most of the fundamental work on powder compaction has been carried out on one-component powders. It is, however, of obvious interest to derive knowledge that enables the prediction of the compactability of mixtures of powders from the information from the compaction behaviour of the individual components. In this context, powder mixtures of two components, i.e. binary mixtures, have been the system of choice in pharmaceutical studies. Binary mixtures can be of two types: simple physical mixtures, i.e. nearly randomized mixtures of particles, and interactive (ordered) mixtures. Most of the studies in this context are empirical, although models for the compaction of binary powder mixtures have been derived.

Concerning simple binary mixtures, the importance of the relative proportions of the ingredients has been studied in relation to the compactability of

Fig. 27.38 Overview of proposed physical granule properties of importance for the compactability of granules.

the respective single component. The mixture can show a change in compactability, as can be predicted proportionally from the compactability of the single powders, but deviations from such a simple linear relationship, both positively and negatively, have also been reported. Such non-linear behaviour has been explained in terms of differences between the components in their mechanical and adhesive properties.

Interactive mixtures, especially their compactability after the admixture of lubricants and dry binders, have been the subject of study. Concerning the tablet strength-reducing effect of a lubricant mixed with solid particles, it depends on the surface coverage of the lubricant film obtained during mixing, on the compaction properties of the lubricant per se, and on the compression behaviour of the substrate particles. Lubricant sensitivity, also referred to as dilution capacity, seems to be strongly related to the fragmentation propensity of the substrate particles, as discussed earlier.

Concerning the tablet-strength increasing effect of a dry binder mixed with solid particles, similar factors seem to control the compactability of the dry binder mixture as for the lubricant mixture, i.e. the degree of surface coverage of the substrate particle, the binding capacity and deformability of the dry binder, and the fragmentation propensity of the substrate particles (Fig. 27.39).

The dilution capacity of interactive mixtures between granules and lubricants or dry binders seems to be related to the degree of deformation the granules undergo during compression, i.e. a high degree of deformation will give a lower sensitivity to a lubricant but also a less positive effect of a dry binder.

REFERENCES

Adams, M.J., Mullier, M.A., Seville, J.P.K. (1994) Agglomerate strength measurement using a uniaxial confined compression test. *Powder Technol.*, **78**, 5.

Eriksson, M. and Alderborn, G. (1995) The effect of particle fragmentation and deformation on the interparticulate bond formation process during powder compaction. *Pharm. Res.* **12**, 1031.

Hiestand, E.N. (1996) Rationale for and the measurement of tableting indices. In: Pharmaceutical Powder Compaction Technology (eds. Alderborn, G. and Nyström, C.), p. 219, Marcel Dekker Inc., New York.

Kendall, K. (1988) Agglomerate strength. *Powder Metall.*, **31**, 28.

Leuenberger, H. (1982) The compressibility and compactability of powder systems. *Int. J. Pharm.* **12**, 41.

Roberts, R. and Rowe, R. (1985) The effect of punch velocity of the compaction of a variety of materials. *J. Pharm. Pharmacol.*, **37**, 377.

Sebhatu, T. and Alderborn, G. (1999) Relationships between the effective interparticulate contact area and the tensile strength of tablets of amorphous and crystalline lactose of varying particle size. *Eur. J. Pharm. Sci.* **8**, 235.

BIBLIOGRAPHY

Alderborn, G. and Nyström, C. (1996) *Pharmaceutical Powder Compaction* Technology. Marcel Dekker Inc., New York.

Alderborn, G., Pasanen, K., and Nyström, C. (1985) Studies on direct compression of tablets. XI. Characterization of particle fragmentation during compaction by permeametry measurements of tablets, *Int. J. Pharm.*, **23**, 79.

Al-Nasassrah, M.A., Podczeck, F. and Newton, J.M. (1998) The effect of an increase in chain length on the mechanical properties of polyethylene glycols. *Eur. J. Pharm. Biopharm.* **46**, 31.

Armstrong, N.A. (1982) Causes of tablet compression problems. *Mfg Chem.* October 62.

Banakar, U.V. (1992) *Pharmaceutical Dissolution Testing.* Marcel Dekker, Inc., New York.

Chien, Y.W. (1992) *Novel Drug Delivery Systems*, 2nd edition. Marcel Dekker, Inc., New York.

Chulia, D., Deleuil, M. and Pourcelot, Y. (1991) *Powder Technology and Pharmaceutical Processes* (Handbook of Powder Technology, vol. 9). Elsevier, Amsterdam.

Duberg,. M. and Nyström, C. (1986) Studies on direct compression of tablets. XVII. Porosity–pressure curves for the characterization of volume reduction mechanisms in powder compression. *Powder Technol.* **46**, 67.

Fig. 27.39 The tensile strength of tablets formed from three substrate substances of different fragmentation propensities in binary mixtures with some fine particulate dry binders i.e. microcrystalline cellulose, methylcellulose and polyvinylpyrrolidone of different particle size. The dotted lines represent the tensile strength of tablets formed from the single substrate substances. (From Nyström, C. and Glazer, M. Int. J. Pharm. 23, 255, 1985.)

Eriksson, M. and Alderborn, G. (1994) Mechanisms of post-compaction changes in tensile strength of sodium chloride compacts prepared from particles of different dimensions. *Int. J. Pharm.* **109**, 59.

European Pharmacopoeia 3rd edition 1997. Council of Europe, Strasbourg.

Hölzer, A.H. and Sjögren, J. (1981) Evaluation of some lubricants by the comparison of friction coefficients and tablet properties. *Acta Pharm. Suec.* **18**, 139.

Lieberman, H.A., Lachman, L. and Schwartz, J.B. (1989) *Pharmaceutical Dosage Forms: Tablets* (2nd edition, volumes 1–3). Marcel Dekker, Inc, New York.

Nyström, C. and Glazer, M. (1985) Studies on direct compression of tablets. XIII. The effect of some dry binders on the tablet strength of compounds with different fragmentation propensity. *Int. J. Pharm.* **23**, 255.

Podczeck, F. (1998) *Particle–particle Adhesion in Pharmaceutical Powder Handling*. Imperial College Press, London.

Sandell, E. (1993) *Industrial Aspects of Pharmaceutics*. Swedish Pharmaceutical Press, Stockholm.

Stanley-Wood, N.G. (1983) *Enlargement and Compaction of Particulate Solids*. Butterworths, London.

28

Coating of tablets and multiparticulates

John Hogan

DEFINITION

Tablet coating is the application of a coating material to the exterior of a tablet with the intention of conferring benefits and properties to the dosage form over the uncoated variety.

In its widest sense the technology is also applicable to multiparticulate systems intended for modified-release applications. To a much lesser extent coatings may also be applied to hard-shell and soft elastic capsules.

Types of tablet coating

Three main types are in use:

- Film coating
- Sugar coating
- Press coating.

Of these, film coating is the major technique: virtually all new coated products introduced on to the market are film coated. Sugar coating is the more traditional technology and has seen no real developments in recent years. As a proportion of the total output of coated tablets on a global basis, though, it is still of some economic importance.

Reasons for coating tablets

The reasons why tablets are coated are varied. The major ones can be summarized as follows:

1. Ingredients may need protection from the environment, particularly light and moisture.
2. Many drugs have a bitter or otherwise unpleasant taste: coating is an efficient way to mask such tastes. Tablets that are coated are also somewhat easier to swallow than uncoated tablets.

3. Coloured coatings also mask any batch differences in the appearance of raw materials and hence allay patient concern over tablets of differing appearance.

Factors 2 and 3 aid patient compliance with dosage schemes.

4. Coatings may be optimized with respect to colouration and gloss to aid in their sales appeal or to reinforce a marketing brand identification.
5. Coloured coatings aid in the rapid identification of product by the manufacturer, the dispensing pharmacist and the patient.
6. Coating tablets facilitates their handling on high-speed automatic filling and packaging equipment. Very often coating confers an added mechanical strength to the tablet core. Cross-contamination is also reduced in the manufacturing plant, as 'dusting' from tablets is eliminated by coating.
7. Functional film coatings are used to impart enteric or controlled-release properties to the coated tablet or, more usually, to coated multiparticulates (see later).

FILM COATING

This is the more modern and generally used technology in tablet coating. Nearly all newly launched coated products are film coated rather than sugar coated, for the reasons given in Table 28.1.

Process description

Film coating involves the deposition, usually by a spray method, of a thin film of polymer surrounding the tablet core. It is possible to use conventional panning equipment, but more usually specialized equipment is employed to take advantage of the fast coating times and high degree of automation possible.

The coating liquid (solution or suspension) contains a polymer in a suitable liquid medium together with other ingredients such as pigments and plasticizers. This solution is sprayed on to a rotating, mixed tablet bed or fluid bed. The drying conditions permit the removal of the solvent so as to leave a thin deposition of coating material around each tablet core.

Coating suspension formulation

Typically this comprises:

- Polymer
- Plasticizer
- Colourants
- Solvent.

Ideal characteristics of a film coating polymer

Solubility

For conventional film coating the polymer should have good solubility in aqueous fluids to facilitate the dissolution of the active ingredient from the finished dosage form. However, where a modified-release

Table 28.1 Major differences between sugar and film coating		
Features	Sugar coating	Film coating
Tablets		
Appearance	Rounded with high degree of polish	Retains contour of original core. Usually not as shiny as sugar coat types
Weight increase due to coating materials	30–50%	2–3%
Logo or 'break' lines	Not possible	Possible
Other solid dosage forms	Coating possible but little industrial importance	Coating of multiparticulates very important in modified release forms
Process		
Stages	Multistage process	Usually single stage
Typical batch coating time	Eight hours, but easily longer	1.5–2 hours
Functional coatings	Not usually possible apart from enteric coating	Easily adaptable for controlled release

action is required then a polymer system of low water solubility or permeability will be chosen.

Viscosity

In general, polymers should have a low viscosity for a given concentration. This will permit the easy, trouble-free spraying of their solutions in industrial film coating equipment.

Permeability

Film coating can be used to optimize the shelf-life of a tablet preparation, as some polymers are efficient barriers against the permeability of water vapour or other atmospheric gases. These properties vary widely between the individual polymers.

Mechanical properties

The particular polymer chosen for a film coat formulation must be one with adequate strength to withstand the impact and abrasion encountered in normal handling. Insufficient coating strength will be demonstrated by the development of cracks and other imperfections in the coating.

It should be mentioned that the polymer chosen must also comply with the relevant regulatory and pharmacopoeial requirements current in the intended marketing area.

Types of polymer available

Cellulose derivatives

Most are substituted ethers of cellulose.

Hydroxypropyl methylcellulose is the most widely used of the cellulosic polymers (Fig. 28.1). It is soluble in aqueous media and forms films which are mechanically tough and relatively easy to apply. The resultant film can be clear or coloured with permitted pigments. The polymer is the subject of monographs in the major international pharmacopoeia.

Other cellulosic derivatives used in film coating include methylcellulose and hydroxypropyl cellulose.

Methacrylate amino ester copolymers

Basically these polymers are insoluble in water below pH 4, but in neutral or alkaline media the films achieve solubility by swelling and increased permeability. For simple formulations the disintegration of the coating can be optimized by the incorporation of water-soluble materials and also by starches. Chemically an example is the polymer poly(butylmethacrylate) (2-dimethylaminoethyl) methacrylate methylmethacrylate.

For coatings designed to confer a modified-release aspect to the final dosage form, more water-insoluble polymers are used. These include ethylcellulose and the ammonio methacrylate copolymers. Yet another group of polymers is designed to provide an enteric protection to the dosage form. This effect is achieved by a pH selectivity of the polymer where it is insoluble at the low pH environment of the stomach yet becomes soluble as the higher pH of the duodenum and the distal portion of the gastrointestinal system is reached.

Aqueous polymer dispersions

Industrially, specialized dispersions of water-insoluble polymers such as ethylcellulose and ammonio methacrylate copolymers for use in aqueous media are frequently encountered in the coating of beads and granules for use in modified-release preparations (Zhang et al 1989). The advantage of these materials is that they permit the aqueous processing of otherwise water-insoluble polymers, with the consequent benefits of this method of processing (see 'Solvents', below).

Fig. 28.1 Hydroxypropyl methylcellulose.

Plasticizers

Plasticizers are generally added to film coating formulations to modify the physical properties of the polymer to make it more usable. One important property is their ability to decrease film brittleness. It is generally accepted that the mechanism by which polymers exert their action is for them to interpose themselves on a molecular scale between the polymer strands. In doing so they permit these strands to move more freely and allow the polymer to act in a more pliable fashion.

Examples of plasticizers are:

- polyols, such as polyethylene glycol 400
- organic esters, such as diethyl phthalate
- oils/glycerides, such as fractionated coconut oil.

In general, only water-miscible plasticizers can be used for aqueous-based spray systems.

Colourants

Any permitted colourants in a film coat formula are invariably water-insoluble colours (pigments). Pigments have certain advantages over water-soluble colours: they tend to be more chemically stable towards light, provide better opacity and covering power, and optimize the impermeability of a given film to water vapour.

Examples of colourants are:

- iron oxide pigments
- titanium dioxide
- aluminium Lakes.

Solvents

After the early development of film coating in the 1950s the polymers used were invariably dissolved in an organic solvent. Modern techniques now rely on water as a solvent because of the significant drawbacks that readily became apparent with the use of organic solvents. The disadvantages of organic solvents for the process can be listed below (see also Hogan 1982).

1. *Environmental*: the venting of untreated organic solvent vapour into the atmosphere is ecologically unacceptable, and efficient solvent vapour removal from gaseous effluent is expensive.
2. *Safety*: organic solvents provide explosion, fire and toxic hazards to plant operators.
3. *Financial*: the use of organic solvents necessitates the building of flame- and explosion-proof

facilities. Ingredient cost is also comparatively high, and the associated costs of storage and quality control must also be taken into consideration.
4. *Solvent residues*: for a given process the amount of residual organic solvent in the film must be investigated. With increasing regulatory pressure this will become an area for additional control in the future.

Process details

The vast majority of film-coated tablets are produced by a process which involves the atomization (spraying) of the coating solution or suspension on to a bed of tablets.

Some examples of equipment suitable for film coating include:

- Accela Cota – Manesty Machines, Liverpool, UK
- Hi-Coater – Freund Company, Japan
- Driacoater – Driam Metallprodukt GmbH, Germany
- HTF/150 – GS, Italy
- IDA – Dumoulin, France.

Examples of units that function on a fluidized-bed principle include:

- Aeromatic-Fielder, Switzerland and UK
- Glatt AG, Switzerland and Germany

Figure 28.2 shows one of the most widely used pieces of equipment for film coating, the Accela Cota.

Basic process requirements for film coating

These fundamental requirements are more or less independent of the actual type of equipment being used and include:

1. adequate means of atomizing the spray liquid for application to the tablet cores;
2. adequate mixing and agitation of the tablet bed. Spray coating relies upon each core passing through the area of spraying. This is distinct from sugar coating, where each application is spread from tablet to tablet prior to drying;
3. sufficient heat input in the form of drying air to provide the latent heat of evaporation of the solvent. This is particularly important with aqueous-based spraying;
4. good exhaust facilities to remove dust- and solvent-laden air.

Fig. 28.2 Accela Cota.

Ideal characteristics of film-coated tablets

Film-coated tablets should display an even coverage of film and colour. There should be no abrasion of tablet edges or crowns. Logos and break lines should be distinct and not filled in. The tablet must also be compliant with finished product specifications and any relevant compendial requirements.

Coating faults

These arise from two distinct causes:

1. *Processing*: for example, inadequate drying conditions will permit coating previously deposited on the tablet surface to stick against neighbouring tablets. When parted, this will reveal the original core surface underneath.
2. *Formulation faults*: film cracking or 'bridging' of break lines are examples of this type. After taking due account of the mechanical properties of the film, reformulation will almost certainly be successful in overcoming the problem (Rowe 1981).

SUGAR COATING

Sugar coating may be considered the traditional method of coating tablets. It involves the successive application of sucrose-based solutions to tablet cores in suitable coating equipment. Conventional panning equipment with manual application of syrup has been extensively used, although more specialized equipment and automated methods are now making an impact on the process. A comparison between sugar coating and film coating has been given in Table 28.1.

Stages involved in the production of sugar-coated tablets

Sugar coating is a multistage process and can be divided into the following steps:

1. Sealing of the tablet cores
2. Subcoating
3. Smoothing
4. Colouring
5. Polishing
6. Printing.

Initially the tablet cores to be sugar coated are sealed against the entry of water by the application of a water-impermeable polymer. Shellac has traditionally been used for this purpose and is indeed still used a great deal today, although more reliable materials, such as cellulose acetate phthalate and polyvinyl acetate phthalate, also find favour.

To attain the typically rounded profile of a sugar-coated tablet the sealed tablet core must be built up

445

to gain the desired profile. This process of subcoating is usually performed by adding bulking agents such as calcium carbonate or talc to the applied sucrose solutions. A gum such as acacia is also added to the applied suspension.

After the correct profile has been obtained the subcoated tablets will almost certainly have a rough surface, which will have to be made smooth before the next stage can be commenced. This is accomplished by the application of a few coats of sucrose syrup.

Nearly all sugar-coated tablets are coloured, as aesthetic appearance is usually considered to be of great importance with this dosage form. The pigments used are those permitted by the national legislation of the country where the products are to be marketed.

After the colour-coating stage the tablets will require a separate polishing stage for them to acquire an acceptable appearance. Several methods can be used, but commonly beeswax and carnauba wax are used in the process.

To facilitate identification sugar-coated tablets are usually printed with a manufacturer's logo or code. The use of indented monograms for this purpose, as for film-coated tablets, would not be feasible as the considerable thickness of sugar coating would obliterate any core markings. The printing process used is an offset gravure in conjunction with special edible inks, although the inkjet process is starting to make an impact.

Process details

Typically tablets are sugar coated by a panning technique. The simplest form would be a traditional sugar-coating pan with a supply of drying air (preferably of variable temperature and thermostatically controlled) and a fan-assisted extract to remove dust- and moisture-laden air.

Methods of applying the coating syrup include manually using a ladle, and, automatic control. In modern equipment some form of automatic control is available for the application of coating syrups.

In general, the equipment listed under film coating can, with suitable modification, be used for sugar-coating techniques.

Ideal characteristics of sugar-coated tablets

First the tablets must comply with finished product specifications and any appropriate compendial requirements. Sugar-coated tablets should ideally be of a perfectly smooth rounded contour with even colour coverage. Most manufacturers take advantage of the aesthetic appeal of a sugar-coated tablet and polish to a high gloss. Any printing should be distinct, with no smudging or broken print.

Coating faults

These are usually associated with process defects, such as splitting of the coat on storage, caused by inadequate drying during the coating application.

PRESS COATING

The technology of press coating differs radically from the previously described film- and sugar-coating techniques. Press coating involves the compaction of granular material around an already preformed core (Fig. 28.3) using compressing equipment similar to that used for the core itself, e.g. Manesty Drycota.

Today press coating is used mainly to separate chemically incompatible materials, one or more being placed in the core and the other(s) in the coating layer. However, there is still an interface of contact left between the two layers. In cases where even this is important then the process of press coating can be taken one stage further. It is possible to apply two press coatings to a tablet core using suitable equipment, e.g. Manesty Bicota. This equipment produces press-coated tablets with perfect separation between active core and coating, as the two can be separated by an inert middle layer.

The formulation and processing of the coating layer requires some care. Large or irregularly sized agglomerates of granules will cause the core to tilt in the second die used for compression of the coating. Thus there is the possibility of an incomplete coating, with the core being visible at the tablet surface.

The disadvantages of the process arise from the relative complexities of the mechanism used in the compressing equipment.

Fig. 28.3 Compaction of granular material around an already preformed core.

FUNCTIONAL COATINGS

All the coatings described above have been designed as a taste mask, as an identification aid, or indeed for many of the reasons previously discussed for coating tablets. There are, however, tablet coatings that perform a pharmaceutical function, such as conferring controlled or enteric release on the dosage form.

Controlled-release coatings

Film coating provides an extremely effective way of conferring a controlled-release aspect to a tablet or, more usually, a multiparticulate system. After coating these particles are filled into hard gelatin shells, or occasionally compressed directly into tablets by a process which permits minimal rupture of the applied film. The coatings involved use polymers with restricted water solubility or permeability, and include ethylcellulose and modified acrylate derivatives.

Multiparticulates, commonly referred to as 'pellets' or 'beads', find favour over conventional non-disintegrating tablets for controlled release use, owing to a number of factors:

1. Their small size (typically 0.7–2.00 mm) allows them to pass through the constricted pyloric sphincter and distribute themselves along the gastrointestinal tract. This tends to overcome the disadvantage that whole tablets have of a rather irregular passage through the gastrointestinal tract and consequent irregular absorption
2. Whole, non-disintegrating tablets can be liable to lodge in restrictions within the gastrointestinal tract, and this can lead to ulcerative damage to the gastric mucosa as the drug solution is leached out from the tablet. Because of their small size, this is not a problem with multiparticulates.
3. Should an individual bead or pellet fail and release all of its contents at once the patient would not be exposed to any undue risk. This is certainly not the case if a non-disintegrating tablet failed, when the consequences would potentially be serious.

Types of multiparticulate

Extruded/spheronized granules

These are produced in modified granulating equipment, with the drug granulation extruded through a mesh or other device under pressure to form small granulates which are subsequently spheronized.

Non-pareils

These are sucrose spheres which are coated with the drug plus an adhesive yet water-soluble polymer (Fig 28.4). After their formation and any necessary intermediate steps such as drying, they may be coated with the controlled-release coating.

Mechanisms of drug release from multiparticulates

Subsequent to the release of the coated pellets from the hard-shell capsule or tablet, the drug is released in a predetermined fashion with respect to time. The mechanisms described below postulate how this may be achieved (for further detail, see Chapter 20).

Diffusion

On contact with the aqueous fluids of the gastrointestinal tract, water will enter the interior of the particle by diffusion. Dissolution of the drug will occur and drug solution will diffuse across the controlled-release coat to the exterior. The kinetics of the process will depend upon which is the rate-controlling step, the dissolution of the drug or the diffusion of the drug solution through the coating.

Erosion

Some coatings can be designed to erode gradually with time, thereby releasing the drug contained within the pellet.

Osmosis

In allowing water to enter under the right circumstances, an osmotic pressure can be built up within

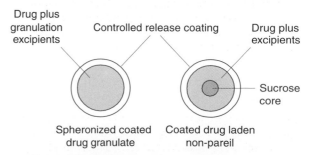

Fig. 28.4 Differences between multiparticulate types.

the interior of the pellet. Should the coating contain micro-imperfections and cracks the drug solution will be forced out of the pellet to the exterior.

Enteric coating

This technique is used to protect the tablet core from disintegration in the acid environment of the stomach for one or more of the following reasons:

1. Prevention of acid attack on active constituents unstable at low pH;
2. To protect the stomach from the irritant effect of certain drugs;
3. To facilitate absorption of a drug that is preferentially absorbed distal to the stomach.

The following polymers are among those commonly used for the purposes of enteric coating:

- Cellulose acetate phthalate
- Polyvinyl acetate phthalate
- Suitable acrylic derivatives.

Because they possess free carboxylic acid groups on the polymer backbone, they exhibit a differential pH solubility profile. They are almost insoluble in aqueous media at low pH, but as the pH rises they experience a sharp, well defined increase in solubility at a specific pH, e.g. pH 5.2 for cellulose acetate phthalate.

Enteric coating is possible using both sugar- and film-coating techniques.

Enteric film coating

The enteric polymers listed are capable of forming a direct film in a film-coating process. Sufficient weight of enteric polymer must be used to ensure an efficient enteric effect. This is normally two or three times that required for a simple film coating.

Enteric sugar coating

The sealing coat is modified to comprise one of the enteric polymers in sufficient quantity to pass the enteric test for disintegration. The subcoating and subsequent coating steps are then as for conventional sugar coating.

STANDARDS FOR COATED TABLETS

The European Pharmacopoeia has similar requirements for coated and uncoated tablets, the differences being:

1. Film-coated tablets must comply with the uniformity of mass test *unless otherwise justified and authorized*.
2. Film-coated tablets comply with the disintegration test for uncoated tablets except that the apparatus is operated for 30 minutes. The requirement for coated tablets other than film coated is modified to include a 60-minute operating time. Furthermore, the test may be repeated using 0.1 N HCl in the event that any tablets fail to disintegrate in the presence of water.

REFERENCES

Hogan, J.E. (1982) Solvent versus aqueous film coating. *Int. J. Pharm. Tech. Prod. Mfr*, **3**, 7.

Rowe, R.C. (1981) The cracking of film coatings on film coated tablets – a theoretical approach with practical implications. *J. Pharm. Pharmacol.*, **33**, 423.

Zhang, G., Schwartz, J.B., Schnaare, R.L. (1989) 6th Int. Symp. Controlled Release of Bioactive Materials, Chicago.

BIBLIOGRAPHY

Aulton, M.E., Abdul-Razzak, M.H., Hogan. J.E. (1981) The mechanical properties of hydroxypropyl methycellulose films derived from aqueous systems. Part 1: The influence of plasticisers. *Drug Dev. Ind. Pharm.*, **7**, 649.

Cole, G., Hogan, J.E., Aulton, M., eds (1995) *Pharmaceutical Coating Technology*. Taylor & Francis.

Hogan, J.E. (1983) Additive effects on aqueous film coatings. *Mfg. Chem.*, **54**, 43.

Porter, S.C. (1981) Tablet coating. *Drug Cosmetic Ind.*, May 46, June 44, Aug. 40, Sept. 50.

Rowe, R.C. (1983) Coating defects – causes and cures. *Mfg Chem.*, **54**, 49.

Melia, C.D., Washington, N., Wilson, C.C. (1994). *Multiparticulate Controlled Release Oral Dosage Forms*. Scottish Academic Press.

European Pharmacopoeia, 3rd edn. Suppl. 2000. Council of Europe, Strasbourg.

29

Hard gelatin capsules

Brian Jones

INTRODUCTION

The word capsule is derived from the Latin *capsula*, meaning a small box. In current English usage it is applied to many different objects, ranging from flowers to spacecraft. In pharmacy the word is used to describe an edible package made from gelatin or other suitable material which is filled with medicines to produce a unit dosage, mainly for oral use. There are two types of capsule, 'hard' and 'soft'; better adjectives would be 'two-piece' instead of hard, and 'one-piece' instead of soft. The hard capsule consists of two pieces in the form of cylinders closed at one end: the shorter piece, called the 'cap', fits over the open end of the longer piece, called the 'body'.

RAW MATERIALS

The raw materials used in the manufacture of both types of capsule are similar. Both contain gelatin, water, colourants and optional materials such as process aids and preservatives; in addition, soft capsules contain various plasticizers. The major pharmacopœiæ (European, Japanese and US) permit the use of gelatin or other suitable material, and in recent years hard capsules have been manufactured also from hydroxypropyl methylcellulose in order to produce a shell with a low moisture content (Ogura and Matsuura 1998).

Gelatin

Gelatin is the major component of the capsule and has been the material from which they have traditionally been made. The reason for this is that gelatin possesses five basic properties:

1. It is non-toxic, widely used in foodstuffs, and acceptable for use worldwide.

449

2. It is readily soluble in biological fluids at body temperature.
3. It is a good film-forming material, producing a strong flexible film. The wall thickness of a hard gelatin capsule is about 100 μm.
4. Solutions of high concentration, 40% w/v, are mobile at 50°C. Other biological polymers, such as agar, are not.
5. A solution in water or in a water–plasticizer blend undergoes a reversible change from a sol to a gel at temperatures only a few degrees above ambient. This is in contrast to other films formed on dosage forms, where either volatile solvents or large quantities of heat are required to cause this change of state, e.g. tablet film coating. These films are formed by spraying and have a structure that could be described as formed of overlapping plates, whereas the gelatin films are homogenous in structure, which gives them their strength.

Gelatin is a substance of natural origin that does not occur as such in nature. It is prepared by the hydrolysis of collagen, which is the main protein constituent of connective tissues (Jones 1987). Animal skins and bones are the raw materials used for the manufacture. There are two main types of gelatin: type A, which is produced by acid hydrolysis, and type B, which is produced by basic hydrolysis. The acid process takes about 7–10 days and is used mainly for animal skins, because they require less pretreatment than do bones. The basic process takes about 10 times as long and is used mainly for bovine bones. The bones must first be decalcified by washing in acid to give a soft sponge-like material, called ossein; calcium phosphates are produced as a byproduct. The ossein is then soaked in lime pits for several weeks.

After hydrolysis the gelatin is extracted from the treated material using hot water. The first extracts contain the gelatin with the highest physical properties, and as the temperature is raised the quality falls. The resulting weak solution of gelatin is concentrated in a series of evaporators and then chilled to form a gel. This gel is than extruded to form strands, which are then dried in a fluidized-bed system. The dried material is graded and then blended to meet the various specifications required. The properties of gelatin that are most important to the capsule manufacturers are the Bloom strength and the viscosity. The Bloom strength is a measure of gel rigidity. It is determined by preparing a standard gel (6.66% w/v) and maturing it at 10°C. It is defined as the load in grams required to push a standard plunger 4 mm

into the gel. The gelatin used in hard capsule manufacture is of a higher bloom strength (200–250 g) than that used for soft capsules (150 g) because a more rigid film is required for the manufacturing process.

Many materials used in the manufacture of pharmaceuticals are manufactured from raw materials of bovine origin, e.g. stearates and gelatin. The outbreak of BSE, which started in the UK, has led to strict rules being introduced by the EU to minimize the risk of transmitting animal spongiform encephalopathy agents (TSEs). All parts of the bovine animals have been rated for infectivity and the high-risk parts, such as the brain and spinal cord, are removed before any processing takes place. The EU rules specify that the animals used must come from herds free from BSE, be subjected to pre- and postmortem veterinary inspection, and be processed by defined manufacturing processes by quality assured companies. No animal material from the UK, Eire, Switzerland or Portugal is permitted to be used. Pharmaceuticals and medicines are controlled specifically through a guidance document (CPMP/BWP/1230/98) issued by the European Agency for the Evaluation of Medicines Products (EMEA).

Colourants

The colourants that can be used are of two types: water-soluble dyes or insoluble pigments. To make a range of colours dyes and pigments are mixed together as solutions or suspensions. The dyes used are mostly synthetic in origin and can be subdivided in the azo dyes – those that have an –N=N– linkage – and the non-azo dyes, which come from a variety of chemical classes. Most dyes used currently are of the non-azo class, and the three most widely used are erythrosine (E127), indigo carmine (E132) and quinoline yellow (E104). Two types of pigment are used: iron oxides (E172), black, red and yellow, and titanium dioxide (E171), which is white and used to make the capsule opaque. The colourants that can be used to colour medicines are governed by legislation, which varies from country to country despite the fact that it is based on toxicological testing (Jones 1993). In the last few years there has been a move away from soluble dyes to pigments, particularly the iron oxides, because they are not absorbed on ingestion.

Process aids

The USNF describes the use of gelatin containing not more than 0.15% w/w of sodium lauryl sulphate for use in hard gelatin capsule manufacture. This functions as a wetting agent, to ensure that the lubricated metal moulds are uniformly covered when dipped into the gelatin solution.

Preservatives were formerly added to hard capsules as an in-process aid in order to prevent microbiological contamination during manufacture. Manufacturers operating their plants to GMP guidelines no longer use them. In the finished capsules the moisture levels, 13.0–16.0% w/v, are such that they will not support bacterial growth because the moisture is too strongly bonded to the gelatin molecule.

MANUFACTURE

The process in use today is the same as that described in the original patent of 1846 (Jones 2000). Metal moulds at room temperature are dipped into a hot gelatin solution which gels to form a film. This is dried, cut to length, removed from the moulds and the two parts are joined together. The difference today is that the operation is now fully automated, carried out as a continuous process on large machines housed in air-conditioned buildings. There are only a comparatively few specialist companies that manufacture empty capsule shells for supply to the pharmaceutical and health-food industries, who fill them with their own products. Two companies, which have done most of the pioneering work in the field, have been making capsules for 100 years: Shionogi Qualicaps (formerly Eli Lilly & Co.) since 1897, and Warner Lambert's Capsugel (formerly Parke Davis) since 1902.

The first step in the process is the preparation of the raw materials. A concentrated solution of gelatin, 35–40%, is prepared using demineralized hot water, 60–70°C, in jacketed pressure vessels. This is stirred until the gelatin has dissolved and then a vacuum is applied to remove any entrapped air bubbles. Aliquots of this solution are then dispensed into suitable containers and the required amounts of dye solutions and pigment suspensions added. The viscosity is measured and adjusted to a target value by the addition of hot water. This latter parameter is used to control the thickness of the capsule shells during production: the higher the viscosity the thicker the shell wall produced. The prepared mixes are then transferred to a heated holding hopper on the manufacturing machine.

The manufacturing machines are approximately 10 m long, 2 m wide and 3 m high. They consist of two parts, which are mirror images of each other: on one half the capsule cap is made and on the other the capsule body. The machines are also divided into two levels, an upper and a lower. The moulds, commonly referred to as 'pins', are made of stainless steel and are mounted in sets on metal strips, called 'bars'. There are approximately 40 000 mould pins per machine. The machines are housed in large rooms where the humidity and temperature are closely controlled.

The sequence of events in the manufacturing process is shown in Figure 29.1. At the front end of the machine is a hopper, called a 'dip pan' or 'pot'. This holds a fixed quantity of gelatin at a constant temperature, between 45° and 55°C. The level of solution is maintained automatically by a feed from the holding hopper. Capsules are formed by dipping sets of moulds, which are at room temperature, 22°C, into this solution. A film is formed on the surface of each mould by gelling. The moulds are slowly withdrawn from the solution and then rotated during their transfer to the upper level of the machine, in order to form a film of uniform thickness. Groups of 'pin bars' are then passed through a series of drying kilns, in which large volumes of controlled humidity air are blown over them. When they reach the rear of the machine the bars are transferred back to the lower level and pass through further drying kilns until they reach the front of the machine. Here the dried films are removed from the moulds, cut to the correct length, the two parts joined together and the complete capsule delivered from the machine. The mould pins are then cleaned and lubricated for the start of the next cycle.

The machines are normally operated on a 24-hour basis 7 days per week, stopping only for maintenance. The output per machine is about 1 million capsules per day, depending upon the size: the smaller the capsule the higher the output.

The assembled capsules are not fully closed at this stage and are in a 'prelocked' position, which prevents them falling apart before they reach the filling machine. The capsules now pass through a series of sorting and checking processes, which can be either manual, mechanical or electronic, to remove as many defective ones as possible. The quality levels are checked through the process using standard statistical sampling plans based on the Military Inspection Standards. If required, capsules can be printed at this stage. This is done using an offset gravure roll printing process using an edible ink based on shellac. The information printed is typically either the product name or strength, a company name or logo, or an identification code. The capsules are finally packed for shipment in moisture-proof liners, preferably heat-sealed aluminium foil bags, in cardboard cartons. In these containers they can be

.Fig. 29.1 The sequence of two-piece hard gelatin capsule shell manufacture.

stored for long periods without deterioration in quality, provided they are not subjected to localized heating or sudden temperature changes that will affect their moisture content and dimensions.

Empty capsule properties

Empty capsules contain a significant amount of water that acts as a plasticizer for the gelatin film and is essential for their function (Jones 2000). During industrial filling and packaging operations they are subjected to mechanical handling, and because the gelatin walls can flex these forces can be absorbed without any adverse effect. The standard moisture content specification for hard gelatin capsules is between 13.0% and 16.0% w/w. This value can vary depending upon the conditions to which they are exposed: at low humidities they will lose moisture and become brittle, and at high humidities they will gain moisture and soften. The moisture content can be maintained within the correct specification by storing them in sealed containers at an even temperature.

Capsules are readily soluble in water at 37°C. When the temperature falls below this their rate of solubility decreases. At below about 30°C they are insoluble and simply absorb water, swell and distort. This is an important factor to take into account during disintegration and dissolution testing. Because of this most Pharmacopœiae have set a limit of $37° \pm 1°C$ for the media for carrying out these tests. Capsules made from HPMC have a different solubility profile, being soluble at temperatures as low as 10°C (Chiwele et al 2000).

Capsule filling

Capsule sizes

Hard gelatin capsules are made in a range of fixed sizes; the standard industrial sizes in use today for human medicines are from 0 to 4 (Table 29.1). For a powder the simplest way in which to estimate the fill weight is to multiply the body volume by its tapped bulk density (Jones 1998). For liquids, the fill weight is calculated by multiplying the specific

Table 29.1 Capsule size and body fill volumes	
Capsule size	Body volume (mL)
0	0.67
1	0.48
2	0.37
3	0.28
4	0.20

gravity of the liquid by the capsule body volume × 0.8.

To accommodate special needs some intermediate sizes are produced, termed 'elongated sizes', that typically have an extra 10% of fill volume over the standard sizes, e.g. for 500 mg doses of antibiotics elongated size 0 capsules are commonly used. The shape of the capsule has remained virtually unchanged since its invention over 150 years ago, except for the development of the self-locking capsule. These were introduced during the 1960s, when automatic filling and packaging machines were introduced. Filled capsules were subjected to vibration during this process, causing some to come apart and spill their contents. To overcome this, modern capsule shells have a series of indentations on the inside of the cap and on the external surface of the body which, when the capsule is closed after filling, form an interference fit sufficient to hold them together during mechanical handling. The manufacturer of the empty shells can be identified from the types of indent, which are specific to each one.

Capsule shell filling

Hard gelatin capsules can be filled with a large variety of materials of different physicochemical properties. The limitations in the types of material that can be filled are shown in Table 29.2. Gelatin is a relatively inert material. The substances to be avoided are those which are known to react with it, e.g. formaldehyde, which causes a crosslinking reaction that makes the capsule insoluble, or those that interfere with the integrity of the shell, e.g. substances containing free water, which can be absorbed by the gelatin causing it to soften and distort.

The materials that have been filled into hard gelatin capsules are given in Table 29.3. The reason that such a range of materials can be handled is the nature of the capsule-filling process. Empty hard gelatin capsules are supplied in bulk containers. First, it is necessary for the filling machine to orientate them so that they are all pointing in the same

Table 29.2   Limitations in properties of materials for filling into capsules

Must not react with gelatin
Must not contain a high level of 'free' moisture
The volume of the unit dose must not exceed the sizes of capsule available

Table 29.3   Types of material for filling into hard gelatin capsules

Dry solids
Powders
Pellets
Granules
Tablets
Semisolids
Thermosoftening mixtures
Thixotropic mixtures
Pastes
Liquids
Non-aqueous liquids

direction, i.e. body first. To do this they are loaded into a hopper and from there pass down through tubes to a rectification section. Here the capsules are held in tight-fitting slots. Metal fingers strike them in the middle, and because the bodies have the smaller diameter, they rotate away from the direction of impact. Next the capsules are sucked through bushings that trap the caps, because of their greater diameter, separating them from the bodies. The bodies are then passed under the dosing mechanism and filled with material. Thus providing a substance can be measured and dosed, it can be filled into capsules. The caps are then repositioned over the bodies and metal fingers push the bodies up into them to rejoin the two parts.

Capsule-filling machines

The same set of basic operations is carried out whether capsules are being filled on the bench for extemporaneous dispensing or on high-speed automatic machines for industrial products. The major difference between the many methods available is the way in which the dose of material is measured into the capsule body.

Filling of powder formulations

Bench-scale filling

There is a requirement for filling small quantities of capsules, from 50 to 10 000, in community pharmacy, in hospital pharmacy, or in industry for special prescriptions or trials. There are several simple pieces of equipment available for doing this, e.g. the 'Feton' from Belgium or the 'Labocaps' from Denmark. These consist of sets of plastic plates which have predrilled holes to take from 30 to 100 capsules of a specific size. Empty capsules are fed into the holes, either manually or with a simple loading device. The bodies are locked in their plate by means of a screw and the caps in their plate are removed. Powder is placed on to the surface of the body plate and is spread with a spatula so that it is filled into the bodies. The uniformity of fill weight is very dependent upon good flow properties of the powder. The cap plate is then repositioned over the body one and the capsules are rejoined using manual pressure.

Fig. 29.2 An auger filling machine using the ring system, Model No. 8 (from Jones 2001, with permission).

Industrial-scale filling

The machines for the industrial-scale filling of hard gelatin capsules come in great variety of shapes and sizes, varying from semi- to fully automatic and ranging in output from 5000 to 15 000 per hour. Automatic machines can be either continuous in motion, like a rotary tablet press, or intermittent, where the machine stops to perform a function and then indexes round to the next position to repeat the operation on a further set of capsules.

The dosing systems can be divided into two groups:

- *Dependent*: dosing systems that use the capsule body directly to measure the powder. Uniformity of fill weight can only be achieved if the capsule is filled completely.
- *Independent*: dosing systems where the powder is measured independently of the body in a special measuring device. Weight uniformity is not dependent on filling the body completely. With this system the capsule can be part filled.

Dependent dosing systems

The auger Empty capsules are fed into a pair of ring holders (Fig. 29.2), the caps being retained in one half and the bodies in the other. The body holder is placed on a variable-speed revolving turntable; the powder hopper is pulled over the top of this plate, which revolves underneath it. In the hopper a revolving auger forces powder down into the capsule bodies. The weight of powder filled into the body is dependent mainly upon the time the body is underneath the hopper during the revolution of the plate holder.

These machines are semiautomatic in operation, requiring an operator to transfer the capsule holders from one operation to the next. It was the first developed for large-scale use at the beginning of the 20th century and is still widely used in many countries.

The contact parts of these machines were originally made from cast iron, but are now made from stainless steel to comply with GMP requirements. The machines are manufactured by many different makers, but are all based on the original Colton Model No. 8 design. Their output varies between 15 000 and 25 000 per hour and is dependent upon the skill of the operator.

Independent dosing systems Most industrial machines in use in Europe and the USA are fully automatic and use dosing mechanisms that form a 'plug' of powder. This is a soft compact formed at low compression forces – between 10 and 100 N – which are significantly less than those used in tabletting. The reason the plug is soft is because it is not the final dosage form, unlike the tablet, as the material will be contained inside a capsule shell. There are two types of plug-forming machine: those that use a 'dosator' system and those that use a 'tamping finger and dosing disc' system.

Dosators This consists of a dosing tube inside which there is a movable spring-loaded piston, thus forming a variable-volume chamber in the bottom of the cylinder (Fig. 29.3). The tube is lowered open end first into a bed of powder, which enters the tube to fill the chamber and form a plug. This can be further consolidated by applying a compression force with the piston. The assembly is then raised from the powder bed and positioned over the capsule body. The piston is lowered, ejecting the powder plug into the capsule body. The weight of powder filled can be adjusted by altering the position of the piston inside the tube, i.e. increasing or decreasing the volume, and by changing the depth of the powder bed.

This system is probably the most widely used in the world and is the one that is described the most in the literature. Examples of machines that use this system are:

Fig. 29.3 A dosing tube or dosator-type machine, Zanasi RM63 (from Jones 2001, with permission).

- *Intermittent motion*: Zanasi (IMA), Pedini, Macophar and Bonapace. Their outputs range from 5000 to 60 000 per hour.
- *Continuous motion*: MG2, Matic (IMA). Their outputs range from 30 000 to 150 000 per hour.

Tamping finger and dosing disc The dosing disc forms the bottom of a revolving powder hopper (Fig. 29.4). This disc has in it a series of sets of accurately drilled holes in which powder plugs are

Fig. 29.4 A dosing disc and tamping finger machine, Höfliger & Karg (from Jones 2000, with permission).

formed by several sets of tamping fingers – stainless steel rods that are lowered into them through the bed of powder. At each position the fingers push material into the holes, building up a plug before they index on to the next position. At the last position the finger pushes the plug through the disc into a capsule body. The powder fill weight can be varied by the amount of insertion of the fingers into the disc, by changing the thickness of the dosing disc, and by adjusting the amount of powder in the hopper.

The machines that use this system are all intermittent in motion. Examples are the Höfliger and Karg, manufactured by Robert Bosch, and the Shionogi Qualicaps F-80.

Instrumented capsule-filling machines and simulators

Unlike tablet machines, few workers have instrumented capsule-filling machines. This is for a variety of reasons. Capsules are used only in the pharmaceutical and health-food industries, as opposed to tablets, which are widely used by many other industries and for which there is therefore more incentive to do fundamental research. The tablet press is simple to quantify: there are two punches and a die that holds a specific volume of material. On a capsule-filling machine there are a variety of moving parts involved in dosing, which occurs in an unconfined bed of powder. The forces involved are small. As a result of this, comparatively few papers have been published on the topic. Machines that use the dosator system have been studied the most (Augsburger 1988). Strain gauges have been fixed to the piston that have enabled the compression forces – 10–250 N – and ejection forces – 1–20 N – in lubricated products to be measured. Distance transducers have been used to measure the relative movements of the piston and dosator. Simulators have also been built to overcome the problem of the machine parts moving, but to date these have had limited application (Britten et al 1995).

Pellet filling

Preparations formulated to give modified-release patterns are often produced as granules or coated pellets. They are filled on an industrial scale using machines adapted from powder use. All have a dosing system based on a chamber with a volume that can easily be changed. Pellets are not compressed in the process and may have to be held inside the measuring devices by mechanical means, e.g. either by inverting the dosator or by applying a suction to the dosing tube. In calculating the weight of particles that can be filled into a capsule it is necessary to make an allowance for their size. Unlike powders, which have a much smaller size, they cannot fill all the available space within the capsule because of packing restrictions. The degree of this effect will be greater the smaller the capsule size and the larger the particle diameter.

Tablet filling

Tablets are placed in hoppers and allowed to fall down tubes, at the bottom of which is a gate device that will allow a set number of tablets to pass. These fall by gravity into the capsule bodies as they pass underneath the hopper. Most machines have a mechanical probe that is inserted into the capsule to check that the correct number of tablets has been transferred. Tablets for capsule filling are normally film coated to prevent dust, and are sized so that they can fall freely into the capsule body.

Semisolid and liquid filling

Liquids can easily be dosed into capsules using volumetric pumps (Jones 2001). The problem after filling is to stop leakage from the closed capsule. This can be done in one of two ways, either by formulation or by sealing of the capsule. Semisolid mixtures are formulations that are solid at ambient temperatures and can be liquefied for filling by either heating thermosoftening mixtures, or by stirring thixotropic mixtures. After filling they cool and solidify, or revert to their resting state in the capsule to form a solid plug. Both types of formulations are filled as liquids using volumetric pumps. These formulation are similar to those that are filled into soft gelatin capsules, but differ in one important respect: they can have melting points higher than 35°C, which is the maximum for soft gelatin capsules because this is the temperature used by the sealing rollers during their manufacture. Non-aqueous liquids, which are mobile at ambient temperatures, require the capsules to be sealed after filling. The industrially accepted method for this is to seal the cap and body together by applying a gelatin solution around the centre of the capsule after it has been filled. When this has been dried it forms a hermetic seal that prevents liquid leakage, contains odours inside the shell and significant reduces oxygen permeation into the contents, protecting them from oxidation. An example of such equipment is the Shionogi Qualicaps Hicapseal machines, which have outputs ranging from 10 000 to 100 000 per hour.

FORMULATION

All formulations for filling into capsules have to meet the same basic requirements:

1. They must be capable of being filled uniformly to give a stable product.
2. They must release their active contents in a form that is available for absorption by the patient.
3. They must comply with the requirements of the Pharmacopœiæ and regulatory authorities, e.g. dissolution tests.

In order to formulate rationally it is necessary to take into account the mechanics of the filling machines and how each type of product is handled.

Powder formulation

The majority of products for filling into capsules are formulated as powders. These are typically mixtures of the active ingredient together with a combination of different types of excipients (Jones 1995; Table 29.4). The ones selected depend upon several factors:

- The properties of the active drug
- Its dose, solubility, particle size and shape
- The size of capsule to be used.

The latter factor defines the free space inside the capsule that is available to the formulator (Jones 1998). The easier active compounds to formulate are low-dose potent ones, which in the final formulation occupy only a small percentage of the total volume – <20% – and so the properties of the mixture will be governed by the excipients chosen, whereas those compounds with a high unit dose, e.g. 500 mg of an antibiotic, leave little free space within the capsule and excipients must be chosen that exert their effect at low concentrations, <5%, and the properties of the mixture will be governed by that of the active ingredient.

Table 29.4   Types of excipient used in powder-filled capsules
Diluents, which give plug-forming properties
Lubricants, which reduce powder to metal adhesion
Glidants, which improve powder flow
Wetting agents, which improve water penetration
Disintegrants, which produce disruption of the powder mass
Stabilizers, which improve product stability

Formulation for filling properties

There are three main factors in powder formulation:

- Good flow, (using free-flowing diluent and glidant)
- No adhesion (using lubricant)
- Cohesion (plug-forming diluent).

The factor that contributes most to the uniform filling of capsules is good powder flow. This is because the powder bed, from which the dose is measured, needs to be homogeneous and packed reproducibly in order to achieve uniform fill weights. Packing is assisted by mechanical devices on the filling machines. Low-dose actives can be made to flow well by mixing them with free-flowing diluents, e.g. lactose. The diluent is chosen also for its plug-forming properties: the most frequently used ones are lactose, maize starch and microcrystalline cellulose. When space is limited then either glidants, which are materials that reduce interparticulate friction, such as colloidal anhydrous silica, or lubricants, which are materials that reduce powder to metal adhesion, e.g. magnesium stearate, are added, enabling the dosing devices to function efficiently. Both of these types of material exert their effect by coating the surfaces of the other ingredients, and thus the mixing of these into the bulk powder has a significant effect on their functioning.

Formulation for release of active ingredients

The first stage in active ingredient release is disintegration of the capsule shell. When capsules are placed in a suitable liquid at body temperature, (37°C) the gelatin starts to dissolve and within 1 minute the shell will split, usually at the ends. With a properly formulated product the contents will start to empty out before all the gelatin has dissolved. The official tests for disintegration and dissolution were originally designed for tablets. Capsules have very different physical properties, and after the contents have emptied out the gelatin pieces remaining will adhere strongly to metal surfaces and may confuse the end-point of the test.

The literature shows that the rate-controlling step in capsule disintegration and product release is the formulation of the contents, which ideally should be hydrophilic and dispersible (Jones 1987). The factors that can be modified to make the active ingredients readily available depend upon their properties and those of any excipients being used. The active ingredients have a fixed set of physico-chemical properties which, except for the particle size, are out of the control of the formulator.

It has been shown that the particle size influences the rate of absorption for several compounds. For sulfisoxazole (Fig. 29.5) three different particle sizes were filled into capsules and administered to dogs; the smallest particle gave the highest peak blood level. This can be explained simply by the fact that the solution rate is directly proportional to the surface area of the particles: the smaller the particle the greater the relative surface area. However, this is not a panacea for formulation problems because small particles tend to aggregate together and the effect is lost. It has been shown that the important factor with particle size was the 'effective surface area', which is the area of the active available to the dissolution fluid. This is related to the packing of particles and is a measure of how well the fluid can penetrate into the mass.

Diluents are the excipients that are usually present in the greatest concentration in a formulation. They were classically defined as inert materials added to a mixture to increase its bulk to a more manageable quantity. Although they are relatively inert chemically, they do play a role in release. The case that first demonstrated this happened in Australia in the late 1960s. A capsule was reformulated that contained diphenylhydantoin, which is used for the treatment

Fig. 29.5 Effect of particle size on bioavailability (after Fincher et al 1965, with permission).

of epilepsy and is taken chronically. The diluent used was changed from calcium sulfate to lactose. In the months following this change there was an upsurge in reports of side-effects similar to overdosing of product. It was demonstrated that the change had had a significant effect on the bioavailability of the active (Fig. 29.6). The change to lactose gave much higher blood levels of the drug, which was probably due to the fact that it is readily soluble whereas calcium sulfate is not.

Since this occurrence the phenomenon has been shown to occur with other actives. The diluent used should be chosen in relationship to the solubility of the active. If a soluble diluent such as lactose is added to a poorly or insoluble compound it will make the powder mass more hydrophilic, enabling it to break up more readily on capsule shell disintegration. The converse is also true: actives that are readily soluble are best mixed with insoluble diluents such as starch or microcrystalline cellulose, because they help the powder mass to break up without interfering with their solubility in the medium.

Some excipients, such as lubricants and glidants, are added to formulations to improve their filling properties, and these can sometimes have an effect on release. The important thing to avoid in formulations are materials that tend to make the mass more hydrophobic. The most commonly used lubricant for both encapsulation and tabletting is magnesium stearate. Simmons et al (1972) studied the dissolution rate of chlordiazepoxide formulations with three levels of magnesium stearate, 0%, 1% and 5% (Fig. 29.7). They found that the dissolution rate was greatly reduced at the highest level of magnesium stearate, which they explained was due to the poor wetting of the powder mass. However, hydrophobic additives are

Fig. 29.7 Effect of lubricant on release of active ingredient (after Simmons et al 1972, with permission).

not always deleterious because they reduce the cohesiveness of the powder mass. This was first demonstrated by Nakagawa et al (1980), who were studying the dissolution of different particle sizes of rifampicin with and without magnesium stearate (Fig. 29.8). They found that for the larger particles (180–355 μm) the addition of magnesium stearate reduced the rate, but for the smaller particles (<75 μm) it increased the rate. This is because magnesium stearate reduces the cohesiveness of the small particles so that they spread more rapidly through the dissolution medium than the unlubricated material. Augsburger et al (1988) studied the system hydrochlorthiazide, microcrystalline cellulose and various levels of magnesium stearate (Fig. 29.9). They filled capsules on an instrumented machine using the same compression force, and found that as the concentration of magnesium stearate increased the dissolution rate improved to a maximum value at about 1.0% w/v, after which it fell. They correlated this to the hardness of the powder plug, which followed a similar pattern, becoming

Fig. 29.6 Effect of diluent on bioavailability (after Tyrer et al 1970, with permission).

Fig. 29.8 Effect of lubricant on in vitro release of rifampicin (after Nakagama et al 1980, with permission).

Fig. 29.9 Effect of lubricant on in vitro release of hydrochlorthiazide (after Botzolakis et al 1982, with permission).

softer – i.e. easier to break apart – as the concentration of lubricant increased. Above 1.0% the plug becomes too hydrophobic for the increase in 'softness' to compensate for this.

The increase in the use of dissolution testing for control purposes has led to products being formulated for this factor. This has been achieved in two ways: by the addition of either surfactants or disintegrants. The addition of a wetting agent, sodium lauryl sulphate, has been studied by several workers. For poorly soluble drugs the use of a soluble diluent together with 1% sodium lauryl sulphate gave the best results. Disintegrants were formerly never added to capsule formulations because starch, which was the most widely used tabletting disintegrant, does not function well in this context. This is because the powder plug is much less compacted than a tablet and the starch swells insufficiently to disrupt it. In more recent times '*superdisintegrants*' have been introduced that either swell many fold on absorbing water, e.g. sodium starch glycolate and croscarmellose, or that act as wicks, attracting water into the plug, e.g. crospovidone. These actions are sufficient to help break up the capsule plug. The choice of disintegrant is dependent upon the solubility of the active and the diluent, which governs whether either swelling or wicking is the main disruptive force required (Botzolakis and Augsburger 1988).

Formulation optimization

The formulator has to produce a product that complies with the three formulation goals. Sometimes these are contradictory: for example, extra hydrophobic lubricant is required for filling machine performance, which could interfere with release. Therefore, in the development stage the formulation needs to be optimized so that it can meet the product specification. This can be done by using various statistical tools based on analysis of variance experiments that can identify the contribution of each excipient and process operation to the product performance, e.g. uniformity of fill weight and content, dissolution rate, disintegration, yield etc. (Armstrong and James 1996).

The latest computer-based systems to aid the formulator are 'expert systems', which are based on neural networks coupled to a knowledge base (Lai et al 1996). The systems are set up using rules that have been established through experience and research. They enable a formulator to enter into the system the characteristics of the active ingredient and the type of product they would like to produce. The system then comes back with suggested formulations to try. This can significantly reduce the development time for a new product.

To summarize, the main factors in powder formulation release are:

• Active ingredient, optimum particle size
• Hydrophilic mass, relating solubility of active to excipients
• Dissolution aids, wetting agent, superdisintegrant
• Optimum formulation for filling and release.

Formulation for position of release

Many products are formulated to release their contents in the stomach. However, this may not always be the best place for the absorption of the active ingredient, and capsule formulation can be readily manipulated to release their contents at various positions along the gastrointestinal tract (Jones 1991).

A common problem with oral dosage forms is making them easy to swallow. Certain people have great difficulty with this because the process is not a reflex and is controlled by the central nervous system. The capsule is a good shape for swallowing because the tongue will automatically align it with its long axis pointing towards the throat. Many tablets are now made this shape – called a 'caplet' – in order to facilitate swallowing. Patients who have difficulty swallowing should be instructed to do it either standing or sitting, in order to make full use of gravity, and to take a drink of water to lubricate the throat. They should drink a little water and hold it in the mouth. The capsule should be placed in the mouth and the head tilted forward. The capsule will now float on the water towards the back of the mouth and when the head is lifted the bolus of water and the capsule will go straight down the throat to the stomach.

In the stomach the release of the active ingredient can be modified in a number of ways. It has been suggested that for some compounds the best way to improve their absorption is for the dosage form to be retained in the stomach so that it will dissolve slowly, releasing a continuous flow of solution into the intestines. 'Floating capsules' have been made which contain various hydrophilic polymers, such as methylcellulose, that swell on contact with water and form a mass that can float on the gastric liquids. Some compounds are destroyed at acid pHs, and an enteric product can be made by either coating the filled capsule with an enteric film in a similar manner to a tablet, or by formulating the contents as pellets and coating them with an enteric polymer.

Much has been written in the literature about the advantages or disadvantages of making prolonged-release dosage forms as monolithic or as multiparticulate systems. The current consensus is that multiparticulates are better because they will be released in a stream from the stomach when the capsule shell disintegrates, and will not be retained for variable periods of time as would a monolithic product. They also avoid the risk of the dose being dumped at one point, which could cause problems of local gastric irritation.

Certain compounds are absorbed only at specific locations along the intestines. If this window of absorption is known then a formulation can be made to release its contents in that region. There is currently an interest in targeting compounds to the distal parts of the intestines. This has been achieved in two ways. Products can be formulated to give a prolonged release and filled into a capsule that is enteric coated, e.g. Colpermin (Pharmacia Upjohn), an enteric-coated capsule filled with a prolonged-release formulation of peppermint oil. The capsule disintegrates in the duodenum and the contents slowly release the peppermint oil, which acts as a smooth muscle relaxant as it passes through the remainder of the tract. Products have also been prepared that have been coated with polymers that are enteric and are soluble only at higher pHs, 6–7. This pH is not reached until further along the small intestine, and so the contents are delivered to the more distal parts. Currently many new chemical entities are proteins or polypeptides, and to make an oral dosage form it is necessary to deliver them to the colon, thereby avoiding the proteolytic enzymes in the stomach and small intestine. The release mechanisms for these capsules are based on specific colonic conditions, e.g. coatings that are disrupted by colon-specific enzymes or by pressure (Nagata and Jones 2001).

Not all capsules administered by the oral route are intended for the gastrointestinal tract. Capsules have been used successfully for many years for products for inhalation. The active ingredient, which is micronized, is filled into the capsule either 'as is' or dispersed on a carrier particle. The weight filled into a capsule is much lower than for other types of product, typically less than 25 mg. These formulations are filled on automatic machines that have microdosing devices, and the product is administered by using a special inhaler. A capsule is placed in the device and the powder is released either by the halves of the capsule being forced apart or by the capsule wall being punctured by sharp pins. The device is breath actuated. When the patient breathes in a turbulent airflow dislodges the carrier particles (if present) and the active powder is inhaled into the lungs. The system has the added advantage over an aerosol device in that the patient can see how many doses they have taken by counting the number of capsules remaining.

REFERENCES

Armstrong, N.A. and James, K.C. (1996) *Pharmaceutical experimental design and interpretation.* Taylor & Francis, London.

Augsburger, L.L. (1988) S.T.P. *Pharma,* **4**, 116–122.

Botzolakis, J.E. and Augsburger, L.L. (1988) *J. Pharm. Pharmacol.,* **36**, 77–84.

Britten, J.R., Barnett, M.I., Armstrong, N.A. (1995) *Pharm. Res.,* **12**, 196–200.

Chiwele, I., Jones, B.E., Podczeck, F., *Chem. Pharm. Bull.,* 2000 (in press).

Fincher, J.H., Adams, H.M. and Beal, H.M. (1965) *J. Pharm. Sci.,* **54**, 704–708.

Jones, B.E. (1987) S.T.P. *Pharma,* **3**, 777–783.

Jones, B.E. (1991) S.T.P. *Pharma Pratiques,* **2**, 128–134.

Jones, B.E. (1993) *Pharm. Tech. Int.* **5(4)**, 14–20.

Jones, B.E. (1995) *Pharm. Tech. Europe,* **7(10)**, 25, 28–30, 34.

Jones, B.E. (1998) S.T.P. *Pharma Sci.,* **8(5)**, 277–283.

Jones, B.E. (2001) Hard capsules. In: Swarbrick, J. and Boylan, J.C. (eds) *Encyclopedia of Pharmaceutical Technology,* 2nd edn. Vol. 1 Marcel Dekker, New York.

Jones, R.T. (1987) Gelatin structure and manufacture and Gelatin physical and chemical properties. In: Ridgway K. (ed) *Hard Capsules, Development and Technology.* Pharmaceutical Press, London, Chs 2 & 3.

Lai, S., Podczeck, F., Newton, J.M., Daumesnil, R. (1996) *Pharm. Tech. Europe,* **8(9)**, 60, 62, 64, 66, 68.

Nagata, S. and Jones, B.E. (2001) *Eur. Pharm. Rev.* **5(2)**, 41–46.

Nakagawa, H., Mohri, K., Nakashima, K., Sugimoto, I. (1980) *Yakugaku Zasshi,* **100**, 1111–1117.

Ogura, T. and Matsuura, S. (1998) *Pharm. Tech. Europe,* **10(11)**, 32, 34, 36, 40, 42.

Simmons, D.L., Frechette, M., Ranz, R.J. Chen, W.S. and Patel, N.K. (1972) *Can. J. Pharm. Sci.,* 7, 62–65.

Tyrer, J.M., Eacke, M.J., Sutherland, J.M., Hopper, W.D. (1970) *Br. Med. J.,* **IV**, 271–273.

30

Soft gelatin capsules

Keith Hutchison, Josephine Ferdinando

INTRODUCTION

The term 'soft gelatin capsules' is commonly abbreviated to 'softgels', and although the terms are interchangeable 'softgels' will be used throughout this chapter for the sake of convenience and consistency.

When pharmaceutical formulation scientists are faced with the challenge of designing a solid oral dosage form for drug compounds, they have a number of choices. Over recent years, new drug molecules have tended to be more hydrophobic and therefore less soluble in aqueous systems. In the case of drugs for oral administration, it is becoming more difficult to formulate poorly water-soluble drugs into products from which the drug is fully released and well absorbed. One of the best methods to overcome this problem is to make a liquid formulation containing the drug. In order to convert this liquid formula into a solid dosage form, it may be encapsulated into soft gelatin capsules.

This chapter explains the reasons why soft gelatin capsules are selected for formulation development, how they are formulated, and how they are manufactured.

DESCRIPTION OF THE SOFT GELATIN CAPSULE DOSAGE FORM (SOFTGELS)

Softgels consist of a liquid or semisolid matrix inside a one-piece outer gelatin shell (Fig. 30.1). Ingredients that are solid at room temperature can also be encapsulated into softgels, provided they are at least semisolid below approximately 45°C. The drug compound itself may be either in solution or in suspension in the capsule-fill matrix. The characteristics of the fill matrix may be hydrophilic (for example polyethylene glycols) or lipophilic (such as triglyceride vegetable oils). Indeed, in many formulations, the matrix may be a mixture of both hydrophilic and lipophilic ingredients.

Significant advances have been made in recent years in the formulation of softgel fill matrices (Fig. 30.1). These include microemulsions and nanoemulsions encapsulated as preconcentrates in softgels. The term 'preconcentrate' means that the softgel fill matrix is a combination of lipophilic and hydrophilic liquids as well as surfactant components, which after oral administration disperse to form, for example, a microemulsion. If the dispersion results in even smaller droplets in the nanoparticle range, then the dispersion is known as a nanoemulsion.

The softgel capsule shell consists of gelatin, water and a plasticizer. It may be transparent or opaque, and can be coloured and flavoured if desired. Preservatives are not required owing to the low water activity in the finished product. The softgel can be coated with enteric-resistant or delayed-release material. Although virtually any shape softgel can be made, oval or oblong shapes are usually selected for oral administration.

Softgels can be formulated and manufactured to produce a number of different drug delivery systems:

- Orally administered softgels containing solutions or suspensions that release their contents in the stomach in an easy to swallow, convenient unit dose form (Fig. 30.2). This is the most common type of softgel, already described above;
- Chewable softgels, where a highly flavoured shell is chewed to release the drug liquid fill matrix. The drug(s) may be present in both the shell and the fill matrix;
- Suckable softgels, which consist of a gelatin shell containing the flavoured medicament to be sucked and a liquid matrix or just air inside the capsule;
- Twist-off softgels, which are designed with a tag to be twisted or snipped off, thereby allowing access to the fill material. This type of softgel can be very useful for unit dosing of topical

Fig. 30.2 Swallowable softgel capsules.

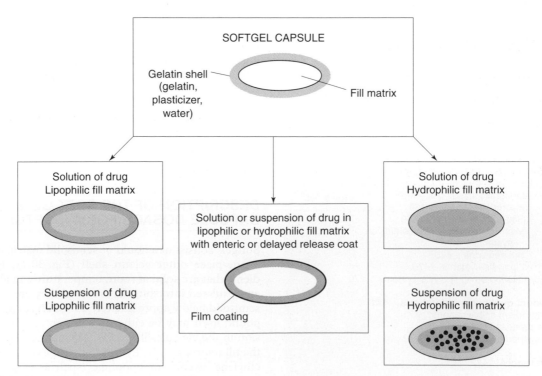

Fig. 30.1 Schematic diagram of different softgel formulations.

Fig. 30.3 Twist-off softgel capsules.

medication, inhalations, or indeed for oral dosing of a paediatric product (Fig. 30.3);

- Meltable softgels, designed for use as 'patient-friendly' pessaries or suppositories.

RATIONALE FOR THE SELECTION OF SOFTGELS AS A DOSAGE FORM

There are a number of reasons why softgels may be selected as the most suitable dosage form. These are summarized in Table 30.1. In the majority of cases improved drug absorption is the primary reason (Ferdinando 2000). However, the other features listed should also be remembered because, either individually or collectively, they are important factors that determine the selection of this drug delivery system.

Improved drug absorption

Increased rate of absorption

Major advances have been made in the development of softgel formulations to address particular drug absorption issues. One of the best methods is

presentation of the drug to the gastrointestinal tract in the form of a solution from which it can be rapidly absorbed. This can be achieved using a drug–solution matrix in a softgel formulation whereby absorption is significantly faster than from other solid oral dosage forms, such as compressed tablets. This is because absorption of a poorly soluble drug from a tablet formulation is rate-limited by the need for disintegration into granules, then drug dissolution into gastrointestinal fluid. With the solution–softgel approach, the shell ruptures within minutes to release the drug solution, which is usually in a hydrophilic or highly dispersing vehicle that aids the rate of absorption. This may be a valuable attribute (a) for therapeutic reasons, such as the treatment of migraine or acute pain, or (b) where there is a limited absorptive region or 'absorption window' in the gastrointestinal tract. Figure 30.4 shows the faster absorption that can

Fig. 30.4 Pharmacokinetic evaluation of softgels and tablets containing 400 mg ibuprofen (in 12 volunteers) (Saano 1991).

Table 30.1 Summary of the key features and advantages of the softgel dose form	
Features	Advantages
Improved drug absorption	Improved rate and extent of absorption and/or reduced variability, mainly for poorly water-soluble drugs
Patient compliance and consumer preference	Easy to swallow. Absence of poor taste or other sensory problem. Convenient administration of a liquid-drug dosage form
Safety – potent and cytotoxic drugs	Avoids dust handling problems during dosage form manufacture: better operator safety and environmental controls
Oils and low melting-point drugs	Overcomes problems with manufacture as compressed tablet or hard-shell capsules
Dose uniformity for low-dose drugs	Liquid flow during dosage form manufacture is more precise than powder flow. Drug solutions provide improved homogeneity over powder or granule mixtures
Product stability	Drugs are protected against oxidative degradation by lipid vehicles and softgel capsule shells

be achieved using a solution–softgel formulation compared to a tablet.

Increased bioavailability

As well as increasing the rate of absorption, softgels may also improve the extent of absorption. This can be particularly effective for hydrophobic drugs with a relatively high molecular weight. An example of such a product is the protease inhibitor saquinavir, which has been formulated as a solution–softgel product (Perry and Noble 1988). The solution–softgel formulation provided around three times the bioavailability of saquinavir as measured by the area under the plasma–time curve (AUC), compared to a hard-shell capsule formulation.

In some cases a drug may be solubilized in a vehicle that is capable of spontaneously dispersing into an emulsion on contact with gastrointestinal fluid. This is known as a self-emulsifying system. In other cases a drug may be dissolved in an oil/ surfactant vehicle that produces a microemulsion or a nanoemulsion on contact with gastrointestinal fluids. A nanoemulsion of progesterone has been developed that provides a good example of this type of formulation. The vehicle, consisting of oils and surfactants in appropriate proportions, when in contact with aqueous fluids, produces an emulsion with an average droplet size less than 100 nm. The solubility of the drug is maintained as long as possible, delivering solubilized drug directly to the enterocyte membrane. This produces increased bioavailability compared to formulations where the drug is dosed in the solid state. Figure 30.5 shows the plasma concentration–time profile for progesterone absorbed from the nanoemulsion formulation.

Softgel formulations may contain excipients, for example one or more surfactants which can aid the stability, wettability or even permeability of the drug (Aungst 2000).

Decreased plasma variability

High variability in drug plasma levels is a common characteristic of drugs with limited bioavailability. By dosing drug optimally in solution, the plasma level variability of such drugs can be significantly reduced. The cyclic polypeptide drug cyclosporine (Sandimmun Neoral®) benefits from such an approach by using a microemulsion preconcentrate in a softgel (Drewe et al 1992, Meinzer 2000).

Patient compliance and consumer preference

A number of self-medicating consumer preference studies have been carried out in an attempt to gauge the relative perception of softgels compared to hard-shell capsules and tablets. The results showed consistently that softgels were perceived to be appealing dosage forms to most consumers, and outperformed all other dosage forms in answering patient needs. Consumers expressed their preference for softgels in terms of (a) ease of swallowing, (b) absence of taste and (c) convenience.

One further aspect of improved compliance is that if, by using a drug solution in a softgel delivery system, its bioavailability is enhanced, it may be possible to reduce the dose administered in order to achieve therapeutic effectiveness. In this way it may also be possible to reduce the capsule size, which will further improve patient compliance.

Fig. 30.5 Pharmacokinetic evaluation of progesterone comparing a softgel nanoemulsion solution of progesterone with a softgel containing a suspension of the drug in an oil following single-dose administration in 12 healthy human volunteers (Ferdinando 2000).

Safety for potent and cytotoxic drugs

The mixing, granulation and compression/filling processes used in preparing tablets and hard-shell capsules can generate a significant quantity of air-borne powders. This can be of great concern for highly potent or cytotoxic compounds in terms of the operator and environmental protection required for satisfactorily safe product manufacture.

By preparing a solution or suspension of drug, where the active component is essentially protected from the environment by the liquid, such safety concerns can be significantly reduced.

Oils and low melting-point drugs

When the pharmaceutical active is an oily liquid, has a melting point less than about 75°C or proves difficult to compress, liquid filling of softgels is an obvious approach to presenting a solid oral dosage form. If the drug is an oily liquid, then it can be encapsulated directly into a softgel without adding a further diluent. Other low melting-point drugs may be formulated with a diluent oil in order to ensure satisfactory liquid flow and dosing into softgels.

Dose uniformity of low-dose drugs

In pharmaceutical manufacture liquid dosing avoids the difficulties of poor powder flow and therefore poor content uniformity. This is an important benefit for formulations containing drug doses in the microgram region. Attempts to produce adequate mixtures of small quantities of a low-dose drug in larger quantities of powdered excipients for tabletting or hard-shell filling are often unsatisfactory. In contrast, improved homogeneity is achieved by dissolving the drug in a liquid and then encapsulating the liquid matrix in a softgel.

Product stability

If a drug is subject to oxidative or hydrolytic degradation, the preparation of a liquid-filled softgel may prove beneficial. The liquid is prepared and encapsulated under a protective nitrogen atmosphere and the subsequently dried shell has very low oxygen permeability. By formulating in a lipophilic vehicle and packaging in well designed blister packs using materials of low moisture transmission, the drug can be protected from moisture. Conversely, it is well accepted that, in a solution, the drug may be more reactive than in the dry state and therefore potentially less stable. The appropriate choice of excipients, an understanding of the drug degradation pathways and appropriate preformulation studies are vital to achieving a stable product.

MANUFACTURE OF SOFTGELS

Softgel capsules were used in the 19th century as a means of administering bitter-tasting or liquid medicines. These were manufactured individually by preparing a small sack of gelatin and allowing it to set. Each sack, or gelatin shell, was then filled with the medication and heat-sealed. This method of manufacture was improved using a process that involved sealing two sheets of gelatin film between a pair of matching flat brass dies. Each die contained pockets into which the gelatin sheet was pressed and into which the medication was filled. The pressure between the two plates enabled individual capsules to be cut out from the die mould, and these capsules were subsequently dried.

However, it was not until the invention of the rotary die encapsulation machine by Robert Pauli Scherer in 1933 that liquid-fill capsules could be manufactured on a production scale. The rotary die process involves the continuous formation of a heat seal between two ribbons of gelatin, simultaneous with dosing of the fill liquid into each capsule. Although the speed and efficiency of the manufacturing process have improved greatly in recent years, the basic manufacturing principle remains essentially unchanged. The overall layout of a soft gelatin encapsulation machine is shown in Figure 30.6.

Before the encapsulation process takes place, there are two subprocesses that are often carried out simultaneously, yielding the two components of a softgel. These are (a) the gel mass which will provide the softgel shell, and (b) the fill matrix for the contents.

The gel mass is prepared by dissolving the gelatin in water at approximately 80°C and under vacuum, followed by the addition of the plasticizer, for example glycerol. Once the gelatin is fully dissolved then other components, such as colours, opacifier, flavours and preservatives, may be added. The hot gel mass is then supplied to the encapsulation machine through heated transfer pipes by a casting method that forms two separate gelatin ribbons, each approximately 150 mm wide. During the casting process the gelatin passes through the sol–gel transition and the thickness of each gel ribbon is controlled to ± 0.1 mm, in the range of about 0.5–1.5 mm. The thickness is checked regularly during the manufacturing process.

Fig. 30.6 Diagram of a soft gelatin encapsulation machine.

The two gel ribbons are then carried through rollers (at which a small quantity of vegetable oil lubricant is applied) and onwards to the rotary die encapsulation tooling (Fig. 30.7). Each ribbon provides one half of the softgel. It is possible to make bicoloured softgels using gel ribbons of two different colours.

Fig. 30.7 Detail of a soft gelatin encapsulation machine.

The liquid fill matrix containing the active drug substance is manufactured separately from preparation of the molten gel. Manufacture of the active fill matrix involves dispersing or dissolving the drug substance in the non-aqueous liquid vehicle using conventional mixer–homogenizers.

A number of different parameters are controlled during the preparation of the active fill matrix, depending on the properties of the drug substance. For example, oxygen-sensitive drugs are protected by mixing under vacuum and/or inert gas; and in some cases an antioxidant component may be added to the formulation. Also, if the drug substance is present as a suspension in the liquid fill matrix then it is important to ensure that particle size of the drug does not exceed approximately 200 μm. By doing this it is possible to ensure that drug particles do not become trapped within the capsule seal, potentially leading to loss of integrity of the softgel.

Rotary die encapsulation is the process by which the gel ribbon and the unit dose of liquid fill matrix are combined to form the softgel. The process involves careful control of three parameters:

1. Temperature. This controls the heat available for capsule seal formation.
2. Timing. The timing of the dosing of unit quantities of fill matrix into the softgel during its formation is critical.
3. Pressure. The pressure exerted between the two rotary dies controls the softgel shape and the final cut-out from the gel ribbon.

Figure 30.8 is a simplified diagram representing the mechanism of softgel formation using contrarotating dies and the wedge-shaped fill-matrix injection system.

Accurately metered volumes of the liquid fill matrix are injected from the wedge device into the space between the gelatin ribbons as they pass between the die rolls. The wedge-shaped injection system is itself heated to approximately 40°C. The injection of liquid between the ribbons forces the gel to expand into the pockets of the dies, which govern the size and shape of the softgels. The ribbon continues to flow past the heated wedge injection system and is then pressed between the die rolls. Here the two softgel capsule halves are sealed together by the application of heat and pressure. The capsules are cut automatically from the gel ribbon by raised rims around each die on the rollers.

After manufacture the capsules are passed through a tumble drier and then, to complete the drying process, spread on to trays and stacked in a tunnel drier that supplies air at 20% relative humidity. The tunnel drying process may take 2 or 3 days, or possibly as long as 2 weeks, depending on the specific softgel formulation. Finally, the softgels are inspected and packed into bulk containers in order to prevent further drying and for storage.

FORMULATION OF SOFTGELS

Gelatin shell formulation

Typical softgel shells are made up of gelatin, plasticizer, and materials that impart the desired appearance (colourants and/or opacifiers), and sometimes flavours. The following sections describe each of these materials, their functions, types, and amounts most often used in manufacturing softgel shells.

Gelatin

A large number of different gelatin shell formulations are available, depending on the nature of the liquid fill matrix. Most commonly the gelatin is alkali- (or base-) processed (type B) and it normally constitutes 40% of the wet molten gel mass. Type A acid-processed gelatin can also be used.

Plasticizers

Plasticizers are used to make the softgel shell elastic and pliable. They usually account for 20–30% of the wet gel formulation. The most common plasticizer used in softgels is glycerol, although sorbitol and propylene glycol are also frequently used, often in combination with glycerol. The amount and choice of the plasticizer contribute to the hardness of the final product and may even affect its dissolution or disintegration characteristics, as well as its physical and chemical stability. Plasticizers are selected on

Fig. 30.8 Softgel formation mechanism.

the basis of their compatibility with the fill formulation, ease of processing, and the desired properties of the final softgel, including hardness, appearance, handling characteristics and physical stability.

One of the most important aspect of softgel formulation is to ensure that there is minimum interaction or migration between the liquid fill matrix and the softgel shell. The choice of plasticizer type and concentration is important in ensuring optimum compatibility of the shell with the liquid fill matrix.

Water

The other essential component of the softgel shell is water. Water usually accounts for 30–40% of the wet gel formulation and its presence is important to ensure proper processing during gel preparation and softgel encapsulation. Following encapsulation, excess water is removed from the softgels through controlled drying. In dry softgels the equilibrium water content is typically in the range 5–8% w/w, which represents the proportion of water that is bound to the gelatin in the softgel shell. This level of water is important for good physical stability, because in harsh storage conditions softgels will become either too soft and fuse together, or too hard and embrittled.

Colourants/opacifiers

Colourants (soluble dyes, or insoluble pigments or lakes) and opacifiers are typically used at low concentrations in the wet gel formulation. Colourants can be either synthetic or natural, and are used to impart the desired shell colour for product identification. An opacifier, usually titanium dioxide, may be added to produce an opaque shell when the fill formulation is a suspension, or to prevent photodegradation of light-sensitive fill ingredients. Titanium dioxide can either be used alone to produce a white opaque shell or in combination with pigments to produce a coloured opaque shell.

Properties of soft gelatin shells

Oxygen permeability

The gelatin shell of a softgel capsule provides a good barrier against the diffusion of oxygen into its contents. The quantity of oxygen (*q*) that passes through the gelatin is governed by the area (*A*), thickness (*h*), particle pressure difference ($p_1 - p_2$), time of diffusion (*t*) and the permeability coefficient (*P*) of the shell by the following equation:

$$q = \frac{PAt\,(p_1 - p_2)}{h} \tag{30.1}$$

The permeability coefficient (*P*) is related to the diffusion coefficient (*D*) and the solubility coefficient (*S*) by the equation $P = DS$. This relationship, described by Henry's Law, assumes no interaction between the gas and the polymeric film, but *P* is clearly affected by the formulation of the gelatin shell, as shown in Figure 30.9.

Figure 30.9 shows the relationship between oxygen permeability coefficient and the glycerol concentration in the gelatin shell of softgels at room temperature and relative humidity values from 31 to 80%. The oxygen permeability decreases with the % RH and the glycerol content in the gelatin shell formulation. For maximum protection against the ingress of oxygen, the gelatin shell should be dry and formulated to contain about 30–40% glycerol.

Residual water content

Softgels contain little residual water, and compounds which are susceptible to hydrolysis are protected if dissolved or dispersed in an oily liquid fill material and encapsulated as a soft gelatin capsule. Figure 30.10 shows the relationship between the equilibrium water content and the concentration of glycerol in the gelatin shell of a softgel capsule, stored at room temperature and environmental relative humidities of between 31 and 80%. The data show, for example, that the minimum water values are found at glycerol levels in the shell of

Fig. 30.9 Relationship between oxygen permeability coefficient and the glycerol concentration in the shell of softgels at room temperature and a range of relative humidity values. From Hom, F.S., Veresh, S.A. and Ebert, W.R. (1975) *J. Pharm. Sci.*, **64(5)**, 851–857.

Fig. 30.10 The relationship between equilibrium water content and the concentration of glycerol in the shell of soft gelatin capsules at room temperature and a range of relative humidity values. (See Hom et al (1975), as Fig. 30.9.)

between 30 and 40%. Such a formulation dried at 31% relative humidity has a water content in the shell of about 7% and a water content in the fill in equilibrium with the atmosphere. The residual water content of most pharmaceutical compounds stored at 20% relative humidity (the drying condition for softgels) is low, and the water levels in the fills of softgels are therefore very small.

Formulation of softgel fill materials

In terms of formulation requirements, the softgel should be considered as a biphasic dosage form: a solid-phase capsule shell and a liquid-phase fill matrix. Although it is possible to incorporate a drug in the shell of a softgel, the overwhelming majority of products have the active ingredient(s) within the fill matrix. The liquid-phase fill matrix is selected from components with a wide range of different physicochemical properties. The choice of components is made according to one or more of a number of criteria, including the following:

- Capacity to dissolve the drug;
- Rate of dispersion in the gastrointestinal tract after the softgel shell ruptures and releases the fill matrix;
- Capacity to retain the drug in solution in the gastrointestinal fluid;
- Compatibility with the softgel shell;
- Ability to optimize the rate, extent and consistency of drug absorbed.

Types of softgel fill matrices

Lipophilic liquids/oils Triglyceride oils, such as soya bean oil, are commonly used in softgels. When used alone, however, their capacity to dissolve drugs is limited. Nevertheless, active ingredients such as hydroxycholecalciferol and other vitamin D analogues, plus steroids such as oestradiol, can be formulated into simple oily solutions for encapsulation in softgels.

Hydrophilic liquids Polar liquids with a sufficiently high molecular weight are commonly used. Polyethylene glycol (PEG) is the most frequently used, for example PEG 400, which has an average molecular weight of approximately 400 Da. Smaller hydrophilic molecules, such as ethanol or indeed water, can be incorporated in the softgel fill matrix in low levels, typically below 10% by weight.

Self-emulsifying oils A combination of a pharmaceutical oil and a non-ionic surfactant such as polyoxyethylene sorbitan mono-oleate can provide an oily formulation which disperses rapidly in the gastrointestinal fluid. The resulting oil/surfactant droplets enable rapid transfer of the drug to the absorbing mucosa and subsequent drug absorption.

Microemulsion and nanoemulsion systems A microemulsion of a lipid-surfactant–polar liquid system is characterized by its translucent single-phase appearance. The droplet size is in the submicrometre range, and light scattering by these droplets results in a faint blue colouration known as the Tyndall effect.

A nanoemulsion is a similar system but contains emulsion droplets in the 100 nm size range. Microemulsion and nanoemulsion systems have the advantage of a high capacity to solubilize drug compounds and to retain the drug in solution even after dilution in gastrointestinal fluids.

In order to produce a microemulsion or nanoemulsion in the gastrointestinal tract a 'preconcentrate' is formulated in the softgel fill matrix. In other words, the preconcentrate fill matrix contains a lipid component and one or more surfactants, which

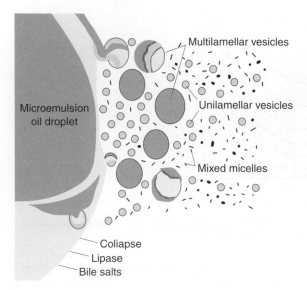

Fig. 30.11 Diagram of proposed nanoemulsion/microemulsion dissolution mechanism.

spontaneously form a microemulsion or a nano-emulsion on dilution in an aqueous environment, such as in gastrointestinal fluid (Fig. 30.11). The resulting microemulsion or nanoemulsion is often stable for prolonged periods.

Suspensions   Drugs that are insoluble in softgel fill matrices are formulated as suspensions. The continuous phase may be any of the vehicles described above. Suspension formulations provide significant advantages for certain low-solubility drugs which are very poorly absorbed after oral administration. With the appropriate choice of excipients, softgel suspensions can have improved bioavailability compared to compressed tablets or hard-shell capsules, or even dilute aqueous solutions.

Lipolysis systems   The advantage of the microemulsion approach lies in the high surface area presented by the microemulsion particles, which are essentially surfactant micelles swollen with solubilized oil and drug. This high surface area facilitates the rapid diffusion of drug from the dispersed oil phase into the aqueous intestinal fluids, until an equilibrium distribution is established. Thereafter, as drug is removed from the intestinal fluids via enterocyte absorption, it is quickly replenished by the flow of fresh material from the microemulsion particles.

Formulation using the lipolysis systems

In addition to promoting the solubility of drug compounds, lipid formulations can also facilitate dissolu-tion by taking advantage of lipolysis. This is because the lipid components of a softgel fill matrix, which comprise triglycerides or a partial (mono-/di-) glyc-eride, are often subject to intestinal fat digestion or lipolysis. Lipolysis is the term used to describe the action of the enzyme pancreatic lipase on triglycerides and partial glycerides, to form 2-monoglycerides and fatty acids. These 2-monoglycerides and fatty acids, known as lipolytic products, then interact with bile salts to form small droplets, or vesicles. These vesicles are broken down into smaller and smaller vesicles, ultimately resulting in the formation of mixed micelles that are approximately 3–10 nm in size.

If a drug compound possesses higher solubility in lipolytic products than in triglyceride oils, then it is advantageous for lipolysis to occur in the intestinal lumen. In this way, the process of lipolysis promotes the formation of an excellent dissolution medium for the drug, namely lipolytic products. On the other hand, the absorption of a drug compound may be adversely affected by the presence of bile salt, and in such a case it may be advantageous for lipolysis to be reduced or blocked completely. It has been found that certain hydrophilic and lipophilic surfactants have the ability to block or promote lipolysis respec-tively (MacGregor et al 1997). These hydrophilic and lipophilic surfactants are often used in softgel fill matrix formulations.

It is possible to measure the rate and extent of lipolysis for a softgel fill matrix formulation. This is done by an in vitro pH stat measurement technique. The experimental conditions for this model are as shown in Table 30.2.

In this model, lipolysis is quantified by the amount of free fatty acids liberated by enzymatic digestion of the lipids in the softgel fill matrix. The quantity of 1.0 M sodium hydroxide titrant is directly propor-tional to the extent of lipolysis.

The mixed intestinal micelles produced as a result of this lipolysis process are physiologically important

---

Table 30.2   An in vitro lipolysis model

- 100 mL pH 6.5 *tris*-maleate buffer at 37°C

- 2.4 % w/w triglyceride oil in a softgel fill matrix formulation

- 20 TBUs* per mL of porcine pancreatic lipase–colipase

  * 1 TBU (tributyrin unit) = 1 μmol butyric acid per minute

- 8 mM bile salt (sodium taurocholate)

- 1.5 mM lecithin, 5 mM $CaCl_2 \cdot 2H_2O$, 150 mM NaCl

- pH maintained at 6.5 using I.0 M NaOH via continuous titration (pH-stat) because they can transport high concentrations of hydrophobic molecules across the aqueous boundary layer that separates the absorptive membrane from the intestinal lumen. Thus, lipolytic products (e.g. fatty acids and monoglycerides) – and hydrophobic drug, if present – reside in the hydrophobic core regions of mixed intestinal micelles. In contrast, the surface of the micelles remains hydrophilic and this facilitates rapid micellar diffusion across the aqueous boundary layer to the intestinal membrane. In the microclimate adjacent to the intestinal membrane the pH is lower than in the intestinal lumen. This promotes demicellization, leading to the formation of a supersaturated solution of lipolytic products (and hydrophobic drug, if present) in close proximity to the enterocyte surface. These materials are then readily absorbed across the cell membrane by passive diffusion.

Mixed intestinal micelles comprising bile salts and lipolytic products can enhance the bioavailability of hydrophobic drugs whose absorption is normally dissolution-rate limited. This is because mixed intestinal micelles can be very potent solubilizing agents for a wide range of hydrophobic drugs, much more so than simple bile salt micelles formed in the absence of lipolytic products. For example, under simulated physiological conditions the aqueous solubility of cinnarizine in simple bile salt micelles is $4 \mu g/mL$, compared to $0.5 \mu g/mL$ in aqueous buffer. However, in the presence of mixed micelles the solubility of cinnarizine is further enhanced to approximately $44 \mu g/mL$ (Embleton et al 1995).

Taking cinnarizine as an example, it would be advantageous to formulate a softgel fill matrix that allows lipolysis to occur in the intestinal lumen because of the high drug solubility in lipolytic products. If the inhibition by a hydrophobic surfactant were allowed to occur, then it is highly likely that cinnarizine absorption would be impaired because of the reduced flow of drug into mixed micelles. However, if certain lipophilic surfactants, with a HLB less than 10, are added to the formulation, then the inhibitory effects of hydrophilic surfactants on lipolysis can be reduced or eliminated.

Two formulations containing cinnarizine, a hydrophobic drug whose absorption is normally dissolution-rate limited, have been compared (Embleton et al 1995). Formulation [A] was prepared as a lipolysing formulation and [B] as a non-lipolysing formulation, as demonstrated by the in vitro model. Formulation [A] was composed of a digestible triglyceride oil, a hydrophilic surfactant and a lipophilic surfactant, which was chosen for its ability to overcome the inhibitory effects of the hydrophilic surfactant on the in vitro triglyceride lipolysis. In vitro this formulation exhibited 79% lipolysis after 60 minutes, compared to the digestible oil alone. In contrast, the non-lipolysing formulation contained a lipophilic surfactant that did not overcome the inhibitory effects of the hydrophilic surfactant on the lipolysis of the triglyceride oil, and was shown to lipolyse to an extent of only 3%. It is proposed that the oil in formulation [A], which forms a fine oil-in-water emulsion on aqueous dilution, is rapidly digested, forming mixed intestinal micelles with endogenous bile. These micelles transport the drug to the intestinal membrane, where the pH of the microclimate promotes micellar breakdown, facilitating enterocyte transport to the systemic circulation. In contrast, on dilution with aqueous fluids, formulation [B] forms a translucent microemulsion (as indicated by a blue tinge resulting from the Tyndall effect). As a result of this formulation failing to lipolyse and thereby remaining unaffected by enzymic activity, the drug is maintained within the oil phase, inhibiting the production of mixed intestinal micelles and restricting drug absorption.

The significance of the lipolysis process in enhancing the bioavailability of hydrophobic drugs was investigated further with an in vivo study (Fig. 30.12). This compared the bioavailability of cinnarizine (30 mg) administered orally as the lipolysing formulation [A] and non-lipolysing formulation [B] with a commercially available tablet, formulation [C], to six beagle dogs. The AUC(0–24 h) for formulation [A] was significantly increased by 64% ($P < 0.01$) compared to the tablet preparation, and by 48% ($P < 0.001$) compared to formulation [B]. The C_{max} of formulation [A] was approximately 75% higher than both formulations [B], ($P < 0.001$) and [C] ($P < 0.01$).

The results of this study have given a valuable insight into the effect of microemulsion formulation on the absorption of a hydrophobic drug in the gastrointestinal tract, and new information as to how the lipolysis process may influence bioavailability (Lacy et al 2000).

PRODUCT QUALITY CONSIDERATIONS

Ingredient specifications

All of the ingredients of a softgel are controlled and tested to ensure compliance with pharmacopoeial specifications. However, additional specification tests may be added for certain excipients in order to ensure the manufacture of a high-quality softgel product. For example, it is important to limit certain trace impurities, such as aldehydes and peroxides

Fig. 30.12 Plasma concentration versus time curves for three formulations of cinnarizine in the dog (*n*=6) (Embleton 1995).

which may be present in polyethylene glycol. The presence of high levels of these impurities gives rise to cross-linking of the gelatin polymer, leading to insolubilization through further polymerization. On prolonged storage this can lead to slow dissolution of the capsule shell and subsequent retarded drug release.

The ingredient requiring the most careful control is gelatin itself. Once a particular grade of gelatin is used in a softgel formulation the quality is controlled using parameters such as the viscosity of a hot solution and the bloom strength of the gel (bloom strength is a measure of the hardness of a gel).

In-process testing

During the encapsulation process the four most important tests are:

- The gel ribbon thickness;
- Softgel seal thickness at the time of encapsulation;
- Fill matrix weight and capsule shell weight;
- Softgel shell moisture level and softgel hardness at the end of the drying stage.

Appropriate control levels for these parameters are established during process development for each softgel product, and are applied in routine production scale manufacture.

Finished product testing

Finished softgels are subjected to a number of tests in accordance with compendial requirements for unit dose capsule products. These normally include capsule appearance, active ingredient assay and related substances assay, as well as fill weight, content uniformity and microbiological testing.

REFERENCES

Aungst B.J. (2000) Mini Review Intestinal Permeation Enchancers. *J. Pharm. Sci.* **89(4)**: 429–442.

Drewe J., Meier R., Vonderscherer J., et al. (1992) Enhancement of the oral absorption of cyclosporin in man. *Br. J. Clin. Pharmacol.* **34**: 60–64.

Embleton J., Hutchison K.G., Lacy J., et al. (1995) The effect of in-vivo lipolysis in improving the bioavailability of orally administered cinnarizine in self-emulsifying oily vehicles. American Association of Pharmaceutical Sciences Conference, Miami Beach.

Ferdinando J.C. (2000) Formulation Solutions – Softgels. Manufacturing and Packaging; 69–73.

Lacy J.E., Embleton J.K., Perry E.A. (2000) Delivery systems for hydrophobic drugs: US Patent 6,096,338.

MacGregor K.J., Embleton J.K., Lacy J.E, et al. (1997) Influence of lipolysis on drug absorption from the gastrointestinal tract. *Advd Drug Del. Rev.* **25**: 33–46.

Meinzer A. (1993) Sandimmun Neoral Soft Gelatin Capsules. International Industrial Pharmaceutical Research Conference. Wisconsin USA.

Perry C.M., Noble S. (1998) Saquinavir Softgel Capsule Formulation. *Drugs* **55:(3)**.

Saano V., Paronen P., Peura P., et al. (1991) Relative pharmacokinetics of three oral 400 mg ibuprofen dosage forms in healthy volunteers. *Int. J. Clin. Pharmacol. Ther. Toxicol.* **29(10)**: 381–385.

31

Pulmonary drug delivery

Kevin Taylor

INHALED DRUG DELIVERY

Drugs are generally delivered to the respiratory tract for the treatment or prophylaxis of airways diseases, such as bronchial asthma and cystic fibrosis. The administration of a drug at its site of action can result in a rapid onset of activity, which may be highly desirable, for instance when delivering bronchodilating drugs for the treatment of asthma. Additionally, smaller doses can be administered locally compared to delivery by the oral or parenteral routes, thereby reducing the potential incidence of adverse systemic effects and reducing drug costs. The pulmonary route is also useful where a drug is poorly absorbed orally, e.g. sodium cromoglycate, or where it is rapidly metabolized orally, e.g. isoprenaline. The avoidance of first-pass metabolism in the liver may also be advantageous, although the lung itself has some metabolic capability.

The lung may be used as a route for delivering drugs having systemic activity, because of its large surface area, the abundance of capillaries and the thinness of the air–blood barrier. This has been exploited in the treatment of migraine with ergotamine, and studies have demonstrated the potential for delivering proteins and peptides such as insulin and growth hormone via the airways.

Lung anatomy

The lung is the organ of external respiration, in which oxygen and carbon dioxide are exchanged between blood and inhaled air. The structure of the airways also prevents the entry of and promotes efficient removal of airborne foreign particles, including microorganisms.

The respiratory tract can be considered as comprising conducting (central) regions (trachea, bronchi, bronchioles, terminal and respiratory bronchioles) and respiratory (peripheral) regions (respiratory bronchioles and alveolar regions), although there is no clear demarcation between them (Fig. 31.1). The upper respiratory tract comprises the nose, throat, pharynx and larynx; the lower tract comprises the trachea, bronchi, bronchioles and the alveolar regions. Simplistically, the airways can be described by a symmetrical model in which each airway divides into two equivalent branches or generations. In fact, the trachea (generation 0) branches into two main bronchi (generation 1), of which the right bronchus is wider and leaves the trachea at a smaller angle than the left, and hence is more likely to receive inhaled material. Further branching of the airways ultimately results in terminal bronchioles. These divide to produce respiratory bronchioles, which connect with alveolar ducts leading to the alveolar sacs (generation 23). These contain approximately $2-6 \times 10^8$ alveoli, producing a surface area of about 70–80 m^2 in an adult male.

The conducting airways are lined with ciliated epithelial cells. Insoluble particles deposited on the airways walls in this region are trapped by the mucus and swept upwards from the lungs by the beating cilia and swallowed.

Inhalation aerosols and the importance of size distribution

To deliver a drug into the airways it must be presented as an **aerosol**. In pharmacy this is defined as a two-phase system of solid particles or liquid droplets dispersed in air or other gaseous phase, having sufficiently small size to display considerable stability as a suspension.

The deposition of a drug/aerosol in the airways is dependent on four factors: the physicochemical properties of the drug, the formulation, the delivery/liberating device and the patient (breathing patterns and clinical status).

The most fundamentally important physical property of an aerosol for inhalation is its size. The particle size of an aerosol is usually standardized by calculation of its **aerodynamic diameter**, d_a, which is the physical diameter of a unit density sphere which settles through air with a velocity equal to the particle in question. Therapeutic aerosols are heterodispersed (polydispersed), and the distribution of sizes is generally represented by the geometric standard deviation (GSD or σ_g), when size is log-normally distributed.

For approximately spherical particles

$$d_a = d_p \times \sqrt{\rho/\rho_o} \qquad (31.1)$$

where d_p is physical diameter, ρ is particle density and ρ_o is unit density, i.e. 1 g/cm^3.

When d_p is the mass median diameter (MMD), d_a is termed the mass median aerodynamic diameter (MMAD).

The influence of environmental humidity on particle size

As a particle enters the respiratory tract, the change from ambient to high relative humidity (approximately 99%) results in condensation of water on to the particle surface, which continues until the vapour pressure of the water equals that of the surrounding atmosphere. For water-insoluble materials this results in a negligibly thin film of water; however, with water-soluble materials a solution is formed on the particle surface. As the vapour pressure of the solution is lower than that of pure solvent at the same temperature, water will continue to condense until an equilibrium between vapour pressures is reached, i.e. the particle will increase in size. The final equilibrium diameter reached is constrained by the Kelvin effect, i.e., the vapour pressure of a droplet solution is higher than that for a planar surface, and is a function of the particle's original diameter (Pritchard, 1987). Hygroscopic growth will affect the deposition of particles, resulting in deposition higher in the respiratory tract than would have been predicted from measurements of their initial size.

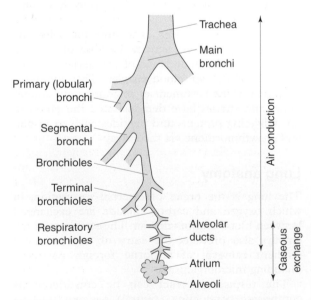

Fig. 31.1 Schematic representation of the human airways. (Reproduced with permission from Wilson and Washington 1989.)

Particle deposition in the airways

The efficacy of a clinical aerosol is dependent on its ability to penetrate the respiratory tract. To penetrate to the peripheral (respirable) regions, aerosols require a size less than about 5 or 6 μm, with less than 2 μm being preferable for alveolar deposition. Literature values for 'respirable' size vary and must be considered alongside the environmental changes in size described above and the heterodispersed nature of inhalation aerosol size distributions. Larger particles or droplets are deposited in the upper respiratory tract and are rapidly cleared from the lung by the mucociliary action, with the effect that drug becomes available for systemic absorption and may potentially cause adverse effects. Steroid aerosols of sufficiently large size may deposit in the mouth and throat, with the potential to cause oral candidiasis. The size of aerosolized drug may be especially important in the treatment of certain conditions where penetration to the peripheral airways is particularly desirable, for instance the treatment and prophylaxis of the alveolar infection *Pneumocystis carinii* pneumonia.

There are three main mechanisms responsible for particulate deposition in the lung: gravitational sedimentation, impaction and diffusion.

Gravitational sedimentation

From Stokes' law, particles settling under gravity will attain a constant terminal settling velocity, U_t:

$$U_t = \frac{\rho g d^2}{18\eta} \qquad (31.2)$$

where ρ is particle density, g is the gravitational constant, d is particle diameter and η is air viscosity.

Thus, gravitational sedimentation of an inhaled particle is dependent on its size and density, in addition to its residence time in the airways. Sedimentation is an important deposition mechanism for particles in the size range 0.5–3 μm, in the small airways and alveoli, for particles that have escaped deposition by impaction.

Inertial impaction

Where a bifurcation occurs in the respiratory tract, the airstream changes direction and particles within the airstream, having sufficiently high momentum, will impact on the airways' walls rather than follow the changing airstream. This deposition mechanism is particularly important for large particles having a diameter greater than 5 μm, and particularly greater than 10 μm, and is common in the upper airways,

being the principal mechanism for deposition in the nose, mouth, pharynx and larynx and the large conducting airways. With the continuous branching of the conducting airways, the velocity of the airstream decreases and impaction becomes a less important mechanism for deposition.

The probability of impaction is proportional to:

$$\frac{U_t U \sin\theta}{gr} \qquad (31.3)$$

where θ is the change in airways direction, U is airstream velocity and r is the airway's radius.

Brownian diffusion

Collision and bombardment of small particles by molecules in the respiratory tract produce Brownian motion. The resultant movement of particles from high to low concentrations causes them to move from the aerosol cloud to the airways walls. The rate of diffusion is inversely proportional to the particle size, and thus diffusion is the predominant mechanism for particles smaller than 0.5 μm.

Other methods of deposition

Although impaction, sedimentation and diffusion are the most important mechanisms for drug deposition in the respiratory tract, other mechanisms may occur. These include ***interception***, whereby particles having extreme shapes, such as fibres, physically catch on to the airways' walls as they pass through the respiratory tract, and ***electrostatic attraction***, whereby an electrostatic charge on a particle induces an opposing charge on the walls of the respiratory tract, resulting in attraction between particle and walls.

Different deposition mechanisms are important for differently sized particles. Those greater than 5 μm will deposit predominantly by inertial impaction in the upper airways. Particles sized between 1 and 5 μm deposit predominantly by gravitational sedimentation in the lower airways, especially during slow, deep breathing, and particles less than 1 μm deposit by Brownian diffusion in the stagnant air of the lower airways. Particles of approximately 0.5 μm are inefficiently deposited, being too large for effective deposition by Brownian diffusion and too small for effective impaction or sedimentation, and they are often immediately exhaled. This ***size of minimum deposition*** should thus be considered during formulation, although for the reasons of environmental humidity discussed previously, the equilibrium diameter in the airways may be significantly larger than the original particle size in the formulation.

Breathing patterns

Patient-dependent factors, such as breathing patterns and lung physiology, also affect particle deposition. For instance, the larger the inhaled volume the greater the peripheral distribution of particles in the lung, whereas increasing inhalation flow rate enhances deposition in the larger airways by inertial impaction. Breath-holding after inhalation enhances the deposition of particles by sedimentation and diffusion. Optimal aerosol deposition occurs with slow, deep inhalations to total lung capacity, followed by breath-holding prior to exhalation. It should be noted that changes in the airways resulting from disease states, for instance airways' obstruction, may affect the deposition profile of an inhaled aerosol.

Clearance of inhaled particles and drug absorption

Particles deposited in the ciliated conducting airways are cleared within 24 hours and ultimately swallowed. Insoluble particles penetrating to the alveolar regions, and which are not solubilized in situ, are removed more slowly. Alveolar macrophages engulf such particles and may then migrate to the bottom of the mucociliary escalator, or alternatively particles may be removed via the lymphatics.

Hydrophobic compounds are usually absorbed at a rate dependent on their oil/water partition coefficients, whereas hydrophilic materials are poorly absorbed through membrane pores at rates inversely proportional to molecular size. Thus, the airways' membrane, like the gastrointestinal tract, is preferably permeable to the unionized form of a drug. Some drugs, such as sodium cromoglycate, are partly absorbed by a saturable active transport mechanism. The rate of drug absorption, and consequently drug action, can be influenced by the formulation. Rapid drug action can generally be achieved using solutions or powders of aqueous soluble salts, whereas slower or prolonged absorption may be achieved using suspension formulations, powders of less soluble salts, or novel drug delivery systems such as liposomes and microspheres.

FORMULATING AND DELIVERING THERAPEUTIC INHALATION AEROSOLS

There are currently three main types of aerosol-generating device for use in inhaled drug therapy: metered-dose inhalers, dry powder inhalers and nebulizers.

Metered-dose inhalers

Metered-dose inhalers (MDIs), introduced in the mid-1950s, are the most commonly used inhalation drug delivery devices. In MDIs, drug is either dissolved or suspended in a liquid propellant mixture together with other excipients, including surfactants, and presented in a pressurized canister fitted with a metering valve (Fig. 31.2). A predetermined dose is released as a spray on actuation of the metering valve. When released from the canister the formulation undergoes volume expansion in the passage within the valve and forms a mixture of gas and liquid before discharge from the orifice. The high-speed gas flow helps to break up the liquid into a fine spray of droplets.

Containers

Pharmaceutical aerosols may be packaged in tin-plated steel, plastic-coated glass or aluminium containers. In practice, MDIs are generally presented in aluminium canisters, produced by extrusion to give seamless containers with a capacity of 10–30 mL. Aluminium is relatively inert and may be used uncoated where there is no chemical instability between container and contents. Alternatively, aluminium containers with an internal coating of a chemically resistant organic material, such as an epoxy resin, can be used.

Propellants

The propellants used in MDI formulations are liquefied gases, traditionally chlorofluorocarbons (CFCs) and increasingly hydrofluoroalkanes (HFAs). At room temperature and pressure these are gases, but they are readily liquefied by decreasing

Fig. 31.2 The metered-dose inhaler. (Reproduced with permission from Morén 1981.)

temperature or increasing pressure. The head space of the aerosol is filled with propellant vapour, producing the saturation vapour pressure at that temperature. On spraying, medicament and propellant are expelled and the head volume increases. To re-establish the equilibrium, more propellant evaporates and so a constant pressure system with consistent spray characteristics is produced. The CFCs currently employed in MDI formulations are trichlorofluoromethane (CFC-11), dichlorodifluoromethane (CFC-12) and dichlorotetrafluoroethane (CFC-114). Formulations generally comprise blends of CFC-11 and CFC-12 or CFC-11, CFC-12, and CFC-114 (Table 31.1.), together with a surfactant such as a sorbitan ester, oleic acid or lecithin, which acts as a suspending agent and lubricates the valve.

CFCs and HFAs are numbered using a universal system. The first digit is the number of carbon atoms minus 1 (omitted if zero), the second is the number of hydrogen atoms plus 1, and the third is the number of fluorine atoms. Chlorine fills any remaining valencies, given the total number of atoms required to saturate the compound. If asymmetry is possible, this is designated by a letter. The symmetrical isomer is assigned the number described above; of the asymmetrical isomers, that designated the letter a is the most symmetrical, b the next most symmetrical, and so on. The CFCs are perfectly miscible with each other and suitable blends give a useful intermediate vapour pressure, usually about 450 kPa. The vapour pressure of the mixture of propellants is given by Raoult's law, i.e. the vapour pressure of a mixed system is equal to the sum of the mole fraction of each component multiplied by its vapour pressure:

$$P = p_a + p_b \tag{31.4}$$

where P is the total vapour pressure of the system and p_a and p_b are the partial vapour pressures of the components, a and b:

$$p_a = x_a p_a^0 \tag{31.5}$$

$$p_b = x_b p_b^0 \tag{31.6}$$

where x_a and x_b are the mole fractions and p_a^0 and p_b^0 are the partial vapour pressures of components a and b, respectively.

The reaction of CFCs with the ozone in the earth's stratosphere, which absorbs ultraviolet radiation at 300 nm, and their contribution to global warming is a major environmental concern. CFCs pass to the stratosphere, where in the presence of UV they liberate chlorine, which reacts with ozone. The depletion of stratospheric ozone results in increased exposure to the UV-B part of the UV spectrum, resulting in a number of adverse effects, in particular an increased incidence of skin cancer. The Montreal Protocol of 1987 was a global ban on the production of the five worst ozone-depleting CFCs by the year 2000. This was amended in 1992, so that production of CFCs in developed countries was phased out by 1 January 1996. In the European Union, all ozone-depleting CFCs had been banned by the end of 1995. Pharmaceutical aerosols are currently exempted, but this exemption is reviewed annually. In household and cosmetic aerosols CFCs have been replaced by hydrocarbons such as propane and butane. Alternatively, compressed gases such as nitrogen dioxide, nitrogen and carbon dioxide may be used, for instance in food products. However, compressed gases do not maintain a constant pressure within the canister throughout its use, as the internal pressure is inversely proportionate to the head volume, and so product performance changes with age. For reasons of toxicity and inflammability, hydrocarbons are not considered appropriate alternatives to CFCs for inhalation products, and so non-ozone depleting alternatives to CFCs are being developed.

Propellants HFA-134a (trifluoromonofluoroethane) and HFA-227 (heptafluoropropane) are non-ozone depleting, non-flammable HFAs, also called hydrofluorocarbons (HFCs), which have been widely investigated as alternatives to CFC-12 (Table 31.2). However, these gases contribute to global warming and further replacements will no doubt be required in the future.

HFA-134a and HFA-227 have some physical properties, including density, which are similar to

Table 31.1	Formulae and physicochemical properties of chlorofluorocarbons (CFCs) used in MDI formulations			
Number	Formula	Boiling point (°C)	Vapour pressure (kPa at 20°C)	Density (g/mL at 20°C)
11	CCl_3F	23.7	89 (0.89 bar)	1.49
12	CCl_2F_2	−29.8	568 (5.68 bar)	1.33
114	$C_2Cl_2F_4$	3.6	183 (1.83 bar)	1.47

Table 31.2 Formulae and physicochemical properties of hydrofluoroalkanes (HFAs) used in MDI formulations

Number	Formula	Boiling point (°C)	Vapour pressure (kPa at 20°C)	Density (g/mL at 20°C)
134a	$C_2F_4H_2$	−26.5	660 (6.6 bar)	1.23
227	C_3F_7H	−17.3	398 (3.98 bar)	1.41

those of CFC-12 and, to a lesser extent, CFC-114. However, they present major formulation problems: in particular they are poor solvents for the surfactants commonly used in MDI formulation and no alternative to CFC-11 is currently available. Ethanol is approved for use in formulations containing HFAs to allow dissolution of surfactants, and is included in marketed non-CFC MDI products. However, ethanol has low volatility and may consequently increase the droplet size of the emitted aerosols.

Metering valve

The metering valve of an MDI permits the reproducible delivery of small volumes (25–100 μL) of product. Unlike the non-metering continuous-spray valves of conventional pressurized aerosols, the metering valve in MDIs are used in the inverted position (Fig. 31.3). Depression of the valve stem allows the contents of the metering chamber to be discharged through the orifice in the valve stem and made available to the patient. After actuation, the metering chamber refills with liquid from the bulk and is ready to dispense the next dose. A corollary of this is that the MDI needs to be primed, i.e. the metering chamber filled, prior to the first use by a patient. MDI valves are complex in design and must protect the product from the environment, while also protecting against product loss during repeated use. The introduction of HFA propellants with different solvent properties has necessitated the development of new valve elastomers. The valve stem fits into the actuator, which is made of polyethylene or polypropylene. The dimensions of the orifice in the actuator plays a crucial role, along with the propellant vapour pressure, in determining the shape and speed of the emitted aerosol plume.

Formulating metered-dose inhalers

Pressurized aerosols may be formulated as either solutions or suspensions of drug in the liquefied propellant. Solution preparations are two-phase systems. However, the propellants are poor solvents for most drugs. Cosolvents such as ethanol or isopropanol may be used, although their low volatility retards propellant evaporation. In practice, pressurized inhaler formulations have, until recently, been almost exclusively suspensions. These three-phase systems are harder to formulate and all the problems of conventional suspension formulation, such as caking, agglomeration, particle growth etc. must be considered. Careful consideration must be given to the particle size of the solid (usually micronized to between 2 and 5 μm), valve clogging, moisture content, the solubility of active compound in propellant (a salt may be desirable), the relative density of propellant and drug, and the use of surfactants as suspending agents, e.g. lecithin, oleic acid and sorbitan trioleate (usually included at concentrations between 0.1 and 2.0% w/w). These surfactants are very poorly soluble (<< 0.02% w/w) in HFAs, and so either ethanol must be used as a cosolvent or alternative surfactants such as fluorinated polymers must be developed (Byron et al 1994). Recently solution formulations of beclomethasone dipropionate have been marketed. Evaporation of HFA propellant following actuation of these formulations results in smaller particle sizes than with conventional suspension formulations of the same drug, with consequent changes in its pulmonary distribution and bioavailability.

Blind end

Metering chamber

Opening for emptying of metering chamber

Valve stem

Opening to actuator seat

Fig. 31.3 The metering valve. (Reproduced with permission from Morén 1981.)

Filling metered-dose inhaler canisters

Canisters are filled by liquefying the propellant at reduced temperature or elevated pressure.

In *cold filling*, active compound, excipients and propellant are chilled and filled at about −30°C. Additional propellant is then added at the same temperature and the canister sealed with the valve. In *pressure filling*, a drug/propellant (CFC-11) concentrate is produced and filled at effectively room temperature and pressure (in fact, usually slightly chilled to below 20°C). The valve is crimped on to the canister and additional propellant (e.g. CFC-12) is filled at elevated pressure through the valve, in a process known as gassing. Pressure filling is most frequently employed for inhalation aerosols. However, no ozone-sparing replacement propellant has the properties (high boiling point: 23.7°C) of CFC-11, which is a major problem for the pharmaceutical industry.

Once filled, the canisters are leak tested by placing them in a water bath at elevated temperature, usually 50–60°C. Following storage to allow equilibration of the formulation and valve components, the containers are weighed to check for further leakage, prior to spray testing and insertion into actuators.

Advantages and disadvantages of metered-dose inhalers

The major advantages of MDIs are their portability, low cost and disposability. Many doses (up to 200) are stored in the small canister and dose delivery is reproducible. The inert conditions created by the propellant vapour, together with the hermetically sealed container, protects drugs from oxidative degradation and microbiological contamination. However, MDIs have disadvantages. They are inefficient at drug delivery. On actuation, the first propellant droplets exit at a high velocity, which may exceed 30 m/s. Consequently, much of the drug is lost through impaction of these droplets in the oropharyngeal areas. The mean emitted droplet size typically exceeds 40 μm, and propellants may not evaporate sufficiently rapidly for their size to decrease to that suitable for deep lung deposition. Vaporization of the droplets is hindered by the low volatility of CFC-11, which is present in concentrations of at least 25% in most CFC-based formulations. Evaporation, such that the aerodynamic diameter of the particles is close to that of the original micronized drug, may not occur until 5 seconds after actuation.

An additional problem with MDIs, which is beyond the control of the formulator and manufacturer, is their incorrect use by patients. Reported problems include:

- Failure to remove the protective cap covering the mouthpiece, the inhaler being used inverted;
- Failure to shake the canister;
- Failure to inhale slowly and deeply;
- Inadequate breath-holding;
- Poor inhalation/actuation synchronization.

Correct use by patients is vital for effective drug deposition and action. Ideally, the MDI should be actuated during the course of slow, deep inhalation, followed by a period of breath-holding. Many patients find this difficult, especially children and the elderly. The misuse of MDIs through poor inhalation/actuation coordination can be significantly reduced with appropriate instruction and counselling. However, it should be noted that even using the correct inhalation technique only 10–20% of the stated emitted dose is delivered to the site of action.

Spacers and breath-actuated metered-dose inhalers

Some of the disadvantages of MDIs, namely inhalation/actuation coordination and the premature deposition of large propellant droplets high in the airways, can be overcome by using extension devices or 'spacers' positioned between the MDI and the patient (Fig. 31.4). The dose from an MDI is discharged directly into the reservoir prior to inhalation. This reduces the initial droplet velocity, permits efficient propellant evaporation and removes the need for actuation/inhalation coordination. The disadvantage of spacers is that they may be cumbersome, e.g. Fisonair (Rhône-Poulenc Rorer), Nebuhaler (AstraZeneca), and Volumatic (Glaxo SmithKline). Alternatively, extension tubes may be built into the design of the MDI itself, e.g. Syncroner (Rhône-Poulenc Rorer) and Spacer Inhalers (AstraZeneca). The Autohaler (3M) is an MDI with

Fig. 31.4 The Nebuhaler spacer device, fitted with a face mask for use by a child. Courtesy of AstraZeneca.

an inspiratory demand valve. This breath-actuated device overcomes the coordination problems of a conventional MDI without adding bulk to the device. However, a substantial inspiratory flow rate is required for its operation.

Dry powder inhalers

In dry powder inhaler (DPI) systems, drug is inhaled as cloud of fine particles. The drug is either preloaded in an inhalation device or filled into hard gelatin capsules or foil blister discs which are loaded into a device prior to use. DPIs have several advantages over MDIs. DPI formulations are propellant free and do not contain any excipient, other than a carrier (see below) – which is almost invariably lactose. They are breath actuated, avoiding the problems of inhalation/actuation coordination encountered with MDIs, and consequently they are particularly useful for young children. DPIs can also deliver larger drug doses than MDIs, which are limited by the volume of the metering valve and the maximum suspension concentration that can be employed without causing valve clogging. However, DPIs have several disadvantages. Liberation of powders from the device and the deaggregation of particles are limited by the patient's ability to inhale, which in the case of respiratory disease may be impaired. An increase in turbulent air flow created by an increase in inhaled air velocity increases the deaggregation of the emerging particles, but also increases the potential for inertial impaction in the upper airways and throat, and so a compromise has to be found. Further, DPIs are exposed to ambient atmospheric conditions, which may reduce formulation stability. For instance, elevated humidity may cause powders to clump. Finally, DPIs are generally less efficient at drug delivery than MDIs, such that twice the dose is usually required for delivery from a DPI than from the equivalent MDI (Melchor et al 1993).

Formulating dry powder inhalers

To produce particles of a suitable size (preferably less than 5 μm), drug powders for use in inhalation systems are usually micronized. The high-energy powders produced have poor flow properties because of their static, cohesive and adhesive nature. The flowability of a powder is affected by physical properties, including particle size and shape, density, surface roughness, hardness, moisture content and bulk density.

To improve their flow properties, poorly flowing drug particles are generally mixed with larger 'carrier' particles (usually 30–60 μm) of an inert excipient, usually lactose. This not only improves liberation of the drug from the inhalation device by improving powder flow, but also improves the uniformity of capsule or device filling. Once liberated from the device, the turbulent air flow generated within the inhalation device should be sufficient for the deaggregation of the drug/carrier aggregates. The larger carrier particles impact in the throat, whereas smaller drug particles are carried in the inhaled air deeper into the respiratory tract.

The success of DPI formulations depends on the adhesion of drug and carrier during mixing and filling of devices or hard gelatin capsules, followed by the ability of the drug to desorb from the carrier during inhalation such that free drug is available to penetrate to the peripheral airways. Adhesion and desorption will depend on the morphology of the particle surfaces and surface energies, which may be influenced by the chemical nature of the materials involved and the nature of powder processing. The performance of DPI systems is thus strongly dependent on formulation factors, and also on the construction of the delivery device and the inhalation technique.

Unit-dose devices with drug in hard gelatin capsules

The first DPI device developed was the Spinhaler (Rhône-Poulenc Rorer) for the delivery of sodium cromoglycate (Fig. 31.5). Each dose, contained in a hard gelatin capsule, is loaded individually into the device. The capsule, placed in a loose-fitting rotor, is pierced by two metal needles an either side of the capsule. Inhaled air flow though the device causes a

Fig. 31.5 The Spinhaler. (Modified from Bell et al 1971, with the permission of the American Pharmaceutical Association.)

turbovibratory air pattern as the rotor rotates rapidly, resulting in the powder being dispersed to the capsule walls and out through the perforations into the air. A minimum air flow rate of 35–40 L/min through the device is required to produce adequate vibrations by the rotor. The occurrence of lactose intolerance and local irritation, coughing and bronchoconstriction caused by the inhalation of large amounts of lactose has led to the development of an aggregated, carrier-free sodium cromoglycate capsule formulation for use in the Spinhaler.

Another unit-dose DPI is the Rotahaler (Glaxo SmithKline), which is a simple two-piece device (Fig. 31.6). The gelatin capsule is inserted into an orifice at the rear of the device and when the two sections are rotated a fin on the inner barrel pulls the two halves of the capsule apart. During inhalation, the freed half of the capsule spins, dispersing its contents, which are inhaled through the mouthpiece. The resistance to air flow is lower than that of the Spinhaler and therefore a lower inspiratory velocity is required.

Other hard gelatin capsule-based devices, working on similar principles, are available for the delivery of drug/carrier mixes. These include the Aerohaler (Boehringer Ingelheim) and the Cyclohaler (Du Pont).

Multidose devices with drug in foil blisters

The main disadvantage of hard gelatin capsule-based devices, namely the individual loading of each dose, was overcome with the development of the Diskhaler (Glaxo SmithKline). In this system, drug is mixed with a coarse lactose carrier and filled into an aluminium foil blister disc which is loaded, by the patient, into the device on a support wheel (Fig. 31.7). Each disc contains four or eight doses of drug and the blisters are pierced with a needle as a result of mechanical leverage on the lid. Air flow through the blister causes the powder to disperse as

Fig. 31.7   The Diskhaler (Reproduced with permission from Sumby et al 1993.)

the patient inhales through the mouthpiece. The foil blisters are numbered, so that the patient knows the number of doses remaining.

Multidose devices with drug preloaded in inhaler

The evolution of the Diskhaler led to the production of the Accuhaler or Diskus Inhaler (Glaxo SmithKline), in which drug/carrier mix is preloaded into the device in foil-covered blister pockets containing 60 doses (Fig. 31.8). The foil lid is peeled off the drug-containing pockets as each dose is advanced, with the blisters and lids being wound up separately within the device, which is discarded at the end of operation. As each dose is packaged separately and only momentarily exposed to ambient conditions prior to inhalation, the Diskhaler and Accuhaler are relatively insensitive to humidity compared to hard gelatin capsule-based systems.

An alternative approach is a *reservoir* type of device, in which a dose is accurately measured and delivered from a drug reservoir. In the Clickhaler DPI (Innovata Biomed), a drug blend is stored in a reservoir. Metering cups are filled by gravity from this reservoir and delivered to an inhalation passage, from which it is inhaled. The device is capable of holding up to 200 doses and incorporates a dose counter, which informs patients when the device, which is discarded after use, is nearly empty.

The Turbohaler (AstraZeneca), has overcome the need for both a carrier and the loading of individual doses (Fig. 31.9). The device contains a large number of doses (up to 200) of undiluted, loosely aggregated micronized drug, which is stored in a reservoir from which it flows on to a rotating disc in

Fig. 31.6   The Rotahaler (Modified with permission from Kjellman 1981.)

Fig. 31.8 The Accuhaler/Diskus Inhaler, showing (a) a schematic diagram and (b) a cross-sectional representation of the device. (Reproduced with permission from Prime et al 1996.)

Fig. 31.9 The Turbohaler. (Reproduced with permission from Wetterlin 1987.)

the dosing unit. The fine holes in the disc are filled and the excess drug is removed by scrapers. As the rotating disc is turned, by moving a turning grip back and forth, one metered dose is presented to the inhalation channel, and this is inhaled by the patient,

with the turbulent air flow created within the device breaking up any drug aggregates. A dose indicator is incorporated. The Turbohaler requires a higher inspiratory effort than the Diskhaler, owing to its higher internal resistance, and is more sensitive to humidity if not closed quickly after each use.

Non-breath actuated devices

Devices are currently under development which reduce or eliminate the reliance on the patient's inspiratory effort to disperse the drug (Rubsamen 1997). Such inspiratory effort may be affected by the patient's age and/or clinical condition. For instance, a device that uses a battery-powered impeller to deaggregate the drug powder is being developed. The device is breath actuated, but deaggregation is independent of the patient's inspiratory flow rate. Inhale Therapeutic Systems have produced a device in which compressed air is used to disperse drug from a unit-dose package into a large holding chamber, from which it is inhaled by the patient.

Nebulizers

Nebulizers deliver relatively large volumes of drug solutions and suspensions and are frequently used for drugs that cannot be conveniently formulated into MDIs or DPIs, or where the therapeutic dose is too large for delivery with these alternative systems. Nebulizers also have the advantage over metered-dose and dry powder systems in that drug may be inhaled during normal tidal breathing through a mouthpiece or face-mask, and thus they are useful for patients such as children, the elderly and patients with arthritis, who experience difficulties with MDIs.

There are two categories of commercially available nebulizer: jet and ultrasonic.

Jet nebulizers

Jet nebulizers (also called air-jet or air-blast nebulizers) use compressed gas (air or oxygen) from a compressed gas cylinder, hospital air-line or electrical compressor to convert a liquid (usually an aqueous solution) into a spray. The jet of high-velocity gas is passed either tangentially or coaxially through a narrow Venturi nozzle, typically 0.3–0.7 mm in diameter. An area of negative pressure, where the air jet emerges, causes liquid to be drawn up a feed tube from a fluid reservoir by the Bernoulli effect (Fig. 31.10). Liquid emerges as fine filaments, which collapse into droplets owing to surface tension. A proportion of the resultant (primary) aerosol

leaves the nebulizer directly; the remaining, large, non-respirable droplets impact on baffles or the walls of the nebulizer chamber and are recycled into the reservoir fluid.

Nebulizers are operated continuously, and because the inspiratory phase of breathing constitutes approximately one-third of the breathing cycle a large proportion of the emitted aerosol is not inhaled but is released into the environment. Open-vent nebulizers, incorporating inhalation and exhalation valves, e.g. the Pari LC nebulizer (Pari) have recently been developed in which the patient's own breath boosts nebulizer performance, with aerosol production matching the patient's tidal volume and greatly enhancing drug delivery. On exhalation, the aerosol being produced is generated only from the compressor gas source, thereby minimizing drug wastage.

The rate of gas flow driving atomization is the major determinant of the aerosol droplet size and rate of drug delivery for jet nebulizers: for instance, there may be up to a 50% reduction in the mass median aerodynamic diameter (MMAD, see below) when the flow rate is increased from 4 to 8 L/min, with a linear increase in the proportion of droplets less than 5 μm (Clay et al 1983).

Ultrasonic nebulizers

In ultrasonic nebulizers the energy necessary to atomize liquids comes from a piezoelectric crystal vibrating at high frequency. At sufficiently high ultrasonic intensities a fountain of liquid is formed in the nebulizer chamber. Large droplets are emitted from the apex and a 'fog' of small droplets is emitted from the lower part (Fig. 31.11). Some models have a fan to blow the respirable droplets out of the device, whereas in others the aerosol only becomes available to the patient during inhalation.

Fig. 31.10 Schematic diagram of a jet nebulizer. Compressed gas passes through a Venturi nozzle, where an area of negative pressure is created. Liquid is drawn up a feed tube and is fragmented into droplets. Large droplets impact on baffles (b), and small droplets are carried away in the inhaled airstream. (Reproduced with permission from Newman 1989.)

Fig. 31.11 Schematic diagram of an ultrasonic nebulizer. (Reproduced with permission from Atkins et al 1992.)

Formulating nebulizer fluids

Nebulizer fluids are formulated in water, occasionally with the addition of cosolvents such as ethanol or propylene glycol, and with the addition of surfactants for suspension formulations. Because hypoosmotic and hyperosmotic solutions may cause bronchoconstriction, as may high hydrogen ion concentrations, iso-osmotic solutions of pH greater than 5 are usually employed (Snell 1990). Stabilizers such as antioxidants and preservatives may also be included, although these may also cause bronchospasm, and for this reason sulphites in particular are generally avoided as antioxidants in such formulations. Although chemically preserved multidose preparations are commercially available, nebulizer formulations are generally presented as sterile, isotonic unit doses (usually 1–2.5 mL) without a preservative.

Whilst most nebulizer formulations are solutions, suspensions of micronized drug are also available for delivery from nebulizers. In general suspensions are poorly delivered from ultrasonic nebulizers, whereas with jet nebulizers the efficiency of drug delivery increases as the size of suspended drug is decreased, with little or no release of particles when they exceed the droplet size of the nebulized aerosol.

As the formulation of fluids for delivery by nebulizers is relatively simple, these devices are frequently the first to be employed when investigating the delivery of new entities to the human lung. Recently, they have been used for the delivery of peptides and liposomes. In general, ultrasonic nebulizers have not been successful for delivering either peptides or liposomes, because of denaturation resulting from the elevated temperatures produced. Consequently, ultrasonic nebulizers are expressly excluded for the delivery of recombinant human deoxyribonuclease in the management of cystic fibrosis. Jet nebulizers have been successfully used to deliver some peptide and liposome formulations, although the shearing forces that occur in the nebulizer may produce time-dependent damage to some materials (Niven and Brain 1994).

Physicochemical properties of nebulizer fluids

The viscosity and surface tension of a liquid being nebulized may affect the output of nebulizers, as energy is required to overcome viscous forces and to create a new surface. However, the size-selectivity of the nebulizer design and dimensions, with more than 99% of the primary aerosol mass being recycled into the reservoir liquid, means that changes in the size distribution of the primary aerosol resulting from changes in the properties of the solution being atomized may not always be reflected in the size distribution of the emitted aerosol. In general, the size of aerosol droplets is inversely proportional to viscosity for jet nebulizers and directly proportional to viscosity for ultrasonic nebulisers (McCallion et al 1995), with more viscous solutions requiring longer to nebulize to dryness and leaving larger residual volumes in the nebulizer following atomization. Surface tension effects are more complex, but usually a decrease in surface tension is associated with a reduction in mean aerosol size.

Temperature effects during nebulization

The aerosol output from a jet nebulizer comprises drug solution and solvent vapour, which saturates the outgoing air. This causes solute concentration to increase with time and results in a rapid decrease in the temperature of the liquid being nebulized by approximately 10–15°C.

This temperature decrease may be important clinically, as some asthma sufferers experience bronchoconstriction on inhalation of cold solutions. Further, the cooling effect within the reservoir fluid will reduce drug solubility and result in increased liquid surface tension and viscosity. Precipitation is uncommon with bronchodilators, which have high aqueous solubility, but problems may arise with less soluble drugs. In such instances the use of an ultrasonic nebulizer may be appropriate, as the operation of such devices increases solution temperature by approximately 10–15°C.

Duration of nebulization and 'dead volume'

Clinically, liquids may be nebulized for a specified period of time, or more commonly, they may be nebulized to 'dryness', which may be interpreted as *sputtering time*, which is the time when air is drawn up the feed tube and nebulization becomes erratic, although agitation of the nebulizer permits treatment to be continued; *clinical time*, which is the time at which therapy is ceased following sputtering; or *total time*, which is the time at which the production of aerosol ceases.

Regardless of the duration of nebulization, not all the fluid in the nebuliser can be atomized. Some liquid, usually about 1 mL, remains as the 'dead' or 'residual' volume, associated with the baffles, internal structures and walls of the nebulizer. The proportion of drug retained as 'dead' volume is more marked for smaller fill volumes, hence for a 2 mL fill volume, approximately 50% of fluid will remain associated with the nebulizer and be unavailable for delivery to the patient. This reduces to approximately 25% with a 4 mL fill volume, although there is a commensurate increase in the time necessary to nebulize to dryness.

Variability between nebulizers

Many different models of nebulizer and compressor are commercially available, and the size of aerosols produced and the dose delivered can vary enormously. For instance, in a study of 18 different commercially available jet nebulizers, operated according to the manufacturers' guidelines, aerosols were produced with MMADs ranging from 0.9 to 7.2 μm (Waldrep et al 1994). Variability may not only exist between different nebulizers but also between individual nebulizers of the same type, and repeated use of a single nebulizer may cause variability due to baffle wear and non-uniformity of assembly. Nebulizers, unlike the DPI and MDI devices, are not manufactured by the producers of nebulizer solutions and suspension. The choice of nebulizer employed for their delivery is thus usually beyond the influence of the pharmaceutical manufacturer.

METHODS OF AEROSOL SIZE ANALYSIS

The regional distribution of aerosols in the airways can be measured directly using gamma scintigraphy, by radiolabelling droplets or particles, usually with the short half-life gamma emitter technetium-99m(^{99m}Tc). However, more commonly in vitro measurements of aerosol size are used to predict clinical performance. The principal methods that have been employed for size characterization of aerosols are microscopy, laser diffraction and cascade impaction.

Optical methods of measuring the physical size of deposited aerosols using microscopy are laborious and do not give an indication of their likely deposition within the humid airways while being carried in an airstream. With methods of analysis based on laser Fraunhofer diffraction, aerosolized droplets or particles are sized as they traverse a laser beam to give a volume median diameter. Again the aerodynamic properties of an aerosol are not being measured. In addition, spraying droplets into a beam exposes them to ambient conditions of temperature and humidity, which may result in solvent evaporation.

Cascade impactors and impingers

Cascade impactors comprise a series of progressively finer jets and collection plates, allowing fractionation of aerosols according to their MMAD as the aerosol is drawn through the device at a known flow rate. Traditional cascade impactors are constructed from metal. The most commonly used comprises eight stages, with metal collection plates followed by a terminal filter. Multistage liquid impingers, working on the same principle, are constructed from glass or glass and metal and have three, four or five stages, with wet sintered glass collection plates followed by a terminal filter. Large dense particles will deposit higher in the impactor, whereas smaller, less dense particles will follow the air flow and only deposit when they have been given sufficient momentum as they are accelerated through the finer jets lower in the impactor (Fig. 31.12). The first stage of the impactor is usually preceded by a 90° bend of metal or glass to mimic the human throat. The cut-off diameters for each stage at a particular air-flow rate can be determined using monodisperse aerosols or calculated using calibration curves. When determining the size of an aerosol, cumulative percentage undersize plots of deposited aerosol on each stage are plotted against the cut-off diameter for that stage to allow calculation of the MMAD.

The five-stage liquid impinger (MSLI) (Fig. 31.13), with an appropriate induction port and mouthpiece adapter, is used to determine the aerodynamic size of DPIs (USP and EP), MDIs and nebulizers (EP). The MSLI may be operated at a flow rate between 30 and 100 L/min. At 60 L/min (i.e. 1 L/s) the effective cut-off diameters of stages 1, 2, 3 and 4 are 13.0, 6.8, 3.1 and 1.7 μm, respectively. The fifth stage comprises an integral filter which captures particles smaller than 1.7 μm. When testing DPIs to USP requirements, an airflow rate (Q) calculated to produce a pressure drop of 4.0 kPa over the inhaler is employed. If this exceeds 100 L/min, then 100 L/min is used. The cut-off diameters of each stage at flow rate (Q) can be calculated from:

$$D_{50'Q} = D_{50'Qn}(Q_n/Q)^{\frac{1}{2}} \qquad (31.7)$$

Fig. 31.12 Illustration of aerodynamic particle size separation by an impactor stage. (Reproduced with permission from Jaegfeldt et al 1987.)

Impaction nozzle or jet

Streamlines

Impaction plate

Fig. 31.13 The multistage liquid impinger. Courtesy of AstraZeneca.

where $D_{50'Q}$ is the cut-off diameter at the flow rate Q and n refers to the nominal cut-off values determined when Q_n is 60 L/min (values given above).

The use of cascade impaction methods to determine the size of aerosols has a number of disadvantages. The high flow rates employed (typically 28.3–60 L/min) result in rapid solvent evaporation, and droplets may be re-entrained in the airstream whereas particles may 'bounce off' metal collection plates, although this latter effect may be reduced by coating the collection surface, for instance with a silicone fluid or glycerol. These effects can result in a significant decrease in the measured aerosol size. Also, these measuring devices are operated at a constant air-flow rate. However, the dispersion of dry powder formulations and the deposition profile of inhaled aerosols will very considerably with flow rate. To overcome the limitations of measurement at a single flow rate the Electronic Lung (The Technology Partnership) has been developed, which uses a computer-controlled piston to draw air through the inhaler and into an impaction sizer,

following a predetermined inhalation profile (Brindley et al 1994).

Cascade impactor methods are invasive, laborious and time-consuming, but necessary to derive information about median aerosol size and the polydispersity of the aerosol. To ensure that inhalation products are likely to be clinically effective, quality control measurements usually involve measurement of the emitted dose and the 'fine particle fraction', (that fraction of the emitted dose less than a stated size, often 5 or 6.4 μm), which are combined to give a 'useful' or 'respirable' dose or mass (Ganderton, 1995). For routine analysis, a simplified two-stage (twin) impinger is frequently employed (Fig. 31.14). Aerosol collected in the throat and the upper stage (stage 1) is considered 'non-respirable', whereas that collected in the lower stage (stage 2) is considered 'respirable'. For this glass device, the cut-off diameter for stage 2 is 6.4 μm, i.e. aerosols collected in this stage have an aerodynamic diameter less than 6.4 μm and are for this measurement technique considered 'respirable'. This twin impinger is included in the BP as a method for determining the emitted dose from MDIs and DPIs.

Fig. 31.14 The two-stage impinger. (Reproduced with permission from Hallworth and Westmoreland 1987.)

REFERENCES

Atkins, P.J, Barker, N.P., Mathisen, D. (1992) The design and development of inhalation drug delivery systems. In: *Pharmaceutical Inhalation Aerosol Technology*. (Ed. A.S.J. Hickey) Marcel Dekker, New York, pp155–185.

Bell, J.H., Hartley, P.S. and Cox, J.S.G. (1971) Dry powder aerosols I: a new powder inhalation device. *J. Pharm Sci.*, **60**, 1559–1564.

Brindley, A., Sumby, B.S., Smith, I.J. (1994) The characterisation of inhalation devices by an inhalation simulator: the electronic lung. *J Aerosol Med.*, **7**, 197–200.

Byron, P.R., Miller, N.C., Blondino, F.E., Visich, J.E., Ward, G.H. (1994). Some aspects of alternative propellant solvency. *Respir. Drug Del. IV*, 231–242.

Clay, M.M., Pavia, D., Newman, S.P., Lennard-Jones, T., Clarke, S.W. (1983) Assessment of jet nebulisers for lung aerosol therapy. *Lancet*, **ii**, 592–594.

Ganderton, D. (1995) In-vitro testing of inhalation products. *Drug Delivery to the Lungs VI*. The Aerosol Society, Bristol, pp 85–88.

Hallworth, G.W., Westmoreland, D.G. (1987) The twin impinger: a simple device for assessing the delivery of drugs from metered dose pressurised aerosol inhalers. *J. Pharm. Pharmacol.*, **39**, 966–972.

Jaegfeldt, H., Andersson, J.A.R., Trofast, E., Wetterlin, K.I.L. (1987) Particle size distribution from different modifications of Turbohaler. In: *A New Concept In Inhalation Therapy*. (Eds. S.P. Newman, F. Morén and G.K. Crompton). Medicom Europe, Bussum, pp 90–99.

Kjellman, N-I.M. (1981) Letter to the Editor *Allergy*, **36**, 437–438.

McCallion, O.N.M., Taylor, K.M.G., Thomas, M., Taylor A.J. (1995) Nebulization of fluids of different physicochemical properties with air-jet and ultrasonic nebulizers. *Pharm. Res.*, **12**, 1682–1688.

Melchor, R., Biddiscombe, M.F., Mak, V.H.F., Short, M.D., Spiro, S.G. (1993) Lung deposition patterns of directly labelled salbutamol in normal subjects and in patients with reversible airflow obstruction. *Thorax*, **48**, 506–511.

Morén, F. (1981) Pressurised aerosols for oral inhalation. *Int. J. Pharm.*, **8**, 1–10.

Newman, S.P. (1989) *Nebuliser Therapy: Scientific and Technical Aspects*. AB Draco, Lund.

Niven, R.W. and Brain, J.D. (1994) Some functional aspects of air-jet nebulizers. *Int. J. Pharm.*, **104**, 73–85.

Prime, D., Slater, A.L., Haywood, P.A., Smith, I.J. (1996) Assessing dose delivery from the Flixotide Diskus Inhaler – a multidose powder inhaler. *Pharm. Tech. Europe*, **8 (3)**, 23–34.

Pritchard, J.N. (1987) Particle growth in the airways and the influence of airflow. In: *A New Concept In Inhalation Therapy*. (Eds. S.P. Newman, F. Morén and G.K. Crompton). Medicom Europe, Bussum, pp 3–24.

Rubsamen, R. (1997) Novel aerosol peptide drug delivery systems. In: *Inhalation Delivery of Therapeutic Peptides and Proteins*. (Eds. A.L. Adjei and P.K. Gupta). Marcel Dekker, New York, pp 703–731.

Snell, N.J.C. (1990) Adverse reactions to inhaled drugs. *Respir. Med.*, **84**, 345–348.

Sumby, B.S., Churcher, K.M., Smith, I.J., Grant, A.C., Truman, K.G., Marriott, R.J., Booth, S.J. (1993) Dose reliability of the Serevent Diskhaler system. *Pharm. Tech. Int.*, **6 (5)**, 20–27.

Waldrep, J.C., Keyhani, K., Black, M., Knight, V. (1994) Operating characteristics of 18 different continuous flow jet nebulizers with beclomethasone dipropionate liposome aerosol. *Chest*, **105**, 106–110.

Wetterlin, K.I.L. (1987) Design and function of Turbohaler. In: *A New Concept In Inhalation Therapy*. (Eds. S.P. Newman, F. Morén and G.K. Crompton). Medicom Europe, Bussum, pp 85–89.

Wilson, C.G. and Washington N. (1989) *Physiological Pharmaceutics: Biological Barriers to Drug Absorption*. Ellis Horwood, Chichester, p157.

BIBLIOGRAPHY

Adjei, A.L. and Gupta, P.K. (eds) (1997) *Inhalation Delivery of Therapeutic Peptides and Proteins*. Marcel Dekker, New York.

Farr, S.J, Kellaway, I.W. and Taylor, G. (1990). Drug delivery to the respiratory tract. In: *Routes of Drug Administration*. (Eds. A.T. Florence and E. Salole). Wright, London, pp 48–77.

Hickey, A.S.J. (ed) (1992) *Pharmaceutical Inhalation Aerosol Technology*. Marcel Dekker, New York.

McCallion, O.N.M. and Taylor, K.M.G. (1999) Ultrasonic nebulizers. In: *Encyclopaedia of Pharmaceutical Technology*. (Eds J. Swarbrick and J.C. Boylan). Marcel Dekker, New York, pp339–352.

McCallion, O.N.M., Taylor K.M.G., Bridges, P.A., Thomas, M., Taylor A.J. (1996) Jet nebulisers for pulmonary drug delivery. *Int. J. Pharm.*, **130**, 1–11.

Morén, F. (1981) Pressurised aerosols for oral inhalation. *Int. J. Pharm.*, **8**, 1–10.

Sciarra, J.J. (1996) Pharmaceutical Aerosols. In: *Modern Pharmaceutics*. 3rd edn., (Eds. G.S. Banker and C.T. Rhodes), Marcel Dekker, New York, pp 547–574.

Sciarra, J.J. and Cutie A.J. (1990) Aerosols. In: *Remington's Pharmaceutical Sciences*. 18th ed. (Eds. A.R. Gennaro et al). Mack Publishing Company, Easton, pp 1694–1712.

Timsina, M.P., Martin G.P., Marriott, C., Ganderton, D., Yianneskis, M. (1994) Drug delivery to the respiratory tract using dry powder inhalers. *Int. J. Pharm.*, **101**, 1–13.

Wilson, C.G. and Washington N. (1989) *Physiological Pharmaceutics: Biological Barriers to Drug Absorption*. Ellis Horwood, Chichester.

32

Nasal drug delivery

Peter Taylor

INTRODUCTION

The nasal cavity has been considered as a route of drug administration for many decades, often for topical therapies such as decongestants. Recently, however, there has been a great deal of research investigating the nose as a route for systemic therapies, especially for peptides and proteins (see Tables 32.1 to 32.3 for examples of topical nasal preparations, systemic preparations on the market, and systemic preparations under investigation).

There are many potential benefits to nasal administration: it is convenient, there is a useful area for absorbing drugs, and there is a good systemic blood supply – but, as with many other routes of delivery, there are also factors working against efficient drug absorption. The aim of this chapter is to review the relevant features of nasal anatomy and physiology, outline the various factors that influence drug absorption and, finally, discuss the various formulation strategies and delivery systems that can be used for nasal drug delivery.

THE ANATOMY AND PHYSIOLOGY OF THE NOSE

The outermost part of the nose is the nasal vestibule, which runs for about 15 mm from the nostrils to the nasal valve (Fig. 32.1). Behind the nasal valve is the nasal cavity, with a length of about 60 mm and a volume of 20 mL, and this passes into the nasopharynx. The nasal cavity is divided vertically for most of its length by the nasal septum, and each wall of the cavity contains three folds or indentations known as the nasal turbinates (or conchae). This folding means that the nasal cavity has a relatively large surface area for its volume – approximately 160 cm^2 (Chien 1992, Lee and Baldwin 1992, Mygind and Dahl 1998).

Table 32.1 Examples of topical nasal preparations (taken from the British National Formulary 39)

Drug	Drug class	Use	Delivery system
Levocabastine	Antihistamine	Allergic rhinitis	Aqueous spray (pump)
Beclomethasone dipropionate	Corticosteroid	Allergic and vasomotor rhinitis	Metered spray (pressurized) of aqueous suspension
Sodium cromoglycate	Cromoglycate	Allergic rhinitis	Aqueous spray (pump)
Ephedrine HCl	Sympathomimetic	Decongestant	Drops
Chlorhexidine HCl	Antimicrobial	Staphylococcal infections (nostrils)	Cream

Table 32.2 Examples of marketed systemic nasal preparations (taken from the British National Formulary 39 and Behl et al 1998a)

Drug	Drug class	Use	Delivery system
Desmopressin	Pituitary hormone	Diabetes insipidus	Metered spray
Buserelin	Gonadorelin analogue	Prostate cancer, endometriosis and others	Metered spray (pump)
Nafarelin	Gonadorelin analogue	Prostate cancer, endometriosis and others	Metered spray
Sumatriptin	Serotonin agonist	Migraine	Unit dose spray
Dihydroergotamine mesylate	Ergot alkaloid	Migraine	4-application spray
Nicotine	–	Cessation of smoking	Metered spray
Salmon calcitonin	Calcium regulator	Postmenopausal osteoporosis	Metered spray

Table 32.3 Examples of drugs under investigation for nasal delivery (taken from Behl et al 1998a)

Drug	Use	Stage of investigation
Cyanocobalamin (Vitamin B_{12}) Gel	Vitamin B_{12} deficiency	NDA submitted (USA)
17-β-oestradiol	Relief of menopausal symptoms	Human studies
Glucagon	Treatment of hypoglycaemia	Human studies
Interferon	Antiviral agent	Human studies
Insulin	Treatment of diabetes	Human studies
Metoclopramide HCl	Antiemetic	Human studies
Vaccines	Influenza, measles, polio etc.	Human studies

The normal functioning of the nose is closely related to its anatomy, for not only is it a sensory organ, it also conditions inspired air, heating and humidifying it before it reaches the lungs. Air passes through the constriction of the nasal valve with a high linear velocity, but the sharp change in direction of the flow into the nasal cavity and the presence of the turbinates (see Fig. 32.1) cause turbulent flow, bringing the air into close contact with the nasal lining. The large surface area of the nasal cavity and the rich underlying vasculature cause rapid heat and moisture transfer to the air; these are also factors that predispose the nasal cavity to being a good site for drug absorption.

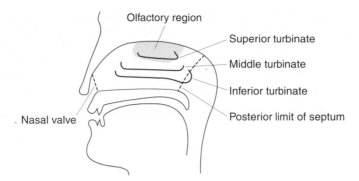

Fig. 32.1 Cross-section of human nasal cavity, showing major structures relevant to nasal drug administration.

Nasal mucosa and mucociliary clearance

The anterior part of the nose, from the nasal vestibule to the turbinates, consists of squamous epithelium. The upper part of the cavity, accounting for about 5% of the total area, is olfactory membrane. The latter contains the sensory olfactory cells as well as serous and mucosal cells; it is so placed because a large proportion of inspired air passes over this region. Most of the nasal cavity, however, is lined with mucous membrane containing a mixture of columnar cells, goblet cells and basal cells. The columnar cells in the forward third of the epithelium are non-ciliated; the remainder are covered with cilia. Cilia are hair-like projections on the exposed surface of epithelial cells. Each cell has about 300 cilia, measuring between 5 and 10 μm in length and 0.1–0.3 μm in diameter. The cilia beat in regular waves, with a frequency of 10 Hz. Their role is to facilitate the movement of mucus from the nasal cavity to the nasopharynx, and ultimately to the GI tract, the combined effect being known as mucociliary clearance (Marttin et al 1998, Schipper et al 1991).

Mucociliary clearance is a non-specific defensive function which also presents a barrier to drug absorption. The mucous layer is normally 5–20 μm thick, consisting mostly of water containing glycoproteins, ions and various other proteins, such as enzymes and immunoglobulins. Glycoproteins give the mucus its viscous character, which causes foreign particles to become trapped, cleared to the GI tract and ultimately eliminated from the body. The mucus is actually divided into two layers, the one closest to the cell surface being a less viscous, watery substance. This aids clearance by lubricating the passage of the mucus over the cell surfaces and easing the action of cilia. The cilia work in a ratchet-like way by engaging the viscous outer gel layer of the mucus, moving it towards the nasopharynx, and then disengaging and returning to their starting position through the serous inner layer. The turnover time for mucus is variously quoted as approximately 10–15 minutes in total (Lee and Baldwin 1992) and 20 minutes for the half-life of mucociliary clearance (Schipper et al 1991).

Mucus presents a diffusional barrier to drug absorption, and any formulation must be able to overcome this, as well as remain in the region long enough to allow drug release and absorption. Various strategies for achieving these goals are given later, but it is important that any interruption to mucociliary clearance, whether from drug or excipient, should be minimal and temporary.

Nasal metabolism

The nasal route of administration avoids hepatic first-pass metabolism, but nasal mucosa does possess enzymatic activity as a protective mechanism against exogenous chemicals. Although not widely investigated yet, there is sufficient evidence to suggest that nasal first-pass metabolism may be a significant factor in the absorption of some drugs (Sarkar 1992). For example, there is a high content of cytochrome P450 enzymes; P450 monooxygenases can oxidize many nasally administered drugs, such as nasal decongestants and anaesthetics. Progesterone and testosterone have been found to be metabolized extensively in vitro, although in vivo they have nasal bioavailabilities approaching 100% (relative to i.v. administration). Uneven distribution of enzymes is thought to be the reason for this apparent anomaly, greater activity being found in the olfactory mucosa used in the in vitro studies, whereas in vivo the steroids were probably absorbed rapidly by the less active respiratory mucosa.

There are many other types of enzyme in the nasal mucosa which can act on conventional drugs. Examples include dehydrogenases, hydroxylases, carboxylesterases, carbonic anhydrase and various phase II conjugative enzymes. Although these enzymes have usually been investigated for toxicological reasons, they may interfere with the efficient absorption of drugs. This is especially true for peptide- and protein-based drugs, as various enzymes, such as aminopeptidases, can significantly decrease the drug's bioavailability. It is now recognized that proteins and peptides are faced with substantial enzymatic, as well as physical, barriers to absorption across mucosal surfaces (Lee et al 1992).

The development of new nasal dosage forms should therefore include some consideration of the nature, extent and location of the drug's metabolism in the nose. Not all metabolism is undesirable, however, and certain enzymes, such as esterases, open the possibility of using prodrugs as a means of improving nasal delivery.

PHYSICOCHEMICAL FACTORS INFLUENCING DRUG ABSORPTION IN THE NASAL CAVITY

Investigation of how the physicochemical properties of various drugs influence their nasal absorption has provided some insight into the various mechanisms and routes of drug absorption. The most important properties are probably the size of the drug molecule, its charge and its degree of hydrophilicity (or lipophilicity).

Molecular size and weight

McMartin et al (1987) compiled literature data for over two dozen compounds ranging in molecular weight from 160 to 34 000 Da. Wherever possible, comparisons were made between absorption of the same compound after delivery by the nasal route in humans and rats and oral administration in humans. All three models showed similar effects: the absorption of small compounds (approx. 100 Da) was high, at around 80%, but this decreased markedly as molecular weight increased. Nasal absorption of a drug with a given molecular weight was slightly higher in rats than in humans, but the greatest difference was seen between oral absorption and nasal absorption in humans. Drug absorption after nasal administration was very much higher than after oral delivery of a particular compound. Also, the molecular weight cut-off, beyond which absorption was negligible, was about two orders of magnitude better for nasal administration (about 20 000 Da compared to around 200 Da for peroral delivery).

These data, even though they relate to a small group of compounds, show the utility of the nasal route, and they led to the proposal that the drugs (which tended to be hydrophilic) were absorbed by non-specific diffusion through aqueous channels between the cells, although other routes were a possibility. The molecular weight cut-off occurs because only molecules that are smaller than the channels can diffuse through them. The hypothesis that transport can occur through aqueous channels has received support in other studies using homologous series of hydrophilic compounds, such as poly(ethylene glycols) (Donovan et al 1990) and labelled dextrans with molecular weights between 1260 and 45 500 Da (Fisher et al 1992).

The effect of pH and the partition coefficient

Although molecular size is undoubtedly an important factor in influencing nasal absorption, the evidence in the preceding section tends to be based upon water-soluble compounds. More lipophilic compounds are likely to travel through one of the alternative routes, probably by partitioning across the mucosal cell membranes and diffusing through the cells at a rate slower than through intercellular channels. Most drugs can be ionized, and their partition coefficients are dependent upon environmental pH (unionized compounds will have a higher oil/water partition coefficient than ionized ones).

The pH at the surface of the mucosal cells has been reported to be 7.39 (Hirai et al 1981a); the mucus layer is slightly acidic, at pH 5.5–6.5 (Chien 1992). It should be mentioned that the local pH can be modified by a nasal formulation. Hirai et al (1981a) studied absorption in a perfused rat model of two model drug compounds at various pHs, a base (aminopyrine) and an acid (salicylic acid). The rate of absorption for both drugs increased as they became less ionized. Aminopyrine is absorbed more quickly at higher pHs, and the curve of absorption rate versus pH closely followed the degree of ionization versus pH curve. This suggests that the more lipophilic, unionized form of the drug is absorbed by passive diffusion through the mucosal cells. The salicylic acid was also absorbed more quickly in its unionized form (at low pH); the rate of absorption did not correspond with the degree of ionization: instead, it was higher than predicted. In this case it was suggested that there was another mechanism working alongside the slower diffusion through the cells, possibly the salicylic acid enhancing its own absorption. It is worth noting that despite both of the model compounds being relatively small, there was no suggestion in this study of a fast absorption through intercellular channels.

Other mechanisms of drug absorption are also present in the nose. The absorption of benzoic acid decreases as pH increases, but there was still appreciable absorption at pHs where the acid is completely ionised (Huang et al 1985), suggesting the existence of two methods of absorption. It is possible that low pHs can have a direct action on the nasal mucosa: the absorption of secretin was greater at low pHs, and histological examination of the epithelial cells found changes in their structure at pH 3 (Ohwaki et al 1987).

The effect of pH on peptide drugs is more complex than on conventional drugs, as peptides have a large number of ionizable groups of either charge. Peptides are characterized by their isoelectric point, the pH at which they have no net charge and where their solubility is often lowest. The nasal absorption of insulin (isoelectric point at pH 5.4), as measured by the reduction in blood sugar in dogs, was greatest at a solution pH of 3.1 (net positive charge on insulin) and lowest at pH 6.1, near its isoelectric point. The absorption mechanisms of peptides are however, complex, owing to their size and structure, and it is unlikely that the effect of pH on insulin absorption is due to a more favourable partitioning of the protein. Indeed, there could well have been direct effects on the epithelial cells at pH 3.1.

The role of the partition coefficient so far has largely been inferred from the relative proportions of the ionized to the unionized forms of the drug, but this relationship is not pronounced. The absorption of a series of barbiturates was studied at pH 6.0, when they would be largely unionized, and only a fourfold variation in absorption was found despite a nearly 50-fold range in the chloroform/water partition coefficient (Huang et al 1985). An investigation into the dependence of the absorption of a series of progesterone derivatives on their octanol/water partition coefficients gave a similar finding: absorption increased with partition coefficient, but to a markedly lower extent (Corbo et al 1989). The latter workers determined partition coefficients in a nasal mucosa–buffer system and found a much better correlation with absorption than the conventional oil/water models give. It is clear from these findings that an appropriate measure of partitioning must be used in order to determine the role of partitioning in nasal absorption, but in general it appears that partitioning is rarely the only factor controlling absorption.

Other physicochemical factors affecting nasal absorption

The solubility of the drug and its dissolution rate are important, especially if it is presented as a solid dosage form (e.g. a powder), as it must be able to cross the mucous layer before it can be absorbed by the epithelial cells. In addition, powder morphology and particle size influence the deposition of the drug inside the nasal cavity. All of these factors must be considered in the design of formulations and will be addressed later in this chapter.

Physicochemical properties and mechanisms of absorption – a summary

The above discussion has shown that the influence of various properties on the absorption of drugs can provide valuable indicators about the mechanisms of drug absorption. It is also clear that the nasal absorption of drugs is a complicated affair, and there is rarely a single way in which a drug can be absorbed. Chien (1992) has written about the various absorption mechanisms; the summary given below is a broad generalization.

Aqueous channels between the cells provide a relatively good route for water-soluble compounds, with absorption being limited mostly by molecular size. Other drugs are absorbed by passive diffusion, possibly using a transcellular route, and there is evidence for active transport of some amino acids. Whatever the mechanism, combined literature data suggest that molecules with a molecular weight up to about 1000 Da should have a relatively good systemic bioavailability without the need for absorption promoters. Absorption promoters could increase this molecular weight limit to about 6000 Da, but beyond this weight it is unlikely that large molecules could be absorbed without causing unacceptable damage to the nasal cavity.

STRATEGIES FOR IMPROVING DRUG AVAILABILITY IN NASAL ADMINISTRATION

There are three main ways to maximize the systemic bioavailability of drugs administered nasally:

- Improve nasal residence time
- Enhance nasal absorption
- Modify drug structure to change physicochemical properties.

Increasing nasal residence time

Mucociliary clearance acts to remove foreign bodies and substances from the nasal mucosa as quickly as possible. One way of delaying clearance is to apply the drug to the anterior part of the nasal cavity, an effect which is largely determined by the type of dosage form used. The preparation could also be formulated with polymers such as methylcellulose, hydroxypropylmethylcellulose or polyacrylic acid (Carbopol), which increase the viscosity of the formulation and act as bioadhesives with the mucus (Schipper et al 1991). Increasing the residence time does not necessarily lead to increased absorption. This can be illustrated by considering insulin solutions with similar viscosities containing carboxymethylcellulose or Carbopol. The carboxymethylcellulose solutions do not enhance the absorption of insulin (Duchene et al 1988), whereas Carbopol solutions do (Morimoto et al 1985). Increasing the viscosity of solutions will decrease the rate of diffusion of molecules through them – hence the apparent lack of effect of carboxymethylcellulose – but the polymer may have other enhancing actions, such as opening the intercellular junctions, as has been suggested for Carbopol (Junginger 1990).

An interesting formulation development for lengthening residence time is the use of microspheres (Pereswetoff-Morath 1998). The absorption of insulin is increased by degradable starch microspheres which, although insoluble, swell in water and form a viscous, bioadhesive mass (Illum et al 1987). Subsequent studies indicate a more direct action of the microspheres on epithelial cells, whereby the swelling of the microspheres causes a temporary dehydration and shrinkage of the cells, followed by opening of the tight intercellular junctions (Edman et al 1992).

Enhancing nasal absorption

Absorption enhancers work by increasing the rate at which drugs pass through the nasal mucosa. Many act by altering the structure of the epithelial cells in some way, but they should accomplish this while causing no damage or permanent change. General requirements of an ideal absorption enhancer at its concentration in use are:

- It should give an effective increase in the absorption of the drug.
- It should not cause permanent damage or alteration to the tissues.
- It should not otherwise be irritant or toxic, either to the local tissues or to the rest of the body.

- It should be effective in small quantities.
- The enhancing effect should occur when absorption is required (i.e. there should not be a lag in its effect).
- The effect should be temporary and reversible.
- The enhancer should fulfil all other expectations of formulation excipients (e.g. stability and compatibility).

The major reason for developing and testing enhancers is to increase the absorption of peptides and proteins, because their size leads to a relatively poor bioavailability. There is a large body of work investigating enhancers for nasal delivery. Much of this is focused on peptide delivery, and the interested reader is directed to reviews such as those written by Behl et al (1998b), Chien (1992) and Hinchcliffe and Illum (1999) for more detail on the various classes of enhancer.

Surfactants and bile salts have received considerable attention. Hirai et al (1981b) investigated surfactants of many types, including non-ionic ethers and esters, and anionic surfactants, for their effect on insulin absorption and found them to be particularly effective enhancers. Unfortunately, the enhancement usually correlates with mucosal damage, as the surfactants associate with cellular components such as membrane lipids and proteins. In some cases the association is so severe as to cause extraction of lipids or proteins and loss of epithelial cells. Surfactants are therefore unsuitable for therapeutic use as enhancers, although Hinchcliffe and Illum (1999) suggest they are experimentally useful as reference compounds guaranteed to cause enhancement.

Bile salts have greater potential as they appear to possess much of the enhancing activity but less of the damage potential of surfactants (bile salts possess some surface activity and can form micelles). Commonly studied bile salts include sodium cholate, sodium deoxycholate, sodium glycocholate and glycodeoxycholate, sodium taurocholate and taurodeoxycholate, all of which can cause enhancement at concentrations of 10–20 mM (Behl et al 1998b).

Several mechanisms have been proposed for the enhancing action of bile salts:

- Increasing cell membrane permeability by forming temporary channels through the lipid structure;
- Forming intercellular aqueous pores by opening the tight junctions between cells;
- Increasing the lipophilicity of charged drugs by forming ion pairs;
- Inhibition of proteolytic enzymes.

The most likely of these mechanisms for increasing the absorption of peptides is the opening of intercellular channels, rather than increasing cell permeability; the latter would probably require massive disruption of the cell before substantial quantities of peptide could pass. Although bile salts are claimed to be safer than surfactants they can still cause damage to epithelial cells. Again there is a positive correlation between their enhancing activity and the damage caused.

Merkus et al (1993) have documented the damage potential of a number of bile salts and surfactants, using an index of morphological damage and a measurement of toxicity on the cilia (specifically the ciliary beat frequency, CBF). Decreases in CBF correspond to cellular damage, and measurement of CBF has the advantage of providing a relatively easy quantitative measure of toxicity which can be used to show the change in toxicity with time, including any reversal. Ciliotoxicity can also furnish another explanation for increased absorption, because a lower CBF tends to increase nasal residence time.

Sodium tauro-24,25-dihydrofusidate (STDHF) is an enhancer with a structure similar to bile salts that has been widely studied as an enhancer for proteins. It has good aqueous stability and solubility (>10% w/v) and is surface active, forming micelles at a critical micelle concentration of 2.5 mM. One study has found an approximately tenfold increase in the bioavailability of human insulin and increases in the bioavailability of labelled dextrans ranging from about fourfold (40 000 Da dextran) up to 72 times (4000 Da) (Lee and Baldwin 1992). The degree of penetration enhancement depends on the concentration of the STDHF, reaching a maximum at around 0.3%. As this is over the critical micelle concentration, any further increase in STDHF concentration will see a rise in the number of micelles, not individual enhancer monomers. It can be concluded that the monomer concentration is more important for producing the enhancing effect than the number of micelles. The same authors claim that STDHF produces only a temporary increase in absorption and causes relatively little cell damage, although Merkus et al (1993) show that STDHF is ciliotoxic at its optimum enhancing concentration. It should be noted, however, that the ciliotoxicity depends on the model used, with a much lower degree of toxicity in human tissue than in the animal model used (chicken trachea).

Another group of surface-active materials is the phosphatidylcholines, for example lysophosphatidylcholine. These are similar to compounds that occur naturally as part of cell membranes and, as might be expected, one mechanism of action of phosphatidylcholines is to disrupt the cell membrane and increase its permeability. They may also inhibit proteolytic enzymes, and lysophosphatidylcholine is mucolytic. They are effective enhancers of protein absorption and, despite their proposed mechanism of action, do not cause the expected damage to the nasal lining. Dodecanoyl-L-α-phosphatidylcholine (DPPC) is one derivative which has been developed with a high activity and low toxicity profile. It is undergoing development as an enhancer for insulin. Early studies showed that DPPC increases the absorption of insulin in humans with little or no irritation to the nose, although more recent work suggests that the amount of insulin absorbed by this route may not be therapeutically useful (Hinchcliffe and Illum 1999).

Cyclodextrins (CD) are hollow cylindrical molecules made up of glucose units in a cyclic arrangement: α-CD has six glucose units, β-CD has seven and γ-CD has eight. These compounds have found a wide range of pharmaceutical uses, from solubility enhancement to taste masking, because of their ability to form 'inclusion complexes'. Here, part or all of a drug molecule inserts itself in the hollow central cavity of the cyclodextrin molecule. The complexed drug molecule takes on some of the physicochemical properties of the cylcodextrin molecule. Derivatives of the cyclodextrins can be used to modify these properties. Cyclodextrins have polar outer surfaces and less polar interiors, so they tend to be water-soluble but have the ability to accommodate hydrophobic molecules as part of the inclusion complex. This results in an increased aqueous solubility for the included species.

Cyclodextrins increase the bioavailability of lipophilic compounds by increasing their aqueous solubility, and hence their availability, at the surface of the nasal epithelium (Merkus et al 1999). As an example, dimethyl-β-cyclodextrin (DMβCD) gives an absolute bioavailability for oestradiol of 95% in rats and 67% in rabbits, a three- to five-fold increase compared with a control preparation. This has been supported by clinical data in humans showing that nasally administered oestradiol is effective as an oestrogen-replacement therapy in ovariectomized postmenopausal women.

Data are available to show the enhancement of absorption of other lipophilic compounds and even hydrophilic drugs. Hydrophilic drugs which have an enhanced absorption include peptides (e.g. buserelin) and proteins (e.g. calcitonin). The bioavailability of insulin is not increased to a therapeutic level. Insulin is one of the major goals for therapeutic administration via the nose, but this has yet to be achieved at sufficient levels even with the use of enhancers. The mechanism of enhancement of hydrophilic drug absorption by cyclodextrins has yet to be fully elucidated, but it is probably the result of a direct action on the nasal epithelium rather than a modification of the drug's physicochemical properties.

One of the main benefits of using cyclodextrins according to Merkus et al (1999) is their lack of toxicity, expressed as direct damage to the nasal cells, ciliotoxicity, or more systemic effects. Particularly useful are the methylated-β-cyclodextrins, which exhibit a combination of high activity and low toxicity.

The enhancers reported so far all act directly on the nasal epithelium, with a consequent risk of irritation and cellular damage. Alternative molecules, such as chitosan (a polysaccharide derived from the shells of crustacea) that have different mechanisms of delivery, have been studied (Illum 1998).

It is unlikely that there will be a single universal absorption enhancer and currently many of the most effective enhancers also cause damage to the nose. However, the volume of research and development work that has been conducted on these enhancers will make the nasal delivery of many drugs feasible.

Modifying drug structure

Structural modifications to the drug molecule are usually made in order to bestow more favourable physicochemical properties to the drug, for example increasing its aqueous solubility or improving its partitioning characteristics. Cyclodextrins can perform some of these functions, although they do not actually change the drug's structure. Some structural changes will be permanent, either by altering substituent groups on the molecule or by using different salt forms. However, they run the risk of changing the drug's therapeutic and toxicological profile and thus require regulatory approval, with its associated costs and lengthy studies.

An alternative is to use prodrugs, whereby the prodrug has favourable properties for absorption but is changed to the active drug on passing through the nasal epithelium. An example is the use of an ester (thereby increasing the drug's lipophilicity) that can be metabolized to the active drug by the esterases present in the nasal mucosa. Peptide and protein drugs especially may benefit from the formation of prodrugs (Krishnamoorthy and Mitra 1998).

NASAL DELIVERY SYSTEMS AND THEIR FORMULATION

General formulation issues

Nasal dosage forms must fulfil the functions of any other type of formulation. They must:

- be effective
- have an acceptable safety and stability, both chemical and microbiological
- be acceptable to the patient to ensure compliance.

If the formulation is a liquid it may commonly contain:

- antimicrobial preservatives (e.g. benzalkonium chloride)
- antioxidants (e.g. butylated hydroxytoluene)
- solubilizing agents or cosolvents (e.g. glycol derivatives)
- salts for adjusting pH and tonicity
- humectants, to minimize irritation to the nose (e.g. glycerol)
- viscosity-increasing agents (e.g. methylcellulose), and
- absorption enhancers.

Types of nasal dosage form and delivery system

The final dosage form used for nasal drug delivery is chosen after consideration of a wide range of issues, covering patient convenience, efficiency of drug delivery and formulation reasons. The specifics of the dosage form or delivery system plays a major role in the absorption of the drug by influencing its deposition. For example, as mentioned above, drugs deposited in the anterior part of the nasal cavity will be better absorbed than those applied further back.

Deposition mechanisms

There are three main ways of depositing inhaled particles on the nasal lining: impaction, sedimentation and diffusion (Kublik and Vidgren 1998).

Impaction Impaction occurs when there is a change in direction of the airflow – as happens when inspired air passes through the nasal valve – and the inertia of large or fast-moving particles carries them in their original direction. This is usually the main way of depositing particles in the turbulence caused by fast flow rates, or with particles larger than 0.5–1 μm. Varying the flow rate from the device or the aerodynamic particle size are the means by which the formulator can influence this type of deposition.

Sedimentation Sedimentation happens when the air is moving slowly and the particles settle slowly under the force of gravity. This mode of deposition is described by Stokes' equation. The only control the formulator can have over this practically is to ensure a slow flow rate and by modifying the drug particle size or formulation droplet size.

Diffusion The final method of deposition, diffusion, occurs by Brownian motion and is thus limited to very small particles (< 0.5 μm). Normally diffusion is not important, as the inspired particles are too large.

Nasal dosage forms

Nasal dosage forms will usually contain the drug in a liquid or powder formulation delivered by a pressurized or pump system. There have been several studies that have looked at the influence of dosage form and delivery system on the deposition and absorption of drugs, and useful summaries are given by Kublik and Vidgren (1998) and Su (1991).

Liquid formulation Liquid formulations are usually aqueous solutions of the drug and thus have the general benefits and drawbacks of pharmaceutical solutions. They are relatively simple to develop and manufacture compared to solid dosage forms, but often have a lower microbiological and chemical stability, requiring the use of various preservatives.

The liquid form can be soothing to the nasal lining but this may be countered by the excipients, such as the antimicrobial preservatives, which can cause irritation or ciliotoxicity. The simplest way to give a liquid is by nose drops, but their cheapness and convenience are usually outweighed by the inaccuracy of dosing volume and the likelihood of too-rapid clearance by the liquid running straight into the oesophagus. Dosing accuracy can be improved by using unit-dose packs containing a predetermined volume, but it is still the case that accurate placing of the drops requires some skill and dexterity on the part of the user.

Squeezed bottles Squeezed bottles are often used for nasal decongestants and work by spraying a partially atomized jet of liquid into the nasal cavity. They give a better absorption of drug by directing the formulation into the anterior part of the cavity and covering a large part of the nasal mucosa. Deposition and volume are still subject to the technique of the user – whether the patient squeezes the bottle smoothly or in a series of vigorous squirts, for example. This type of delivery system, where the formulation is expelled through a plain orifice without any type of valve system, is subject to contamination by 'suck-back', as external material can be drawn back into the container as the pressure on it is released.

Metered-dose pump systems Metered-dose pump systems offer greater control over dosing than any of the previous systems. They can deliver solutions, suspensions or emulsions, with a predetermined volume between 25 and 200 μL, thus offering deposition over a large area. The formulation scientist is able to incorporate a high degree of control over the size and localization of the dose by changing various factors, such as the rheological and surface tension characteristics of the formulation and the design and geometry of the pump.

The interactions between these factors are complex, but one example will show the type of control that is available. The angle at which the spray leaves the nozzle (the cone angle) will affect where the formulation is deposited. A small cone angle (about 35°) tends to be deposited towards the back of the nasal cavity and larger angles (tending towards 90°) will go further forward.

Metered-dose systems are also available as pressurized products. These permit the delivery of solid particulate preparations and present special formulation challenges because of the requirement to form a stable dispersion of the drug in the propellant system. Pressurized metered-dose systems give a good distribution of the formulation in the nasal cavity, but there is evidence that it is not as even as the distribution from metered-dose pumps.

Particle size and dose volume are two important factors for controlling delivery from metered-dose systems. The optimum particle size for deposition in the nasal cavity is 10 μm (mass median diameter; Su 1991). In addition, particulate formulations tend to have a longer residence time in the nasal cavity than liquids, because they are removed more slowly by mucociliary clearance.

The volume of formulation that can be delivered is obviously limited by the size of the nasal cavity, and larger volumes tend to be cleared faster despite covering a larger area. Better absorption is often achieved by administering two doses, one in each nostril, rather than a single large dose (e.g. two 80 μL doses rather than one 140 μL; Kublik and Vidgren 1998).

CONCLUDING REMARKS

The nasal route is one of many which is receiving a large amount of attention as a way of delivering drugs into the systemic circulation. Attention is focused particularly on peptide and protein drugs, and several have reached the market. Delivery systems for these drugs will often need to incorporate absorption enhancers or some means of increasing the time that the drug is in contact with the nasal lining.

Recent advances uphold the promise of the nasal route as a convenient way to administer a wide range of drugs.

REFERENCES

Behl, C.R., Pimplaskar, H.K., Sileno, A.P., deMeireles, J., Romeo, V.D. (1998a) Effects of physicochemical properties and other factors on systemic nasal drug delivery. *Adv. Drug Del. Rev.*, **29**, 89–116.

Behl C.R., Pimplaskar H.K., Sileno A.P., Xia W.J., Gries W.J. deMeireles J., Romeo V.D. (1998b) Optimization of systemic nasal drug delivery with pharmaceutical excipients. *Adv. Drug Del. Rev.*, **29**, 117–133.

British National Formulary 39, March 2000. British Medical Association and Royal Pharmaceutical Society of Great Britain, London.

Chien, Y., (1992) *Novel Drug Delivery Systems*, 2nd edn, Marcel Dekker, New York, Ch 5 Nasal drug delivery.

Corbo, D.C., Huang, Y.C., Chien, Y.W. (1989) Nasal delivery of progestational steroids in ovariectomised rabbits 2. Effect of penetrant hydrophilicity. *Int. J. Pharm.*, **50**, 253–260.

Donovan, M., Flynn, G., Amidon, G. (1990) Absorption of polyethylene glycols 600 through 2000: the molecular weight dependence of gastrointestinal and nasal absorption. *Pharm. Res.* 7, 863–868.

Duchene, D., Touchard, F., Peppas, N.A. (1988) Pharmaceutical and medical aspects of bioadhesive systems for drug administration. *Drug Dev. Indus. Pharm.* **14**, 233–318.

Edman, P., Björk, E., Rydén, L. (1992) Microspheres as a nasal delivery system for peptide drugs. *J. Controlled Release*, **21**, 165–172.

Fisher, A., Illum, L., Davis, S., Schacht, E. (1992) Di-iodo-L-tyrosine labelled dextrans as molecular size markers of nasal absorption in the rat. *J. Pharm. Pharmacol.*, **44**, 550–554.

Hinchcliffe, M., Illum, L. (1999) Intranasal insulin delivery and therapy. *Adv. Drug Del. Rev.* **35**, 199–234.

Hirai, S., Yahika, T., Matsuzawa, T., Mima. H. (1981a) Absorption of drugs from the nasal mucosa of rat. *Int. J. Pharm.* 7, 317–325.

Hirai, S., Yashiki, T., Mima, H. (1981b) Mechanisms for the enhancement of the nasal absorption of insulin by surfactants. *Int. J. Pharm.*, **9**, 173–184.

Huang, C., Kimura, R., Nassar, R., Hussain, A.A. (1985) Mechanism of nasal absorption of drugs I: Physicochemical parameters influencing the rate of in-situ nasal absorption of drugs in rats. *J. Pharm. Sci.*, **74**, 608–611.

Illum, L. (1998) Chitosan and its use as a pharmaceutical excipient. *Pharm. Res.* **15**, 1326–1331.

Illum, L., Jorgensen, H., Bisgaard, H. (1987) Bioadhesive microspheres as a potential nasal drug delivery system. *Int. J. Pharm.*, **39**, 189–199.

Junginger, H.E. (1990) Bioadhesive polymer systems for peptide delivery. *Acta Pharm. Tech.*, **36**, 110–126.

Krishnamoorthy, R., Mitra, A.K. (1998) Prodrugs for nasal drug delivery. *Adv. Drug Del. Rev.*, **29**, 135–146.

Kublik, H., Vidgren, M.T. (1998) Nasal delivery systems and their effect on deposition and absorption. *Adv. Drug Del. Rev.*, **29**, 157–177.

Lee, W.A., Baldwin, P.A. (1992) Nasal membranes: structure and permeability. In: Junginger H.E. (ed) *Drug Targeting and Delivery: Concepts in Dosage Form Design*. Ellis Horwood, New York, Ch 16.

McMartin, C., Hutchinson, L.E.F., Hyde, R., Peters, G.E. (1987) Analysis of structural requirements for the absorption of drugs and macromolecules from the nasal cavity. *J. Pharm. Sci.* 76, 535–540.

Marttin, E., Schipper, N.G.M., Verhoef, J.C., Merkus, F.W.H.M. (1998) Nasal mucociliary clearance as a factor in nasal drug delivery. *Adv. Drug Del. Rev.* **29**, 13–38.

Merkus, F.H.W.M., Schipper, N.G.M., Hermans, W.A.J.J., Romeijn, S.G., Verhoef, J.C. (1993) Absorption enhancers in nasal drug delivery: Efficacy and safety. *J. Controlled Release*, **24**, 201–208.

Merkus, F.H.W.M., Verhoef, J.C., Marttin, E., Romeijn, S.G., van der Kuy, P.H.M., Hermens, W.A.J.J., Schipper, N.G.M. (1999) Cyclodextrins in nasal drug delivery. *Adv. Drug Del. Rev.*, **36**, 41–57.

Morimoto, K., Morisaka, K., Kamanda, A. (1985) Enhancement of nasal absorption of insulin and calcitonin using polyacrylic acid gel. *J Pharm. Pharmacol.*, **37**, 134–136.

Mygind, N., Dahl, R. (1998) Anatomy, physiology and function of the nasal cavities in health and disease. *Adv. Drug Del. Rev.* 29, 3–12.

Ohwaki, K., Ando, H., Kakimoto, F., Useugi, K., Watanabe, S., Miyake, S., Kayano, M. (1987) Effects of dose, pH, osmolarity on nasal absorption of secretin in rats: histological aspects of the nasal mucosa in relation to the absorption variation due to the effects of pH and osmolarity. *J. Pharm. Sci.*, **76**, 695–698.

Pereswetoff-Morath, L. (1998) Microspheres as nasal drug delivery systems. *Adv. Drug. Del. Rev.*, **29**, 185–194.

Sarkar, M.A. (1992) Drug metabolism in the nasal mucosa. *Pharm. Res.*, **9**, 1–9.

Schipper, N.G.M., Verhoef, J.C., Merkus, F.W.H.M. (1991) The nasal mucociliary clearance: relevance to nasal drug delivery. *Pharm. Res.*, 7, 807–814.

Su, K.S.E. (1991) Nasal delivery. In Lee, V.H.L. (ed) *Peptide and Protein Drug Delivery*. Marcel Dekker, New York, Ch 13.

33

Transdermal drug delivery

Brian Barry

CHAPTER CONTENTS

The main purpose of this chapter is to show how the physicochemical properties of a drug in a topical dosage form affect that drug's transdermal delivery (or percutaneous absorption). This process, and the drug's topical bioavailability, depend on the medicament leaving a formulation (cream, ointment, patch etc.) and penetrating through the stratum corneum into the viable epidermis and dermis. Within the living tissues the molecule usually produces its characteristic pharmacological response before the blood or lymph circulations remove it (possibly to produce a systemic effect). The ultimate aim in dermatological biopharmaceutics is to design active drugs, or prodrugs, and to incorporate them into vehicles or devices that deliver the medicament to the active site in the biophase at a controlled rate.

The plan of the chapter is:

- to introduce the reader to the structure, functions and topical treatment of human skin;
- to deal with the principles of membrane diffusion, skin transport, the properties influencing transdermal delivery, permeation with and without stratum corneum control, and the methods for studying these processes;
- to consider how to maximize the bioavailability of a topical drug;
- to review the philosophy of transdermal patches;
- to close with a brief discussion of dermatological vehicles and a protocol for producing a dermatological formulation.

The reader may then see that skin therapy is a paradox. At first sight it appears to be a simple form of treatment, yet closer examination reveals that sound dermatological design represents one of the most difficult aspects of the science of pharmaceutical formulation.

STRUCTURE, FUNCTION AND TOPICAL TREATMENT OF HUMAN SKIN

The skin combines with the mucosal linings of the urogenital, digestive and respiratory tracts to protect the internal body structure from a hostile external environment of varying pollution, temperature, humidity and radiation. The skin safeguards the internal organs, limits the passage of chemicals into and out of the body, stabilizes blood pressure and temperature, and mediates the sensations of heat, cold, touch and pain. It expresses emotions (such as the pallor of fear, the redness of embarrassment and anger, and the sweating of anxiety). The integument identifies individuals through the characteristics particular to humans, e.g. colour, hair, odour and texture.

Skin damages easily: mechanically, chemically, biologically and by radiation. Thus the tissue suffers cuts, bruises, burns, bites and stings; detergents, chemical residues, organic solvents and pollutants attack and penetrate the surface; and micro-organisms and plants deliver contact allergens.

Topical and systemic drugs, toiletries and cosmetics and many diseases may all harm the skin.

Anatomy and physiology

The human skin comprises three tissue layers: the stratified, avascular, cellular epidermis, the underlying dermis of connective tissue, and the subcutaneous fat (Fig. 33.1(a)). Hairy skin contains hair follicles and sebaceous glands; the glabrous skin of

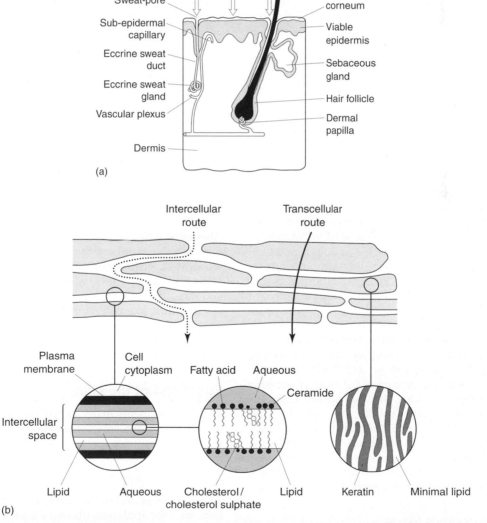

Fig. 33.1 Simplified diagram of skin structure and routes of drug penetration. (a) Macroroutes: (1) via the sweat ducts; (2) across the continuous stratum corneum; or (3) through the hair follicles with their associated sebaceous glands. (b) Representation of the stratum corneum membrane, illustrating two possible microroutes for permeation.

the soles and palms produces a thick epidermis with a compact stratum corneum, but there are no hair follicles or sebaceous glands.

The epidermis

The multilayered epidermis varies in thickness, ranging from about 0.8 mm on the palms and soles to 0.006 mm on the eyelids. The cells of the basal layer (stratum germinativum) divide and migrate upwards to produce the stratum corneum or horny layer. Humans survive in a non-aqueous environment because of the almost impermeable nature of this dead, dense layer, which is crucially important in controlling the percutaneous absorption of drugs and other chemicals. The stratum corneum may be only 10 μm thick when dry but swells severalfold in water. There are two main types of horny layer: the pads of the palms and soles, which are adapted for weight bearing and friction, and the remaining flexible, rather impermeable membranous layer. The basal cell layer also includes melanocytes, which produce and distribute melanin granules to the keratinocytes. Langerhans' cells (important in defence mechanisms operated by the immune system) are prominent in the epidermis.

The dermis

The dermis (or *corium*), at 3–5 mm thick, consists of a matrix of connective tissue woven from fibrous proteins (collagen, elastin and reticulin) that are embedded in an amorphous ground substance of mucopolysaccharide. Nerves, blood vessels and lymphatics traverse the matrix and skin appendages (eccrine sweat glands, apocrine glands, and pilosebaceous units) pierce it. The dermis needs an efficient blood supply to convey nutrients, remove waste products, regulate pressure and temperature, mobilize defence forces and contribute to skin colour. Branches from the arterial plexus deliver blood to sweat glands, hair follicles, subcutaneous fat and the dermis itself. This supply reaches to within 0.2 mm of the skin surface, so that it quickly absorbs and systematically dilutes most compounds passing the epidermis. The generous blood volume in the skin usually acts as a 'sink' for diffusing molecules reaching the capillaries, keeping penetrant concentrations in the dermis very low, maximizing epidermal concentration gradients, and thus promoting percutaneous absorption.

The subcutaneous tissue

The subcutaneous fat (*subcutis, hypoderm*) provides a mechanical cushion and a thermal barrier; it synthesizes and stores readily available high-energy chemicals.

The skin appendages

The *eccrine sweat glands* (2–5 million) produce sweat (pH 4.0–6.8) and may also secrete drugs, proteins, antibodies and antigens. Their principal function is to aid heat control, but emotional stress can also provoke sweating (the clammy palm syndrome).

The *apocrine sweat glands* develop at the pilosebaceous follicle to provide the characteristic adult distribution in the armpit (axilla), the breast areola and the perianal region. The milky or oily secretion may be coloured and contains proteins, lipids, lipoproteins and saccharides. Surface bacteria metabolize this odourless liquid to produce the characteristic body smell.

Hair follicles develop over all skin except the red part of the lips, the palms and soles, and parts of the sex organs. One or more *sebaceous glands*, and in some body regions an apocrine gland, open into the follicle above the muscle that attaches the follicle to the dermoepidermal junction.

Sebaceous glands are most numerous and largest on the face, the forehead, in the ear, on the midline of the back and on anogenital surfaces; the palms and soles usually lack them. These holocrine glands produce sebum from cell disintegration; its principal components are glycerides, free fatty acids, cholesterol, cholesterol esters, wax esters and squalene. Abnormal sebaceous activity may lead to seborrhoea (excess sebum), gland hyperplasia without clinical seborrhoea, obstruction of the pilosebaceous canal (acne and comedones – whiteheads or blackheads), and other types of dysfunction – the dyssebacias.

The *nails*, like hair, consist of 'hard' keratin with a relatively high sulphur content, mainly as cysteine. Unlike the stratum corneum, the nail behaves as a hydrophilic matrix with respect to its permeability.

Functions of the skin

The skin performs many varied functions but here we need consider only some aspects of its containment and protective roles.

Mechanical function

The dermis provides the mechanical properties of skin, with the epidermis playing a minor part. Skin is elastic, but once it has taken up its initial slack it extends further only with difficulty. With age, the skin wrinkles and becomes more rigid. The thin horny layer is quite strong and depends for its pliability on a correct balance of lipids, water-soluble hygroscopic substances (the natural moisturising factor – NMF) and particularly water. The tissue requires some 10–20% of moisture to act as a plasticizer and so maintain its suppleness.

Protective function

Microbiological barrier The stratum corneum provides a microbiological barrier and the sloughing of groups of corneocytes (squames), with their adhering microorganisms, aids the protective mechanism. However, microbes penetrate superficial cracks and damaged stratum corneum may allow access to the lower tissues, where infection may develop. The so-called acid mantle (produced by sebaceous and eccrine secretions, at pH 4.2–5.6) probably does not defend the skin against bacteria via its acidity, as was once thought. However, skin glands also secrete short-chain fatty acids that inhibit bacterial and fungal growth. Nitric oxide, produced from nitrates in sweat, may help to prevent infections from skin pathogens, just as acidified nitrite has an antimicrobial action in the oral and gastrointestinal tracts. Bacteria are unlikely to enter the tiny opening of the inner duct of the eccrine gland; the entrances to the apocrine gland and the hair follicle are much wider, and these appendages may become infected.

Chemical barrier An important function of human skin is to bar the entry of unwanted molecules from outside while controlling the loss of water, electrolytes and other endogenous constituents. The horny layer is very impermeable to most chemicals and usually contributes the rate-limiting step in transdermal absorption. The intact skin is a very effective barricade because the diffusional resistance of the horny layer is large and the permeable appendageal shunt route provides only a small fractional area (about 0.1%).

Radiation barrier For skin exposed to sunlight, ultraviolet light of 290–400 nm is the most damaging. Three main acute reactions follow irradiation: erythema, pigmentation and epidermal thickening. Ultraviolet light stimulates melanocytes to produce melanin, which partially protects the skin. In a severe photosensitive disease such as xeroderma pigmentosum, sunlight may induce changes even in patients whose intense racial pigmentation makes them less susceptible to sunburn. Chronic reactions to sunlight include skin 'ageing', premalignancy and malignancy. Sun-damaged skin may produce solar keratoses, progressing to a squamous cell carcinoma. Bowen's disease, malignant melanoma and basal cell carcinoma may evolve.

Heat barrier and temperature regulation The stratum corneum is so thin over most body areas that it does not effectively protect the underlying living tissues from extremes of cold and heat; it is not an efficient heat insulator. The skin, however, is the organ primarily responsible for maintaining the body at 37 °C. To conserve heat, the peripheral circulation shuts down to minimize surface heat loss; shivering generates energy when chilling is severe. To lose heat, blood vessels dilate, eccrine sweat glands pour out their dilute saline secretion, water evaporates, and removal of the heat of vaporization cools the body.

Electrical barrier In dry skin, resistance and impedance are much higher than in other biological tissues.

Mechanical shock An acute violent blow bruises and blisters the skin; friction may blister or thicken the epidermis, producing callosities and corns. Accidental minor trauma to patients on corticosteroids may severely damage their skin, when the collagen is thinned by drug overuse.

Rational approach to drug delivery to and via the skin

There are three main ways to attack the problem of formulating a successful topical dosage form:

1. We can manipulate the barrier function of the skin: for example, topical antibiotics and antibacterials help a damaged barrier to ward off infection; sunscreen agents and the horny layer protect the viable tissues from ultraviolet radiation; and emollient preparations restore pliability to a desiccated horny layer.
2. We can direct drugs to the viable skin tissues without using oral, systemic or other routes of therapy.
3. The third approach uses skin delivery for systemic treatment. For example, transdermal therapeutic systems provide systemic therapy for conditions such as motion sickness, angina and pain.

Dermatologists aim at five main target regions: skin surface, horny layer, viable epidermis and upper dermis, skin glands and systemic circulation (Figs. 33.1 and 33.2).

Surface treatment

We care for the skin surface mainly by using a simple camouflage or cosmetic application, by forming a

Fig. 33.2 The macroroutes by which drugs penetrate the skin and examples of treatments appropriate to disorders of the various strata (Reproduced with permission from Barry (1983).)

protective layer, or by attacking bacteria and fungi. Some examples include protective films, sunscreens, and barriers that hinder moisture loss and so avert chapping. For topical antibiotics, antiseptics and deodorants, the surface microorganisms are the target. Then, effective surface bioavailability requires that the formulation should release the antimicrobial so it can penetrate the surface skin fissures and reach the organisms. Developmental studies should at least

confirm that the formulation releases and does not bind the medicament.

Stratum corneum treatment

The main therapies aimed at the horny layer improve emolliency by raising water content, or stimulate sloughing (keratosis) with, for example, salicylic acid. The insertion of moisturizing agents or keratolytics into the stratum corneum involves their release from the vehicle and penetration into the tissue. Ideally, the medicament should not enter viable skin, but this is difficult to prevent.

Skin appendage treatment

We may reduce hyperhydrosis of the sweat glands with antiperspirants such as aluminium or other metal salts. In acne we use topical exfolients such as salicylic acid, tretinoin (retinoic acid) or isotretinoin, and benzoyl peroxide and antibiotics such as erythromycin and clindamycin. Other topical antibiotics applied in skin treatment include framycetin and neomycin sulphates, fusidic acid, polymyxins and mupirocin. Depilatories usually contain strontium or barium sulphides, or thioglycolates; male-pattern baldness may be treated with minoxidil and finasteride. Topical imidazoles (clotrimazole, econozole, miconazole, ketoconazole and sulconazole), amoralfine and terbinafine treat fungal diseases of the nails, stratum corneum and hair.

Delivering the medicament to the diseased site is a problem with appendage treatment. For example, it is difficult to achieve a high antibiotic concentration in a sebaceous gland when, as in acne, a horny plug blocks the follicle. When delivered through the skin, the drug may not be sufficiently hydrophobic to partition from the water-rich viable epidermis and dermis into the sebum-filled gland.

Viable epidermis and dermis treatment

We can treat many diseases provided that the preparation delivers drug to the receptor efficiently. However, many potentially valuable drugs cannot be used topically as they do not readily cross the stratum corneum. Hence, investigators may use stratagems such as adding penetration enhancers to diminish this layer's barrier function (see later). Another approach develops prodrugs, which reach the biological receptor and release the pharmacologically active fragment. The efficacy of many topical steroids depends partly on molecular groups that promote percutaneous absorption but which may not enhance drug-receptor binding.

Drug examples include topical steroidal and non-steroidal anti-inflammatory agents; corticosteroids may also be used in psoriasis. Antibiotics include those listed above. Anaesthetic drugs such as benzocaine, amethocaine and lignocaine reduce pain, and antipruritics and antihistamines alleviate itch, but they may cause sensitization. Topical 5-fluorouracil and methotrexate eradicate premalignant and some malignant skin tumours, and treat psoriasis. The psoralens (particularly in conjunction with ultraviolet light – PUVA therapy) mitigate psoriasis; and 5-aminolaevulinic acid (with visible light irradiation – photodynamic therapy) treats skin cancer.

Transcutaneous immunization

The skin has a highly effective immunological surveillance and effector system. A new therapy involves developing transcutaneous immunization via the topical application of vaccine antigens. The process uses an adjuvant such as cholera toxin added to a vaccine antigen (e.g. diphtheria toxoid) to induce antibodies to the diphtheria toxoid. The adjuvant and the antigen target Langerhans' cells, potent antigen-presenting cells in the epidermis. Simple application of the vaccine formulation to the skin of experimental animals and human volunteers has produced positive responses.

Systemic treatment via transdermal absorption

Generally, in the past healthy skin has not been used as a drug route during systemic attacks on disease, with the noteworthy exceptions of nitroglycerin and antileprotics. The body absorbs drugs slowly and incompletely through the stratum corneum, and much of the preparation is lost by washing, by adherence to clothes and by shedding with stratum corneum scales. Other problems include marked variations in skin permeability with regard to subject, site, age and condition, which make control difficult. However, in recent years considerable scientific work has led to the route being used to treat several conditions by means of transdermal patches (see later).

Figure 33.2 illustrates drug penetration routes and examples of treatments appropriate to various skin strata.

DRUG TRANSPORT THROUGH THE SKIN

Basic principles of diffusion through membranes

A useful way to study percutaneous absorption is first to consider how molecules penetrate inert (artificial) membranes, and then move on to the special situation of skin transport. An understanding of the basic principles of permeation through membranes is also valuable in all other areas of biopharmaceutics: oral, buccal, rectal, nasal, lung, vaginal, uterine, injection or eye. The underlying mathematics are also relevant to dosage form design, particularly sustained- or controlled-release formulations and drug targeting.

The diffusion process

In passive diffusion matter moves from one region of a system to another, following random molecular motions. The basic hypothesis underlying the mathematical theory for isotropic materials (which have identical structural and diffusional properties in all directions) is that the rate of transfer of diffusing substance per unit area of a section is proportional to the concentration gradient measured normal to the section. This is expressed as Fick's first law of diffusion:

$$J = -D \frac{\partial C}{\partial x} \qquad (33.1)$$

where J is the rate of transfer per unit area of surface (the flux), C is the concentration of diffusing substance, x is the space coordinate measured normal to the section, and D is the diffusion coefficient. The negative sign indicates that the flux is in the direction of decreasing concentration, i.e. down the concentration gradient. In many situations D is constant, but in more complex materials D depends markedly on concentration; its dimensions are $(length)^2$ $(time)^{-1}$, often specified as $cm^2 \, s^{-1}$.

Fick's first law contains three variables, J, C and x, of which J is additionally a multiple variable, dm/dt, where m is amount and t is time. We therefore usually employ Fick's second law, which reduces the number of variables by one. For the common experimental situation in which diffusion is unidirectional, i.e. the concentration gradient is only along the x-axis, Eqn 33.2 expresses Fick's second law as:

$$\frac{\partial C}{\partial t} = D \frac{\partial^2 C}{\partial x^2} \qquad (33.2)$$

Many experimental designs employ a membrane separating two compartments, with a concentration gradient operating during a run and 'sink' conditions (essentially zero concentration) prevailing in the receptor compartment. If we measure the cumulative mass of diffusant, m, which passes per unit area through the membrane as a function of time, we obtain the plot shown in Figure 33.3. At long times the plot approaches a straight line and from its slope we obtain the steady flux dm/dt (Eqn 33.3):

$$\frac{dm}{dt} = \frac{DC_0 K}{h} \qquad (33.3)$$

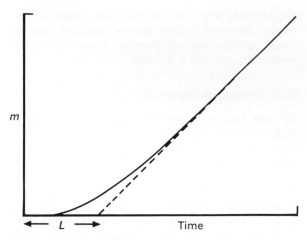

Fig. 33.3 The time course for absorption for the simple zero-order flux case obtained by plotting m, the cumulative amount of diffusant crossing unit area of membrane, as a function of time. Steady state is achieved when the plot becomes linear; extrapolation of the linear portion to the time axis yields the lag time L.

Here C_0 is the constant concentration of drug in the donor solution, K is the partition coefficient of the solute between the membrane and the bathing solution, and h is the thickness of the membrane.

If a steady-state plot is extrapolated to the time axis, the intercept so obtained at $m = 0$ is the lag time, L:

$$L = \frac{h^2}{6D} \qquad (33.4)$$

From Eqn 33.4, D is estimated provided that the membrane thickness, h, is available. Knowing these parameters and C_0, and measuring dm/dt, Eqn 33.3 provides one way of assessing K. Equation 33.3 shows why this permeation procedure may be referred to as a zero order process. By analogy with chemical kinetic operations, Eqn 33.3 represents a zero-order process with a rate constant of DK/h.

Sometimes with biological membranes (such as skin) we cannot separate the value of D from that of K. We then often use a composite parameter, the permeability coefficient, P, where $P = KD$ or $P = KD/h$. The latter definition is used when h is uncertain, e.g. diffusion through skin.

Complex diffusional barriers

Barriers in series The treatment above deals only with the simple situation in which diffusion occurs in a single isotropic medium. However, skin is a heterogeneous multilayer tissue and in percutaneous absorption the concentration gradient develops over several strata. We can treat skin in terms of a laminate, each layer of which contributes a diffusional resistance, R, which is directly proportional to the layer thickness h and indirectly proportional to the product of the layer diffusivity D and the partition coefficient K with respect to the external phase. The total diffusional resistance of all the layers in a three-ply membrane such as skin (stratum corneum, viable epidermis and dermis) is given by the expression:

$$R_T = \frac{1}{P_T} = \frac{h_1}{D_1 K_1} + \frac{h_2}{D_2 K_2} + \frac{h_3}{D_3 K_3} \quad (33.5)$$

Here R_T is the total resistance to permeation, P_T is the thickness-weighted permeability coefficient, and the numerals refer to the separate skin layers.

If one segment has a much greater resistance than the other layers (e.g. the stratum corneum compared to the viable epidermis or dermis) then the single high-resistance phase determines the composite barrier properties. Then $P_T = K_1 D_1/h_1$, where the subscript 1 refers to the resistant phase.

Barriers in parallel Human skin is pierced by shunts and pores, such as hair follicles and sweat glands (Fig. 33.1). Investigators often idealize this complex structure and consider the simple situation in which the diffusional medium consists of two or more diffusional pathways linked in parallel. Then the total diffusional flux per unit area of composite, J_T, is the sum of the individual fluxes through the separate routes. Thus:

$$J_T = f_1 J_1 + f_2 J_2 \ldots \quad (33.6)$$

where f_1, f_2 etc. denote the fractional areas for each diffusional route and J_1, J_2 etc. are the fluxes per unit area of each separate route. In general, for independent linear parallel pathways during steady-state diffusion

$$J_T = C_0 (f_1 P_1 + f_2 P_2 + \ldots) \quad (33.7)$$

where P_1, P_2 ... represent the thickness-weighted permeability coefficients.

If only one route allows diffusant to pass, i.e. the other routes are impervious, then the solution reduces to the simple membrane model with the steady-state flux determined by the fractional area and the permeation rate through the open channel.

Skin transport

The skin is very effective as a selective penetration barrier. The epidermis provides the major control element – most small water-soluble non-electrolytes diffuse into the capillary system 1000 times more rapidly when the epidermis is absent, damaged or

diseased. Furthermore, in the intact skin substances penetrate at rates that may differ 10 000-fold. It is important that pharmaceutical scientists predict and control this selective permeability by relating the physiological and physicochemical attributes of the skin to the properties of the penetrant in a vehicle. We need to correlate the intrinsic properties of the skin barrier with the molecular requirements for breaching it, as modified by interactions with the components of topical vehicles. The eventual aim in dermatological biopharmaceutics is to design drugs with selective penetrability for incorporation into vehicles or devices that deliver the medicament to the active site, at a controlled rate and concentration, for the necessary time.

Routes of penetration

When a molecule reaches intact skin it contacts cellular debris, microorganisms, sebum and other materials. The diffusant then has three potential entry routes to the viable tissue: through the hair follicles with their associated sebaceous glands, via the sweat ducts; or across the continuous stratum corneum between these appendages (see Fig. 33.1). We can summarize the relevant features before arriving at a general conclusion.

Sebum and surface material

The layer of sebum mixed with sweat, bacteria and dead cells is thin (0.4–10 μm), irregular and discontinuous; it hardly affects transdermal absorption. This lack of significant effect may seem surprising, particularly as over 300 volatile compounds have been detected on the skin surface, as well as many non-volatiles.

Skin appendages

Their fractional area available for absorption is small (about 0.1%) and this route usually does not contribute appreciably to the steady-state flux of a drug. However, the route may be important for ions and large polar molecules that cross intact stratum corneum with difficulty. Skin appendages may also act as shunts, important at short times prior to steady state diffusion, e.g. in bioassays that use pharmacological reactions. Thus minute concentrations of nicotinates or corticosteroids penetrating rapidly down the shunt route may quickly trigger erythema or blanching, respectively.

Although we usually ignore the hair follicle route for molecular flux under steady-state conditions, very large molecules and particles of colloidal dimensions can target the follicle. Thus, 'naked' DNA has been used for immunization by topical application. It was speculated that normal follicles have efficient mechanisms for inducing immune responses to proteins in the follicle. A preparation made from antibodies from transgenic plants, when rubbed into the scalp, neutralized the hair-loss effects of toxic chemicals used in cancer chemotherapy. Colloidal particles, such as liposomes and small crystals, are useful for targeting the hair follicle. In general, particles larger than 10 μm remain on the skin surface, those between approximately 3 and 10 μm concentrate in the hair follicle, and when less than 3 μm they penetrate follicles and stratum corneum alike.

Epidermal route

The epidermal barrier function thus resides mainly in the stratum corneum. This has a 'bricks and mortar' structure, analogous to a wall (Fig. 33.1(b)). The corneocytes, consisting of hydrated keratin, comprise the 'bricks'. These are embedded in the 'mortar', which is composed of a complex lipid mixture of ceramides, fatty acids, cholesterol and cholesterol esters, formed into multiple bilayers. Most molecules penetrating through the skin use this intercellular microroute.

Because stratum corneum is dead, it is assumed that there are no active transport processes and no fundamental differences between in vivo and in vitro permeation processes. However, there may be discrepancies in how some substances permeate excised skin and skin in vivo. These differences may arise because we manipulate the skin to insert it into the diffusion apparatus, including possibly damaging it.

Topically applied agents such as steroids, hexachlorophane, griseofulvin, sodium fusidate and fusidic acid may form a depot or reservoir by binding within the stratum corneum.

Diseases that disrupt the horny layer, such as eczema and exfoliative dermatitis, may allow easier access.

The viable layers (particularly the epidermis) may metabolize and inactivate a drug, or activate a prodrug. The dermal papillary layer contains so many capillaries that the average residence time of a drug in the dermis may only be about a minute before it is washed away. Usually, the deeper dermal layers do not influence transdermal absorption, although drugs such as non-steroidal anti-inflammatory agents reach as far down as muscle.

However, the dermis may bind a hormone such as testosterone, decreasing its systemic removal. If the penetrant is very lipophilic it crosses the horny layer to meet an aqueous phase, in which it is poorly soluble. The chemical potential immediately below the barrier may then become high, approaching that in the barrier. The potential gradient (stratum corneum to viable tissue) thus falls, together with the flux. The rate-determining step in percutaneous absorption then becomes barrier clearance, not barrier penetration.

Conclusions

The stratum corneum develops as a thin, tough, relatively impermeable membrane which usually provides the rate-limiting step in transdermal drug delivery. The entire horny layer, not just some specialized region, provides the diffusional resistance. The membrane allows no drug to pass readily, but nearly all low molecular weight molecules penetrate to some extent. The lipid bilayers of the intercellular route provide the main pathway. Diffusion is passive, governed by physicochemical laws in which active transport plays no part.

For electrolytes and large molecules with low diffusion coefficients, such as polar steroids and antibiotics, and for some colloidal particles, the appendages may provide the main entry route.

Once past the horny layer, molecules permeate rapidly through the living tissues and sweep into the systemic circulation.

The fraction of a drug that penetrates the skin via any particular route depends on:

- the physicochemical nature of the drug, particularly its size, solubility and partition coefficient;
- the timescale of observation;
- the site and condition of the skin;
- the formulation;
- how vehicle components temporarily change the properties of the stratum corneum.

PROPERTIES THAT INFLUENCE TRANSDERMAL DELIVERY

When a preparation is applied to diseased skin the clinical result arises from a sequence of processes:

1. Release of the medicament from the vehicle;
2. Penetration through the skin barriers;
3. Activation of the pharmacological response.

Effective therapy optimizes these steps as they are affected by three components, the drug, the vehicle and the skin.

Figure 33.4, which represents the movement of drug molecules arising from, for example, a transdermal drug delivery system with a rate-controlling membrane, illustrates the complexity of percutaneous absorption. Any drug particles must first dissolve so that molecules may diffuse towards the membrane within the patch. The penetrant partitions into the membrane, diffuses across the polymer and partitions into the skin adhesive. The molecules diffuse towards the vehicle/stratum corneum interface. They then partition into the stratum corneum and diffuse through it. Some drug may bind at a depot site; the remainder permeates further, meets a second interface, and partitions into the viable epidermis. For a lipophilic species this partition coefficient may be unfavourable, i.e. less than 1. Within the epidermis, enzymes may metabolize the drug or it may interact at a receptor site. After passing into the dermis, additional depot regions and metabolic sites may intervene as the drug moves to a capillary, partitions into its wall and out into the blood for systemic removal. A fraction of the diffusant may partition into the subcutaneous fat to form a further depot. A portion of the drug can reach deep muscle layers, as illustrated by, for example, the efficacy of non-steroidal anti-inflammatory drugs.

However, there are further complications. The following factors may be important: the non-homogeneity of the tissues; the presence of lymphatics; interstitial fluid; hair follicles and sweat glands; cell division; cell transport to and through the stratum corneum; and cell surface loss. The disease, the healing process, the drug and vehicle components may progressively modify the skin barrier. As vehicle ingredients diffuse into the skin, cellular debris, sweat, sebum and surface contaminants pass into the dermis, changing its physicochemical characteristics. Emulsions may invert or crack when rubbed in, and volatile solvents may evaporate.

To discuss this complicated process in a simple fashion, we review the material under the headings of biological factors and physicochemical factors. However, because transdermal delivery is a dynamic process it should be borne in mind that, as one variable changes, it usually causes several effects on drug flux. The various factors are separated for convenience, but in practice this is an artificial distinction, useful for discussion (and learning) purposes.

Biological factors

Skin condition

The intact, healthy skin is a tough barrier but many agents can damage it. Vesicants such as acids and alkalis injure barrier cells and thereby promote penetration, as do cuts, abrasions and dermatitis. In heavy industry, workers' skins may lose their reactivity or 'harden' because of frequent contact with irritant chemicals.

Many solvents open up the complex dense structure of the horny layer. Mixtures of non-polar and polar solvents, such as chloroform and methanol, remove the lipid fraction, forming artificial shunts through which molecules pass more easily.

Disease commonly alters skin condition; fortunately, for biopharmaceutical purposes we need only an elementary understanding of the gross changes in deranged skin. We are interested mainly in visible damage. Is the skin inflamed, with loss of stratum corneum and altered keratinization? Then

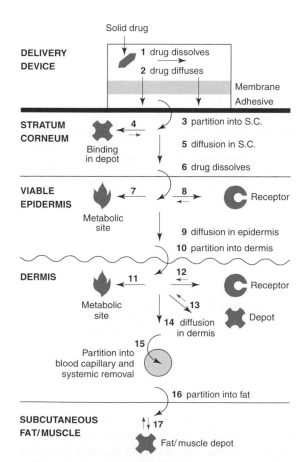

Fig. 33.4 Some stages in drug delivery from a transdermal patch. (Modified from Barry (1983), with permission.)

permeability increases. Is the organ thickened, with corns, calluses and warts, or as in ichthyosis? Drug permeation should now decrease. In diseases characterized by a defective stratum corneum, percutaneous absorption usually increases. Thus, a psoriatic plaque may take up twice as much 8-methoxypsoralen as does uninvolved skin.

After injury or removal of the stratum corneum, within 3 days the skin builds a temporary barrier that persists until the regenerating epidermis can form normal keratinizing cells. Even the first complete layer of new stratum corneum cells formed over a healing layer can markedly reduce permeation.

Skin age

It is often assumed that the skin of the young and the elderly is more permeable than adult tissue, but there is little evidence for any dramatic difference. Children are more susceptible to the toxic effects of drugs and chemicals, partly because of their greater surface area per unit body weight; thus potent topical steroids, boric acid and hexachlorophane have produced severe side-effects and death. Premature infants may be born with no stratum corneum. This can be turned to advantage by treating breathing difficulties with caffeine or pain with buprenorphine, via simple topical application instead of intravenous injection through tiny, delicate veins.

Blood flow

Theoretically, changes in the peripheral circulation could affect transdermal absorption; an increased blood flow could reduce the amount of time a penetrant remains in the dermis, and also raise the concentration gradient across the skin. Usually the effect is not clinically important (although it can be shown experimentally). In clinically hyperaemic skin, any increase in absorption almost always arises because the disease damages the skin barrier. Potent rubefacients, such as nicotinic acid esters, would also only have a significant effect after damaging the skin. Potent vasoconstricting agents, such as topical steroids, could reduce their own clearance rate or that of another drug.

Regional skin sites

Variations in cutaneous permeability around the body depend on the thickness and nature of the stratum corneum and the density of skin appendages. However, the absorption rate varies widely for a specific substance passing through identical skin sites in different healthy volunteers; the most permeable regions in some individuals compare with the least permeable sites in others. Investigators produce different rank orders for the permeabilities of skin sites in general; such permeabilities depend on both the intrinsic resistance to permeation per unit thickness of stratum corneum and the overall thickness of the tissue. As an example, plantar and palmar callus may be 400–600 μm thick compared to 10–20 μm for other sites. However, despite this greater thickness the tissue is less resistant **per unit thickness**, so that the flux of diffusing drug is not so decreased compared to other sites, as might be expected.

Because of the relatively high permeability and ease of access of the site, the hyoscine Transderm system employs the postauricular skin (i.e. behind the ear) to insert drugs into the bloodstream. Originally this site was selected because it was thought that the layers of stratum corneum are thinner and less dense, there are more sweat and sebaceous glands per unit area, and many capillaries reach closer to the surface, increasing its temperature by 4–6°C relative to the thigh. However, facial skin in general is more permeable than other body sites, such as the limbs or torso.

Skin metabolism

The skin metabolizes steroid hormones, chemical carcinogens and some drugs. Such metabolism may determine the therapeutic efficacy of topically applied compounds (particularly prodrugs) and the carcinogenic responses in the skin. It has been estimated that the skin can metabolize some 5% of candidate topical drugs.

Species differences

Mammalian skins differ widely in characteristics such as horny layer thickness, sweat gland and hair follicle densities, and pelt condition. The capillary blood supply and the sweating ability differ between humans and common laboratory animals. Such factors affect the routes of penetration and the resistance to permeation. Subtle biochemical differences between human and animal skins may alter reactions between penetrants and skin. Frequently, mice, rats and rabbits are used to assess percutaneous absorption, but their skins have more hair follicles than human skin and they lack sweat glands. Comparative studies on skin penetration indicate that, in general, monkey and pig skins are most like that of humans. Hairless mouse skin has some similar characteristics: it has been widely used, but its stratum corneum is fragile; hairless rat and fuzzy guinea pig may be better models for humans.

Snake skin has also been selected as it has the benefits that no sacrifice is required (the snake sheds its skin), it is readily available, and there is little leaching of chemicals to confuse UV assays.

Animal skin has been much used to obtain skin penetration data but it is best to use human skin whenever possible.

Physicochemical factors

Skin hydration

When water saturates the skin the tissue swells, softens and wrinkles and its permeability increases markedly. In fact, hydration of the stratum corneum is one of the most important factors in increasing the penetration rate of most substances that permeate skin. Hydration may result from water diffusing from underlying epidermal layers, or from perspiration that accumulates after the application of an occlusive vehicle or dressing. A dramatic example is the use of occlusive plastic films in topical steroid treatment, when the penetration of the steroid often increases tenfold. Occlusion decreases in the order: occlusive films = transdermal patches > lipophilic ointments > w/o cream > o/w cream. Powders, applied either as dusting powders or in lotions, provide a large surface area for evaporation and therefore dry the skin.

Commercial products are often promoted as skin softeners, with the presumption that they increase the skin's moisture content. However, they may contain humectants such as glycerol, propylene glycol or polyethylene glycol and emulsifiers that actually withdraw moisture from the skin.

Table 33.1 summarizes the effects that skin delivery systems may exert on stratum corneum hydration and permeability.

Temperature and pH

The penetration rate of material through human skin can change tenfold for a large temperature variation, as the diffusion coefficient decreases as the temperature falls. However, adequate clothing on most of the body would usually prevent wide fluctuations in temperature and penetration rates. Occlusive vehicles increase skin temperature by a few degrees, but any consequent increased permeability is small compared to the effect of hydration.

According to the simple form of the pH–partition hypothesis, only unionized molecules pass readily across lipid membranes. Now weak acids and bases dissociate to different degrees, depending on the pH and their pK_a or pK_b values. Thus, the proportion of unionized drug in the applied phase mainly determines the effective membrane gradient, and this fraction depends on pH. However, ionized molecules do penetrate the stratum corneum to a limited extent. Because they usually have a much greater

Table 33.1 Expected effects of skin delivery systems on horny layer hydration and skin permeability – in approximate order of decreasing hydration

Delivery system	Examples/constituents	Effect on skin hydration	Effect on skin permeability
Occlusive dressing	Plastic film, unperforated waterproof plaster	Prevents water loss; full hydration	Marked increase
Occlusive patch	Most transdermal patches	Prevents water loss; full hydration	Marked increase
Lipophilic material	Paraffins, oils, fats, waxes, fatty acids and alcohols, esters, silicones	Prevents water loss; may produce full hydration	Marked increase
Absorption base	Anhydrous lipid material plus water/oil emulsifiers	Prevents water loss; marked hydration	Marked increase
Emulsifying base	Anhydrous lipid material plus oil/water emulsifiers	Prevents water loss; marked hydration	Marked increase
Water/oil emulsion	Oily creams	Retards water loss; raised hydration	Increase
Oil/water emulsion	Aqueous creams	May donate water; slight hydration increase	Slight increase?
Humectant	Water-soluble bases, glycerol, glycols	May withdraw water, decreased hydration	Can decrease or act as penetration enhancer
Powder	Clays, organics, inorganics, 'shake' lotions	Aid water evaporation, decreased excess hydration	Little effect on stratum corneum

aqueous solubility than the neutral species, in saturated or near-saturated solutions, they may make a significant contribution to the total flux (i.e. although K may be small for ionized species, C_0 may be very high – see Eqn 33.3).

The stratum corneum is remarkably resistant to alterations in pH, tolerating a range of 3–9.

Diffusion coefficient

The diffusional speed of a molecule depends mainly on the state of matter of the medium. In gases and air, diffusion coefficients are large because the void space available to the molecules is great compared to their size, and the mean free path between molecular collisions is large. In liquids the free volume is much smaller, mean free paths are decreased and diffusion coefficients much reduced. In skin, the diffusivities drop progressively and reach their lowest values within the compacted stratum corneum matrix. For a constant temperature, the diffusion coefficient of a drug in a topical vehicle or in skin depends on the properties of the drug and the diffusion medium and on the interaction between them.

However, the **measured** value of D may reflect influences other than intrinsic mobility. For example, some drug may bind and become immobilized within the stratum corneum, and this process affects the magnitude of D as determined from the lag time (Eqn 33.4). However, regardless of such complications, the value of D measures the penetration rate of a molecule under specified conditions and is therefore useful to know.

Drug concentration

It was seen previously that the flux of solute is proportional to the concentration gradient across the entire barrier phase (Eqn 33.3). Thus, drug permeation usually follows Fick's law. One requirement for maximal flux in a thermodynamically stable situation is that the donor solution should be saturated. A formulator can optimize the solubility of a drug such as a corticosteroid by controlling the solvent composition of the vehicle. Then a saturated solution may be obtained at a selected concentration of the drug by experimenting with a series of solvents or, more usually, by blending two liquids to form a miscible binary mixture with suitable solvent properties.

Although the concentration differential is usually considered to be the driving force for diffusion, the chemical potential gradient or activity gradient is actually the fundamental parameter. Often the distinction is unimportant, but sometimes we must consider it. Thus, the thermodynamic activity of a penetrant in the donor phase or the membrane may be radically altered by, for example, pH change, complex formation, or the presence of surfactants, micelles or cosolvents. Such factors also modify the effective partition coefficient.

Partition coefficient

The partition coefficient (K, see Chapter 2) is important in establishing the flux of a drug through the stratum corneum (Eqn 33.3). When the membrane provides the sole or major source of diffusional resistance, then the magnitude of the partition coefficient is very important: this can differ by a factor of 10^8, drug to drug or (for one penetrant) vehicle to vehicle. The stratum corneum-to-vehicle partition coefficient is then crucially important in establishing a high initial concentration of diffusant in the first layer of the membrane.

Once it was incorrectly thought that good skin penetration required a K close to unity. However, many congeneric series of molecules display an **optimal K**, well below which they are too water soluble to partition well into the horny layer. At higher values the compounds are so lipid soluble that they do not readily pass from the stratum corneum into the water-rich viable tissue. For a drug series this behaviour produces a parabolic or bilinear relation between pharmacological activity and partition coefficient.

Topical steroids provide a good example of the importance of the partition coefficient. Thus, triamcinolone is five times more active systemically than hydrocortisone, but it exhibits only about one-tenth the topical activity. Triamcinolone acetonide, with a more favourable K value, shows a 1000-fold increase in cutaneous activity. Betamethasone possesses only 10 times the topical potency of hydrocortisone, although it is some 30 times stronger systemically. Of the 23 esters of betamethasone tested, the 17-valerate has the highest topical activity and this coincides with the most balanced lipid/water partition coefficient. The anti-inflammatory responses to hydrocortisone and its C-21 esters behave similarly. As the side chain lengthens from 0 to 6 carbon atoms, the partition coefficient increases, as does the anti-inflammatory index. Thereafter the activity declines as the homologous series extends and the partition coefficient further increases.

Polar cosolvent mixtures, such as propylene glycol with water, may produce saturated drug solutions and so maximize the concentration gradient across the stratum corneum. However, the partition coefficient of a drug between the membrane and the solvent mixture generally falls as the solubility in the solvent system rises. Thus, these two factors – increase in solubility and decrease in the magnitude of the partition coefficient – may oppose each other in promoting flux through the membrane, when the system is not saturated. Hence it is important not to oversolubilize a drug if the aim is to promote penetration: the formulation should be at or near saturation.

Surface activity and micellization affect transdermal delivery. There are two main complicating situations in membrane transport, one where the drug is surface active and forms micelles, and the other where additional surfactant is present. When the drug micellizes its total apparent solubility increases dramatically but the apparent partition coefficient decreases. However, the free monomer concentration remains constant, as does the true (monomer) partition coefficient. Then, if the micelle cannot cross the membrane this aggregate has little effect on the permeation process other than by serving as a reservoir to replace monomers as they leave to enter the skin, and by maintaining a constant donor concentration.

When drug and surfactant are present, the effect of surfactant on drug transport is complicated. The drug in the surfactant solution partitions between the micellar and the non-micellar pseudophases. The skin absorption of micellar drug may be negligible and the effective concentration of the unassociated diffusing species may be so lowered that its flux falls drastically. However, all these effects are more important for more permeable membranes such as gastrointestinal or buccal tissue.

Surfactants also have effects on skin that relate to the lowering of interfacial tension at the skin surface and in hair follicles, and changes in protein conformation and disruption of intercellular lipid packing in the stratum corneum. They then function as penetration enhancers – see later.

Complex formation is analogous in many ways to micellar solubilization in the manner in which it affects drug permeation. Thus, when complexes form, the apparent solubility and the apparent partition coefficient of the drug change. An increase in the apparent partition coefficient may promote drug absorption, e.g. some caffeine–drug complexes.

Molecular size and shape

Absorption is apparently inversely related to molecular weight: small molecules penetrate faster than large ones. However, the specific effect of the size of the penetrating molecule on the flux could only be determined if the effect of size could be separated from the resultant change in solubility characteristics. This is difficult to do, as the role of the partition coefficient is so dominant. With rare exceptions, we cannot experimentally increase the size of a molecule without also dramatically changing its partition coefficient.

It is even more difficult to determine the effect of molecular shape, separated from partition coefficient domination, and so nothing is known about this factor in skin permeation.

Ideal molecular properties for drug penetration

From the above considerations, we can deduce the ideal properties that a molecule would require so as to penetrate the stratum corneum well. In brief, these are:

- A low molecular mass, preferably less than 600 Da, when the diffusion coefficient will tend to be high;
- An adequate solubility in oil and water, so that the concentration gradient in the membrane can be high;
- A balanced partition coefficient;
- A low melting point; this correlates with good ideal solubility.

These features explain why transdermal patches can deliver adequate amounts of nicotine to be effective in smoking cessation therapy – this drug illustrates all these requirements well.

DRUG PERMEATION THROUGH SKIN

Stratum corneum rate controlling

It is useful here to summarize the basic concepts used in considering transdermal drug delivery, when the drug, the skin and the vehicle interact. Usually the relative impermeability of the stratum corneum provides the rate-limiting step in percutaneous absorption. The assumptions made in analysing relevant data include:

- Stratum corneum provides the rate-limiting step.
- Skin is a homogenous intact membrane; appendages are unimportant.
- Only a single non-ionic drug species is important, dissolving to form an ideal solution unaffected by pH, and dissolution is not rate limiting.

- Only drug diffuses from the vehicle. Formulation components neither diffuse nor evaporate, and skin secretions do not dilute the vehicle.
- Diffusion coefficient is constant with time or position in the vehicle or horny layer.
- Penetrant reaching viable tissue sweeps into the circulation, maintaining sink conditions below the stratum corneum.
- Donor phase depletes negligibly, i.e. constant drug concentration in the vehicle.
- Vehicle does not alter skin permeability during an experiment by, for example, changing stratum corneum hydration or by acting as a penetration enhancer.
- Drug remains intact and unaltered.
- Flux estimates are steady-state values.

Most analyses use Eqn 33.3, assume that h, the stratum corneum thickness, is constant, and relate changes in the penetration rate to variations in the other three parameters.

An important alternative form of Eqn 33.3 uses thermodynamic activities. Thus:

$$\frac{dm}{dt} = \frac{aD}{\gamma h} \qquad (33.8)$$

where a is the thermodynamic activity of the drug in its vehicle and γ is the effective activity coefficient in the skin barrier. To obtain the maximum rate of penetration, we see that we should use the drug at its highest thermodynamic activity. Now the dissolved molecules in a saturated solution are in equilibrium with the pure solid (which by definition is at maximum thermodynamic activity). The solute molecules are also thus at maximum activity. (It is useful in this context to think of thermodynamic activity as 'escaping tendency', i.e. the drive for the drug to escape from the vehicle and enter the skin). The conclusion, therefore, is that all vehicles that contain the drug as a finely ground suspension (in which the solute activity is maximal and equal to that of the solid) should produce the same penetration rate, *provided that the assumptions above remain valid*. (The effect of supersaturation is dealt with later.)

If we use the placebo vehicle to dilute, for example, an ointment containing a drug in suspension, the drug flux (and hence the clinical efficacy) will not fall until the concentration decreases below the saturation value. This is why many extemporaneously diluted preparations have essentially the same therapeutic activity as their undiluted form – the dilution process never reached subsaturation.

Stratum corneum not rate controlling

Next we consider situations in which the impermeability of the stratum corneum is **not** important, i.e. we are concerned only with drug and vehicle interactions. Then the release of the drug from the vehicle provides the rate-limiting step and the skin functions as a sink. This could happen in a patient with a disrupted or absent horny layer, or when drug diffusion in the vehicle is exceptionally slow. The vehicle also provides the rate-controlling mechanism in many release studies that use either no membrane or an artificial porous membrane. Such experiments may correlate with clinical treatment only for patients with severely damaged skin.

When diffusion within the vehicle provides the rate-controlling step, our mathematical treatment assumes that the skin is a sink. Thus, it maintains essentially zero concentration of the penetrating material by passing it rapidly to the circulation. Then the concentration gradient develops solely in the applied formulation. Two important situations are absorption from solution and from suspension.

Absorption from solution: skin a perfect sink

We can deduce an equation that applies to the release of penetrant from one side of a layer of vehicle on the skin, under the following conditions:

1. Only a single drug species is important, it is in true solution, and it is initially uniformly distributed throughout the vehicle.
2. Only the drug diffuses out of the vehicle. Other components do not diffuse or evaporate, and skin secretions do not pass into the vehicle.
3. The diffusion coefficient does not alter with time or position within the vehicle.
4. When the penetrant reaches the skin, it absorbs instantaneously.

Under these limitations, Eqn 33.9 represents the relationship between m, the quantity of drug released to the sink per unit area of application, and C_0, the initial concentration of solute in the vehicle, D_v, the diffusion coefficient of the drug in the vehicle, and t, the time after application.

$$m \approx 2C_0 \sqrt{\frac{D_v t}{\pi}} \qquad (33.9)$$

Differentiating this equation provides the release rate dm/dt:

$$\frac{dm}{dt} \approx C_0 \sqrt{\frac{D_v}{\pi t}} \qquad (33.10)$$

Figure 33.5 illustrates plots of a typical release experiment for betamethasone 17-benzoate dissolved at various concentrations in a polar gel and diffusing into a chloroform sink. According to Eqn 33.9, a plot of m versus $t^{1/2}$ should provide a straight line, as Figure 33.6 illustrates. A relationship such as Eqn 33.9, or a modification in which m is still proportional to $t^{1/2}$, often fits data outside the limits used originally to define the equation, i.e. up to 65% release instead of only about 30%.

According to these equations we may alter the release rate of a drug from solution, and hence its bioavailability, by changing the drug concentration or the diffusion coefficient.

Absorption from suspensions: skin a perfect sink

The amount and rate of release of a drug suspended in a vehicle, such as an ointment, may be related to time and to the variables of the system. The relevant equations are derived for a simple model system under the following conditions:

1. The suspended drug is micronized so that particle diameters are much smaller than the vehicle layer thickness.
2. The particles are uniformly distributed and do not sediment in the vehicle.
3. The total amount of drug, soluble and suspended, per unit volume (A) is much greater than C_s, the solubility of the drug in the vehicle.

Fig. 33.6 In vitro release of betamethasone 17-benzoate from gel formulations as a function of the square root of time: steroid strength indicated on the plots. (Reproduced with permission from Barry (1983).)

4. The surface to which the vehicle is applied is immiscible with the vehicle, i.e. skin secretions do not enter the vehicle.
5. Only the drug diffuses out of the vehicle; vehicle components neither diffuse nor evaporate.
6. The receptor, which is the skin, operates as a perfect sink.

We can then obtain an equation that relates m to t in the form:

$$m = \sqrt{D_v t(2A - C_s)C_s} \qquad (33.11)$$

Fig. 33.5 In vitro release of betamethasone-17-benzoate from gel formulations as a function of time: steroid strength indicated on plots. (Reproduced from Barry (1983), with permission.)

This equation holds essentially for all times less than that corresponding to complete depletion of the suspended phase. If we differentiate Eqn 33.11 with respect to time, we obtain the instantaneous rate of release, dm/dt, given by:

$$\frac{dm}{dt} = \frac{1}{2}\sqrt{\frac{D_v(2A - C_s)C_s}{t}} \qquad (33.12)$$

For a common condition in which the solubility of the drug in the vehicle is very small and A is appreciable (i.e. $A \gg C_s$), Eqn. 33.11 simplifies to:

$$m \approx \sqrt{2AD_vC_st} \qquad (33.13)$$

Then Eqn 33.12 becomes:

$$\frac{dm}{dt} \approx \sqrt{\frac{AD_vC_s}{2t}} \qquad (33.14)$$

These equations indicate that the formulator can manipulate drug bioavailability from ointment suspensions by altering the diffusion coefficient, the total concentration or the solubility. However, Eqn 33.14 predicts that $dm/dt \propto A^{1/2}$; doubling A only increases dm/dt by about 40%.

For obvious reasons Eqns 33.9–33.14 are often referred to as 'square root of time' relationships; they may also be called Higuchi equations, after the pharmaceutical scientist who developed them. The amount of drug released is proportional to the square route of time; the flux is an inverse function of time$^{1/2}$.

METHODS FOR STUDYING TRANSDERMAL DRUG DELIVERY

Experiments in percutaneous absorption may be designed to answer many questions, such as:

1. What is the drug flux through the skin and how do the apparent diffusion coefficient, partition coefficient, and structure–activity relationships control it?
2. What is the main penetration route – across the stratum corneum or via the appendages?
3. Which is more important clinically or toxicologically – transient diffusion (possibly down the appendages) or steady-state permeation (usually across the intact stratum corneum)?
4. Does the drug bind to the stratum corneum, the viable epidermis or the dermis; does it form a depot in the subcutaneous fat or penetrate to the deep muscle layers?

5. What is the rate-limiting step in permeation – drug dissolution or diffusion within the vehicle or patch; partitioning into, or diffusion through, the skin layers; or removal by the blood, lymph or tissue fluids?
6. How do skin condition, age, site, blood flow and metabolism affect topical bioavailability? Are differences between animal species important?
7. How do vehicles modify the release and absorption of the medicament? What is the optimal formulation for a specific drug – an aerosol spray, a solution, suspension, gel, powder, ointment, cream, paste, tape or delivery device?
8. Are vehicle components inert, or do they modify the permeability of the stratum corneum, if only by changing its hydration state?
9. To increase drug flux, should we use stratagems such as penetration enhancers, iontophoresis etc.?
10. Is the formulation designed correctly to treat intact stratum corneum, thickened epidermis or damaged skin?
11. Should the experimental design produce a pharmacokinetic profile, measuring absorption, distribution, metabolism and excretion in vivo?

No single method can answer all questions and provide a full picture of the complex process of transdermal absorption. We will therefore deal with the important general techniques, dividing them into in vivo and in vitro procedures. The former uses the skins of living humans or experimental animals in situ, whereas the latter employs isolated membranes and includes simple release studies.

In vitro methods

These are valuable techniques for screening and for measuring fluxes, partition coefficients and diffusion coefficients because the investigator can closely control laboratory conditions.

Excised skin

Excised skins from rats, mice and guinea pigs (normal and hairless), rabbits, hamsters, pigs, hairless dogs, snake, monkeys etc. have been mounted in diffusion cells. However, mammalian skin varies widely in stratum corneum properties and the number density of appendages. Thus, it is best to obtain human skin from autopsies, amputations or cosmetic surgery. Investigators use either stratum corneum, epidermis, dermatomed skin or whole skin clamped in a diffusion cell. They measure the compound passing from the stratum corneum side through to a fluid bath. We can consider two main situations and illustrate just some of the many types of diffusion cell used.

In diffusion cells designed to examine steady-state flux and deduce fundamental parameters, a well-stirred donor solution at constant concentration releases penetrant through a membrane into an agitated 'sink' receptor liquid simulating the blood supply (Fig. 33.7). Figure 33.8 shows how three important quantities vary with time: the amount entering the membrane, that passing through (see

also Fig. 33.3 and Eqns 33.3 and 33.4) and that remaining in the membrane.

Diffusion cells aimed more at simulating in vivo or clinical conditions use an agitated receptor solution to correspond to the blood and an unmixed donor phase to represent the formulation (Fig. 33.9). The donor compartment may be closed or open to ambient conditions or to controlled temperature and humidity; the skin may be washed, or materials added during an experiment. The test formulation may be a solid deposited from a volatile solvent, a liquid, a semisolid, a film or a drug device.

A technique known as attenuated total reflectance spectroscopy may also be used to measure passage across stratum corneum to determine the diffusion

Fig. 33.7 Diffusion cells for zero-order or steady-state flux experiments (not to scale). (a) Bank of two cells drilled from a Perspex block. (b) Simple glass diffusion cell suitable for human skin. (c) Glass cell with continuously circulating donor and receptor solutions. (d) Glass cell used for determining vapour diffusion through the skin. D, donor compartment; R, receptor compartment; M, membrane; P, sampling port; BM, bar magnet; SS, stainless steel support; TS, Teflon support; W, well; Dr, drierite. (Reproduced with permission from Barry (1983).)

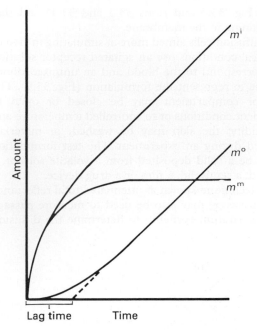

Fig. 33.8 Amount of penetrant entering the membrane (m^i), diffusing through (m^o) and being sorbed (m^m) under zero-order flux conditions. (Reproduced with permission from Barry (1983).)

coefficient of the penetrating molecule. The measuring technique may employ infrared or Raman spectroscopy.

Artificial membranes

Because human skin is variable and difficult to obtain, workers often use other materials, for example cellulose acetate, silicone rubber or isopropyl myristate; or lamellar systems designed to mimic the intercellular lipid of the stratum corneum. However, these membranes are not as complex as human skin and care must be taken if the results of such experiments are to be extrapolated to the clinical situation.

Release methods without a rate-limiting membrane

These procedures record drug release to a simple immiscible phase. They measure only those drug/vehicle interactions that affect release characteristics, and they do not determine skin absorption. Such procedures are mainly valuable in quality control protocols. Typical arrangements are shown in Figure 33.10; Eqns 33.9–33.14 may be used to analyse results.

Fig. 33.9 Diffusion cells for simulation of in vivo conditions (not to scale). (a) Teflon and glass cell. (b) Glass cell with stainless steel support for the membrane. (c) Stainless steel cell with flow through receptor solution. D, donor compartment; R, receptor compartment; M, membrane; P, sampling port; BM, bar magnet; S, polyethylene sail; SS, stainless steel support. (Reproduced with permission from Barry (1983).)

In vivo methods

Often, in vivo methods use animals. However, most animals differ significantly from humans in features that affect percutaneous absorption: the thickness and nature of the stratum corneum, the density of hair follicles and sweat glands, the nature of the pelt, the papillary blood supply and biochemical aspects. Only a few techniques produce animal diseases that are similar to human afflictions. Thus animal models are valuable for studying the anatomy, physiology and biochemistry of skin, for screening topical

Fig. 33.10 Release methods without a rate-limiting membrane (not to scale). (a) Stirrer agitates three phases, which represent the formulation, the skin and the blood supply. (b) Release from an open container to a stirred immiscible receptor phase. (c) Release through a simple dialysis membrane. (Reproduced with permission from Barry (1983).)

agents, for detecting possible hazards, and for preliminary biopharmaceutical investigations. However, experience with animals cannot fully substitute for human studies; regulatory bodies will usually request additional data from human studies before granting a product licence.

Histology

Experimenters may try to locate skin penetration routes from microscopic sections; however, the cutting, handling and development of skin sections encourages leaching and the translocation of materials away from their original sites, a problem with histological methods in general.

Histochemical techniques have been used for those few compounds that produce coloured end-products after chemical reaction. A mistake in the past was to colour a penetrant with a dye and examine skin sections to locate the penetrant. However, each chemical species partitions and diffuses separately, and so the dyed complex dissociates and results are valid only for the dye itself. Added dye, or other different tracer molecules, should not be used.

A few compounds fluoresce, revealing their behaviour by microscopy, e.g. vitamin A, tetracycline and benzpyrene. Tumours fluoresce in photodynamic therapy when treated with 5-aminolaevulinic acid.

Microscopic autoradiography is difficult to apply to diffusable substances without modification.

Substances emit α and β rays, and there may be considerable scattering on the autoradiogram; reducing substances reacting with the photographic emulsion – or an incorrect technique – can produce shadowing. Tritium-labelled isotopes are useful because of their weak emissions; strong β emitters darken areas up to 2 or 3 mm away, a great distance at the cellular scale.

Confocal microscopy can provide information at different depths in the skin.

Surface loss

In theory, we should be able to determine the flux of material into skin from the loss rate from the vehicle. However, because of skin impermeability, the concentration decrease in the vehicle would generally be small and analytical techniques would have to be sensitive and accurate. Also, those differences that could be detected would probably arise because the vehicle changed by evaporation or by dilution with sweat or transepidermal water, and not simply by drug partitioning into the skin. Alternatively, any drug decrease may only reflect deposition on the skin surface or combination with the stratum corneum, rather than penetration to the systemic circulation. Loss techniques have in the past been used mainly to monitor radioactive species; advances in HPLC analysis have made the methods more widely applicable.

Microdialysis

Microdialysis probes are inserted in the dermis and perfused with buffer. Drug molecules pass from the extracellular fluid into the buffer through pores in the membrane, which exclude large molecules, particularly proteins. The resulting drug solution is collected and analysed. For highly protein-bound drugs the technique requires very sensitive methods of analysis, as the drug concentrations in the samples are reduced accordingly.

Analysis of body tissues or fluids

When urinary analysis is used, the entire drug penetrating the skin should be accounted for by 'calibrating' the subject with a slow intravenous injection and a simultaneous determination of blood levels. This procedure allows for the pharmacokinetic factors inherent in drug absorption, distribution, storage, metabolism and excretion. Analysis of circulating blood can present difficulties with dilution, extraction and detection, although we may now routinely detect nanogram drug quantities. Faeces analysis alone has limited use. Sometimes the drug has an affinity for an animal organ, which can be removed and analysed, e.g. for iodine, iodides and mercury. Tissue biopsies may be analysed and even individual sections measured. Adhesive tape can strip sequential layers of the stratum corneum; the individual strips are then analysed for drug content.

Observation of a pharmacological or physiological response

If the drug stimulates a reaction in the viable tissues, we may use this to determine penetration kinetics. Local allergic, toxic or physiological reactions include sweat gland secretion, pigmentation, sebaceous gland activity, vasodilatation, vasoconstriction, vascular permeability, epidermal proliferation and keratinization. The most productive biopharmaceutical technique has been the vasoconstrictor or blanching response to topical steroids. For example, Figure 33.11 illustrates the blanching profiles of betamethasone benzoate in a quick-break aerosol foam, in the foam concentrate and in semisolids, compared with Betnovate Cream. The superiority of the aerosol foam and the inferiority of the benzoate cream are apparent. We use the vasoconstrictor test to screen novel synthetic steroids and develop topical formulations, to test marketed products for bioavailability and clinical efficacy, to perform fundamental studies in percutaneous absorption and to develop dosage regimens.

Fig. 33.11 Blanching response to betamethasone benzoate formulations containing 0.025% steroid and 0.1% betamethasone 17-valerate (B 17-V) cream. (Reproduced with permission from Barry (1983).)

Other response methods include changes in blood pressure (e.g. topical application of nitroglycerin), reduction in pain threshold, and the production of convulsions.

Physical properties of the skin

Relevant methods include the measurement of transepidermal water loss, thermal determinations (particularly differential scanning calorimetry), mechanical analysis, use of ultrasound, classification of function and dimension, spectral analysis (infrared and Raman), and the use of photoacoustic and electrical properties.

Bioassays

Many specialized bioassays screen topical formulations prior to clinical trial, including those for antibacterials, antifungals, antiyeast preparations, antimitotics, antiperspirants, sunscreen agents, antidandruff, anaesthetic–analgesic formulations, antipruritics, antiwart, poison oak/ivy dermatitis, antiacne and psoriasis. Topical corticosteroid bioassays are the most sophisticated and refined of all such bioassays (see previously in this chapter); other steroid bioassays include antigranuloma, thymus involution, inflammation, cytological techniques and psoriasis bioassays.

MAXIMIZING THE BIOAVAILABILITY OF DRUGS APPLIED TO SKIN

Most drugs penetrate human skin poorly, and many major research efforts have attempted to maximize the input of such drugs. The great challenge for the future is to deliver the therapeutic peptides and proteins arising from the biotechnology revolution. The fundamental problem has two major aspects: not only is the stratum corneum a resistant barrier to penetration, but there is great biological variability in its impermeability. This section will therefore consider some ways in which pharmaceutical scientists have attempted to circumvent the horny layer barrier.

Drug or prodrug selection

The simplest way to consider factors that affect the permeation rate of a drug through the stratum corneum is via the simple equation for steady-state flux (Eqn 33.3). When, as is usual, the stratum corneum provides the major source of diffusional resistance of the skin, the partition coefficient of the drug is crucially important in establishing a high initial concentration in the first layer of this membrane. If the drug does not possess the correct physicochemical properties (usually it has too low a partition coefficient), we may be able to design a prodrug with an optimal partition coefficient for entering the skin barrier. After absorption and diffusion to the viable tissues, enzymes convert the prodrug to the active species. Very many steroid derivatives have topical anti-inflammatory activity greater than that of their parent steroids; with their optimized partition coefficients they act as prodrugs (see earlier in this chapter).

Chemical potential adjustment

One scheme for optimizing the bioavailability of a topical medicament is to ensure that the drug exhibits its maximum chemical potential, and thus its maximum thermodynamic activity, within the vehicle (Eqn 33.8).

Under *ideal conditions*, the drug flux through the skin should be directly proportional to the drug activity in the vehicle, provided that D, γ and h remain constant. This has the important conse-

quence that all saturated solutions of a specific drug in any vehicle (providing it does not modify the properties of the stratum corneum) should provide the same maximal flux.

However, it is possible to produce **supersaturated** solutions, either deliberately or via mixed vehicles evaporating on the skin. The theoretical maximum flux appropriate to thermodynamically stable vehicles may then increase manyfold using such supersaturated systems. Because supersaturated preparations are inherently unstable, manufacturers find it difficult to formulate them. An alternative is to employ controlled supersaturation in the rather special environments of transdermal patches; it is thought that this may offer the best hope of success. In practice, therefore, patients usually only meet the effects of supersaturation from volatile systems evaporating on their skin.

Hydration

Hydration of the stratum corneum is one of the most important factors in increasing the penetration rate of most substances: water opens up the compact layer of the horny layer. Moisturizing factors, occlusive films, hydrophobic ointments and transdermal patches all enhance skin bioavailability (see earlier, Skin hydration, and Table 33.1).

Ultrasound (phonophoresis)

This technique, used primarily in physiotherapy and sports medicine, involves placing the topical preparation on the skin over the area to be treated and massaging the site with an ultrasound source. The ultrasonic energy disturbs the lipid packing in the intercellular spaces of the stratum corneum by heating and cavitation effects, and thus enhances drug penetration into the tissue. A problem with the technique is, of course, the need for an ultrasonic probe, correctly focused to work in the stratum corneum. The method is therefore not readily suitable for home use.

Iontophoresis

Iontophoresis, the electrical driving of charged molecules into tissue, has applications in dentistry, ophthalmology, surgery and general medicine. As usually practised, the procedure involves passing a small direct current (approximately 0.5 mA/cm^2) through a drug-containing electrode in contact with the skin. A grounding electrode placed elsewhere on the body completes the electrical circuit. The transport of the charged molecules is driven primarily by electrical repulsion from the driving electrode. However, polar neutral molecules can also be delivered by a current-induced convective flow of water (electro-osmosis). Considerable interest is now being shown in the possible transdermal delivery of therapeutic peptides and proteins, as well as many other drugs.

A problem with the technique is that, although the apparent current density per unit area is low, nearly all the current penetrates via the low-resistance route, i.e. the appendages, particularly the hair follicles. Thus the *actual* current density in the follicle may be high enough to damage growing hair. There is also concern about other possible irreversible changes to the skin.

As with ultrasound there is the problem of home use, although considerable work has been done on miniaturizing systems for patient use, e.g. paper batteries and wristwatch-like devices.

Electroporation

Electroporation is the creation of aqueous pores in the lipid bilayers by the application of short (micro- to millisecond) electrical pulses of approximately 100–1000 V/cm. Flux increases of up to 10 000-fold have been obtained for charged molecules. Again, there is the problem of instrumentation for home use for this potent technique.

Electroporation may combine with iontophoresis to enhance the permeation of peptides such as vasopressin, LHRH (luteinizing hormone-releasing hormone), neurotensin and calcitonin.

Stratum corneum removal

Laser ablation uses high-powered pulses from a laser to vaporize a section of the horny layer so as to produce permeable skin regions. The apparatus is costly and requires expert operation to avoid damage such as burns – it is hardly appropriate for home use. Hot needles have also been proposed.

Adhesive tape can remove the horny layer prior to drug application, as can controlled mechanical dermal abrasion. One other method forms a bleb (blister) by suction, an epidermatome removes the raised tissue, after which a morphine solution delivered directly to the exposed dermis produces fast pain relief.

Photomechanical wave

A drug solution is placed on the skin, covered by a black polystyrene target, and irradiated with a laser pulse. The resultant photomechanical wave produces stresses in the horny layer that enhance drug delivery. The technique is likely to remain experimental.

Needle array

The stratum corneum can be simply bypassed by an injection, and one development of this approach is a device consisting of 400 microneedles to insert drug just below the barrier. The feel to the skin is rather like a cat's tongue, or sharkskin. The solid silicon needles (coated with drug) or hollow metal needles (filled with drug solution) penetrate the horny layer without breaking and without stimulating nerves in the deeper tissues. Flux increases of up to 100 000-fold are claimed. The technique may also be combined with iontophoresis.

Penetration enhancers

Substances exist which temporarily diminish the impermeability of the skin. Such materials, known also as *accelerants* or *sorption promoters*, if they are safe and non-toxic, can be used clinically to enhance the penetration rate of drugs and even to treat patients systemically by the dermal route. The attributes of the ideal penetration enhancer are:

1. The material should be pharmacologically inert.
2. It should be non-toxic, non-irritating and non-allergenic.
3. The action should be immediate and the effect should be suitable and predictable.
4. Upon removal of the material, the skin should immediately and fully recover its normal barrier property.
5. The enhancer should not cause loss of body fluids, electrolytes or other endogenous materials.
6. It should be compatible with all drugs and excipients.
7. The substance should be a good solvent for drugs.
8. The material should be cosmetically acceptable (good spreadability and skin 'feel').
9. The chemical should formulate into all the variety of preparations used topically.
10. It should be odourless, tasteless, colourless and inexpensive.

No single material possesses all these desirable properties. However, very many substances exhibit several of these attributes and they have been investigated clinically or in the laboratory. A sample summary includes:

- Water
- Sulphoxides (especially dimethylsulphoxide) and their analogues
- Pyrrolidones
- Fatty acids and alcohols
- Azone and its derivatives
- Surfactants – anionic, cationic and non-ionic
- Urea and its derivatives
- Alcohols and glycols
- Essential oils, terpenes and derivatives
- Synergistic mixtures.

For safety and effectiveness, the best penetration enhancer of all is water. Most substances penetrate better through hydrated stratum corneum than through the dry tissue. Thus, any chemical which is pharmacologically inactive, non-damaging, and which promotes horny layer hydration, can be considered as a penetration enhancer. Examples include the natural moisturizing factor and urea.

The literature on the use of skin penetration enhancers is voluminous – entire books have been devoted to considering various theories and examples. One simple way to classify enhancer actions is via the *lipid–protein–partitioning* concept. This hypothesis suggests that accelerants act in one or more ways selected from three main possibilities (see Fig. 33.1(b)).

Lipid action The enhancer interacts with the organized intercellular lipid structure of the stratum corneum so as to disrupt it and make it more permeable to drug molecules. Very many enhancers operate in this way. Some solvents may act by extracting the lipid components, thus making the horny layer more permeable.

Protein modification Ionic surface active molecules in particular tend to interact well with the keratin in the corneocytes, to open up the dense keratin structure and make it more permeable. However, the intracellular route is not usually important in drug permeation, although *drastic* reductions to this route's resistance could open up an alternative pathway for drug penetration.

Partitioning promotion Many solvents can enter the stratum corneum, change its solvent properties, and thus increase the partitioning of a second molecule into the horny layer. This molecule may be a drug, a coenhancer or a cosolvent. For example, ethanol has been used to increase the penetration of the drug molecules nitroglycerin and oestradiol. Propylene glycol is also widely used, particularly to provide synergistic mixtures with molecules such as Azone, oleic acid and the terpenes, i.e. to raise the concentration of these enhancers in the horny layer.

Ion pairs

Charged molecules do not readily penetrate the stratum corneum, so investigators have borrowed a technique used in analytical science. This is to form a lipophilic ion pair by adding a suitable species of a charge opposite to that of the drug ion. The complex formed then readily partitions into the lipid of the stratum corneum, as the charges temporarily neutralize each other. The ion pair diffuses across the horny layer to meet the aqueous viable epidermis. There the complex dissociates into its component charged species, which are readily soluble in water and thus partition into the epidermis and diffuse onward. However, the magnitude of the enhancement obtained is not great, typically being only about twofold.

Complex coacervates

Complex coacervation is the separation of oppositely charged ions into a dense coacervate oil phase, which is rich in the ionic complex. A coacervate may be thought of in this context as a further development of ion pairs. Similarly to ion pairs, the coacervate partitions into the stratum corneum, where it behaves as ion pairs, diffusing, dissociating and passing into the viable tissues. As for simple ion pairs, the flux enhancement obtained is similarly modest.

Liposomes and transfersomes

Liposomes are colloidal particles, typically consisting of phospholipids and cholesterol, to which other ingredients may be added. These lipid molecules form concentric bimolecular layers in the form of vesicles, that may be used to entrap and deliver drugs to and through the skin. How well they transport drugs *through* the skin is controversial, although significant enhanced fluxes, compared to saturated aqueous solution (maximum thermodynamic activity), have been obtained for several drugs. For example, the flux of oestradiol has been increased 20-fold using a variety of liposomes. The same vesicles increased 10-fold the deposition of this hormone within the stratum corneum.

Transfersomes are a special type of liposome that incorporate so-called 'edge activators' – molecules such as sodium cholate. The inventors claim that such vesicles are ultradeformable (up to 10^5 times that of an unmodified liposome). As such they can squeeze through pores in the stratum corneum which are less than one-tenth the diameter of the liposome. Thus, sizes up to 200–300 nm can penetrate intact skin. Two particular features are claimed to be important when using transfersomes: they require a hydration gradient to encourage skin penetration, so that they only exhibit their marked delivery abilities when applied to the skin under non-occluded conditions. Then the hydration gradient operating from the (relatively) dry skin surface towards the waterlogged viable tissues drives the transfersomes through the horny layer (Fig. 33.12). Secondly, they work best under in vivo conditions.

Truly remarkable results are claimed for transfersomes. Data indicate that as much as 50% of a topical dose of a protein or peptide (such as insulin) penetrates the skin in vivo in 30 minutes.

High-velocity particles

The PowderJect system fires solid particles through the stratum corneum into the lower skin layers, using a supersonic shockwave of helium gas travelling at Mach 2–3. The claimed advantages of the system include:

- pain-free delivery – the particles are too small to trigger the pain receptors in the skin;
- improved efficacy and bioavailability;
- targeting to a specific tissue, such as a vaccine delivered to epidermal cells;
- sustained release, or
- fast release;
- accurate dosing;
- overcomes needle phobia;
- safety – the device avoids
  - skin damage
  - infection from needles or splashback of body fluids, particularly important for HIV and hepatitis B virus.

Fig. 33.12 Ultradeformable *transfersome* squeezing through minute pores in the stratum corneum, driven by the water concentration gradient. The modified liposome thus penetrates from the horny layer surface (relatively dry) to the wet viable tissues.

However, there have been problems with bruising of the skin and particles bouncing off the skin surface.

A similar device is the Intraject, which is a development of the vaccine gun designed to deliver liquids through the skin without the use of needles.

TRANSDERMAL THERAPEUTIC SYSTEMS

Probably the most innovative practical step in the science of transdermal delivery in recent years has been the introduction into medicine of skin patches.

The original Transdermal Therapeutic System (TTS) or Transdermal (Drug) Delivery System (T(D)DS) was introduced as a device that would release drug to the skin at a controlled rate, well below the maximum the tissue can accept. Thus, the device, not the stratum corneum, would control the rate at which a drug diffuses through the skin, as the intended flux would be much lower than the maximum skin flux.

A TTS tries to provide systemic therapy in a more convenient and effective way than parenteral or oral therapy. The claimed advantages for the percutaneous over the oral route include:

1. Drug administration through the skin eliminates variables that influence gut absorption, such as changes in pH along the gastrointestinal tract, food and fluid intake, stomach emptying time and intestinal motility and transit time, and the presence of human and bacterial enzymes.
2. Drug enters the systemic circulation directly, eliminating the 'first-pass' effect of enzymes in the gut and the liver, the body's main metabolizing organ (but note that skin has its own enzymes and may thus metabolize some 5% of drug types).
3. Transdermal input may provide controlled, constant drug administration, displaying a single pharmacological effect. The continuity of input may permit the use of drugs with short half-lives and improve patient compliance.
4. Percutaneous administration could eliminate pulse entry into the circulation. Peaks in plasma concentrations often produce undesirable effects and troughs may be subtherapeutic.
5. The transdermal route can use drugs with a low therapeutic index.
6. Patches may be readily removed, although there is a reservoir effect and blood levels do not fall immediately to zero after TTS removal.

Transdermal systems usually contain potent drugs that should not irritate or sensitize the skin; they must be stable and have the correct physicochemical properties to partition into the stratum corneum and permeate to the vasculature.

Device design

Manufacturers design patches in a variety of ways, but for simplicity they may be categorized into one of two main types, the monolith (or matrix) or the rate-limiting membrane configurations. In considering these two designs, it is convenient initially to accept the original assumption that the skin under the patch operates as a perfect sink, even though no TTS produced to date works perfectly on this basis.

Monolith or matrix system

In these patches, the Higuchi square root of time law is usually obeyed. Equations 33.9–33.14 illustrate the relationships when the drug is dissolved in the matrix or exists as a suspension; Figure 33.13 illustrates release profiles, plotted both linearly and as square route functions of time. Figure 33.14 illustrates the fundamental construction for a suspension-type TTS. An occlusive backing layer protects the drug

matrix, which comprises a suspension of drug in equilibrium with its saturated solution (maximum thermodynamic activity). An adhesive layer contains dissolved drug in equilibrium with that in the matrix, and attaches the patch to the skin. A protective strippable film is removed prior to application.

Rate-limiting membrane system

As these patches include a membrane, we might expect that the release profile would follow the simple Fickian conditions considered at the beginning of this chapter. Thus, at steady state we would expect the amount of drug released to the skin to be directly related to time (see Eqn 33.3 and Fig. 33.3). However, such a profile only follows when the membrane is initially free of drug. The lag time then represents the period during which the membrane equilibrates with drug *after application to the sink* (in this case the skin). In practice this does not happen, because the drug equilibrates in all patch components on storage, before the patient receives the patch.

Figure 33.15 illustrates the situation; a typical patch in this category consists of a backing layer, a reservoir containing the drug, the membrane, a skin adhesive and the protective film. On storage, the drug equilibrates into the membrane and adhesive. This portion of the drug more readily releases into the skin, as it does not have to permeate through all of the membrane. The result is to produce a so-called burst effect that leads to the type of plot illustrated in Figure 33.16. Such profiles may be confused with Higuchi plots, i.e. with matrix release plots, as illustrated in the first plot of Figure 33.13. An advantage is that the burst component can provide a quick-acting, priming dose of drug.

Future trends

It gradually became apparent to pharmaceutical scientists how difficult it was to formulate a TTS in

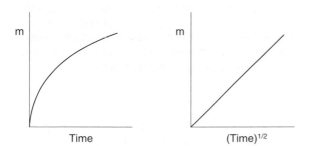

Fig. 33.13 Release profiles, plotted both linearly and as square route function of time, for matrix or monolith patches operating under Higuchi conditions (see Eqn 33.13).

Fig. 33.14 Fundamental construction for a suspension type Transdermal Therapeutic System based on a matrix or monolith design (not to scale).

Fig. 33.15 Transdermal Therapeutic System based on a rate-limiting membrane design (not to scale).

Fig. 33.16 Release profile from rate-limiting membrane patches; effect of increasing amount of drug partitioned into the membrane and adhesive on storage (which provides the 'burst' component).

such a way that the control of delivery remained within the patch and not in the very impervious skin of the patient. It is also expensive to manufacture complex, multilayered patches, particularly those containing membranes. There is thus a trend to concentrate on simple designs that are also thinner and therefore less obtrusive (cosmetically more acceptable). The result is a move towards the simple adhesive matrix patch illustrated in Figure 33.17.

Clinical patches

The following section discusses some examples of TTSs used in therapy. Besides their inherent clinical interest and value, each one exemplifies one or more biopharmaceutical features of importance in this mode of disease management.

Transdermal scopolamine (hyoscine)

The first patch brought to market delivered hyoscine through the thin, relatively permeable postauricular skin, via a rate-controlling membrane. The contact adhesive liberates priming drug to saturate horny layer binding sites and thus reduces the time before the clinical effect arises.

The TTS treats motion sickness and, apart from its value to cruise passengers, it was used by American astronauts. It can control the emetic side-effects of anticancer drugs, inhibit radiation sickness and

Fig. 33.17 Simple drug-in-adhesive patch (not to scale).

control vertigo. Two-thirds of patients still experience a dry mouth, but woodwind instrumentalists in orchestras have turned even this to advantage: they have found that application of the patch suppresses salivation.

This patch provides an excellent example of the original basic philosophy of TDDSs. In the usual dosage form of injections or tablets, hyoscine can produce side-effects such as excitement, confusion and hallucinations, which the controlled input from the TDDS eliminates. About 70% of the control resides in the patch; the variable nature of the patient's skin affects the remainder.

Transdermal nitroglycerin (glyceryl trinitrate, GTN)

A major use of TDDS technology is to deliver nitroglycerin, isosorbide dinitrate and isosorbide mononitrate for the treatment of angina, congestive heart failure and acute myocardial infarction. The nitroglycerin patch can also be valuable for the prophylactic treatment of phlebitis and extravasation secondary to venous cannulation.

The introduction of the first nitroglycerin device led to a vigorous debate as to the relative merits of patches, ointments and tablets. The main arguments revolved around whether or not the patch system delivered suboptimal drug levels to the blood; whether tolerance developed to the nitroglycerin; and if the TDDS or the patient's skin controlled the rate of GTN input. With regard to the last point, it was concluded that only about 50% or less of the control was inherent within the device.

Transdermal oestradiol

Several oestradiol systems treat women for menopausal symptoms or other results of oestrogen deficiency (hormone replacement therapy, HRT). The claimed benefits of transdermal delivery over oral therapy for such patches include:

- First-pass metabolism is avoided; therefore a lower dose is administered.
- Continuous, low-rate transdermal dosing maintains oestrogen plasma levels within physiological limits.
- Such dosing does not affect the blood levels of proteins produced by the liver. In particular, the angiotensin concentration remains the same and therefore the risk of hypertension is minimized. (Oral oestrogen therapy has been likened to hitting the liver with a sledgehammer!) However,

as liver enzymes are not stimulated, the beneficial effects on serum lipids are absent.

- Large increases in oestrone (the major metabolite of oestradiol) are avoided and the oestrone:oestradiol ratio restores to the premenopausal value.

Originally, the oestrogen patch was marketed only for women who had undergone a hysterectomy, because unopposed oestrogen (that which is given alone) can cause endometrial hyperplasia and increase the risk of endometrial cancer. Now women with an intact uterus can use combination patches that deliver oestradiol for 2 weeks, followed by a further 2 weeks of a progestin such as norethysterone acetate or levonorgestrel.

Patches are applied once or twice weekly and are effective in treating menopausal and post-menopausal symptoms such as flushing and vaginal atrophy. They also appear to be valuable in treating osteoporosis. Their contribution to reduction in the risk of cardiovascular disease remains to be clarified.

Transdermal clonidine

This formulation was originally introduced to treat hypertension. It was then reported to ameliorate some of the short-term symptoms associated with stopping smoking (craving, irritability, anxiety, restlessness and hunger).

After its introduction, clinical trials revealed a high incidence of topical irritation to clonidine (up to 50% of patients were affected). This finding emphasizes the importance of screening drug candidates for such side-effects before committing significant resources to a transdermal delivery programme.

Transdermal fentanyl

This opioid analgesic patch treats chronic intractable pain, such as that produced by cancer, over a 72-hour period. A TTS providing 25 μg of fentanyl per hour is approximately equivalent to the oral administration of 90 mg of morphine sulphate daily.

Transdermal nicotine

There are several such patches available and commercial competition is intense because of the huge worldwide market for smoking cessation therapy. Within the first year of introduction, total sales exceeded that for any other drug in history. However, as is common to most forms of antismoking treatment, subsequent yearly sales fell dramatically.

The TTSs provide an alternative to treatment via nicotine chewing gum, lozenges, sublingual tablets, nasal sprays and inhalers. The patches, designed to be worn for 16 or 24 hours, are available in different strengths so as to provide a weaning process. The concept is to try to match the plasma trough levels of nicotine produced by cigarette smoking, but not to mimic the 'hit' arising from inhalation. (A bolus of nicotine reaches the brain within seconds after inhaling from a cigarette – this is the main *physiological* component of addiction).

The nicotine patch can also maintain labour when there is danger of a premature delivery, and a patient with Parkinson's disease has claimed that the device had 'restored him to his pre-Parkinson's self'. Tourette's syndrome is a bizarre disorder characterized by jerky motions, rage and a propensity to utter obscenities: nicotine patches improved the effectiveness of drugs used in the treatment of afflicted children.

Nicotine is an ideal skin penetrant as it has a low molar mass, is liquid (low melting point), has a balanced partition coefficient and is miscible with oil and water (see Ideal properties for drug penetration, earlier in this chapter).

Transdermal testosterone

Hypogonadism (arising from pituitary or testicular disorder) afflicts 1 in 200 men, and testosterone deficiency may also arise from accidents and orchidectomy. The first patch developed was applied to the shaved scrotum, as scrotal skin is the most permeable skin site in males. With developments in formulation, more convenient areas, such as the back, abdomen, thigh or upper arm, may be used.

General conclusions on the usage of transdermal patches

- In recent years the formulation of transdermal patches has been a vibrant developmental area within the pharmaceutical industry.
- However, the original concept that the patch, not the skin, should control drug input to the patient has not been realized; no marketed patch fully controls the drug flux.
- There has been a move from a complex patch structure towards a simpler matrix formulation.
- Future progress will depend on:
  - correct choice of drug
  - synthesis of prodrugs
  - development of suitable penetration enhancers.

- There is a need to solve problems relating to, e.g.:
  - irritancy,
  - sensitization,
  - cutaneous metabolism,
  - localized body load of drug,
  - wearability of the patch for up to 7 days; the device must:
    - be thin, flexible and unobtrusive
    - adhere well when the patient sweats, exercises and bathes
    - not encourage microbial growth
    - not collect dirt around the periphery (where the adhesive contacts the environment).

FORMULATION OF DERMATOLOGICAL VEHICLES

People apply many skin preparations, ranging from powders, through semisolids to liquids. Formulators have often in the past developed such preparations for stability, compatibility and patient acceptability rather than considering the influences that the components may have on drug bioavailability. Modern formulation methods nowadays, however, have to concentrate on biopharmaceutical principles.

A valuable approach in designing a vehicle to produce optimum bioavailability is to use fundamental permeation theories, while remembering that the treatment regimen and the diseased skin usually violate the constraints of simple diffusion theory. However, with our present knowledge, such a formal approach may often limit the investigator to a single-phase system such as a polar gel; multiphase systems usually provide intractable theoretical problems. But physicians usually want a topical application to provide several therapeutic effects, as well as good absorption. These aims include anti-inflammatory efficacy in acute inflammation, symptomatic relief of pain and itch, protection from irritation, cleansing, and lubricant and emollient actions. A single-phase vehicle cannot readily achieve so much: complex multicomponent bases are necessary. Patients also tend to favour creams rather than gels or ointments.

This section considers the formulation of vehicles mainly in terms of *unmedicated* preparations. A good base must foster the remarkable recuperative capability of skin. For minor conditions it is often as important to select a vehicle that promotes healing and does no further damage, as it is to apply a therapeutic agent. A general rule is that for wet lesions the patient should use an aqueous dressing,

and for dry skin a lipophilic base is best. Most vehicles are blended from one or more of three main components – aqueous solvents, powder and oil – together with thickening and emulsifying agents, buffers, antioxidants, preservatives, colours, propellants etc. We shall consider typical examples of the main types of skin preparation.

Dermatological formulations

Liquid preparations

Liquid preparations for external application include simple soaks or baths, applications, liniments, lotions, paints, varnishes, tinctures, and ear drops. A simple soak provides an active ingredient in aqueous solution or suspension, sometimes with water-miscible solvents. Gums and gelling agents may vary the consistency, from mobile liquids to stiff ringing gels. Bath additives such as Oilatum Emollient deposit a layer of liquid paraffin on the stratum corneum in an attempt to maintain its moisture content by occlusion. Applications may be liquid or viscous and often incorporate parasiticides, e.g. dicophane, benzyl benzoate, gamma benzene hexachloride and malathion. Liniments may be alcoholic or oily solutions or emulsions, which should not be applied to broken skin. Lotions are aqueous solutions or suspensions from which water evaporates to leave a thin uniform coating of powder. Evaporation cools and soothes the skin, making lotions valuable for treating acutely inflamed areas. Alcohol enhances the cooling effect and glycerol sticks the powder to the skin. Lotions may also be dilute emulsions, usually of the oil-in-water type. Paints, varnishes and tinctures present solutions of active ingredients in volatile solvents such as water, industrial methylated spirits, acetone or ether. Ear drops are often aqueous solutions, although glycerol and alcohol may also be used.

Gels (jellies)

Gels are two-component semisolid systems rich in liquid. Their one characteristic feature is the presence of a continuous structure providing solid-like properties. In a typical polar gel, a natural or synthetic polymer builds a three-dimensional matrix throughout a hydrophilic liquid. Typical polymers used include the natural gums tragacanth, carrageenan, pectin, agar and alginic acid; semisynthetic materials such as methylcellulose, hydroxyethylcellulose, hydroxypropylmethylcellulose and carboxymethylcellulose; and the synthetic polymer Carbopol (carbomer). Certain clays such as bentonite, Veegum and Laponite may be also used. Provided that the drug does not bind to the polymer or clay, such gels release medicaments well; the pores allow relatively free diffusion of molecules that are not too large.

Powders

Dusting powders for application to skin folds are finely divided (impalpable) insoluble powders which dry, protect and lubricate, e.g. talc, zinc oxide, starch and kaolin. Dusting powders should not contain boric acid, as abraded skin may absorb it in toxic amounts.

Ointments

Ointments are greasy, semisolid preparations, often anhydrous and containing dissolved or dispersed medicaments.

Hydrocarbon bases These usually consist of soft paraffin or mixtures with hard paraffin. Paraffins form a greasy film on the skin, inhibiting moisture loss and improving hydration of the horny layer in dry scaly conditions. This hydration is also a main reason why ointments are so effective in encouraging percutaneous absorption of a drug.

The Plastibases are a series of hydrocarbons containing polyethylene, which forms a structural matrix in systems which are fluid at the molecular scale but are typical dermatological semisolids. They are soft, smooth, homogenous, neutral, colourless, odourless, non-irritating, non-sensitizing, extremely stable vehicles. Plastibases are compatible with most medicaments and they maintain their consistency even at high concentrations of solids and under extremes of temperature. The bases apply easily and spread readily, adhere to the skin, imparting a velvety, non-greasy feel, and can readily be removed.

Soap-based greases may be produced by, for example, incorporating aluminium stearate in a heavy mineral oil. A random arrangement of metallic soap fibres weaves throughout the oil, producing a product which changes its consistency only slightly when heated; the base readily incorporates drugs and the addition of lanolin permits the absorption of a little water.

Fats and fixed-oil bases Dermatological vehicles have frequently contained fixed oils of vegetable origin, consisting essentially of the mono-, di- and triglycerides of mixtures of saturated and unsaturated fatty acids. The most common oils include peanut, sesame, olive, cottonseed, almond, arachis, maize and persic. Such oils can decompose on exposure to air,

light and high temperatures, and may turn rancid. Trace metal contaminants catalyse oxidative reactions which the formulator combats with antioxidants, such as butylated hydroxytoluene, butylated hydroxyanisole or propyl gallate, or with chelating agents such as the salts of ethylenediaminetetraacetic acid (EDTA). However, antioxidants may be incompatible with the drug or they may sensitize some patients.

Silicones Dimethicones, or dimethyl polysiloxanes, have properties similar to hydrocarbon bases. They are water repellent with a low surface tension and are incorporated into barrier creams to protect the skin against water-soluble irritants.

Absorption bases Absorption bases soak up water to form water-in-oil emulsions while retaining their semisolid consistencies. Generally, they are anhydrous vehicles composed of a hydrocarbon base and a miscible substance with polar groups that functions as a water-in-oil emulsifier, e.g. lanolin, lanolin isolates, cholesterol, lanosterol and other sterols, acetylated sterols, or the partial esters of polyhydric alcohols such as sorbitan monostearate or mono-oleate. Bases such as Wool Alcohols Ointment BP and Simple Ointment BP deposit a greasy film on the skin, similar to a hydrocarbon base, but they suppress less the transepidermal water loss. However, they may hydrate the stratum corneum by applying a water-in-oil emulsion, thereby prolonging the time during which the horny layer can absorb moisture. Some individuals are sensitive to lanolin. This may be important because the sensitization occurs unexpectedly and physicians frequently overlook it, especially in atopic patients, who may apply large quantities of lanolin-containing emollients for protracted periods. Modern purified lanolin preparations are less sensitizing.

Emulsifying bases These essentially anhydrous bases contain oil-in-water emulsifying agents which make them miscible with water and so washable or 'self-emulsifying'. There are three types, depending on the ionic nature of the water-soluble emulsifying agents: anionic (e.g. Emulsifying Ointment), cationic (e.g. Cetrimide Emulsifying Ointment) and non-ionic (e.g. Cetomacrogol Emulsifying Ointment). Because they contain surfactants, emulsifying bases may help to bring the medicament into more intimate contact with the skin. The bases mix with aqueous secretions and readily wash off the skin; thus they are useful for scalp treatments.

Water-soluble bases Formulators prepare water-soluble bases from mixtures of high and low molecular weight polyethylene glycols (macrogols, Carbowaxes). Suitable combinations provide products with an ointment-like consistency, which soften or melt on skin application. They are non-occlusive, mix readily with skin exudates and do not stain sheets or clothing; washing quickly removes any residue. The macrogols do not hydrolyse, deteriorate, support mould growth or irritate the skin. Examples include Macrogol Ointment and Polyethylene Glycol Ointment; because they are water-soluble, they will not take up more than 8% of an aqueous solution before losing their desirable physicochemical characteristics. To enable a base to incorporate more water stearyl alcohol can be substituted for some of the macrogol component. Macrogol bases are used with local anaesthetics such as lignocaine, but they are incompatible with many chemicals, including phenols, iodine, potassium iodide, sorbitol, tannic acid, and the salts of silver, mercury and bismuth. The bases diminish the antimicrobial activity of quaternary ammonium compounds and methyl and propyl parahydroxybenzoates, and rapidly inactivate bacitracin and penicillin.

Creams

Creams are semisolid emulsions for external application. Oil-in-water emulsions are most useful as water-washable bases, whereas water-in-oil emulsions are emollient and cleansing. Patients often prefer a w/o cream to an ointment because the cream spreads more readily, is less greasy, and the evaporating water soothes the inflamed tissue. O/w creams ('vanishing' creams) rub into the skin; the continuous phase evaporates and increases the concentration of a water-soluble drug in the adhering film. The concentration gradient for drug across the stratum corneum therefore increases, promoting percutaneous absorption. To minimize drug precipitation, a formulator may include a less volatile, water-miscible cosolvent. An o/w cream is non-occlusive because it does not deposit a continuous film of water-impervious liquid. However, such a cream can deposit lipids and other moisturizers on and into the stratum corneum and so restore the tissue's hydration ability, i.e. the preparation has emollient properties.

It is difficult to predict the role that an emulsion plays in percutaneous absorption. This is because, added to all the physiological and physicochemical considerations already discussed, the following must also be considered:

- Partitioning of the medicament between the emulsion phases;
- The addition of preservatives;
- Determination of a true viscosity for the diffusing molecules in the vehicle;

- The possibility of phase inversion or cracking of the emulsion when applied to the skin.

Drug may also be trapped in the micelles and the gel and liquid crystalline phases present in the continuous phase. Emulsions are complex systems and so all medicaments must be considered individually with respect to emulsion design. There are few worthwhile formulation guidelines additional to the principles already discussed.

Pastes

Pastes are ointments containing as much as 50% powder dispersed in a fatty base. They may be useful for absorbing noxious chemicals in babies, such as the ammonia that bacteria release from urine. Because of their consistency, pastes localize the action of an irritant or staining material, such as dithranol or coal tar. They are less greasy than ointments because the powder absorbs some of the fluid hydrocarbons. Pastes lay down a thick, unbroken, relatively impermeable film that can be opaque and act as an efficient sun filter. Skiers use such formulations on the face to minimize windburn (excessive dehydration) and to block out the sun's rays.

Aerosols

Aerosols may function as drug delivery systems for solutions, suspensions, powders, semisolids and emulsions.

Solution aerosols are simple products with the drug dissolved in a propellant or a propellant/solvent mixture. Typical agents incorporated are steroids, antibiotics and astringents. The powder aerosol methodology is useful for difficult soluble compounds such as steroids and antibiotics. Semisolid preparations, such as ointments and creams, may be prepared in a flexible bag with compressed nitrogen used for expulsion instead of a volatile propellant. Emulsion systems produce foams that may be aqueous or non-aqueous and stable or quick-breaking. Medicinal stable foams are aqueous formulations used, for example, for preoperative shaving and for contraception. The stable foam, which is similar to a medicated shaving cream, varies in stability depending on the surfactant, solvent and propellant used.

Cosmetic or aesthetic criteria for dermatological formulations

However well designed a topical vehicle for maximum drug bioavailability is, the preparation must still be acceptable to the patient. A product that is poor in appearance may lead to non-compliance. Patients generally prefer a formulation which is easy to transfer from the container, spreads readily and smoothly, leaves no detectable residue, and adheres to the treated area without being tacky or difficult to remove. The dosage of such preparations is typically in the range of 1–5 mg/cm^2 of skin.

Stiff pastes may be hard to rub into the skin or to apply evenly; application to damaged areas may therefore be painful. However, a thick layer of material can occlude the tissue or protect it from mechanical, chemical or light damage. Ointments and pastes do this, and the viscous drag imposed on application may dislodge scales, dead tissue and the remnants of previous doses. The medicament then makes intimate contact with the diseased site. A stiff preparation also helps to delineate the area of treatment.

The sensations of greasiness and tackiness arise from those constituents that form the skin film. For creams, stearic acid and cetyl alcohol produce non-tacky films. Formulations that include synthetic or natural gums should use the minimum amount, as the polymers tend to leave a tacky coating on the skin.

Insoluble solids leave an opaque layer that often appears powdery or crusty. However, as therapy requires such solids in lotions and pastes, the formulator can do little to vary the film's nature and patients accept the residue as part of the treatment.

Physicochemical criteria for dermatological formulations

The developer of dosage forms must note the physical and chemical behaviour of the drug and the dosage form during preformulation studies, throughout bench-scale work, pilot studies and batch processing, at the manufacturing level, and during storage and use of a product. Some general factors that a pharmaceutical scientist evaluates for a new semisolid during developmental studies and storage include:

- Stability of the active ingredients
- Stability of the adjuvants
- Rheological properties – consistency, viscoelasticity, extrudability
- Loss of volatiles, including water
- Phase changes – inhomogeneity, bleeding, cracking
- Particle size distribution of dispersed phase
- Apparent pH
- Particulate contamination.

The first difficulty arises in assessing the chemical stabilities of the drug (in its complex vehicle) and the adjuvants. A general method establishes a shelf-life by using an accelerated stability test at elevated temperatures and the Arrhenius relationship. However, for a multiphase system such as a cream, heat may change the phase distribution and may even crack the emulsion. Thus, the investigator may have to assess the preparation for a long time at the storage temperature. Because of vehicle complexity, it may be difficult to separate the labile components for analysis.

Many dermatologicals contain volatile solvents, and batches may lose some solvent through the walls of plastic containers or through faulty seams or ill-fitting caps.

Heterogeneous systems may suffer phase changes when stored incorrectly. Emulsions may crack and cream, suspensions can agglomerate and cake, and ointments and gels may 'bleed' as their matrices contract and squeeze out constituents. High temperatures can produce or accelerate such adjustments. Multipoint rheological assessments can readily quantify structural changes in colloidal systems; viscoelastic determinations, such as creep and oscillation, are also valuable.

For suspensions and emulsions, a particle size analysis may often detect a potentially unstable formulation long before any other parameter changes markedly. Emulsion globules may grow through coalescence as gel networks break down on storage; crystals may enlarge or change their habit, or revert to a more stable, less active polymorphic form. Such alterations in crystal form may affect the therapeutic activity of the formulation.

The apparent pH of a topical product may change on storage. Although pH measurements of complex vehicles have no fundamental meaning, investigators sometimes use a pH electrode to monitor formulations as they age.

It can be difficult to manufacture creams and ointments completely free from foreign particles. Aluminium and tin tubes may contaminate a topical with 'flashings' – metal slivers and shavings formed during container fabrication. Their presence is particularly undesirable in ophthalmic ointments, and various pharmacopoeial tests limit the extent of such contamination. Plastic tubes are now generally used.

In addition to instrumental tests, the pharmaceutical scientist should note any qualitative changes during product storage. The colour may vary, e.g. natural fats, oils and lanolin brown as they oxidize, becoming rancid with a disagreeable odour. The texture may alter as phase relationships vary.

Microbial contamination and preservation: rancidity and antioxidants

Topical bases often contain aqueous and oily phases, together with carbohydrates and even proteins, and so bacteria and fungi readily attack them. Microbial growth spoils the formulation and is a potential toxic hazard and a source of infection. Conditions that lower immunity, such as injury, debilitating diseases or drug therapy, may encourage organisms that are usually not highly infectious to infect the host, i.e. to become opportunistic pathogens. In 1969, 33 samples of 169 cosmetics and topical drugs surveyed were microbially contaminated, half with Gram-negative organisms which were a health hazard. In the mid-1960s, an outbreak of serious eye infection was traced to an antibiotic ophthalmic ointment contaminated with *Pseudomonas*.

There are many potential sources of microbial contamination. It can occur in raw material and in the manufacturing water, in processing and filling equipment, in packing material, if there is poor plant hygiene or an unclean environment, and if plant operatives fail to comply with good manufacturing procedures.

Because of the complexity of dermatological vehicles and their manufacturing processes there exists no universal preservative, although we can summarize the essential requirements for selecting a material to preserve a specific formulation. The additive must be compatible with all ingredients; it should be stable to heat, prolonged storage and product use conditions; and it must be non-irritant, non-toxic and non-sensitizing to human tissue.

Many prototype pharmaceutical preparations could deteriorate on storage because some components oxidize when oxygen is present. This decomposition can be particularly troublesome in emulsions, because emulsification may introduce air into the product and because of the high interfacial contact area between the phases.

The ideal antioxidant would possess the following properties:

- Effective at low concentrations;
- It and its decomposition products should be non-toxic, non-irritant, non-sensitizing, odourless and colourless;
- Stable and effective over a wide pH range;
- Neutral – should not react chemically with other ingredients;
- Non-volatile.

PROTOCOL FOR DESIGNING, DEVELOPING AND TESTING A DERMATOLOGICAL FORMULATION

Below are listed steps that may help a pharmaceutical scientist to design a satisfactory formulation. The treatment, although condensed, is useful for providing a checklist to control the development programme.

1. Identify the disease or condition to be treated.
2. Determine the site for drug action – skin surface, stratum corneum, viable epidermis, dermis, appendages or systemic circulation. Consider the body region, e.g. scalp, trunk, feet, nails etc.
3. Note the receptor site within the target area (this may be unknown).
4. Estimate the condition of the average patient's skin – thickened (e.g. ichthyosis), broken and inflamed (e.g. acute eczema), pilosebaceous unit blocked (acne), etc. Remember that successful treatment may rapidly change the condition of the skin. For example, a weeping, wet skin without an intact horny layer may heal quickly to produce a few cell layers with a dry surface.
5. Choose the best drug or prodrug for the disorder; consider its pharmacological and pharmacokinetic profiles, toxicity, sensitizing potential, stability, susceptibility to skin enzyme metabolism and physicochemical properties (particularly the diffusion coefficient and partition coefficient relevant to the horny layer).
6. Evaluate the optimum kinetics for drug delivery to the target site. Consider pulsed or steady-state treatment, amount and strength of dosage form and frequency of application.
7. In the light of points 1–6 above, select the type of formulation needed, e.g. cream, ointment, aerosol, delivery device.
8. Decide whether and where there is a rate-limiting step in the treatment, e.g. solely within the vehicle, permeation across the stratum corneum, or clearance from the viable tissues. Concentrate on maximizing this rate.
9. Choose vehicle ingredients that are stable, compatible, and cosmetically and therapeutically acceptable. Be aware that these adjuvants may have their own therapeutic effects, e.g. occlusive vehicles moisturize the skin.
10. If the intention is to promote drug penetration, optimize the formulation to the maximum chemical potential of the drug. Remember that

vehicles often change after application as components evaporate or penetrate the skin and secretions mix with the formulation.

11. If the drug is a poor penetrant consider using a penetration enhancer, but remember that a new enhancer will need a full toxicological screen. Regulatory authorities are particularly cautious about the use of such promoters.

12. Perform in vitro tests with trial formulations using a simple synthetic membrane (or no membrane) and a suitable sink; ensure that the drug releases readily from the vehicle.

13. Repeat 12, preferably with human skin, to monitor permeation. Such experiments may include a steady-state design and a scheme that mimics clinical use (the so-called finite dose design).

14. Conduct in vivo studies in animals and human volunteers to check for efficacy, safety and acceptability; determine the pharmacokinetic profile and the topical bioavailability.

15. Do clinical trials.

16. Throughout the programme, review the physicochemical behaviour and stability of the dosage form and package during preformulation studies, scale-up procedures, manufacture, storage and use.

BIBLIOGRAPHY

Barry, B.W. (1983) *Dermatological Formulations: Percutaneous Absorption*. Marcel Dekker, New York. (Provides additional fundamental information and general background.)

Bronaugh, R.L. and Maibach, H.I. (eds) (1999) *Percutaneous Absorption*, 3rd edn. Marcel Dekker, New York. (A modern multiauthored text with many relevant chapters.)

Chien, Y.W. (1992) *Novel Drug Delivery Systems*. 2nd edn, Chapter 7. Marcel Dekker, New York. (First two chapters provide background on rate-controlled drug delivery.)

Hsieh, D.S. (ed) (1994) *Drug Permeation Enhancement*. Marcel Dekker, New York. (Parts I, II and III deal with drug enhancement through skin.)

Potts, R.O. and Guy, R.H. (eds) (1997) *Mechanisms of Transdermal Drug Delivery*. Marcel Dekker, New York. (Provides information on biophysical methods for determining molecular transport across skin.)

Roberts, M.S. and Walters, K.A. (eds) (1998) *Dermal Absorption and Toxicity Assessment*. Marcel Dekker, New York. (A substantial text with much relevant information.)

Smith, E.W. and Mailbach, H.I. (eds) (1995) *Percutaneous Penetration Enhancers*. CRC Press, Boca Raton. (Chapters deal with chemical and physical enhancement methods and theories, together with analytical techniques.)

Williams, A.C. and Barry, B.W. (1999) Raman spectroscopy. In: *Percutaneous Absorption* 3rd edn. (Bronaugh, R.L. and Maibach, H.I., eds), Marcel Dekker, New York, pp 499–514.

34
Rectal and vaginal drug delivery

Josef Tukker

RECTAL DRUG DELIVERY

Introduction

The administration of drugs by routes other than the oral one has to be considered in several circumstances and for a great many varying reasons. Arguments for choosing the rectal route for drug administration include:

1. The patient is not able to make use of the oral route. This may be the case when the patient have a problem with their gastrointestinal tract, is nauseous or is postoperative (when they may be unconscious or not able to ingest a drug orally). Furthermore, several categories of patients, i.e. the very young, the very old or the mentally disturbed, may more easily use the rectal than the oral route.
2. The drug under consideration is less suited for oral administration. This may be so in cases where oral intake results in gastrointestinal side-effects; also, the drug may be insufficiently stable at the pH of the GI tract, or susceptible to enzymatic attack in the GI tract or during the first passage of the liver after absorption. Also, drugs with an unacceptable taste can be administered rectally without this inconvenience to the patient. The formulation into suppositories of certain drugs that are candidates for abuse, as in suicide, has also been considered.

Besides these apparent advantages, the rectal route also has several drawbacks. Depending on tradition, there are strong feelings of aversion in certain countries, such as the UK and the USA, to rectal administration of drugs, whereas there is complete acceptance on the continent and in Eastern Europe. More rational points in this respect are the slow and sometimes incomplete absorption that has been reported, and the considerable inter- and intrasubject variation. The development of proctitis has also been reported. There are also problems with the large-scale production of suppositories and the achievement of a suitable shelf-life (the latter demanding stringent storage conditions).

It can thus be concluded that rectal administration should certainly not be the route of first choice, but can in certain circumstances be of great advantage to the patient. The rectal route is used in many different therapies, intended either for local or for systemic effect. *Local effect* is desired in the case of pain and itching, mostly due to the occurrence of haemorrhoids. Locally active drugs which are used include astringents, antiseptics, local anaesthetics, vasoconstrictors, anti-inflammatory compounds and soothing and protective agents. Also some laxatives fall into this category. For the attainment of a *systemic effect* all orally given drugs can be used and many are, bearing in mind the limitations discussed above. Antiasthmatic, antirheumatic and analgesic drugs are very much used for this purpose.

Anatomy and physiology of the rectum

Rectal dosage forms are introduced into the body through the anus and are thus brought into the most caudal part of the GI tract, i.e. the rectum. Anatomically the rectum is part of the colon, forming the last 150–200 mm of the GI tract.

The rectum can be subdivided into the anal canal and the ampulla, the latter forming approximately 80% of the organ. It is separated from the outside world by a circular muscle, the anus. The rectum can be considered as a hollow organ with a relatively flat wall surface, without villi and with only three major folds, the rectal valves. The rectal wall is formed by an epithelium which is one cell layer thick, and is composed of cylindrical cells and goblet cells which secrete mucus. A diagram of part of the rectal wall and the rectum's venous drainage is shown in Figure 34.1.

The total volume of mucus is estimated as approximately 3 mL, spread over a total surface area of approximately 300 cm². The pH of the mucous layer is reported as approximately 7.5. Furthermore, there seems to be little buffer capacity. This point will be discussed later in relation to absorption.

Under normal circumstances the rectum is empty; filling provokes a defecation reflex, which is under voluntary control. Data comparing drug absorption from freshly prepared and aged, more viscous suppositories suggest that there is enough motility to provoke the spreading even of rather viscous suppositories.

Fig. 34.1 Venous drainage of the human rectum (after Tondury, 1981): 1 middle rectal vein; 2 tunica muscularis: stratum longitudinale; 3 m. levator ani; 4 inferior rectal vein; 5 m. sphincter ani externus; 6 superior rectal vein; 7 and 8 plexus venosus rectalis (submucosus); 9 skin; 10 v. marginalis.

Absorption of drugs from the rectum

Blood supply, especially venous drainage, is important for the understanding of drug absorption. As can be seen from Figure 34.1, there are three separate veins. The lower and middle haemorrhoidal veins drain directly into the general circulation; the upper one drains into the portal vein, which flows to the liver. This means that drug molecules can enter the general circulation directly or by passing through the strongly metabolizing liver. In the latter case only a proportion of the drug molecules (if they are of the high clearance type) will enter the general circulation intact. Thus the bioavailability may be less than 100%. Compared to the small intestine this situation is still more favourable. Recent investigations have shown that avoiding the first passage through the liver is possible, but the extent of this effect cannot be generalized, as it will depend on the actual part of the rectum through which the drug is absorbed.

Thus keeping the drug in the lower part of the rectum would be advisable.

The insertion of a suppository into the rectum results in a chain of effects leading to the bioavailability of the drug. This is represented in a simplified scheme in Figure 34.2.

Depending on the character of its vehicle (see later) a suppository will either dissolve in the rectal fluid or melt on the mucous layer. Because the volume of rectal fluid is so small, dissolution of the complete vehicle will be difficult and require extra water. Owing to osmotic effects (of the dissolving vehicle) water is attracted, with the unpleasant consequence of a painful sensation for the patient. Independent of the vehicle type, drugs that are dissolved in the suppository will diffuse out towards the rectal membranes. Suspended drugs will first have to leave the vehicle (if it is water immiscible) under the influence of either gravity or motility movements, and can then start dissolving in the rectal fluid. The dissolved drug molecules will have to diffuse through the mucous layer and then into and through the epithelium forming the rectal wall.

The process of absorption will be a passive diffusion process, as it is throughout the whole GI tract for almost all drugs; active transport processes, as shown in the upper regions of the GI tract, have not been shown to be present in the rectal area.

For a generalized discussion on drug absorption the reader is referred to Part Three of this book. However, some specific points concerning rectal absorption will be discussed here. Table 34.1 gives a survey of the physiological factors in rectal absorption.

The quantity of fluid available for drug dissolution is very small (approximately 3 mL, spread in a layer approximately 100 μm thick over the organ). Only under non-physiological circumstances is this volume enlarged, e.g. by osmotic attraction by water-soluble vehicles or by diarrhoea. Thus the dissolution of slightly soluble substances, for example phenytoin, can easily be the slowest step in the absorptive process.

The properties of the rectal fluid, such as composition, viscosity and surface tension, are essentially unknown and have to be estimated from data available for other parts of the GI tract. The pH and the buffer capacity of the rectum were mentioned earlier in this chapter. The rectum is usually empty, except temporarily when faecal matter arrives from higher parts of the colon. This material is either expelled or

Table 34.1 Physiological factors affecting absorption from the rectum

Quantity of fluid available

Properties of rectal mucus

Contents of the rectum

Motility of the rectal wall

RELEASE MECHANISM

Fig. 34.2 Release process of a drug from a suspension suppository.

transported back into the colon, depending on the voluntary control exhibited on the anal sphincter. The rectal wall may exert a pressure on a suppository present in the lumen by two distinct mechanisms. First, the abdominal organs may simply press on to the rectum, especially when the body is upright. This may stimulate spreading and thus promote absorption. The second source of pressure is the motility of the muscles of the rectal wall, which may originate from the normally occurring colonic motor complexes. These are waves of contractions running over the wall of the colon in a caudal direction and are associated with the presence of food residues in the colon.

In contrast with the upper part of the GI tract, in the rectum no esterase or peptidase activity is present, resulting in a much greater stability of peptide-like drugs. Administration of these compounds using the rectal or vaginal route has been satisfactory, but only if absorption enhancers such as surfactants were used concomitantly. All kinds of surfactants seem to do the promoting work, of which polyoxyethylene lauryl alcohol ether appears to be the most powerful. One major drawback of these enhancers, however, is the irritation of the rectal mucosa in the long term; less irritating enhancers are needed to explore this interesting area in greater depth.

Formulation of suppositories

Suppositories are used mainly for the administration of drugs via the rectal route, but not exclusively. Application via other routes, such as the vagina, is less common but of distinct use in the treatment of locally occurring infections. Other suppository-type products (bougies) used through other body orifices, e.g. the ear, nose and urethra, are very uncommon and are not discussed here. Alternative dosage forms for the rectal and or vaginal route are tablets, capsules, ointments and enemas. These will be discussed later, and concentrate first on rectal suppositories. Suppositories are formulated in different shapes and sizes (usually 1–4 g). Their drug content varies widely, from less than 0.1% up to almost 40%. A more detailed description, together with the methods of preparation can be found in *Pharmaceutical Practice* (Winfield and Richards 1998). Generally the suppository consists of a vehicle in which the drug is incorporated, and in some cases additives are coformulated.

The vehicle (suppository base)

There are two main classes of vehicles in use, the glyceride-type fatty bases and the water-soluble ones. Although the ideal vehicle has not been found, the large variety of bases that are available enables a well considered choice for every drug that has to be formulated as a suppository.

Choosing the optimum base requires a lot of practical experience and at present this can only partly be guided by scientifically sound data. Much remains to be learned here. However, some general guidelines can be given.

Requirements of the vehicle There is no doubt that a suppository should either melt after insertion in the body or dissolve in (and mix with) the available volume of rectal fluid. For fatty bases this means a melting range lower than approximately 37°C (one must be aware of the fact that the body temperature might be as low as 36°C at night). The melting range should be small enough to give rapid solidification after preparation, thereby preventing the separation of suspended, especially high-density, drug particles and agglomeration. When the solidification rate is high this may result in fissures, especially when rapid cooling is applied. On the other hand, the melting range should be large enough to permit easy preparation, which on an industrial scale may take a considerable length of time.

During solidification a suppository should exhibit enough volume contraction to permit removal from the mould or plastic former. The viscosity of the molten base plays an important role both from a technological and from a biopharmaceutical point of view. During preparation the viscosity determines the flow into the moulds, but also the separation of drug particles. Clearly a compromise has to be found here. During and after melting in the rectal cavity the suppository mass is forced to spread over the absorbing surface, the rate of which may be determined partly by its viscosity. Drug particles that have to be transported through the base to the interface with the rectal fluid, and have to pass this interface to be released, will evidently also see viscosity as a determining factor in their journey.

A good suppository base should further be chemically and physically stable during storage as a bulk product, and after preparation into a suppository. It should have no incompatibility with drug molecules and should permit an optimal release of the drug it contains.

Clearly this list of requirements cannot always be completely fulfilled, and often an acceptable compromise is the best that one can expect.

Fatty vehicles The fatty vehicles in use nowadays are almost exclusively semi- or fully synthetic ones. Cocoa butter is no longer used because of its many disadvantages, such as its well known polymorphic behaviour, its insufficient contraction at cooling, low softening point, chemical instability, poor water-absorptive power and its price.

The semisynthetic type of fatty vehicles (sometimes termed **adeps solidus**) have few or none of the problems mentioned above. A comparison is made in Table 34.2.

The general composition of both types is mixed triglycerides with C_{12}–C_{18} acids. In the semisynthetic vehicles these acids are saturated, whereas cocoa butter contains a considerable amount of the unsaturated oleic acid (see iodine number in the table, which for reducing drugs should be <0.5). The presence of oleic acid is almost solely responsible for the special properties of this vehicle. The melting range of the (semi)synthetic bases is usually approximately 3°C and higher than that of cocoa butter; the acid content is lower (mostly <0.5), which is one of the reasons that the ageing of aminophylline suppositories is slower when (semi)synthetic vehicles are used. The hydroxyl number in the table refers directly to the amount of mono- and diglycerides present in the fatty base. A high number means that the power to absorb water is high. This may lead to an increased rate of decomposition for drugs that are easily hydrolysed, such as acetylsalicylic acid. It should be realized that this capacity could lead to the formation of a w/o emulsion in the rectum, which is generally to be avoided because of its very low drug release rate. An advantage of a high hydroxyl number is the larger melting and solidifying range, which permits easier manufacture.

Water-soluble vehicles Water-soluble (or miscible) vehicles are much less used, for reasons to be discussed below. They comprise the classic glycerol–gelatin or soap bases, which are used exclusively for laxative purposes or in vaginal therapy.

The macrogols are also used. They consist of mixtures of polyethylene glycols of different molecular weight. The melting point is well over body temperature, which means that they mix with the rectal fluid. For true dissolution the available volume of rectal fluid (1–3 mL) is too small. Because of their high melting point they are especially suited for application in tropical climates, but several disadvantages must be considered. They are hygroscopic and therefore attract water, resulting in a painful sensation for the patient. The incorporation of at least 20% water and moistening before insertion can help to reduce this problem. A considerable number of incompatibilities with various drugs (e.g. phenols, sulphonamides) has been reported. Owing to the solubilizing character of this base (low dielectric constant) drugs may tend to remain in the base and release may be slow.

Choice of vehicle A summary of the points that are important for the choice of a suppository base is given in Table 34.3. The parameters mentioned are evidently not independent of each other, and one interesting parameter can be added to this list, i.e. the volume of the suppository. Usually suppositories for adults are 2 mL and those for children 1 mL. It has been suggested that the larger volume may provoke a reaction in the rectal wall, thus helping to spread the melt over a larger area. Indeed the increase in volume of, for example, paracetamol suppositories, resulted in faster and more complete drug absorption.

The drug

Table 34.4 lists the factors related to the drug substance that are of possible consequence for the quality of suppositories.

Drug solubility in vehicle The drug solubility in the vehicle is of particular interest from the biopharmaceutical point of view, as it directly determines the

Table 34.3 Formulation parameters of suppository bases
Composition
Melting behaviour
Rheological properties

Table 34.2 Some properties of fatty suppository bases				
	Melting range (°C)	Acid content	Hydroxyl number	Iodine number
Cocoa butter	31–34	<5	0	34–38
Adeps solidus	33–37.5	<2	<5–30	<3

Table 34.4 Drug-substance related factors
Solubility in water and vehicle
Surface properties
Particle size
Amount
pK_a

type of product, i.e. solution or suspension suppository. The drug solubility in the rectal fluid determines the maximum attainable concentration and thus the driving force for absorption. When a drug has a high vehicle to water partition coefficient it is likely to be in solution to an appreciable extent (or completely) in the vehicle. This generally means that the tendency to leave the vehicle will be small and so the release rate into the rectal fluid will be low. This is obviously unfavourable for rapid absorption. On the other hand, a certain lipid solubility is required for penetration through the rectal membranes (see above, under Absorption of drugs from the rectum). The optimal balance between these two requirements is usually found using the rules listed in Table 34.5. This table assumes that the release from the dosage form is considered as the rate-limiting step. Thus the tendency to remain in the base should be lowered as much as possible (rules 1 and 2). When the solubility in fat and water are both low no definite rule can be given. It may well be that the dissolution rate will become the controlling step, and thus it seems advisable to use micronized drug particles.

It should be stated as a general rule that emulsion-type suppositories (w/o) are strongly discouraged. The transfer of drug molecules present in dissolved state in the inner phase will be very slow, and so the absorption will be very much retarded.

It seems logical, therefore, that the first choice of a formulation would be a readily water-soluble form of the drug dispersed in a fatty base. This lays special emphasis on the water solubility of drugs and the methods to improve this. The role of pK_a in this respect should also be considered. For a detailed discussion of these points, see Chapters 2, 3, 8 and 17.

Surface properties The surface properties of drug particles are also important, as these particles will be transferred from one phase to another (see Fig. 34.2). This happens first when the drug is brought into contact with the vehicle and air has to be displaced from its surface. When this is not achieved particles may form agglomerates. This adversely affects final content uniformity by creating an increased tendency to separate. If wetting by the vehicle has taken place displacement by rectal fluid will be required to let the drug go into solution, which is the prerequisite for absorption. This is the underlying reason why people have tried the addition of surfactants to their formulation (see below).

Particle size The particle size of the drug is an important parameter, both technologically and biopharmaceutically. To prevent undue sedimentation during or after preparation the particle size should be limited. The available literature data do not allow us to define an exact limit; however, the use of particles smaller than approximately 150 μm is an indication rather than a rule.

It is, of course, assumed that no agglomeration is taking place. The smaller the particles the less the possible mechanical irritation to the patient (esp. < 50 μm) and the higher the dissolution rate, and therefore drugs with a low water solubility will be dispensed in small, preferably micronized, particles. One should, however, be aware of the increased tendency of these particles to agglomerate as a result of strongly increased van der Waals forces in this case. Also, an unnecessary size reduction operation should be avoided if possible.

There are good indications that size reduction is not a good decision for all drugs. It has been shown, especially for readily water-soluble drugs, that large particles give blood levels that are higher than or at least equivalent to small particles. This would lead to the suggestion to use particles in the size range 50–100 μm. The lower limit of 50 μm to increase transport through the molten vehicle (see Fig. 34.2) and the upper limit of 100 μm is a safe protection against undue sedimentation during preparation. There is, however, no clear-cut picture, as to which solubility class this would apply to. For example, paracetamol (solubility in water approximately 15 mg mL^{-1}) gave the best blood levels when the particle size was smaller than 45 μm.

It should also be borne in mind that the spreading suppository mass should drag the suspended particles along to maximize the absorption surface. For heavy compounds it has become clear that this is a problem, but so far little or no proof is available that organic drugs (density usually 1.2–1.4 g cm^{-3}) suffer from this disadvantage when dispersed in, for example, 150 μm sized particles. Principally this may be expected, but care is needed to prevent too-rapid formulation decisions in this respect.

Amount of drug A complicating factor is the amount of drug present in a suppository. If the

Table 34.5 Drug solubility and suppository formulation		
Solubility in		Choice of base
Fat	Water	
Low	High	Fatty base (rule 1)
High	Low	Aqueous base (rule 2)
Low	Low	Indeterminate

number of particles increases, this would also increase the rate of agglomerates formation. This will depend very much on particle size and the presence of additives. The theory describing the agglomeration behaviour of dispersed systems (DLVO theory, see Chapter 6) can be applied in the non-aqueous systems we are dealing with, but certain refinements are necessary. Another consequence of the presence of suspended particles is the increased viscosity of the molten base. Also in this case we have to rely largely on empirical data, rather than on theory. It therefore seems advisable to include a decision on particle size in the development plan for an actual suppository formulation.

Other additives

For several widely varying reasons, formulators of suppositories make use of additives to improve their product. Most of these additions are based on empirical data and will be dealt with in the accompanying volume on dispensing (in preparation). The dispensing aspects include formulations for specific drugs that affect the melting point of the suppository; it may become depressed (by a soluble liquid compound) or increased (by a high amount of soluble high-melting active compound). The important point to consider in these situations is the possible influence of formulation changes on the release characteristics. We will further limit the discussion to fatty suppositories, where this plays a particular role.

The addition of viscosity-increasing additives (e.g. colloidal silicon oxide or aluminium monostearate, both approximately 1–2%) will create a gel-like system with a slower release rate of the drug. Data from the literature are not consistent on this point. In vitro this can be easily established, but whether the actual release in vivo will also be depressed cannot be easily predicted, as rectal motility will in certain cases be able to overcome this problem. The addition of lecithin is a worthy possibility when high amounts of solid drug are used. The reason why has clearly to be found in a decreased attraction between the drug particles, altering the flow properties of the dispersion in the positive sense.

The addition of surface-active agents has been extensively practised but still remains a source of great uncertainty. When these compounds are used to create an emulsion system (thus w/o) this must certainly be discouraged, as the release will be unacceptably slow. It may well be, however, that surfactants act as wetting agents. This can influence the release in a positive sense, but so far very little convincing information is available showing that wetting (i.e. dis-placement of base by rectal fluid) is a real problem. Surfactants may also act as 'deglomerators', which may prevent the formation of cake in the melting suppository, which in turn would certainly slow down drug release. Also here no firm conclusions can be drawn, as very little research work has been performed on agglomeration in non-aqueous media. The role of surfactants as spreading enhancers has never been clarified either, and this factor is strongly related to the occurrence of rectal motility. There are good indications that the presence of surfactants in a concentration higher than the critical micelle concentration can retard drug release from the suppository.

The finished product

Manufacture

Suppositories are manufactured both on a small scale in batches of 10–20 and on a (semi)automatic scale in batches up to 20 000 per hour. Essentially the mode of manufacture is similar in both cases, and involves melting of the vehicle, mixing the drug and the molten vehicle, dispensing in a former, cooling to solidify and, if necessary, packing in the final container. This includes a number of technological processes for which the relevant theory should be considered (see, for example, Chapter 13 for the mixing of semisolids). Most suppositories are nowadays packed individually in a plastic (PVC) or aluminium foil pack. Requirements leading to a good protection against moisture and oxygen can be deduced from the individual needs of the drug and the properties of the packaging material.

Quality control

A list of properties that should be controlled is given in Table 34.6.

The *appearance* of a suppository includes its odour, colour, surface condition and shape. These

Table 34.6 Control parameters of suppositories
Appearance
Weight
Disintegration
Melting (dissolution) behaviour
Mechanical strength
Content of active ingredient
Release

are organoleptically controlled and will be discussed in the accompanying volume (in preparation). The requirements for **weight** and **disintegration** are given in the European and national pharmacopoeias. The melting and dissolution behaviour is in fact reflected in the disintegration test. Many other methods are available, but none of them has been shown to provide more relevant information. The European Pharmacopoeia method proves to be rather insensitive and not too much value should be placed on the passing of this test.

The ***mechanical strength*** can be valuable to avoid problems with formulations in which the melting range has been depressed. This can be tested in several ways, including a tablet-crushing strength tester.

No official requirements are published as yet with regard to **content uniformity**. This has, however, been shown to be a potential problem in the semi-automatic manufacture of batches of a few kilograms, when, owing in particular to sometimes insufficient mixing, the uniformity of content was insufficient. Paying careful attention to the design and control of the filling apparatus could solve most of these problems. However, the beginning and the end of the production process still give poor results, necessitating some degree of rejection.

Drug release from suppositories

Perhaps the most important thing to realize is that for the patient the release characteristics are the determining step towards the success of the therapy. What is really wanted is optimal bioavailability (for details see Part Three), which for the formulator means ensuring optimal and reproducible release in vivo.

Because there are very few ways to obtain in vivo release information this will usually have to be interpreted from in vitro release, which introduces the problem of in vitro/in vivo correlation. Current knowledge does not permit the choice of an in vitro method with a high predictive power for in vivo performance. Some aspects can be discussed, however, to give helpful pointers in this respect. Table 34.7 lists

Table 34.7 **In vitro release parameters**
Temperature
Contact area
Release medium
Movements
Membranes

the parameters to be examined in testing suppository release in vitro.

The ***temperature*** to be chosen for testing rectal dosage forms is easily defined as the body temperature. Although for most practical purposes this can be set at 37°C, this is not the case for especially fatty suppository testing, for example. Most available vehicles have melting ranges below 37°C, but this does not necessarily mean that their viscosity at 37°C is the same. As the body temperature may be as low as 36°C at night, this implies that the release rate at 37°C may be an overestimate. Also, comparing bases at 37°C may lead to erroneous conclusions. The temperature at which testing is performed might be crucial, especially when ageing has occurred. Special attention should therefore be given to the actual testing temperature.

In the set-up shown in Figure 34.3 the temperature at the surface of the water layer inside the tube, where molten suppository material is gathered, may be a few degrees lower than the bulk temperature. By choosing the right dimension and closing the tube on the upper side this problem is eliminated here.

Fig. 34.3 Tube apparatus for sedimentation-controlled release testing from suppositories.

The **contact area** in the rectum over which spreading occurs cannot be standardized without introducing either an over- or an underestimate. In Figure 34.3 the area is relatively small (i.e. approximately 10 cm^2) compared to the total surface area of the rectum (approximately 300 cm^2). This type of apparatus therefore is clearly intended to be used for comparative studies only, and not for a complete in vivo simulation. At present no method is available that closely mimics the in vivo situation.

Another parameter to be considered is the **release medium**. Because not enough information is available on the actual composition and structure of the rectal fluid, a choice is usually made for a relatively large volume of water or buffer solution. As the rate-limiting step in the bioavailability of fatty suppositories is very often drug release from the suppository, it seems reasonable enough not to include mucins that control the viscosity in vivo. The large volume in most in vitro methods would then not be so important either. More difficult is the choice of buffer, and especially its strength, as little is known about this factor in vivo (see above). For water-soluble vehicles the problem is even greater, and essentially no ideal solution has yet been found to the problem of choosing the volume and composition of the release medium. Interest has been created in the inclusion of one or another way of incorporating a **pressure** feature in release testing. It is clear that rectal motility exists and that it may influence bioavailability, but it is not yet clear how to incorporate this knowledge in the design of a release tester. Attempts have been made, but no conclusive answer has yet been found.

Very often **membranes** have been used in release testers, usually to envelop the suppository in a small volume of release medium. This has the enormous drawback that the release as measured in the outer compartment is not equal to the actual release taking place in the inner compartment. Most published results do not take into account that the membrane may form a resistance to passing drug molecules, and that the actual release may be underestimated. By a calculation procedure it is possible to obtain the actual release if certain conditions can be met. It seems advisable, therefore, to avoid membranes in a release tester whenever possible.

The actual true validation of in vitro release testing remains the in vivo performance. Several possibilities exist to obtain such data. Bioavailability determination should consider both rate and extent of absorption. Whenever possible these data should be obtained in humans, as at present no sufficiently reliable animal model is available. For a more detailed discussion on the general aspects of bioavailability testing and in vitro/in vivo correlations, see Chapter 18.

Rectal formulations other than suppositories

Apart from suppositories, many formulations can be used for the rectal administration of drugs. For the treatment of **local** disturbances, such as haemorrhoids, fatty ointments are widely used. In the treatment of rectocolitis large-volume enemas are used, e.g. 100 mL. This enables the drug to reach the upper part of the rectum and the sigmoid colon.

For the **systemic** administration of drugs, delivery forms such as tablets, capsules and microenemas are used. Tablets are not very attractive because they cannot disintegrate rapidly, owing to the small amount of water present in the rectum. Tablets that release CO_2 after insertion can be used, thereby stimulating defecation.

Capsules used to achieve a systemic effect are usually filled with a solution or suspension of the drug in vegetable oil or paraffin. Such capsules are mostly of the soft-shell type. Limited experience has been obtained with this dosage form, but it seems that there are no striking differences between the bioavailability from rectal capsules and that from fatty suppositories.

Microenemas are solutions or dispersions of the drug in a small volume (approximately 3 mL) of water or vegetable oil. This form is supplied in a small plastic container equipped with an application tube. After insertion of the tube, the container is emptied by compressing the bulb. The advantage of this delivery system is obvious, as no melting and dissolution process is necessary before drug release can start, if water is used as a vehicle. Many good results have been obtained with drugs delivered in microenemas, but this form is still of limited applicability because of its relatively high cost compared to suppositories, for example. Moreover, administration cannot be performed easily by patients themselves, and it is rather difficult to deliver the total content of the plastic container.

VAGINAL DRUG DELIVERY

Vaginal administration of drugs

The vaginal route is mainly used for the achievement of local effects, e.g. in the case of *Trichomonas* and *Candida* infections. Some drugs are, however, administered vaginally to achieve systemic effects. In some cases the drugs given by intravaginal route have a higher bioavailability than with the oral route, because the drug enters immediately into the systemic circulation without passing the metabolizing liver (as is the case with drugs absorbed from the lower part of the rectum).

The vaginal wall is very well suited for the absorption of drugs for systemic use, as it contains a vast network of blood vessels. Only a few drugs are administered by this route at present, however. Among these are oestrogens and prostaglandin analogues, which are usually administered as vaginal creams or hydrogels. Progesterone has been given as vaginal suppositories (pessaries) for some years, and better results are obtained in this way than after oral dosing.

Formulation of vaginal dosage forms

Many different types of formulations have been and are applied vaginally, e.g. tablets, capsules, pessaries, solutions, sprays, foams, creams and ointments. Because of the rather low moisture content under normal physiological conditions, additives are used to improve the disintegration of vaginal tablets, e.g. bicarbonate together with an organic acid, which results in CO_2 release. A good filler for vaginal tablets is lactose, as this is a natural substrate for the vaginal microflora, which converts lactose into lactic acid, resulting in a pH value of 4–4.5.

Vaginal suppositories (pessaries) are mostly prepared with glycerol–gelatin bases, as this mixture is well tolerated. Polyethylene glycols are less common because they are said to promote irritation. Also, fatty excipients are not much used. Most delivery forms for vaginal application demand an auxiliary device to obtain deep insertion of the delivery system.

BIBLIOGRAPHY

de Blaey, C.J. and Polderman, J. (1989) Rationales in the design of rectal and vaginal delivery forms of drugs. In: *Drug Design*, Vol. 9 (ed. E.J. Ariëns). Academic Press, New York, pp. 237–266.

de Boer, A.G., Molenaar, F., de Leede, L.G.J., Breimer, D.D. (1982) Rectal drug administration: clinical pharmacokinetic considerations. *Clin. Pharmacokinetics*, 7, 285–311.

Müller, B. (ed) (1986) *Suppositorien*. Wissenschaftliche Verlagsgesellschaft mbH, Stuttgart.

Rytting, J.H. (1990) Rectal route of peptide and protein delivery. In: *Peptide and Protein Drug Delivery* (ed. V.H. Lee). Marcel Dekker, New York, pp 579–594.

Thoma, K. (1980) *Arzneiformen zur rectalen und vaginalen Applikation*. Werbe- und Vertriebsgesellschaft Deutscher Apotheker mbH, Frankfurt am Main, Germany.

Tondury G. (1981) *Angewandte und Topographische Anatomie*, 5th edn. Georg Thieme Verlag, Stuttgart.

Winfield, A.J. and Richards, R.M.E. (1998). *Pharmaceutical Practice*, 2nd ed. Churchill Livingstone, Edinburgh.

35

Delivery of pharmaceutical proteins

Daan Crommelin, Ewoud van Winden, Albert Mekking

INTRODUCTION

Protein structures

Pharmaceutical proteins are built up of amino acids chains (their primary structure). To be pharmacologically active, this amino acid sequence must form a well defined three-dimensional structure. Parts of the protein will fold in locally identifiable, discrete structures such as α helices or β sheets (known as secondary structures). The overall (tertiary) structure of the protein is established by the proper positioning of the different subunits relative to each other. In some cases individual protein molecules form a quaternary structure, in which the individual protein molecules interact and build a larger, well defined structure (e.g. haemoglobin).

The formation and stability of the secondary, tertiary and quaternary structures is based on relatively weak physical interactions (e.g. electrostatic interactions, hydrogen bonding, van der Waals forces and hydrophobic interactions) and not on covalent chemical-binding principles. Repulsive energy between apolar parts of the protein and water are responsible for hydrophobic interactions. The physical forces involved are relatively weak. This means that protein structures can be rather easily changed, leading to a modification or even loss of their pharmacological characteristics.

Amino acid chains can be modified by covalently attaching non-amino acid sections, such as sugar (glycoproteins), phosphate or sulphate groups. In particular, the sugar part can make up a substantial part of the molecular weight of the (glyco)protein. These groups may be essential for the pharmacological effect of a therapeutic protein, not only while acting at its receptor sites, but also to provide the proper pharmacokinetic profile.

Pharmaceutical protein molecules are large and diffusional transport through epithelial barriers such as those encountered in the gastrointestinal tract is slow unless specific transporter molecules are available. Moreover, the conditions in the lumen of the GI tract are extremely hostile to these proteins. (Enzymatic) degradation is fast. Therefore, the large majority of pharmaceutical proteins are delivered via the parenteral route (i.e. by the needle). The issue of alternative routes of administration is discussed later in this chapter.

Conserving the integrity of these large molecules is essential to ensure an optimal therapeutic effect and to minimize effects such as the induction of unwanted immune responses. An immune response may neutralize the therapeutic activity in chronic dosing schedules and cause serious side-effects. Protein stability concerns both their chemical and their physical structure. There are many functional groups in the amino acid chain available for chemical degradation, and the preferred three-dimensional structure is readily irreversibly disturbed (e.g. through heat, changes in pH or ionic strength). Some analytical approaches to monitor the protein structure are discussed later.

The preferred shelf-life for pharmaceutical products is a minimum of 2 years. Most proteins degrade too fast when formulated as aqueous solutions, even when kept in the refrigerator. Therefore, they have to be stored in a dry form and be reconstituted before administration. These delicate structures are usually dried by freeze-drying (see Chapter 26). The choice of the proper excipients (e.g. lyoprotectants) has proved to be extremely important.

Sources of pharmaceutical proteins

Nowadays most proteins used in therapy or under development are produced by recombinant DNA or hybridoma technology (known as biotechnology or biotech products). Examples are human insulin, erythropoietin, monoclonal antibodies, cytokines and interferons. They are all produced in cell cultures by prokaryotic or eukaryotic cells, ranging from *Escherichia coli* to mammalian cells such as Chinese hamster ovary cells, or transgenic animals. From the examples listed, one may conclude that many of the pharmaceutical proteins are basically endogenous products. However, a number of currently used biotech products are not exactly identical to the endogenous product. For example, the glycosylation patterns of the recombinant form may be reproducibly produced on a large scale, but not completely match the endogenous product. Extensive evaluation of these products in clinical trials has proved their efficacy and safety.

Isolation of the expressed protein from the culture medium is a multistep process consisting of several different (chromatographic/filtration) steps. For every protein a 'tailor-made' purification protocol has to be developed to remove impurities while ensuring integrity.

Biotech-derived molecules may make up the majority of protein drugs, but there are still proteins of major therapeutic importance isolated from blood from humans or animals. Examples are albumin, blood clotting factors (such as Factor VIII from blood from human volunteers), and antisera from patients or animals such as horses and sheep. Here again, special purification protocols have to be developed, with particular emphasis on reduction of viral contamination (see later).

Specific challenges

It is clear that pharmaceutical proteins offer special challenges to the pharmaceutical formulator. They are delicate, large molecules with many functional groups. Their structure, being stabilized by relatively weak physical bonds, is readily and irreversibly changed. In vivo this may directly affect the interaction with the receptor, change their pharmacokinetic characteristics, e.g. their clearance, or make them immunogenic. Moreover, their epithelial penetration capability is very low unless the proper transporter molecules are available. Thus, as a rule, pharmaceutical proteins are administered parenterally.

In the sections that follow several issues will be dealt with in more detail.

FORMULATION OF PHARMACEUTICAL PROTEINS FOR PARENTERAL ADMINISTRATION

Stability issues

In the introduction to this chapter it was pointed out that pharmaceutical proteins are high molecular weight molecules with amino acid building blocks that are sensitive to degradation and with a specific three-dimensional structure. Table 35.1 lists the pathways for degradation of proteins.

Physical instability

Degradation rates depend on environmental conditions and the formulator should carefully select conditions for optimal stability. For example,

Table 35.1 Pathways of degradation of proteins.

Fragmentation

H_2N —— Lys — Ala — COOH → H_2N — Lys + Ala — COOH

Isomerization

L-form amino acid → D-form amino acid

Deamidation

H_2N ..... Asn ..... COOH → H_2N ..... Asp ..... COOH + — NH_2

Oxidation

$$\begin{matrix} & & & O \\ & & & || \end{matrix}$$

H_2N ..... Met ..... COOH → H_2N ..... Met ..... COOH

Disulphide scrambling

H_2N ..... Cys ..... Cys ..... Cys ..... COOH ⟷ H_2N ..... Cys ..... Cys ..... Cys ..... COOH

H_2N ..... Cys ..... Cys ..... Cys ..... COOH

Oligomerization

$n(H_2N$ ..... Cys ..... Cys ..... COOH) → $n(H_2N$ ..... Cys ..... Cys ..... COOH)

$n(H_2N$ ..... Cys ..... Cys ..... COOH)

Aggregation

$n(H_2N$ ..... COOH) → $(H_2N$ ..... COOH)$_n$

Cross-linking

$n(H_2N$ ..... COOH) → H_2N ..... COOH

H_2N ..... COOH

Denaturation

elevated temperatures can cause denaturation of proteins in aqueous solution. Interestingly, low temperatures may also induce destabilization. Besides, protein aggregation is often initiated by adsorption of the protein monomer on the walls of the container. Proteins may also aggregate by shaking or by exposure to shear forces. Hydrophobic parts of the molecule are then exposed to hydrophobic interfaces (air/water), the protein unfolds and aggregation occurs.

Chemical instability

Because of the many amino acids involved, full prevention of all chemical degradation reactions is difficult. The formulator should consider which chemical degradation pathways are relevant. Under neutral conditions the peptide bonds between amino acids are stable; only the asparagine–glycine and asparagine–proline bonds are relatively labile.

Deamidation is a rather common degradation reaction in water. Asparagine and glutamine are the amino acids that can be deamidated. Deamidation reaction kinetics depend on pH and neighbouring amino acids.

Oxidation is not limited to methionine and cysteine (Table 35.1): histidine, tryptophan and tyrosine are also sensitive to oxidation reactions. Oxidation is catalysed by traces of transition metal ions. An oxidative milieu may also cause free cysteine units to form disulphide bridges or disulphide bond scrambling.

Naturally occurring amino acids are in the L form. Isomerization to the D form is possible and will change the structure of the protein.

Improper choice of excipients may also cause degradation reactions. For example, sugars are often used as excipients (Table 35.2), but reducing sugars can react with free primary amino groups of the protein molecule via the so-called Maillard reaction (even in the dry state) and form brownish reaction products. Reducing sugars (e.g. lactose) should therefore be excluded from protein-containing formulations.

Excipients used

Table 35.2 lists the excipients used in protein-containing parenteral dosage forms. Not all of the ingredients listed are always needed, e.g. many pharmaceutical proteins are sufficiently soluble in water. This is in particular true for highly glycosylated molecules. In this case no solubility-enhancing substances are needed. However, if solubility enhancement is necessary, the selection of the proper pH conditions should first be considered. Protein solubility depends on its net charge. In general, as with low molecular weight drugs, uncharged protein molecules (at the pH of their isoelectric point, i.e.p.) have the lowest solubility in water. Therefore, choosing pH conditions 'away' from the i.e.p. can solve the protein (and the problem). Some amino acids (e.g. arginine and lysine) increase protein solubility and reduce aggregation reactions by a not-well understood mechanism. Detergents such as polysorbate 20 and 80 or sodium dodecyl sulphate can also be used to prevent aggregation. These compounds prevent the adsorption of proteins to interfaces (air/water and container/water) and thereby interface-induced protein unfolding. Human serum albumin has a strong tendency to adsorb to interfaces and may therefore be added to therapeutic protein formulations as an anti-aggregation agent.

Table 35.2   Excipients used in parenteral dosage forms and their function

Excipient	Function	Examples
Solubility-enhancing substances	Increase solubility of proteins	Amino acids, detergents
Antiadsorbent/aggregation blockers	Reduction of adsorption and aggregation prevention	Albumin, detergents
Buffer components	Stabilizing pH	Phosphate, citrate
Preservatives	Growth inhibition in vials for multiple dosing	Phenol, benzylalcohol, organic Hg-compounds
Antioxidants	Prevent oxidation	Ascorbic acid, sulphites, cysteine
Stabilizers during storage (lyoprotectants)	Preservation of integrity while in dry form	Sugars
Osmotic compounds	Ensure isotonicity	Sugars, NaCl

Oxidation reactions are catalysed by heavy metals. Chelating agents are used to reduce oxidation damage through binding of the ions. This approach cannot be used if the metal ion is necessary as an integral part of the protein structure. Examples are zinc ions in insulin formulations and iron ions in haemoglobin. Then, antioxidants such as sulphites may be added to reduce the oxidation tendency. In the case of vials for multiple dosing, preservatives have to be included in the formulation. Benzyl alcohol and phenol are often used for this purpose.

Buffered aqueous protein solutions may be stable for 2 years under refrigerator conditions. Some monoclonal antibody formulations, for example, are available as aqueous solutions, but the more common situation is that the formulation has to be freeze-dried in the vials to avoid degradation and to ensure that the product can be readily reconstituted.

During freeze-drying (Chapter 26) water is removed by sublimation. In the freeze-drying process three discrete phases can be discerned. The first is freezing of the solution to temperatures typically around -35 to $-40°C$, followed by a sublimation phase with temperatures of around $-35°C$ and low pressures to remove the frozen water (phase 2), and a final, secondary drying stage to remove most residual water. The pressure must remain low, but the temperature can rise up to about $20°C$ without collapse of the porous cake (see below). A lyoprotectant (e.g. sugar) is necessary to stabilize the product as the removal of water may irreversibly affect the protein structure. Moreover, sugar lyoprotectants also happen to form readily reconstitutable porous cakes.

The freezing temperature should be low enough to convert the aqueous solution with the sugar and the protein into a glass. Glass formation in sugar solutions usually occurs around $-30°C$. Just below the glass transition temperature the sublimation process can begin during the lowering of the pressure in the chamber. The sublimated water is collected on a condenser with a considerably lower temperature (typically $-60°C$). As sublimation extracts a large amount of latent heat from the system, the temperature in the vials containing the frozen protein solution could fall even lower than the starting temperature, slowing down sublimation. The vials are therefore heated in a controlled way to keep them at temperatures low enough to preserve their glassy texture, but high enough to let the sublimation process proceed at a sufficiently high speed.

The mechanism(s) of action of lyoprotectants (non-reducing sugars) are not fully understood. The following may play a role:

- Lyoprotectants replace water as stabilizing agent ('water replacement theory') of the protein;
- Lyoprotectants increase the glass transition temperature in the frozen system and in the dried system, avoiding collapse of the porous cake which would slow down water removal from the frozen cake (during freeze drying) and interfere with a rapid reconstitution of the freeze-dried cake;
- Lyoprotectants slow down the secondary drying process and minimize the chances of overdrying of the product in the secondary drying stage.

Microbiological requirements

Typically, pharmaceutical proteins are administered via the parenteral route. This implies that the product should be sterile. In addition, virus and pyrogen removal steps should be part of the purification and production protocol.

Pharmaceutical proteins cannot be sterilized by autoclaving, gas sterilization or ionizing radiation, because these procedures damage the molecules. Therefore, sterilization of the end-product is not possible. This leaves aseptic manufacturing as the only option.

All utensils and components must be presterilized (by heat sterilization, ionizing radiation or membrane filtration) before assembling the final formulation to minimize the bioburden. Protein products are manufactured under aseptic conditions in class 100 areas (fewer than 100 particles > 0.5 μm per cubic foot). This low level contamination is reached by filtration of air through HEPA (high-efficiency particulate air) filters. Finally, the product is filled into the containers through sterile filters with 0.22 μm pores before capping or freeze drying/capping.

Pharmaceutical proteins are produced by living organisms. Viruses can be introduced into the product either by the use of contaminated culture media or via infected (mammalian) production cells. It is therefore important that purification and manufacturing protocols contain viral decontamination steps. Viral decontamination can be accomplished by virus removal and/or by viral inactivation. The problem faced when selecting inactivation techniques is that there is often a narrow window between successful viral inactivation and preservation of the integrity of the pharmaceutical protein structure.

Viruses can be removed by filtration, precipitation or chromatography. For virus inactivation, heat treatment (pasteurization), radiation or crosslinking agents (e.g. β-propiolactone) can be used. As no single process guarantees complete virus removal, often several different decontamination steps are introduced in series in the 'downstream' purification process and in the manufacturing of the final formulation.

Gram-negative host cells, such as *E. coli*, are often used as production cells for non-glycosylated proteins. Gram-negative cells contain large amounts of endotoxins in their membranes. These endotoxins are heat stable, amphipatic, negatively charged lipopolysaccharides and are potent pyrogens. Pyrogens have to be removed in order to meet pharmacopoeial criteria, and this can be done, for example, through anion-exchange chromatography.

ANALYTICAL TECHNIQUES TO CHARACTERIZE PROTEINS

It is clearly important to be able to guarantee the integrity of a protein. As mentioned earlier, a protein

molecule is a complex three-dimensional structure of amino acids, often coupled to saccharide, phosphate or sulphate moieties. The total structure is responsible for the pharmacodynamic (e.g. receptor interaction) and pharmacokinetic (e.g. clearance, targeting) effect. It is not possible to define the structure of a pharmaceutical protein with the same precision as small, low molecular weight molecules, where a combination of analytical techniques provides unequivocal structural evidence.

Therefore, a set of pharmacological, immunological, spectroscopic, electrophoretic and chromatographic approaches is used to characterize the protein as closely as possible. Table 35.3 lists a number of regularly used analytical techniques and the information that is obtained.

Quality assessment used to be based on functional tests in vivo (relevant animal models). An example is the pharmacopoeial test for insulin: the lowering of the blood glucose level in rabbits upon

Table 35.3   Approaches to confirm protein structure

Approach	Information obtained
In vivo tests, use of test animals	Pharmacological effect
In vitro tests (sensitive cells)	Functional test
Immunological tests	
ELISA	Interaction with one epitope on protein
RIA	Interaction with one epitope on protein
Analytical approaches	
Spectroscopic	
UV spectroscopy	Secondary/tertiary structure
fluorimetry	Secondary/tertiary structure
CD spectroscopy	Secondary/tertiary structure
infrared spectroscopy	Secondary/tertiary structure
mass spectrometry	Secondary/tertiary structure
Electrophoretic approaches	
SDS-PAGE	Molecular weight
IEF	Isoelectric point
High-performance liquid chromatography (HPLC)	
GP (gel permeation)	Molecular weight/aggregates
HI (hydrophobic interaction)	Hydrophobic interactions
Affinity chromatography	Interaction with specific ligand
IEC (ion exchange)	Charge patterns
RP (reversed phase)	

CD, circular dichroism;
ELISA, enzyme-linked immunosorbent assay;
IEC, ion-exchange chromatography;
IEF, isoelectric focusing;
HPLC, high-performance liquid chromatography;
MALDI, matrix-assisted laser desorption ionization;
MS, mass spectrometry;
RIA, radioimmunoassay;
SDS-PAGE, sodium dodecyl sulphate polyacrylamide gel electrophoresis;

injection of the insulin product to be tested. These tests do not have the sensitivity to identify small changes in molecular structure or detect early degradation products, and they do not provide information on such things as the presence of product immunogenicity. In vitro cell tests, such as those used for cytokine activity assessment, inform us about the functional activity of the molecule, but not its pharmacokinetic behaviour or immunogenicity. ELISA (enzyme-linked immunosorbent assay) and RIA (radioimmunoassay) belong to the class of immunological tests. Here the interaction of a monoclonal antibody with one epitope region on the protein is determined. The rest of the molecule is not 'probed'.

Electrophoretic techniques such as SDS-PAGE (sodium dodecyl sulphate–polyacrylamide gel electrophoresis) and IEF (isoelectric focusing) are powerful tools to assess product purity and to provide molecular weight and isoelectric point (i.e.p.) information regarding the protein.

Table 35.3 lists a number of chromatographic techniques that elucidate product characteristics. In particular, impurities and degradation products can be picked up at an early stage. Gel chromatography discriminates mainly on the basis of molecular size and is a powerful technique to monitor aggregate formation. Ion-exchange resins separate on the basis of subtle variations in protein charge patterns and are being used to detect oxidation (e.g. methionine) and deamidated (converted glutamine and asparagine) products. Modern mass spectroscopic techniques such as MALDI–TOF (matrix-assisted laser desorption ionization–time of flight) mass spectroscopic analysis, or a combination of HPLC (high-pressure liquid chromatography) with electrospray ionization-induced mass spectrometry give detailed information on amino acid sequence and glycosylation patterns.

In conclusion, to ensure pharmaceutical protein quality one must follow a strict protocol regarding the definition of the protein production cell lines used, the chosen culturing conditions and downstream processing conditions, and the filling/ (drying)/ finishing process. Analytical approaches to confirm the protein structure will always include a long list of approaches, ranging from in vivo tests in animals to information provided by highly sophisticated analytical technologies.

None of these tests tells the whole story; together they tell more, but there is never the situation encountered with many low molecular weight molecules whereby a full description of the drug, including a detailed impurity profile, is available.

ADMINISTRATION OF PHARMACEUTICAL PROTEINS

Routes of administration

As mentioned in the introduction to this chapter, oral administration of a pharmaceutical protein results in a very low bioavailability. The protein is enzymatically attacked in the gastrointestinal tract and, moreover, penetration through the gut wall will be slow and incomplete. Oral vaccines containing antigenic protein material are an exception to the general rule that proteins should not be administered orally. With vaccines, even low uptake levels may still deliver sufficient material to lymphoid tissue just below the epithelium (in the so-called Peyer's patches) to induce a strong (both local and systemic) immune response.

When a protein is delivered intravenously clearance from the blood compartment can be fast, with a half-life of minutes, or slow, with a half-life of several days. An example of a rapidly cleared protein is tissue plasminogen activiator (tPA), with a plasma half-life of a few minutes. On the other hand, human monoclonal antibodies have half-lives of the order of days.

Protein drugs are often administered subcutaneously or intramuscularly. These routes of administration are considered to be more patient friendly and the injection process easier than with the intravenous route. Upon intramuscular (i.m.) or subcutaneous (s.c.) injection the protein is not instantaneously drained to the blood compartment. Studies monitoring the fate of a protein upon s.c. injection demonstrate that passage of a protein through the endothelial barrier lining the local capillaries at the site

Fig. 35.1 Correlation between the molecular weight and the cumulative recovery of recombinant interferon (IFN α-2a), cytochrome C, inulin and 5-Fluoro-2′-deoxyuridine (FudR) in the efferent lymph from the right popliteal lymph node following s.c. administration into the lower part of the right hind leg of sheep (from Crommelin and Sindelar, 1998)

of injection is size dependent. If the protein is too large it will enter the lymphatic system and be transported via the lymph into the blood. Figure 35.1 shows the relationship between molecular size and lymphatic drainage. Lymphatic drainage takes time and a delay in the onset of systemic activity is observed. The protein is also exposed to the local environment containing proteases. Therefore, the bioavailability of protein drugs upon s.c. (and i.m.) administration can be far from 100%. This can have dramatic consequences, e.g. some diabetics become insulin resistant because of high tissue peptidase activity.

There is not always a direct relationship between plasma level and pharmacological response (i.e. no direct pharmacokinetic–pharmacodynamic (PK/PD) relationship). As the mechanism of action of a drug might be complex, involving different sequential steps, fast clearance from the blood compartment may not necessarily mean that drug action is also short-lived. The relationship between a pharmacokinetic profile and the pharmacodynamic result of the presence of the drug can be quite complex. A drug may trigger a reaction, which may result in measurable, pharmacological effects much later. As an example, the cytokine intraleukin-2 (IL-2) (in its PEG-ylated form) is rapidly cleared from the blood compartment and a pharmacological effect (increase

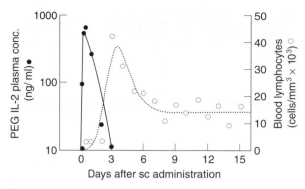

Fig. 35.2 PEG-IL-2 pharmacokinetics and pharmacodynamics (changes in blood lymphocyte count) after subcutaneous adminstration of 10 MIU/kg in rats. PEG = poly(ethylene glycol); (from Crommelin and Sindelar 1998)

in the number of blood lymphocytes) is observed long afterwards (can be days) (Fig. 35.2).

Finding alternatives for the parenteral route has been an area of interest for many years. Table 35.4 lists different possible routes of delivery for proteins.

With the exception of the pulmonary route, all other options have a low bioavailability. Some bioavailability data on the intratracheal administration of proteins in rats are shown in Table 35.5. The extent of absorption depends strongly on the nature

Table 35.4 Alternative routes of administration to the oral route for biopharmaceuticals (adapted from Crommelin and Sindelar 1998)

Route	Relative advantage	Relative disadvantage
Nasal	Easily accessible, fast uptake, proven track record with a number of 'conventional' drugs, probably lower proteolytic activity than in the GI tract, avoidance of first-pass effect, spatial containment of absorption enhancers is possible	Reproducibility (in particular under pathological conditions), safety (e.g. ciliary movement), low bioavailability for proteins
Pulmonary	Relatively easy to access, fast uptake, proven track record with 'conventional' drugs, substantial fractions of insulin are absorbed, lower proteolytic activity than in the GI tract, avoidance of hepatic first-pass effect, spatial containment of absorption enhancers (?)	Reproducibility (in particular under pathological conditions, smokers/non-smokers), safety (e.g. immunogenicity), presence of macrophages in the lung with high affinity for particulates
Rectal	Easily accessible, partial avoidance of hepatic first-pass effect, probably lower proteolytic activity than in the upper parts of the GI tract, spatial containment of absorption enhancers is possible, proven track record with a number of 'conventional' drugs	Low bioavailability for proteins
Buccal	Easily accessible, avoidance of hepatic first-pass effect, probably lower proteolytic activity than in the lower parts of the GI tract, spatial containment of absorption enhancers is possible, option to remove formulation if necessary	Low bioavailability of proteins, no proven track record yet (?)
Transdermal	Easily accessible, avoidance of hepatic first-pass effect, removal of formulation is possible if necessary, spatial containment of absorption enhancers is possible, proven track record with 'conventional' drugs, sustain/controlled release possible	Low bioavailability of proteins

Table 35.5 Absolute bioavailability of a number of proteins (intratracheal vs intravenous) in rats

Molecule	MW (kDa)	No. of amino acids	Absolute bioavailability (%)
α-Interferon	20	165	> 56
PTH-84	9	84	> 20
PTH-34	4.2	34	40
Calcitonin (human)	3.4	32	17
Calcitonin (salmon)	3.4	32	17
Glucagon	3.4	29	< 1
Somatostatin	3.1	28	< 1

PTH, recombinant human parathyroid hormone.
(From Crommelin and Sindelar 1998 with permission)

of the protein. Insulin is a candidate drug for pulmonary delivery to diabetics to mimic the natural physiological response to a meal (postprandial glucose control). Subcutaneous injection gives a relatively slow response; pulmonary uptake is faster. New pulmonary delivery devices (see Chapter 31) not only increase average bioavailability but also reduce variation in uptake.

Three approaches have been followed to improve the bioavailability of pharmaceutical proteins when exploring alternative routes of administration. First, coadministration of protease inhibitors, such as bacitracin, should slow down metabolic degradation. Second, excipients (often with an amphipatic character, such as bile salts) can be added to enhance passage through epithelial barriers. The third approach is to prolong the presence of the protein at the absorption surface, e.g. by the use of mucoadhesives.

Intranasal delivery of chitosan and starch microspheres demonstrated enhanced uptake of coadministered insulin. In humans, intranasal delivery of insulin with chitosan results in absolute bioavailabilities of 7%. In conclusion, bioavailability is indeed strongly enhanced when using these approaches, but safety issues must be addressed before these absorption enhancers can be introduced into marketed products.

Release control

Many therapeutic proteins are short-lived in the blood compartment. Assuming there is a direct relationship between blood level and therapeutic effect, it is important to maintain therapeutically relevant drug concentrations in the bloodstream. Portable pump systems with adjustable pump rates are available for patients. Catheters provide the link between the pump and, for example, the peritoneal cavity. These systems are particularly useful if a constant dose input is required and the drug is needed over a limited period of time. Otherwise, more flexible delivery systems are preferred. For insulin (with a plasma half-life of 5 minutes) different forms of controlled-release systems for s.c. injection are available. Release control is based on different physicochemical appearances (amorphous/crystalline) of insulin itself and on insulin complexes with Zn^{2+} ions or proteins, such as protamine. Zn^{2+} ions tend to slow down the release of insulin. Amorphous insulin plus Zn^{2+} ions results in moderate prolongation of drug action. Crystalline insulin plus Zn^{2+} ions gives a long-acting product. The addition of protamine (at neutral pH a positively charged protein) to insulin and Zn^{2+} ion combinations protracts the insulin effects even more (up to 72 hours; long-acting). Isophane insulin (NPH: neutral protamine Hagedorn) contains insulin and protamine in isophane proportions (no excess of either component), resulting in intermediate-acting formulations.

At present, efforts are being made to build 'closed-loop' systems where insulin administration is controlled by:

- a biosensor permanently monitoring blood glucose levels;
- an infusion pump with adjustable pump rate; and
- an electronic section with an algorithm linking blood glucose levels to insulin need at any time.

In hospitals such equipment is available to stabilize blood glucose in patients for limited periods, but no portable 'patient-friendly' systems for chronic use are yet available.

In even earlier stages of development are 'artificial pancreases'. Isolated insulin-producing β cells from the islets of Langerhans are introduced into the body in a container system with a wall that allows the passage of glucose, insulin and nutrients. However, the container wall keeps the β cells separated from the patient's immune system. Increasing blood glucose levels will stimulate the secretion of insulin by the encapsulated β cells. The excreted insulin will be released from the container and glucose levels will fall until normal blood levels are reached.

Controlled-release systems containing microspheres (with diameters between 10 and 100 μm) for s.c. administration are currently under development. A 30-day action sustained-release system designed on the basis of biodegradable polylactic-glycolic acid has been formulated for human growth hormone. These microspheres are prepared using a double emulsion technique whereby the proteins are exposed to organic solvents, and protein encapsulation efficiency is rather low. Alternatively, a dextran-based microsphere preparation protocol has been developed without the use of organic solvents and with extremely high loading efficiencies.

CONCLUDING REMARKS

Protein drugs are rapidly gaining in importance, and both market volume and market share are expected to rise. Biotechnological techniques permit the design and synthesis of active proteins. It is the task of the pharmaceutical formulation scientist to turn the pure substance into a formulation that can be safely administered to the patient, exerting optimal therapeutic benefits. In this chapter different aspects of this formulation process are described and special attention is given to those aspects where biotech products clearly differ from low molecular weight drugs.

BIBLIOGRAPHY

Baudys, M. and Kim, S.W., eds. (1999) Insulin Delivery. *Adv. Drug Del. Rev.* **35**, 141–335.

Crommelin, D.J.A. and Sindelar R.D. (1998) *Pharmaceutical Biotechnology*. Harwood Academic Publishers, Amsterdam.

Franssen, O., Vandervennet, P. Roders, P. and Hennink, W.E. (1999) Chemically degrading dextran hydrogels: controlled release of a model protein from cylinders and microspheres. *J. Controlled Release*, **59**, 219–228.

Manning, M.C., Patel, K. and Borchardt, R.T. (1989) Stability of proteins, *Pharm. Res.* **6**, 903–917.

Wang, W. (1999) Instability, stabilization and formulation of liquid protein pharmaceuticals. *Int. J. Pharm.* **185**, 129–188.

Van de Weert, M., Hennink, W.E. and Jiskoot, W. (2000) Protein instability in Poly(lactic-co-glycolic acid) microparticles. *Pharm. Res.*, **17**, 1159–1167.

36

Packs and packaging

Dixie Dean

Packaging can be defined as an economical means of providing presentation, protection, identification/information, containment, convenience and compliance for a product during storage, carriage, display and use until such time as the product is used or administered. This total timescale must be within the shelf-life of the product, which is controlled by the selection of the right combination of product and pack. In looking at the above definition emphasis on any one factor may change with time, advancements in science and technology, or trends in product form. For instance, there has been a distinct move from the use of unpleasant oral liquids to the solid dose form, which has recently concentrated on delayed- or sustained-release products. Such changes can have a positive influence on the type of pack used, as shown by the increasing applications of blister and strip packaging. Both sustained-release and these unit-type packs offer obvious patient convenience, as a selected number of units can be readily detached and carried as a day's treatment, possibly leading to improved compliance. However, packaging can offer convenience factors anywhere along its lifecycle, e.g. reel-fed materials used for the production of blisters and strips need relatively little storage space compared to any preformed bottle, which literally wastes space by storing air prior to being filled. Further examples of packs offering patient convenience include a range of unit dose presentations that permit immediate disposal after use, metered dose aerosols and nasal sprays which combine convenience with dosage control, squeeze eyedrop packs (compared to the earlier bottle, dropper and teat assembly) etc.

The role of the pack

The role of the pack and the packaging operation needs emphasis as the shelf-life of all pharmaceutical products, irrespective of whether they are ethicals, semiethicals or proprietaries (over-the-counter or OTC), is largely dependent on certain functions of the pack. The pack must be economical and therefore contribute to overall profitability; it must provide protection against climatic, biological, physical and chemical hazards; it must provide an acceptable presentation which will contribute to or enhance product confidence while at the same time maintaining adequate identification and information; and last but not least it must contribute in terms of convenience and compliance. Each of these aspects has to be considered against the total (shelf) life of the product, which involves periods of storage (static), carriage (motion),

possible display and finally use or administration, directly by a patient or indirectly by a health professional. In certain cases the pack may form part of the administration system, as is seen with aerosols metered dose nasal pumps, prefilled syringes etc. As these total pack requirements become increasingly extensive and sometimes conflicting, it is not surprising to find that the final choice is inevitably a compromise, hence the question 'What is an ideal pack?' rarely has a simple answer. For example, the external image of the pack must not only compliment product confidence, provide clear and concise product identification, adequate information related to the contents (including legal requirements), the route of administration, storage conditions, batch number, expiry date, manufacturer's name and address and product licence number, but also assist in patient compliance. Producing an aesthetically acceptable design is therefore only one stage where compromise has to be exercised.

In addition to this aesthetic requirement the majority of the remaining pack factors are associated with its function. The primary pack consists of those packaging components that form the part of the pack directly containing the product (i.e. bottle, cap, cap liner, label etc.). The main functions of the primary pack are to contain and to restrict any chemical, climatic or biological or occasionally mechanical hazards that may cause or lead to product deterioration. Because the primary pack also represents the pack of 'use', it must also function in the hands of the user as a means of drug administration. The packaging external to the primary pack, known as the secondary packaging, mainly provides the additional physical protection necessary to ensure the safe warehousing and delivery of the product to the point where bulk quantities are broken down into individual or specific units.

THE PACK AS A PROTECTION

Although each function of the pack has to assume a certain level of importance, protection is almost invariably the most critical factor as it controls the total shelf-life of the product. Asking the question 'protection against what?' produces a whole list of possible hazards, many of which are listed below. These are not identified in any particular order of importance as those that are relevant to a specific product will vary in both number and criticality. They cover mechanical, climatic, biological and chemical factors.

Mechanical hazards

Physical or mechanical damage may occur due to the following.

Shock or impact damage

This phrase implies rough handling, where rapid deceleration occurs (drops, impacts). Shock can normally be reduced or overcome by various forms of cushioning, restriction of movement, more careful handling etc. However, it should be noted that damage can occur to the pack or packaging material before it reaches the stage of a packed product.

Compression

Top pressure or loading can distort and crush a pack and damage the product inside. The crushing of a carton can make a product unsaleable even though no damage has occurred to the contents. Although this is most likely to occur during stacking in the warehouse or in transit, where vibration adds a further hazard, compression of the pack can occur in other situations (i.e. capping on a production line, when being carried home by the user etc.).

Vibration

Vibration consists of two variables, frequency and amplitude. These can vary enormously, e.g. a load on a truck may bounce up and down say 0–50 mm, up to 120 times per minute, whereas vibration from aircraft/ships engines may have an extremely low amplitude but a very high frequency. Each extreme may produce different forms of damage to product and/or pack, i.e. components of product may separate, screw caps may loosen, labels or decoration may abrade etc.

Abrasion

Although this results from both regular and irregular forms of vibration it is listed separately as the visual appearance of the product or pack can be affected, e.g. a rectangular bottle in a carton will move up and down and from side to side. A round bottle in the same circumstances will suffer from an additional possibility of rotation. See below under Chemical hazards.

Puncture or piercing

Many materials can suffer penetration from sharp objects. Again this can happen at any stage from basic material supply to the finished pack. Adequate cushioning and/or resistance to penetration helps to reduce the risks. Poor control of forklift trucks is a puncture hazard.

Climatic or environmental hazards

These may be ever-present hazards or hazards which are specific to a local environment. Although climatic conditions are covered by such phrases as arctic, antarctic, temperate, subtropical and tropical, severe conditions can occur elsewhere, i.e. in a deep freeze (−19 to −22°C), in a bathroom or kitchen where conditions can be worse than many tropical areas, displayed under high-wattage bulbs in a shop window, stored near pipes or heaters in a shop or warehouse etc. Climatic hazards therefore include the following.

Moisture

Moisture as liquid or water vapour may cause physical changes (e.g. dulling, softening, hardening etc.) or chemical change (hydrolysis, effervescence, etc.) It may also act as a carrier for other contaminants. Certain materials (including all plastics) are to some degree permeable to moisture, and even screw closures which appear to make a good seal are likely to permit some passage of moisture depending on the sealing medium, the torque, the evenness and shape of the sealing surface, the aperture size and circumferential area of the container etc. It must be emphasized that either moisture loss or moisture gain may be critical to some products.

Temperature

Extremes of temperature (cold and hot) or cycling temperature can cause deterioration to product and/or pack. Although higher temperatures generally represent an acceleration effect occasions can be found where deterioration increases at lower temperatures (certain plastic will become more brittle and crack, for example). A high temperature coupled with a high RH will produce a shower effect if the temperature is lowered sufficiently to reach dew point. Contamination from liquid moisture can then encourage mould and bacterial growth.

Pressure

Air-pressure differentials are frequently seen as a danger for materials sent by air using unpressurized aircraft. Pressurized aircraft are pressurized to the equivalent to about 3000 m above sea level; hence there is a –0.25 bar differential compared to takeoff. Goods filled in factories at sea level and sent to mountainous areas, or vice versa, will suffer from similar patterns, i.e. goods packed in Johannesburg, South Africa, at 2000 m and then sent to Durban at sea level will be exposed both to a positive pressure and probably to a temperature change.

Light

Light consists of wavelengths from the UV zone through the visible to infrared. Although UV is a potential source of photochemical change, such changes may not always be visible. Printed or decorated packaging materials may also suffer from discolouration (white may go yellow, deeper colours may fade), and this may be seen as implying a change in product efficacy or strength. Although light can be excluded by using selected materials, tin plate, foil etc., opacity and/or colour may reduce penetration or filter out selected wavelengths. The additional use of UV absorbers in plastics may also restrict light rays entering the pack. It should also be noted that many products are protected by a carton, outer etc. for a larger proportion of their life. Protection may then only be necessary for a relatively short display or use period when exposure to light occurs.

Atmospheric gases

These include oxygen, carbon dioxide, nitrogen and any other airborne gases. Oxygen leading to oxidation is the more obvious hazard. Carbon dioxide, however, can cause a pH shift (unbuffered solution in plastic bottles, particularly LDPE, which is relatively permeable to CO_2) and/or lead to precipitation of some products. The permeation of the common gases through plastic is typically in the ratio of 1:4:20 for nitrogen, oxygen and carbon dioxide, respectively, the latter being the most permeable.

Odorous gases, or volatile ingredients associated with perfumes, flavours and product formulations may also pass into or out of a pack. If a volatile ingredient is lost from a flavour, an unpleasant odour or taste may result.

Solid airborne contamination (particulates)

Particulates may be carried by or in the atmosphere. In the case of most plastic contamination may be increased by electrostatic attraction under dry conditions whereby particulates are drawn from the atmosphere by electrical charges. The presence of particulates will inevitably increase microbiological contamination risk.

Biological hazards

Microbiological

There is a general tendency towards improved microbial control for all products. This means that the packaging materials must be reasonably clean initially and, when put together to form a finished pack, restrict any further contamination as much as possible. In the case of sterile products the pack and its closure must maintain a 100% effective seal against microbiological ingress, i.e. bacteria, moulds and yeasts. Ingress of yeasts is critical with sugar-based products, e.g. syrups, as fermentation may occur. Mould will also grow on cellulose-based materials, i.e. paper and board, if these are kept under humid conditions.

Other forms of infestation

In common with foods, other sources of infestation that can contaminate pharmaceutical products include attack by insects, termites, vermin, rodents or any other bird- or animal-contaminating source. Although this is more likely to happen under poorly controlled conditions of hygiene and housekeeping, such infestation can still occasionally cause problems even in the UK.

Pilferage and adulteration risks

Pilferage being a human failing is broadly another biological hazard. The example of the Tylenol poisonings, in 1982 has placed greater emphasis on the need for tamper-resistant packs. Prior to this, various seals were used to indicate whether any product had been removed or replaced, rather than as a means of protecting against deliberate adulteration. Security seals, a possibly preferred phrase to tamper evidence, are widely used for pharmaceutical products as a means of increasing and maintaining user confidence in the product and pack.

Chemical hazards

As chemical interaction, if inherent to the formulation, cannot normally be reduced or avoided by pack selection (unless it is associated with exchange between the product and external atmosphere), the main risk must relate to interaction or incompatibility between product and pack. Compatibility investigations must basically cover any exchange that can occur between the product and the pack, and vice versa. These may be associated with interaction or contamination, covering migration, absorption, adsorption, extraction, corrosion, erosion etc, whereby ingredients may be lost or gained. Such exchange may be identifiable as organoleptic changes, increase in toxicity/irritancy, degradation, loss or gain of microbial effectiveness, precipitation, haze, turbidity, colour change, pH shift etc. Again other external influences may catalyse, induce or even nullify chemical changes.

Some examples of chemical interaction between a product and its pack and the resulting contamination are described below.

1. Adsorption of chemical entities on to component surfaces occasionally occurs. Losses of EDTA and certain preservatives (e.g. benzalkonium chloride, thiomersal and other mercurials) have been observed.
2. The more volatile preservatives, e.g. chlorbutol, phenol, 2-phenylethanol, show fairly rapid loss through low-density polythene by absorption and surface evaporation. If an external overwrap, which is not permeable to the preservative, is added, then loss can usually be restricted to relatively low levels, i.e. less than 10%.
3. Other surface-active ingredients which may be found in plastics may also enter the product by dissolution, surface abrasion etc. These include antistatic additives, slip additives, antislip additives, mould release agents, antiblock agents, lubricants etc.
4. Detachment of glass spicules may occur when alkaline solutions of citrates, tartrates, chlorides and salicylates are stored in soda glass containers. This may occasionally occur when treated or even neutral glass is autoclaved in the presence of similar alkaline salts.
5. Organoleptic changes may occur, caused by permeation of volatile or odorous substances through plastic materials, e.g. solvents from printing inks.

STAGES IN THE DEVELOPMENT OF A PACK–PRODUCT COMBINATION

Development stages

To follow the theme that no pharmaceutical excipient, drug entity, intermediate or finished product can exist without a pack means that knowledge of the pack employed is relevant for all developmental stages of a dosage form, from preformulation studies right through to the finally chosen pack. The placing of formulations on test without reference to the packaging material, the closing system, the torque to which a screw cap has to be closed etc. is condemned.

Attempts to accelerate deterioration by the use of excessively high temperatures should also not be employed. In the same way that products may change when exposed to accelerated conditions, packs and packaging materials may similarly suffer changes, e.g. caps can tighten and crack (if plastic) or loosen and become ineffective as closures. It is therefore advised that packs generally should not be exposed to temperatures of more than 45°C, and even at this condition the time period should not exceed 12 months, with a maximum of 6 months being preferable.

With modern analytical techniques, TGA, DTA, GC, GPC, DSC, HPLC, IR, UV, TLC etc., changes in product or pack are becoming easier to detect and define in terms of actual change. It is also interesting to note the change in emphasis from identifying product purity to the identification and quantification of impurity and degradation products which in earlier years would have remained unidentified. These can now be fully quantified by the analytical techniques available. However, the student is warned that total reliance on so-called scientific methods is not enough. Sensual observations related to feel, appearance, texture, colour, smell and taste (where safe) should also be used, as these simple observations can occasionally detect change before any analytical procedure has been developed.

The stages broadly associated with packaging development are as follows.

Preformulation

All preformulation studies need some form of container. It is therefore important to understand the limitations associated with any packaging contact material used to contain or retain the material under test even at this very early stage of product development.

Product formulation

Formulations and any intermediates all require to be contained and stored. It is therefore necessary to make certain that all packaging contact materials are defined and that all pack parameters (torque, heat seal etc.) are identified, controlled and documented (all part of good laboratory practice (GLP) and good pharmaceutical manufacturing practice (GMP)) during formulation studies.

Consideration of container materials

It is important to have a basic knowledge of all packaging materials, their properties, characteristics etc., and the processes by which they are fabricated/ decorated as a packaging container or component, as well as how these and any subsequent processes may affect their properties, e.g. sterilization by ethylene oxide can lead to ethylene oxide and ethylene glycol residues. Gamma irradiation of low-density polyethylene not only marginally reduces material flexibility owing to molecular cross-linkage, but can give rise to formic acid and formaldehyde residues.

Pack feasibility tests

This is the stage where a product (preferably the formulation selected for ultimate sale) is tested in a range of possible packs, usually over a range of conditions from say −20°C to 45°C, together with some cycling conditions covering a temperature–humidity range. Note the weakness of testing under constant temperature conditions, when in actual practice all conditions are cycling and therefore variable. In addition to the storage tests indicated above the immersion of pieces of pack, or pack components if plastic, in the product or a simulant – i.e. an extractive-type test – may also be employed. Extractive tests are usually mandatory for plastics used for injectables and ophthalmic products. All materials used for these tests should be given a provisional specification and thoroughly checked (more rigorous quality control tests) prior to any use. Feasibility tests usually extend over 1–12 months, with 3–6 months normally being the minimum before a decision to proceed with a certain pack is taken. However, decisions based on accelerated conditions are sometimes difficult to interpret, as limited failure at, say, 45°C or severe cycling conditions, e.g. 15–37°C, 50–90% relative humidity (RH) over 12-hourly cycles, does not necessarily mean a pack (or the product) will fail under more realistic climatic conditions.

Formal stability tests

Once sufficient confidence has been generated in the pack–product combination, formal stability tests, on which the shelf-life will be based, can proceed. Test conditions have been specified by the International Conference on Harmonization and adopted by the major regulatory bodies in Europe, the USA and Japan. Normally three large-scale batches of product in each pack variant are stored at 25°C and 60% RH for long-term stability purposes, and at 40°C and 75% RH for accelerated stability, and sampled over a period of 5 years at examination intervals of 0 (initial), 3, 6, 9, 12, 18, 24, 30, 36, 48 and 60 months. The data generated are sent to the regulatory authorities as part of the Marketing Authorization Application.

Ongoing stability

This consists of repeated stability on random batches from production in order to confirm that the shelf-life does not change.

Complaints

This is the final means of monitoring the success of the product and pack. It is somewhat similar to the monitoring and recording of adverse reactions in that it is a safeguard to both the company producing the drug and the person receiving it.

In all the above tests analytical and packaging technological support is essential to check both the product and the pack. Some of the types of test employed are identified in this chapter. The aims quoted earlier bear repeating as without them there is no assurance that a satisfactory product pack has been achieved, i.e.

1. a specifiable product;
2. a specifiable pack;
3. a specifiable series of processes controlling all operations, from raw material to the assembly of the finished pack, as this ultimately becomes the basis for the control of all future production.

To achieve these specifiable parameters requires the cooperation and coordination of virtually all company disciplines so that the final aim of having a successful product which is effective, safe and profitable is met. The pack must therefore carry the product image literally from inception to disposal.

PACK SELECTION

Factors influencing choice of pack

Before a pack can be selected and the relevance of the various hazards considered, it is necessary to establish a thorough background brief which covers consideration of the product, the market, the distribution system, manufacturing facilities and other considerations. These are discussed below.

The product

Product detail must include chemical and physical characteristics of the drug entity, the excipients and the formulation. It must also cover any recognized routes of deterioration or degradation, the dosage and frequency of dosage, the mode of administration and type of patient (baby, child, teenager, adult, elderly, infirm etc.), any of which could influence the product and pack style and any controlling legislative detail. Whether the product is seasonal or has a year-round use may be a further influence on pack selection.

The market

The eventual channels of sale should be considered, i.e. where, when, how and by whom it is to be used or administered (e.g. doctor, dentist, nurse, patient etc.). Where the product may be used (i.e. clinic, home, hospital), whether for home trade and/or export, the quantity per pack and the predicted sales for initial launch and follow-up sales, must all be carefully considered during pack design and selection.

The distribution system

The distribution system should be carefully thought out, for example conventional wholesale/retail outlets, or direct to selected outlets. How a product is to be distributed may be more relevant to export markets where less sophisticated transport systems (mules, donkeys, camels etc.) may be used, and where climatic conditions may be more severe, particularly if intermediate storage facilities are non-existent (e.g. no dockside warehouses) so that the consignment will be directly exposed to the atmosphere.

Manufacturing facilities

The suitability of the manufacturing facilities may have to be considered for a number of reasons, i.e. new pack, increased sales, improvements in GMP, revised product, new product etc. For example, can the envisaged product be manufactured and packed with existing facilities, or are new plant, equipment and buildings required? If the latter applies then the likely profit must be balanced against the likely cost

of the venture. For example, an entirely new facility for the introduction of a packed product by an aseptic or a terminal autoclaving process would be more expensive than that required for a solid or liquid dosage form.

PACKAGING MATERIALS

Packaging types, styles and systems can be broadly defined by the material of construction, e.g. glass, plastic, metal, rubber, paper etc., and the process used for fabrication, e.g. blow moulding, injection moulding etc.

Glass and glass containers

Glass has had a successful history for pharmaceutical products in that it offers transparency, sparkle, easy cleaning, effective closure and reclosure where applicable, high-speed handling, good rigidity and stackability, and depending on the selection of the correct type of glass, is generally inert. The two main disadvantages, fragility and heavy weight, have partially been reduced by surface coatings to increase the surface lubricity and careful design. The latter includes the avoidance of sharp angles and the use of adequate radii. Plastic-coated or plastic-sleeved containers are likely to allow even thinner glass containers to be produced. The specific gravity of glass normally lies between 2.25 and 2.5, whereas most plastics are well below 1.5 (PVC is 1.4–1.45).

Glass is basically of three types: neutral, (type I), surface-treated soda glass (type II) and soda or alkali glass (types III and IV). These materials may be converted into components by pressing, blowing into a mould, or the shaping of glass cane (tubular containers). Typical compositions of type I (neutral) and type III (soda or alkali) glass are as follows (Table 36.1).

Table 36.1 Typical glass compositions (%)

	Type I	Type III
Silica	66–74	66–75
Lime	1–5	6–12
Soda	7–10	12.5–19
Alumina	4–10	1–7
Boric oxide	9–11	—

In type I glass the alkaline element is largely eliminated by the use of boric oxide to neutralize the oxides of potassium and sodium. Neutral glass has a higher melt temperature (around 1750°C) and a narrower working temperature range, which, together with the higher cost of boric oxide and the greater likelihood of imperfections, usually means a cost of two to three times that of soda glass for containers made by the blow-moulding process.

Surface-treated glass (type II) is made by treating the hot surface of type III (soda) glass with sulphur dioxide, ammonium sulphate or, in some countries, ammonium chloride. This neutralizes some of the surface alkali radicals, producing a more neutral surface. The process, which may also be referred to as sulphuring or sulphating, invariably leaves a hazy surface bloom (normally sodium sulphate) and so washing is essential prior to use. Soda glass (type III) is the most widely used material where extraction of alkali metal ions is not critical to the product. Type IV glass has a similar composition to type III, but it cannot be guaranteed to have the same quality. All glass types are available in clear (white flint) and amber, with other colours, including green, being produced as special makings. Although the majority of all glass containers are made by a blow-moulding process, vials, ampoules and cartridge tubes, produced by 'shaping' glass softened by heat from a length cut from glass cane, find wide application for pharmaceutical and cosmetic products.

Metal and metal containers

Metal, mainly as tin plate or aluminium, was at one time widely used for rigid containers for tablets, capsules, pastilles, powders and even liquid products. A significant part of this usage has been lost to other materials over the last 10 years. Light flexible gauges of metal (aluminium, tin and tin-coated lead) were widely used for collapsible tubes. Thin gauges of aluminium are widely used as foil in combination with other support or heat-sealing polymer films. Although all the above uses for metals still exist, there has been a gradual reduction in their use other than for foil and for aerosols. In addition to containers, tin plate, aluminium and aluminium alloy have been widely employed for ancillary components, including closures. Although the use of tin plate and certain types of aluminium screw closures has reduced, the special aluminium alloy developed for rolled-on and rolled-on pilfer-proof closures has remained in use owing mainly to recent events related to security and tamper evidence.

The production of collapsible tubes made by a process known as impact extrusion has been fairly static recently, first because of the growth in plastic tubes, and more recently because of the introduction of a multi-ply lamination, once known as 'Glaminates'. Metal collapsible tubes in the UK are largely made in aluminium (plain or lacquered) with a few in pure tin. As aluminium work hardens during impact extrusion (i.e. it becomes less flexible and more springy) aluminium tubes have to undergo an annealing process to ensure that the metal becomes flexible and capable of being shaped and folded. If any interaction between the product and metal is likely an internal protective lacquer, usually based on vinyl or epoxide resins, can be added. As metal tubes have a shoulder bearing an orifice (which takes a closure) and an open end (through which the contents are filled and after which the metal is folded and crimped), they have in effect two closures and two areas of seal. Whereas the dispensing end can be sealed, with a blind nozzle and/or a screw cap to make a good seal, the folded metal is less reliable in terms of searching or mobile products. The fold can therefore be improved by the addition of a latex or heat-seal band. Although the number of folds in the filling end can also be varied (e.g. saddleback (triple) fold, double fold etc.) the longer tube length required for the former (say + 9 mm) will add to the cost.

Tubes with elongated nozzles and a controlled orifice size are used for eye ointments. Nearly all caps on metal tubes are wadless, being plastic and moulded in polyethylene and polypropylene.

Plastics and plastic containers

Types and uses

Past years have seen a significant expansion in the use of plastics, from a few thermoset caps and the odd container (for menthol cones and shaving sticks) to a point where plastics have become a major packaging material. Plastics now used are related mainly to the thermoplastic resins. The most economic four are polyethylene (low, medium and high densities), polyvinyl chloride (unplasticized and plasticized), polypropylene (homopolymer and copolymer) and polystyrene (general purpose and impact modified). Other selected materials find specialized usages for containers, devices, components, plies or coatings. These include nylon (PA), arcylonitrile butadiene styrene (ABS), styrene acrylonitrile (SAN), polycarbonate (PC), polysulphone, polyvinylidene chloride (PVdC), polymonochlorotrifluoroethylene

(PCTFE), polyester (PET) and polytetrafluoroethylene (PTFE). Plastic resins or polymers offer many attributes, in choice of material and grade, processes of fabrication and decoration, a wide selection in design, and physical and chemical properties, all on an economical basis.

Disadvantages

In theory plastics appear to have certain disadvantages, e.g. possible extraction, interaction, adsorption, absorption, lightness and hence poor physical stability; all are permeable to some degree to moisture, oxygen, carbon dioxide etc; and most exhibit electrostatic attraction, allow penetration of light rays unless pigmented black etc. It is necessary to be aware of other possible negative features. These include:

1. *stress cracking*: a phenomenon related to low-density polythene and certain stress cracking agents such as wetting agents, detergents and some volatile oils;
2. *panelling or cavitation*: whereby a container shows inward distortion or partial collapse owing to absorption of gases from the headspace, absorption causing swelling of the plastic, or dimpling following a steam autoclaving operation;
3. *crazing*: a surface reticulation which can occur particularly with polystyrene and certain chemical substances (isopropyl myristate first causes crazing, which ultimately reaches a state of total embrittlement and disintegration);
4. *poor key of print*: certain plastics, such as the polyolefins, need pretreating before ink will key. Additives that migrate to the surface of the plastic may also cause printing problems;
5. *poor impact resistance*: both polystyrene and PVC have poor impact resistance. This can be improved by the inclusion of impact modifiers, such as rubber in the case of polystyrene and methyl methacrylate butadiene styrene for PVC. However, both increase the permeability of each.

The majority of these effects can be either overcome or minimized by one means or another. An industrial example will illustrate the point.

It was required to pack a nasal spray formulation in a plastic squeeze bottle which was available worldwide. This immediately called for a low-density polyethylene pack. The product, however, contained a volatile preservative system which both dissolved in LDPE and was lost from it by volatilization, thereby immediately suggesting that a conventional squeeze pack was unsuitable. The LDPE bottle was, however, enclosed in a PVC blister impermeable to the volatile preservative and fitted with a peelable foil lid (also impermeable). As a result of this combination the loss of preservative was restricted to less than 5% of the total, i.e. preservative soluble in the LDPE, and preservative in the air space of the PVC blister reached a point where equilibrium was achieved between product, LDPE and the surrounding air space.

Additives

Because plastics still tend to be seen as relatively new materials, those used for ophthalmic solutions and injectables have a specific extractives procedure to pass. However, a knowledge of the constituents that may be found in a plastic material is equally important. The constituents fall into four categories: the polymer, residues associated with the polymerization process, additives (those constituents added to modify the plastic in a specific way) and any processing aids (which are used to assist any part of the process). The list of residues, additives and processing aids varies according to the plastic involved. Natural polyethylenes usually are low in residues and are likely to contain only a small quantity of an antioxidant. Polyvinylchloride, on the other hand, invariably contains a stabilizer to restrict any degradation that may occur during the heat processing.

The residues, additives and processing aids that may be used, and therefore possibly extracted from, a plastic include the following:

Monomer residues	Modifiers
Catalysts	Emulsifiers
Accelerators	Antioxidants
Solvents	Mould-release agents
Extenders	Lubricants
Fillers	Stabilizers
Slip additives	Colourants – pigments and
Antislip additives	dyes
Antistatic agents	Whiteners and opacifiers
Antiblocking	UV absorbers
agents	Flame retardants
Plasticizers	Light excluders (e.g. carbon
Release agents	black)

Most plastics will include only a few of the constituents listed above. However, depending on the additive used, other properties of the plastic can be changed, e.g. fillers such as chalk or talc are likely to increase moisture permeation.

Fabrication of plastics

Unlike glass, plastic containers and components can be fabricated by a far greater number of processes. These include injection moulding, injection and extrusion blow moulding, injection stretch and extrusion stretch blow moulding, thermoforming, scrapless forming process (SFP), reaction injection moulding (RIM) and solid-phase pressure forming (SPPF), all of which relate mainly to thermoplastic resins. Designs, rate of moulding and cost all vary according to the process chosen and the number of moulds involved, i.e. single or multiple cavity. Irrespective of the process, all moulding operations operate to a 'cycle' whereby the basic resin is heated, softened, shaped in a mould or moulds, and cooled to a temperature at which the article can be handled without distortion. Virtually all plastics shrink in the moulding/cooling operation and allowance has to be made for this. After moulding plastics can be decorated or printed by another wide range of processes, i.e. silk screen, dry offset letterpress, hot die stamping, cliche or tampon printing, therimage, letraset, or labelled by heat-sensitive, self-adhesive labels or plain paper labels using a special adhesive. Knowledge of both the fabrication and decoration of plastics is essential when a plastic material is to be used in contact with a pharmaceutical product.

Paper and board

The use of paper-based materials (cellulose fibre) remains a significant part of pharmaceutical packaging in spite of the fact that paper is rarely used on its own for a primary pack. However, the list of paper usages covers labels, cartons, bags, outers, trays for shrink wraps, layer boards on pallets etc., and combinations of paper, plastic and foil which are discussed separately. Cartons are used for a high percentage of pharmaceutical products for a number of reasons, increasing display area, providing better stacking for display of stock items, and the collating of leaflets which would otherwise be difficult to attach to many containers. Cartons also provide physical protection, especially to items such as metal collapsible tubes. Cartons therefore tend to be a traditional part of pharmaceutical packaging. Fibreboard outers, either as solid or as corrugated board, also find substantial application for bulk shipments.

Regenerated cellulose film (trade names Cellophane and Rayophane) are still used as an overwrapping material either for individual cartons or to collate a number of cartons. However, it is being substantially replaced by orientated polypropylene film. Although paper, even when waxed, has relatively poor protective properties against moisture, both paper and board (ointment, pill and tablet boxes) were once widely used for primary packs, particularly for dispensing operations.

Films, foils and laminates

The development of plastic films (early 1950s onwards) as distinct from regenerated cellulose film based on viscose, and the process of laminating two or more plies selected from films, cellulose coatings, foil and paper, has seen an ever increasing use of the various combinations. These materials fall into different roles, such as supportive, barrier, heat seal and decorative. Paper, for example, is usually a supportive ply which can readily be printed to give decorative appeal. Aluminium foil, even in the thinnest gauges (particularly when laminated or coated with a plastic ply), offers the best barrier properties, which are not approached even by the most impermeable plastics. Metallization, a relatively new process whereby particles of metal are laid down on to a surface under vacuum, can significantly improve the barrier properties of a material but these do not approach the properties of pure foil. The reflective properties of both metallization and foil can add to the decorative appeal of a pack. Plastics, as either films or coatings, can be used for decoration, flexibility, to provide various barrier properties, heat sealability, see-through properties (i.e. transparency), and to protect the other plies within the lamination.

In terms of cost, paper/plastic (paper/LDPE or paper/PVdC) or single plies of coated regenerated cellulose film or coated polypropylene represent the more economical materials that can be used for strip packs, sachets, overwraps etc. Although in general costs increase as the number of plies increases, newer techniques such as coextrusion, where a number of plastic plies are extruded in combination, can produce complete laminations cheaper than those produced by individual bonding. However, lamination bonding is still essential for plies containing paper and foil, as these materials cannot be extruded.

Uses for films, foils laminations are numerous, e.g. sachets, diaphragm seals for bottles, strip packs, blister packs, liners for large containers, overwraps, flow wraps, and liners for boxes, either attached (e.g. Cekatainer and Hermetet cartons) or loose bag-in-box systems and bags. Each of the above is likely to use different materials or combinations of materials for a number of reasons. For example, a blister pack consists of a thermoformed tray with a lid made from board, paper, foil or film with coatings, which will either tenaciously adhere to the tray and act as a push-through material or be peelable, so that the lid can be peeled back to gain access to the contents. The thermoformable portion, i.e. the tray, can again be made from a single material, e.g. polystyrene, polyvinyl chloride, polyester etc., or be a combination, e.g. PVC coated with PVdC, PVC/PVdC/PE/PVdC/PVC, PVC/PCTFE (i.e. Aclar).

The thermoforming operation, whereby a heated and softened plastic ply, or sheet is drawn into a cooled mould, can be done by vacuum, positive air pressure, mechanically by a die, or a combination of these. If thicker foil is incorporated into the basic web to give a combination of nylon or polypropylene/40–50 μm foil/PVC or polyethylene, then cold forming, whereby a web is stretched without perforating, can be carried out. Foil blisters, as these are known, when sealed with a foil lid, can provide a hermetic pack, i.e. one that excludes virtually any exchange of gases between the product and the surrounding atmosphere. Similar protection can be achieved by using a foil-bearing laminate for a strip pack. In this case either the foil laminate is stretched by the insertion of an item in the 'pocket area' when it is held against a recess in a heat-sealing roller, or the pocket area is prestretched prior to reaching the intermeshing heat-sealing roller position. In all cases the blister or pocket has to be especially designed for the item to be filled if the maximum economy of material and machine is to be achieved. The volume and area of a blister pack is very product/machine dependent, and although it may be practical to put an item in a larger size of blister or pocket (at additional cost in material and possible slower production speed), it is usually impossible to make packs smaller without technical risks being taken, e.g. product sticking to foil lid in a blister pack; product causing pocket to perforate in a strip pack etc.

Both blister and strip packs appear to offer a reasonable degree of child resistance, particularly if the materials are opaque (opinion based on actual recorded poisonings or accidents).

Rubber-based components

Rubber components may be made from either natural or synthetic sources. The majority of rubber usage is related to the closure of sterile products (aqueous or oil-based and freeze-dried or powdered solids). Although natural rubber is being replaced by synthetics it offers advantages in terms of resealing (multidose injections), fragmentation and coring

(descriptions for the means by which particles are created when a needle is passed through a rubber), but is poorer in respect to ageing, multiple autoclaving, extractives, moisture and gas permeation and the absorption of preservative systems. Synthetic rubbers tend to reverse all of the above properties and some formulations actually contain natural rubber in order to improve resealability, fragmentation and coring. However, most rubber formulations are relatively complex and may contain one or more of the following: vulcanizing agents (many of which are sulphur based), accelerators, fillers, activators, pigments, antioxidants, lubricants, softeners or waxes.

The main types of rubber used for pharmaceutical products include natural rubber, neoprene, nitrile, butyl, chlorobutyl, bromobutyl and silicone. Of these silicone is the most expensive and, although the most inert, is readily permeable to moisture, gases and absorbent to certain preservatives.

As indicated above, rubber components are likely to contain more additives than plastics. They are therefore tested by basically similar extractives and product contact procedures before they are used for injectable or i.v.-type products.

Rubber gaskcts are also found in aerosols and metered-dose pump systems.

CLOSURES

Functions of a closure

Closures may be required to perform any of the following functions:

1. To provide a totally hermetic seal. This is a closure that permits no exchange between the contents and the outside of the pack, e.g. a fused glass ampoule.
2. To provide an effective microbiological seal, e.g. rubber bung and metal overseal. As rubber is permeable to moisture and gases to some degree, a bacteriological seal may not be strictly hermetic.
3. To provide an effective seal which is acceptable to the product, i.e. a closure which is not hermetic or a total guarantee against bacterial ingress, but adequate for the product.

Providing a 'seal' frequently depends on the marriage of a hard material with a softer, more resilient one, so that the former makes a physical impression on the latter. Closures generally require consideration of the following:

1. To be resistant and compatible with the product and the product/air space. NB Product contact will vary according to how the pack is stood: upright, upside down, on side, intermittent contact during transportation, movement etc.;
2. If of a reclosable variety, to be readily openable and effectively resealed;
3. To be capable of high-speed application where necessary for automatic production without loss of seal efficiency;
4. To be decorative and of a shape that blends in with the main container;
5. To offer such additional functions as may be deemed necessary – to aid pouring, metering, administration, child resistance, tamper evidence etc.;
6. To prevent or limit exchange with the outside atmosphere, to a permissible level. As well as moisture exchange, this may have to cover gases, vapours and actual liquid seepage or leakage.

Although a closure can be affected by various basic means, i.e. adhesion, heat sealing, welding, crimping, mechanical impression, interlocking, stapling, sewing etc., the majority of systems are related to physical compression or heat sealing.

The *physical compression systems* include:

1. screw caps – in metal or plastic; prethreaded or rolled on, with or without a wadding system (i.e. wadless);
2. plug in – a friction push-in fit;
3. push over – where a flanged or raised ring portion is pressed over a bead or lip.

Some closure systems endeavour to combine one or more of these systems and thereby achieve a multiple seal: for example, a seal may press externally on a sealing surface and also on an internal bore. Wadless thermoplastic caps using a 'crab's claw' seal or a skirted bore seal are becoming increasingly popular.

Wadded screw caps either contain a wad plus a facing, a disc of resilient plastic, or have a flowed-in plastic compound. The wad may be of compocork, feltboard, pulpboard or expanded polyethylene, faced with such materials as aluminium foil, tin foil (expensive), polyethylene, a vinyl material or PVdC (Saran). The latter, which has good barrier properties and is reasonably inert, is now the most widely used. Foil or waxed foil is slightly preferable if a higher barrier material is required. The wadding materials mentioned above are occasionally used, usually waxed, on their own. Plasticized PVC, polyethylene or foamed polyethylene have also found selective usage. Flowed-in linings, although slightly inferior in barrier properties and inertness, offer production-line advantages in that there is no wad to fall out whereby a pack is left without an effective closure. Wadless caps also have this same advantage. The knowledge required to understand closure systems is frequently underrated.

Rolled-on (RO) and rolled-on pilfer-proof (ROPP) aluminium alloy metal caps have always been popular for the security of export products. The RO and ROPP closure consists of a plain metal shell containing a wadding or flowed-in system, which is placed over the container neck and top pressure applied to give a good impression on the wad. While the pressure is still held, the threads are formed by a mechanical inwards pressure. In the case of the pilfer-proof closure an additional perforated collar is rolled under a lower bead. This type of closure system is capable of maintaining an excellent seal and does not suffer from the occasional tearing of the wad facing that occurs when a conventional screw cap is applied to a substandard bottle finish. In the case of a rubber wad it also avoids any watch-spring affect. However, a RO or ROPP cap does require a slightly higher standard for the quality of the bottle neck.

Determination of closure efficiency

Closure efficiency, i.e. the ability to prevent undesirable exchanges between the product and the outside atmosphere, can be determined by numerous methods:

1. Placing a desiccant in a pack stored under high RH and detecting any moisture gain;
2. Putting liquid inside the pack, storing at high temperature and low RH, and then detecting any moisture loss as a reduction in weight;
3. Holding the empty pack under water, applying a vacuum and observing for leakage or liquid ingress. Adding a dye and a wetting agent to the water may assist the defection of leaks;
4. Putting liquid in the pack, inverting and applying a vacuum. A poor seal is detected by liquid seeping or leaking out;
5. Checking that cap-removal torque (assumes quality of bottle and cap) is satisfactory. Torque can be time–temperature related, particularly on plastic bottles, and so measurement should be made against a standard condition and test period;
6. Checking on compression 'ring' seal in cap liner when the system contains a liner or lining

compound. If indentation by bottle surface on liner is not uniform or continuous, a faulty seal can occur. This can be confirmed by 'painting' the bottle rim before applying the cap to the specified torque; if the liner does not have a continuous ring of the marker paint then closure is incomplete.

The above tests cover those carried out to establish that a closure is satisfactory in a development programme and those that can be used in production monitoring as part of online quality control. Some closuring systems using ratchet tamper evidence closures or rolled pilfer-proof seals have two release torques, one to release the cap from the bottle sealing surface and one to 'break' the tamper-evident feature.

Heat seals

As indicated earlier another widely used method of sealing is heat (direct and indirect). To achieve an effective and permanent heat seal the two sealants must be compatible (partly compatible sealants can be used to give a peelable seal). Four factors have to be controlled: temperature, pressure, dwell (the length of time that temperature and pressure are applied) and the cooling period. Contamination of any area of seal (for example with product) should be avoided, although certain plastics will seal better than others in the presence of a contaminant. The main heat sealants include polyethylene (low density), wax coatings, PVdC, Surlyn ionomer, selected vinyl-based products and certain types of modified polypropylene. Conditions of sealing vary according to the heat sealant, with the majority sealing between 75°C and 150°C. The total effectiveness of the seal is also dependent on other variables, such as seal width, seal pattern, pack shape, and the presence of creases or stress lines (particularly if product area is overfilled or undersize) etc. The seal is usually checked by vacuum (carried out under water, probably containing a dye plus a wetting agent) to see if ingress occurs, and by the force required to pull the seal apart.

Other sealing methods

Plastics can also be sealed by other techniques, such as ultrasonics, high-frequency welding, hot-air welding and by other heat sources (flame, infrared, induction etc.).

Suffice it to say that closure is a most essential part of both primary and secondary packs.

FILLING

Packaging lines

Products packed on production lines include such items as unit and multidose packs, closable and non-reclosable packs, sterile products produced aseptically or by terminal sterilization, or non-sterile products with or without a degree of microbiological control, preformed containers which have to be filled and sealed etc., or those packed by a form fill seal process etc. Packaging lines may be fairly conventional and involve unscrambling, cleaning, filling, closuring, labelling, cartoning (probably with leaflet insertion), outerization and finally palletization, or be selective to a specialist operation, e.g. blister and strip packaging. Additional operations that may be carried out on a production line include printing, batch coding, expiry dating, and the incorporation of administration aids etc. Glass bottles other than those used for the more critical types of product (injections, eye drops or similar sterile products) are normally manufactured and packed clean and then subjected to pressurized air and vacuum as a final cleaning process (for fibres) prior to filling.

The total efficiency and hence profitability of a packed product depends not only on the type of pack and the material selected but also on the production line operation and the packaging equipment chosen. For example, the filling speed for a tablet will depend on its characteristics: the size, shape, fragility, resistance to powdering if uncoated, surface lubricity etc., and the type of pack chosen. For a non-fragile easy-flowing tablet, filling speeds for a wide-mouthed container (100s) could be 20 000 tablets per minute, with 5000 for a blister pack and 2000 for a strip pack. Choosing a narrow-mouthed container irrespective of the material used could reduce the filling speed to below 10 000 tablets per minute.

Organization of packaging lines

The organization of a production line involves several factors which may ultimately affect output. These include labour, planned maintenance, staff training, online quality control (QC), facilities for batch coding and expiry dating where relevant, constant delivery of an adequate supply of materials to the agreed specification on to the line, and removal of the finished product from the line. Also required are clearly defined procedures for cleaning, start-up and close-down of the line, plus full documentation on both procedures and materials to be handled (including reclamation, verification, reconciliation) and environmental control, which all form part of good manufacturing practice (GMP), and of course the actions to take should one piece or part of a machine break down. On a line performing a number of separate functions (i.e. unscrambling, feeding, filling, closing, labelling and cartoning) each following operation should be capable of higher output speeds than the former. Intermediate holding areas, such as a revolving table top, may also be placed between certain functions should, say, the capper unit temporarily need attention. In this way the first part of the filling operation can still continue provided the alteration or adjustment to the capper can be carried out relatively quickly. The rest of the line with the higher-output capability can then cope with the backlog of containers.

Packaging of certain products

The method of packaging obviously depends on the type of material to be packed. **Solid items** such as tablets and capsules are counted by, for example, resolving disc, slat counter, breaking a beam of light etc. **Powder or granular products** may be filled by volume using an auger (powder held in a rotating screw) or a filling cup, or by weight using a bulk feed plus trickle top-up. In the case of very small quantities a dosator which dips into a constant level of powder held in a reservoir can be employed. Whatever the fill process, observations have to be made as to whether it changes the characteristics of the powdered product, e.g. separation due to vibration, impaction due to compression etc. **Cream and ointment-type products** are filled volumetrically either by a piston-type filler or by an auger. **Liquid products** are also widely filled by a piston filler, a volume cup method using a pressure or gravity feed, or, where a rigid non-collapsible container is involved, by vacuum. In this process two tubes are lowered into the bottle and a seal made by a gasket on the container neck. When a vacuum is drawn on the vacuum tube, liquid flows through the filling tube until it reaches the level of the vacuum tube. The flow then cuts off. This process provides a clean fill, detects containers that are faulty (contain holes or have a dipped or uneven sealing surface), and of course operates a no-container no-fill feature. However, it is not ideally suited to frothing or more viscous liquids. A container that would collapse under a relatively low vacuum can be filled by vacuum, provided it is placed in an outer container and then sealed so that a vacuum can be drawn internally and externally to the pack.

Aerosols

Aerosols fall into a category of their own. They use a variety of materials (metal, glass, coated glass or plastic as containers, and combinations of metal, plastic and rubber for the valve) and offer a form of packaging where product and pack cannot be separated. In fact, an aerosol only comes into existence once it has been filled with a product and pressurized with a propellant. The latter may be either an inert gas or a halogenated hydrocarbon. Pharmaceutical aerosols by and large can be divided into metered-dose aerosols, where the total volume usually does not exceed 50 mL, and topical applications with a volume of 100 mL plus.

Metered-dose aerosols, many of which are used to treat asthmatic or bronchial conditions, are required to produce a product with a fine particle size, i.e. significant part of the cloud below 7 μm. This can be achieved by using powder or liquid aerosols where break-up is assisted by the propellant formulation and the valve. Attempts to produce a fine particle cloud using inert gases with a break-up system have so far fallen short of the standard required. The recent criticisms of the use of fluorocarbon propellants and their possible attack on the ozone layer has led to considerable innovation, with trends towards separating the product from the pressurized part of the system. As a result a number of bag-in-can or piston systems have been developed. Although such systems will dispense a solid or liquid product they will now provide sufficient break-up to give a true 'aerosol type' of dispensing.

Parenterals

Parenterals can normally be divided into small volume (SVP), e.g. injections, and large volume (LVP), e.g. i.v. injections and dialysis solutions. Although the size of containers varies between SVP and LVP the range of materials used, i.e. glass, plastic, rubber, is common to each. The background required for the development of a parenteral shares the same phases as other products. However, greater emphasis has to be placed on the packaging material and the sterilization process, hence the points made below.

Glass Glass can be sterilized by dry heat, steam or ethylene oxide, but is discoloured by γ irradiation.

Rubber Rubber can be sterilized by steam ethylene oxide subject to adequate aeration to remove residues, but has to be very carefully checked if irradiation is used as unacceptable physical and chemical changes may occur. Rubber generally will not withstand dry heat.

Plastics Only a few plastics will withstand dry heat.

Sterilization Sterilization is possibly by steam, ethylene oxide, γ-irradiation and a process not previously mentioned – accelerated electrons – which is in essence a milder form of γ-irradiation. This rather sweeping statement has to be supported by adequate testing, as each case must be considered on its own merits. In the case of ethylene oxide treatment, degassing may be a critical stage as residues of ethylene oxide, ethylene glycol (hydrolysed ethylene oxide) and epichlorhydrin (if chloride ions are present) are all toxic in nature. γ-radiation can cause physical (due to molecular crosslinking) and chemical changes to a plastic.

Labelling

If the pack is not already printed, labelling normally follows closuring. Although the preferred labelling system in Europe and the UK is reel-fed self-adhesive labels, with limited use of plain labels and adhesive and heat-seal labels, this is not necessarily the case in other countries. The USA, for example, is more orientated towards heat-sealing (reel-fed and cut singles) than any self-adhesive system.

Both self-adhesive and heat-seal labels contain constituents that may prove to be migratory when adhered to certain plastics. Inactivation of benzalkonium chloride when self-adhesive labels have been applied to LDPE has been recorded.

QUALITY CONTROL OF PACKAGING

In the UK pharmaceutical products are broadly controlled by guidelines related to good manufacturing practice (GMP) and good laboratory practice (GLP). These cover all stages in the discovery, development, production, testing and sale of a pharmaceutical entity, and the means of providing records and documentation. Many of the aspects are related to quality assurance and quality control. However, any approval of a new drug discovery must involve thorough attention to detail, with the effective recording of information through all initial evaluation stages of drug preformulation, formulation, clinical and safety evaluation, packaging development and formal stability, leading to a production/marketing operation. In terms of packaging this should mean that any 'container' used for excipients or drug entities is identified, recorded and cleared for use at all stages. This should also include the storage of intermediates, and all tests irrespective of whether they are investigational or formal in nature, coupled to the procedures that control the pack, e.g. a product is to be stored in a glass bottle with a plastic cap with a liner/facing.

1. Glass bottles should be described by type (amber/white flint), type of glass (I, II, III etc.) and closure type (e.g. screw neck), and cleared as meeting a provisional specification in terms of dimensions, quality etc.
2. The closure should be defined terms of material (black phenol formaldehyde and wadding, i.e. pulpboard faced with 20 gm^{-2} Saran) and identified and cleared in terms of material, dimensions, quality etc.

If these materials are then used for a test at least the on and off torques should be recorded within, say, 1 hour of application. The climatic conditions (temperature and RH) may in certain circumstances need recording, e.g. in the packing of a moisture-sensitive product. This information and the associated documentation – probably a laboratory notebook – is all part of GLP. The recording, examining and passing of bottles prior to acceptance for any type of test is part of quality control. To put testing into perspective, no test should be performed without good knowledge of the pack, the product, and how the two items were assembled. For example, moisture gain by a sensitive product coupled with the finding of loose caps immediately poses the questions 'Were the caps adequately tightened?', 'Are the bottles and caps satisfactory?'. These questions cannot be answered unless a disciplined approach is used and adequate detail recorded. This attitude should apply to all developmental work, as well as the more important items such as clinical trial supplies, human volunteer studies etc. Tests between products and packs which are carried out to define a suitable pack/product are usually termed either feasibility or investigational studies. Once this stage has been completed, coupled with the development of analytical methods and analytical data, usually from accelerated storage tests, there should be a high confidence that the pack product combination chosen has an acceptable shelf-life or stability profile. The final proof that this opinion is correct lies with the formal stability programme, where the product is produced in the pack to be sold (or a near replica of it), by the final product method, and placed on test for a period of up to 5 years. The storage conditions in such a programme may range from 4 to 50°C, with challenges associated with low and high RH, light, etc. with analytical periods of 0 (initial), 3, 6, 9, 12, 18, 24, 30, 36, 48 and 60 months. Regulatory bodies dictate the number of batches to be put on test: usually a minimum of three production-scale batches.

'Analysis' normally involves purity, identification of degradation products, loss or gain of moisture if relevant, microbial levels, effectiveness of preservative system, any exchange, interaction, adsorption, absorption between product and pack, and last but not least assessment of appearance, flavour, smell etc., as these aspects are sometimes more readily quantified by an observer than by a pure chemical analytical method. Specific analytical methods are essential for the main drug entity.

Because certain drugs degrade according to an Arrhenius plot a range of test temperatures can be chosen, i.e. 4°C, 15°C, 25°C, 35°C (or 37°C), 45°C. The temperatures required are 25°C and 40°C to equate with temperate and tropical parts of the world. However, it should be emphasized that most medicines finish up in the bathroom or kitchen (preferably out of the reach of children), and so even home conditions can be particularly severe while the product is being used or simply stored. Although disposal of drugs is recommended for dispensed medicines after the course of treatment has been completed both these and OTC products are inevitably stored for longer periods.

The procedures and controls for drug development are both intense and rigorous, and the same type of control is maintained throughout production, marketing etc., finishing with the monitoring of any complaints and/or adverse reactions. Products once launched are also sampled, say, one batch in 50 and put on a further stability test – known as ongoing or existing product stability – to ensure that the shelf-life profile is maintained. Any change following launch to processes, pack or product is not only similarly monitored but needs further input from packaging expertise.

Packaging development, whether carried out by a formulator or a special packaging section, must be based on a thorough knowledge of all packaging materials, packaging processes, basic test procedures as applied to paper, plastic, glass, metal, laminations etc., and devise programmes that provide the level of confidence that is essential between product and pack. In many cases this will involve packs that act as devices, or separate devices and user/patient type tests designed to establish functional efficiency and/or what will go wrong under conditions of misuse.

The ultimate of all pack clearance procedures is a pack specification that becomes the lead document for purchase and clearance of future deliveries of packaging materials.

Whereas quality assurance is the establishing of procedures that maintain quality, quality control is the actual testing activity. For instance, incoming packaging materials are first examined as a bulk delivery, then sampled on a statistical sampling basis, and finally examined in terms of variables and attributes for critical, major and minor faults to agreed acceptable quality levels (AQLs). As examination covers dimensional, aesthetic and functional aspects plus identification, (particularly relevant with plastics), it ensures that the material specified has been received. As production lines become faster, stoppages due to repairs, malfunction etc. have become more critical as ineffective and inefficient production can significantly affect costs. As an alternative to the statistical sampling of deliveries arriving in house, two other options are:

1. a random sample taken at the point of manufacture which is isolated and identified so that it can be checked by the user;
2. purchasing on warranty certification, which confirms that the quality specified is met as per agreed statistical testing scheme operated by the manufacturer.

With many, items where a high quality of cleanliness is essential sampling of the bulk delivery may lead to an additional risk of particulate or microbial contamination. In such circumstances the alternative schemes indicated above may be used to maintain the integrity of the incoming stock. Inspection and quality control play a further role with ongoing stock inspection, control on production lines, i.e. of the packaged product and the monitoring of finished (saleable) warehoused stock. As mentioned earlier, the final success of any product and its pack can only in the long run be equated to sales and complaints.

Concluding comment

This introduction to the packaging of pharmaceuticals should serve to establish the broad indepth knowledge required by the packaging technologist. The fact that all products only have a shelf-life when packed emphasizes the importance of what has frequently been seen as a minor role in the past. The success of any product depends on an effective marriage between product and pack.

BIBLIOGRAPHY

Briston, J.H. (1983) *Plastics in Packaging*. Properties and Application, Institute of Packaging Melton Mowbray, UK.

Briston, J.H. (1983) *Plastics in Packaging*. Conversion Processes, Institute of Packaging, Melton Mowbray, UK.

Dean, D.A. (1984) Pharmaceutical Packaging–present and future trends. Mang Chem. Aerosol News, March 10th, pp 282–284.

Dean, D.A. (1992) Packaging of pharmaceuticals: packages and closures; Institute of Packaging Melton Mowbray.

Montresor, J.M., Mostyn, H.P. and Paine, F.A. (1983) *Packaging Evaluation*. Institute of Packaging. Melton Mowbray, UK.

Moody, B.E. (1977) *Packaging in Glass*. Hutchinson, London.

Oswin, C.R. (1983) *Packaging Life*. Institute of Packaging, Melton Mowbray, UK.

Remington's Pharmaceutical Sciences (latest edition), Lea and Febiger, New York.

Ross, C.F. (1983) Packaging of pharmaceutical products, sterilisation and safety. Institute of Packaging, Melton Mowbray, UK.

Swinbank, C. *Intermediate Bulk Containers*. Institute of Packaging, Stanmore, Middx.

British and European Pharmacopoeias packaging specifications

BP 2000, Appendix XIX Containers

A Introduction (Ph. Eur. 3.2)
B Glass containers for pharmaceutical use (Ph. Eur. 3.2.1)
C Plastic containers and closures (Ph. Eur. 3.2.2)
D Containers for blood and blood products (Ph. Eur. 3.2.3–3.2.8)
E Rubber closures for containers for aqueous parenteral preparations (Ph. Eur. 3.2.9)

BP 2000, Appendix XX Materials used for manufacture of containers (Ph. Eur. 3.1)

A Materials based on PVC (Ph. Eur. 3.1.1–3.1.2)
B Polyolefines (Ph. Eur. 3.1.3)
C Polyethylene (Ph. Eur. 3.1.4–3.1.5)
D Polypropylene for containers and closures for parenteral and ophthalmic preparations (Ph. Eur. 3.1.6)
F Silicone (Ph. Eur. 3.1.8–3.1.12)
G Plastic additives (Ph. Eur. 3.1.13)
H Rubber for closures for containers for aqueous parenteral preparations and powders for freeze-dried products (Ph. Eur. 3.1.12)

37

Pharmaceutical plant design

Michael Aulton, Andrew Twitchell

This chapter comprises three separate sections relating to the facilities and equipment in which medicinal products are manufactured. The first part discusses manufacturing facilities and describes the selection, design and utilization of a manufacturing facility, and introduces the concept of process validation. The second describes the properties and selection of the materials used in the construction of pharmaceutical facilities. The final part describes the types, causes and prevention of chemical corrosion of pharmaceutical plant.

MANUFACTURING FACILITIES FOR PHARMACEUTICAL PRODUCTS

After a considerable investment of both time and money in developing and testing many new chemical entities and products, some will reach the stage where there is the requirement to manufacture the product in large quantities. This section summarizes some of the factors that need to be taken into consideration when building a facility for producing pharmaceutical products on a large scale. This is only intended as an overview and the reader is referred to the work of Cole (1998) for a more detailed description of the design of pharmaceutical production facilities.

Manufacturing site selection

Pharmaceutical manufacturing facilities require considerable capital expenditure and are likely to be used for many years. It is therefore necessary to think very carefully about where the facility is to be located, as well as how it is constructed. One important consideration is whether the company should develop a new site or refurbish an existing one. Upgrading or redesigning an existing site may often be a more cost-effective option, but may not always be feasible. For example, there may be insufficient space to expand an existing site. It may be 'outdated' and not suitable for upgrading, or the company may be introducing a new product type where there is no existing plant, or the existing site may not be in a suitable location.

Local planning regulations which may delay the development of an existing site also need to be considered, as even small delays in bringing a pharmaceutical product to market can have considerable cost implications.

Considerations when selecting a new site

Most major pharmaceutical companies are multinational and have numerous disciplines contributing to the production of the final product (e.g. chemical synthesis, pharmacological and toxicological testing, product development and product manufacture), which may be located in many different countries. Increasingly, however, there is a tendency to concentrate specific disciplines in a small number of sites, and this may dictate where the production site is located. If this is not the case, then the advantages and disadvantages of locating in different countries need to be considered. Many countries, particularly developing countries, offer incentives to pharmaceutical companies to attract them to build manufacturing facilities in particular areas. These may, for example, take the form of tax incentives, such as no local taxes for a number of years, free land or building grants. Other factors that vary considerably between different countries and which may influence where the site is located include labour costs and availability, energy and construction costs, environmental legislation, likely opposition from the local residents and local employment legislation.

The chosen location must also have an acceptable local infrastructure, including suitable road links, services such as electricity and water, and the availability of a suitably qualified workforce.

Design and utilization of manufacturing facilities

Aims of manufacturing facility design

The major requirements when designing and using manufacturing facilities should be to ensure the following:

1. *Acceptable product quality.*
   - Each unit dose should contain the correct component(s) in the correct concentration and have the desired release properties. There should be negligible cross-contamination between products or chemical contamination from operators. This is particularly important when using highly sensitizing materials (e.g. penicillins) and very potent substances (e.g. hormones and cytotoxic drugs). In these later cases 'dedicated' facilities should ideally be used.
   - The facility must be designed to maximize protection against the entry of insects/animals.

- Microbiological contamination must be acceptably low both to protect the patient and to ensure a satisfactory product shelf-life.
- The factory should be designed to ensure that no unauthorized personnel gain entry to processing or storage areas.
- Each product must be correctly packaged and labelled to ensure the patient takes the correct medication and that it reaches the patient in a satisfactory condition. If the product is not of the required quality this will have considerable cost implications – for example if the batch has to be destroyed. If the batch has to be recalled after distribution, owing to errors such as incorrect labelling, this is very costly both financially and in damage to the company's reputation.

2. *An acceptable working environment.*
- It is the duty of the pharmaceutical company to ensure that the manufacturing area is designed and operated so that the exposure of personnel to drugs, solvents etc. is at an acceptably low level. This may be achieved in some circumstances by controlling the air flow and quality in the area, but with more toxic materials special breathing apparatus with appropriate filters may be necessary.
- Comfortable working conditions should be provided for process operators wherever possible, bearing in mind any particular product requirements, such as the need to prepare a product at a low temperature or humidity.

3. *Manufacturing efficiency.* Correctly designed and located facilities within the manufacturing area will improve the efficiency of the manufacturing process and thus reduce the cost of product manufacture. Careful consideration needs to be given to all the different stages involved in the process and how material will be transferred between stages, so that the production facility layout is optimized. For example, the use of gravity feeding of material between stages might require the facility to be sited on different levels, whereas the use of pneumatic or vacuum systems allow the facility to be sited on one level.

Achievement of manufacturing aims

Environmental conditions Control of the air temperature, relative humidity and particulate and microbial content is important so that the aims of

the manufacturing process can be met. The specific conditions required depend on the product being manufactured. The following are illustrative examples.

- For a tabletting operation, typical environmental conditions might be a temperature of 21°C, a relative humidity of 35–40% and an air filtration target of 95% removal of particles less than 5 μm. These figures are such because powder flow is influenced by both air temperature and, particularly, relative humidity.
- Hard gelatin capsule filling processes, on the other hand, are typically carried out at temperature of 24°C and a relative humidity of approximately 30%. These figures are necessary because capsule shells become brittle and crack if the relative humidity and temperature are too low, and become soft and sticky and tend to jam the capsule filler if the relative humidity and temperature are too high.
- Air relative humidity is also vital when manufacturing deliquescent products, where levels as low as 20% may be required.
- With clean preparation areas the air particulate level is very important and the filtration target may be for more than 99% removal of particles of 1 μm or less.

Typical 'comfortable' working conditions for operators are 18–24°C and 30–60% relative humidity.

The temperature of the air may be controlled either by passing it through a steam-based or electrical heating system, or over refrigerant coils. The relative humidity may be increased by spraying water (of small droplet size) into the airstream, or decreased by using refrigeration systems or desiccant wheels.

In order to maintain the required conditions in the manufacturing area, the stale air must be frequently 'replaced' with 'conditioned' air. The frequency at which this needs to occur will depend on factors such as the nature of the production process, the number of operators present and whether the room is 'in use'. It may vary from approximately 20 changes per hour (typical solid dose production) to 500 (rooms for sterile production).

Architectural considerations Manufacturing areas should be of a suitable size, construction and location to facilitate proper operation, cleaning and maintenance. Any pipework, light fittings or ventilation points should be designed and sited to avoid the creation of recesses which might collect 'dust' and are difficult to clean. If possible, they should be accessible from outside the manufacturing area for maintenance.

Interior surfaces (walls, floors and ceilings) should be smooth, free from cracks and open joints, should not shed particulate matter, and should permit easy and effective cleaning or disinfection. Lighting should be sufficient for easy reading of in-process control systems, equipment dials etc.

Validation of manufacturing facilities

Validation and why it is required

Detailed coverage of validation is beyond the scope of this chapter owing to its complexity and the constantly changing requirements of the regulatory authorities. This section therefore summarizes the scope of validation with respect to manufacturing facilities and explains why it is important. In order to be aware of the latest position, the reader should consult information provided by regulatory authorities or other relevant authoritative sources.

Validation is a component of cGMP (current good manufacturing practice). Numerous definitions exist, including that of the Food and Drug Administration (FDA, USA), which has defined process validation as 'establishing documented evidence which provides a high degree of assurance that a specific process will consistently produce a product meeting its predetermined specifications and quality characteristics'. In other words, validation is proving that a process works.

Essentially, the purpose of validation is to ensure consistent product quality. A new product or an old product manufactured using a modified process or facility cannot be sold until the 'process' has been adequately validated.

The scope of validation

When manufacturing a product all aspects of the 'process' need to be validated. This includes bulk drugs, excipients, suppliers, analytical methods, computer systems and personnel, as well as manufacturing equipment and processes. It must be ensured that the manufacturing equipment complies with the intended specification and that all services and recording equipment function correctly. The manufacturing process must be robust and produce a product with consistent properties. This is usually confirmed by manufacturing three full-scale production batches under specified conditions. In order to minimize cross-contamination between batches, the processes used to clean all equipment in which the product comes into contact must also be validated.

Types of validation

Validation may be divided into four types.

Prospective validation   This is where the validation programme is designed *before* the equipment or facility is used, or before the product manufactured by the process being validated is distributed. This type of validation is employed when producing the data on initial full-scale production batches required to obtain a regulatory authorization for marketing and manufacture of that product.

Retrospective validation   This is achieved by reviewing historical manufacturing and testing data of products or processes which are already in operation and working well.

Concurrent validation   This is ongoing prospective validation or ongoing review and evaluation of historical data.

Revalidation   Revalidation involves repeating all or part of the validation if, for example, a process or facility is modified.

Cost/benefits of validation

The cost of validation is considerable, with significant resources including personnel (from product development, quality assurance and engineering departments) and materials being required. Inadequate validation may, however, lead to the rejection of, or withdrawal of, legal authorization to manufacture and market the product. In other circumstances it may lead to expensive product recalls. Other benefits of well designed validation programmes are likely to include a reduction in process support required, fewer batch failures, greater output and speeding-up of marketing authorizations.

Cleaning as an example of a validation process

It is clearly desirable that a pharmaceutical product contains only those components that are supposed to be present. As most manufacturing equipment will not be used solely in the production of a single product, there is the possibility that, without adequate cleaning procedures, cross-contamination between products may occur. Although this should be detected during quality control tests, and therefore not endanger the public, it will still lead to costly batch wastage.

Cleaning protocols must therefore be validated to ensure that they are suitable. Because equipment can never be 100% clean, the aim of a cleaning procedure is to minimize the possibility of *significant* cross-contamination between batches of different products.

A typical specification would be that the contaminant level in the product taken by a patient is not greater than a 1000th of its lowest daily therapeutic dose.

Once a piece of equipment has been cleaned following a documented procedure, it is 'analysed' to detect the level of any product residue remaining. This may be achieved, for example, by:

- swabbing the equipment over a 100 cm² area at positions likely to be contaminated and analysing the swabs;
- collecting and analysing rinsings from final cleaning water (e.g. for cream manufacturing vessels);
- producing a placebo batch of the product in the cleaned container.
- Visual and tactile inspection is also useful for detecting contamination (except for very potent drugs).

It is a good idea for the product selected to validate the cleaning procedure to be the one that is likely to be the most difficult to clean of those produced in the equipment. Care must also be taken to ensure that any cleaning materials used are pharmaceutically acceptable, and that they are present in suitably low amounts. Once a cleaning process has been validated, operators must *always* follow the designated procedure to ensure a consistently successful process.

MATERIALS OF FABRICATION

Desirable properties and selection

In selecting materials for the construction of satisfactory plant the pharmaceutical engineer encounters problems involving chemical, physical and economic factors. The following brief outline indicates something of the scope and limitations of the choice of materials available.

Chemical factors

Two aspects of chemical action must be considered under this heading, namely, the possible contamination of the **product** by the material of the plant, and any effect on the **material of the plant** by the drugs and chemicals being processed. The importance of the first of these becomes evident when it is realised that impurities often have considerable toxicological effects, and even trace amounts of impurity may initiate decomposition mechanisms in the product. An example of the latter is the inactivating effect of heavy metals on penicillins. The appearance of a product may also be affected by changes in colour due to contamination from the materials of the plant.

It should be remembered that contamination from some materials may be innocuous, the products being non-toxic.

Our increasing knowledge of materials of plant construction is assisting greatly in providing plant that will be resistant to attack and deterioration in use from the effects of acids, alkalis, oxidizing agents etc. Alloys having special physical and chemical properties have been developed, and materials such as plastics have been introduced to meet the problems encountered.

Physical factors

An ideal construction material would satisfy all the following criteria. In practice no material is ideal and the selection procedure must be based on compromise.

Strength Sufficient mechanical strength is an obvious necessity and will be suited to the size of the plant and the stresses to which it will be subjected.

Weight In most cases weight should be reduced to a minimum, other factors being satisfactory, and especially in plant that may have to be moved about from place to place.

Wearing qualities These are particularly important where there is a possibility of friction between moving parts, an extreme case being the material used for the grinding surfaces of size-reduction mills.

Ease of fabrication It must be possible to process the material in order to manufacture the various units of the plant. Properties that enable materials to be cast, welded, bent or machined are of prime importance.

Thermal expansion The design of plant may be greatly complicated by the use of material that has a high coefficient of expansion. This increases the stresses and the risk of fracture with temperature changes, and the temperature range over which the plant will be operated is likely to be considerably restricted.

Thermal conductivity In heat-transfer plant, such as steam or water-heated vessels, good thermal conductivity is desirable. It must be remembered, however, that the bulk of the resistance to heat transfer may lie in the boundary layer films (see Chapter 38).

Cleaning Smooth polished surfaces simplify cleaning processes, and materials that can be 'finished' with such surfaces are ideal when scrupulous cleanliness is necessary.

Sterilization Where sterility is essential the material should be capable of withstanding the necessary treatment, usually steam under pressure. This factor is to some extent bound up with the previous one, as cleaning is a normal preliminary to the sterilization of apparatus and plant equipment.

Transparency This *may* be a useful property where it is necessary to observe the process. Borosilicate glass is used in the construction of pharmaceutical plant.

Economic factors

Cost and maintenance of plant must, of course, be economic. Here the main concern is not simply to obtain the least costly material: better wearing qualities and lower maintenance may well mean that a higher initial cost is more economical in the long run.

MATERIALS USED IN FABRICATION

A brief description of materials which are suitable for the fabrication or construction of pharmaceutical apparatus and manufacturing plant is given below.

Metals

Ferrous metals – steels

The element iron is abundant in nature in the form of its ores and, despite the tendency for the metal to corrode, it is still widely used. Steel consists of iron with added carbon, which may exist in the free state (graphite) or in chemical combination as iron carbide, Fe_3C. The phase diagram for the iron/carbon system is complex. Iron can exist in two allotropic forms. At temperatures below 940°C the stable form is α-iron (ferrite) but the γ form (austenite) can persist at normal temperatures if other metals such as chromium and nickel are alloyed with the iron. When steel is in the molten condition, austenite is able to dissolve carbon. Various eutectics and solid solutions may form on cooling, giving rise to steels of differing properties. These properties depend on the carbon content and any heat treatment that the steel may receive.

Mild steel This is the commonest form of steel for general purposes and has a carbon content between 0.15 and 0.3%. It is ductile and can be welded to give structures of high mechanical strength, but its resistance to corrosion is poor.

Cast iron The effect of increasing the carbon content beyond 1.5% is to lower the melting point of iron so that it can easily be melted and cast into sand moulds to form objects of intricate shape. Cast iron is resistant to corrosion but it reacts with materials such as phenols to give coloured compounds. Most pharmaceuticals are required to pass a limit test for iron, and if they are handled in cast-iron vessels they may fail to comply. Such vessels may be lined with resistant materials to take advantage of the strength of cast iron while shielding the product from the metal.

Cast iron is hard and brittle and can be welded and machined only with great difficulty. The hardness and corrosion resistance can be increased by adding silicon, though such high-silicon iron is extremely brittle.

Stainless steels These steels contain a proportion of nickel and chromium which confer a high degree of corrosion resistance. The stainless steels can be easily fabricated and polished to a high mirror finish. They are extensively used in the food, pharmaceutical, cosmetic and fermentation industries, where their high cost can be fully justified.

The most common type is the so-called austenitic stainless steel, where the nickel and chromium content stabilizes austenite at normal room temperatures. As can be seen from the phase diagram (Fig. 37.1) an alloy containing 18% chromium and 8% nickel (which is more costly than chromium) is the most economical form of austenitic stainless steel. The steel is often stabilized by the addition of 1% titanium or niobium, which prevents 'weld decay'. This can result from the removal of chromium as chromium carbide along the line of any welding that might be performed. Such depleted steel is then prone to corrosion.

Stainless steel owes its resistance to a tenacious oxide layer that forms on the surface. Materials such as nitric acid, which are oxidizing agents, can be handled in it but chlorides can penetrate the film and stainless steel equipment should not be used for hydrochloric acid.

One minor objection to stainless steel is its low thermal conductivity compared to other metals, but this is not usually significant as the main resistance to heat transfer may reside in the boundary layers (see Chapter 38).

Stainless steels can be used for most pharmaceutical plant equipment. Small apparatus commonly made from stainless steel includes funnels, buckets and measuring vessels. Sinks and benchtops are also made of stainless steel where a smooth surface with high corrosion-resisting qualities is necessary.

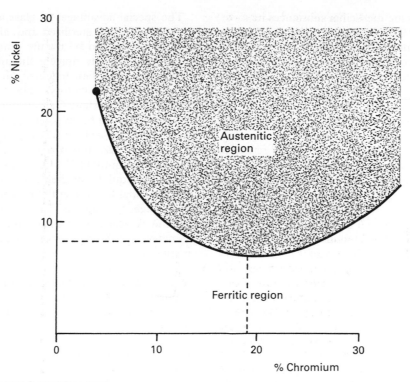

Fig. 37.1   Phase diagram for stainless steel.

The high cost often excludes its use, but often this may be justified even on a very large scale. For example, a great deal of the plant used in the production of penicillin is of this material, as it is by far the most satisfactory, being strong, corrosion-resistant, non-contaminating and readily cleaned and sterilized.

Non-ferrous metals

Copper   Copper is malleable and ductile and thus easily fabricated. It has a thermal conductivity eight times greater than steel but is corroded by a number of substances, particularly oxidizing agents. It is attacked by nitric acid in all concentrations, by hot concentrated hydrochloric and sulphuric acids, and by some organic acids. Ammonia reacts with it readily to form blue cuproammonium compounds. Many drug constituents react with it, and for this reason copper is usually protected by a lining of tin when used for pharmaceutical plant. It was formerly used for evaporators and pans used for sugar coating (Chapter 28). Because of its susceptibility to attack by pharmaceutical materials there is a tendency today to replace it with stainless steel.

Copper piping is easy to make because of the ductility of the metal and it is used extensively for services such as cold water, gas, vacuum, and low-pressure steam. Where necessary, copper piping may be tinned, e.g. for distilled water, but nowadays stainless steel piping is used for this purpose.

Copper alloys   These include alloys with zinc, tin, aluminium, silicon and nickel, all of which have their special uses.

Aluminium   Aluminium has good corrosion resistance to many substances, although it is attacked by mineral acids (it is resistant to strong nitric acid), caustic alkalis, mercury and its salts. Its resistance is often due to the formation of a film on the surface. For example, acetic acid forms a film of gelatinous aluminium subacetate, which is then resistant to acetic acid, and pure strong ammonia solutions form a resistant film of aluminium hydroxide. It is also highly resistant to oxidizing conditions, as it forms a compact oxide film.

Pure aluminium is soft but more corrosion resistant than most of its alloys, such as Duralumin. Alloys combining corrosion resistance with strength are formed with the addition of small percentages of manganese, magnesium or silicon. Plant is easily fabricated and has excellent thermal conductivity.

For plant producing medicinal substances its most valuable property is probably the non-toxicity of its salts, which are, moreover, colourless. As it is also non-toxic to microorganisms it has considerable use in biosynthetic processes, such as the production of citric and gluconic acids, and of streptomycin by deep culture methods. The metal is also suitable for plant used for preparing culture media and for absorption and extraction vessels used in preparing antibiotics. As a result of the formation of resistant film it is used for acetic acid plant and storage vessels for ammonia. Because of its low density it is most useful for transport containers, such as drums and barrels.

Lead Much lead is used in the chemical industry because of its remarkable resistance to corrosion and the great ease with which it can be made into complicated shapes. The lead-chamber process for manufacturing sulphuric acid is one example from many in the heavy chemical industry. It is little used in pharmaceutical practice, however, because of the risk of contamination by traces of poisonous lead salts. Pharmaceutical materials must comply with a limit test for lead.

Tin Tin has a high resistance to a great variety of substances and, as its salts are non-toxic, it is widely used throughout the food industry. It is, however, weak, its main use being to provide a protective coating for steel, copper, brass etc. The coating of other metals with tin has been known for over 2000 years, and today more than half the output of the metal is used for this purpose. 'Tin plate' – sheet steel coated with tin – is used for containers.

Non-metals

Inorganics

Glass Glass is widely used in the laboratory and glass equipment can be obtained for manufacturing on a larger scale. Ordinary soda glass is used for bottles and other cheap articles, but is not satisfactory for large-scale plant or for containers where alkali contamination might be a serious drawback. For these purposes borosilicate glass is used, which has several advantages over soda glass. It is, for example, less brittle. It has a low thermal expansion and can be used safely over wide temperature ranges. However, its thermal conductivity is low and therefore it should be heated gradually to avoid fracturing. Pipeline may be used with pressures up to 8 bar if the pipe diameter is less than 50 mm, and pipelines with larger diameters are used with pressures up to 4 bar.

The special advantages of glass are that it can be easily cleaned and sterilized and, also, that the contents of vessels can be readily examined for colour and clarity. A disadvantage is the difficulty of joining sections of glass plant together. Ground-glass joints are sometimes satisfactory, especially in small-scale apparatus, but are rigid. Gaskets of rubber and plastic are used to form a flexible jointing, but these must be chosen with care as they are normally less resistant to attack than glass. For this reason gaskets are now often made from PTFE, but careful alignment of the sections is required for their successful use.

Glass pipeline is useful for transporting liquids from stage to stage in various operations. Such pipeline is available from 15 mm to 300 mm in diameter, with fittings for the assembly of complete systems.

All-glass stills are used for preparing pharmaceutical quality Water for Injections and other distilled preparations. Vessels up to 100 L are used, and larger tanks can be made by clamping glass plates in frames.

Glass fibres are excellent for heat insulation or refrigeration plant. Woven fibre may be used for filter cloths and glass may be sintered in the preparation of filters.

Fused silica Fused silica (Vitreosil) has an extremely low coefficient of thermal expansion and vessels made from it can be heated to red heat and plunged into cold water without breaking. It has a high melting point and it is difficult to fuse it completely, so that equipment tends to be opaque, although transparent forms are available.

Glass linings and coatings Metal may be coated with glass to give a protective lining. The dangers of such apparatus are those of uneven expansion of metal and glass, and of the glass surface accidentally chipping. Great care must therefore be taken in heating and cooling, and in protecting the glass lining from accidental damage.

Vessels of up to 50 000 L capacity, pipeline and fittings, valves, condensers, columns, pumps, stirrers and mixers are among the many glass-coated items still in use, although they have been largely replaced with stainless steel vessels.

Its high resistance to corrosion and ease of cleaning make glass valuable for pharmaceutical use.

Organics

Plastics The range of materials known collectively as plastics is so wide that only a brief account can be given. It is convenient to group them under the following headings:

- Rigid materials
- Flexible materials
- Coatings and linings
- Cements and filters
- Special cases.

'Keebush' is an example of a rigid material. This is a phenolic resin with various inert fillers selected for their particular purpose. It may be machined, welded, and worked in other ways, and is resistant to such an extent that it can be used for gears, bearings and similar items with a noise reduction of two-thirds compared to metal. It is resistant to corrosion, except that of oxidizing substances and strong alkalis. Any item may be made from this material – vessels, pipes, fittings, valves, pumps, fans, ducts, filter presses and many others.

Polyethylene and polyvinyl chloride (PVC) are similar materials and are either rigid or flexible, depending upon the amount of plasticizer added. They do not withstand high temperatures but are non-resistant only to strong oxidizing acids, halogens and organic solvents.

Rigid or semirigid mouldings may be used for tanks, pipes, ducts and other similar items; slightly flexible funnels, buckets and jugs are made which are almost unbreakable.

Polytetrafluoroethylene (PTFE, Teflon) is a semi-rigid plastic with extreme resistance to all agents other than fluorine or molten alkali metals. It is a slippery non-wettable material but can be bonded to metals as a protective coating. It is also usable at temperatures above 200°C, but it is costly, which prohibits its extensive use.

Metallic surfaces may be protected from corrosion by plastics of the polyethylene or PVC types pre-pared for coating with suitable plasticizers. Perfect adhesion of plastic to metal is sometimes difficult, and other disadvantages are the differences in thermal expansion of plastic and metal and the danger of the coating accidentally chipping.

Uses of these materials include the lining of tanks and vessels and the coatings on stirrers and fans. Plastic cements are used for spaces between acid-resistant tiles and bricks, and for similar purposes.

Special cases include transparent plastic guards for moving parts of machinery, and asepsis screens. Nylon and PVC fibres may be woven into filter cloths.

Rubber Hard rubber may be used for purposes similar to those mentioned for plastics. Soft rubber may be used for linings, coatings and valves. Rubber swells in contact with oils; it is subject to oxidation and is attacked by some organic solvents. Synthetic rubbers that have greater resistance have been developed.

CORROSION

General introduction and theory

Corrosion is a complex form of material deterioration that results from a reaction with its environment. It is the destruction of a material (usually a metal) by means other than mechanical. Most environments are corrosive. Corrosion is not restricted to reactions with strong acids. The following have been shown to cause corrosion:

- Air and moisture
- Rural, urban and industrial atmospheres
- Fresh, salt and distilled water
- Steam and gases, such as chlorine, ammonia, hydrogen sulphide, sulphur dioxide
- Mineral acids, such as hydrochloric acid, sulphuric acid, nitric acid
- Organic acids, such as acetic, citric, formic
- Alkalis
- Soils
- Organic solvents
- Vegetable and petroleum oils.

Importance of corrosion

Corrosion is very important in the chemical and pharmaceutical process industries, for a number of reasons. The possibility of any of the following occurring must be considered.

Safety

- Loss of pharmacologically active or toxic substances
- Loss of inflammable or explosive chemicals
- Sudden loss of material being processed at high temperature or high pressure
- Possibility of burns from acids etc.
- Corroding of equipment is known to have caused fairly harmless compounds to become toxic or explosive.

Financial losses

- Replacement of corroded parts
- Plant shut-down, i.e. stoppage due to unexpected corrosion failures. This leads to loss of revenue
- Loss of expensive chemicals.

Contamination of the product

This is of particular importance in the pharmaceutical industry as the product is usually for human consumption or administration. Metal ions can promote degradation reactions and can be toxic.

Appearance of plant

This is not a minor consideration. Satisfactory factory appearance is an important aspect of good manufacturing practice.

Corrosion mechanisms

The corrosive reaction of metals is generally electrochemical in nature. The relevant points of a simple, acceptable theory of electrochemical corrosion are summarized below.

1. An anode (−) and a cathode (+) form a cell in conjunction with an electrically conducting environment (electrolyte). Anodic and cathodic areas can arise on a single piece of metal because of local differences in the outside environment and in the metal itself. Different stresses, scratches and impurities produce varying electrical potentials. Cells with far greater electrical potentials are formed between different metals or alloys. Anodes and cathodes may be close (local cells) or far apart.

2. Direct current (DC) flows. The current is a flow of electrons within the metal(s) from anode to cathode. Metal ions (positive charge) travel from the anode in the electrolyte; they do not usually reach the cathode, but remain in solution.

Single-metal corrosion

Simple electrochemical corrosion is explained diagrammatically in Figure 37.2. This shows the mechanism for corrosion of a single piece of steel (predominantly iron) in water (dissociated by the presence of dissolved chemicals).

The anodic reaction is:

$$Fe \rightarrow Fe^{2+} + 2e^-$$

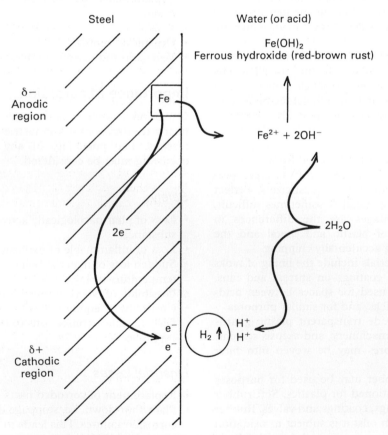

Fig. 37.2   Diagrammatic representation of the electrochemical corrosion of steel (iron) in water.

and the cathodic reaction is:

$$2H^+ + 2e^- \rightarrow H_2$$

The overall reaction is therefore:

$$Fe + 2H_2O \rightarrow Fe(OH)_2 + H_2$$

The important consequence of this reaction is that structurally strong metal leaves the anode as a metal ion in solution. The metal is therefore weakened and the solution contaminated with corrosion product.

Corrosion between metals

This is important because joints, flanges, seals, bolts etc. are often constructed of different metals. A cell is set up between the metals, one becoming the anode and the other the cathode. The potential difference between the metals depends on the electrode potentials of the metals. A knowledge of the electromotive series of metals is therefore important. These are summarized in Table 37.1, from which the following points can be noted:

1. A negative sign in the fourth column implies that the reaction in the direction of element to ion is spontaneous, i.e. it requires negative energy to proceed in that direction.
2. When two metals are coupled or in indirect contact with each other via the electrolyte a metal higher in the series will be the anode and one lower will act as the cathode.
3. Metals high in the table have less corrosion resistance. For example, metals above copper

Table 37.1 The electromotive series of some commonly used metals

	Element	Ion produced	Standard electrode potential (V)
Active end	Na	Na$^+$	−2.71
	Mg	Mg^{2+}	−2.34
	Al	Al^{3+}	−1.67
	Zn	Zn^{2+}	−0.76
	Cr	Cr^{3+}	−0.71
	Fe	Fe^{3+}	−0.44
	Ni	Ni^{2+}	−0.25
	Sn	Sn^{2+}	−0.14
	Pb	Pb^{2+}	−0.13
Reference zero	H	H$^+$	0.000
	Cu	Cu^{2+}	+0.35
	Cu	Cu$^+$	+0.52
	Ag	Ag$^+$	+0.80
	Pt	Pt^{2+}	+1.20
Noble end	Au	Au^{3+}	+1.42

oxidize readily. This also explains why gold and silver are found as free metals in their native state, whereas aluminium and iron are found only combined as oxides.

4. The greater the difference in potential between two metals, the greater will be the rate of corrosion. For example, sodium reacts violently with water, iron slowly rusts, yet lead is not attacked by water.
5. When two metals are in contact, the corrosion rate of the anodic member of the couple is accelerated.
6. A metal will replace another metal in solution if the latter is lower in the series. This is best understood by examination of Figure 37.3.
7. The table therefore indicates whether or not a metal is attacked by acids or water, as metals above hydrogen are attacked because they replace hydrogen in solution,

e.g. Al + HCl(in solution) $\rightarrow$ AlCl$_3$(in solution)

Fe + H$_2$O(in solution) $\rightarrow$ Fe(OH)$_2$(in solution)

Cathodic protection

This term is used to describe the technique whereby a structurally important metal is forced to become wholly cathodic (and therefore protected from corrosion) by attaching a more electronegative second metal to it. An example is galvanization, in which steel is coated with a layer of zinc. The zinc becomes the anode, thereby protecting the steel. The advantage of this technique over normal coatings is that even if the galvanized coating is scratched the exposed metal surface will remain cathodic. Metal objects can be protected in a similar way by attaching to them replaceable pieces of a more electronegative metal (e.g. a small aluminium block attached to a steel object).

Passivity

This is the phenomenon in which a metal appears in practice to be much less reactive than would be predicted by its position in the electromotive series. For example, one would expect aluminium to be extremely reactive, as its electrode potential is −1.67 V, yet it is commonly used in construction because of its lack of reactivity. The explanation is that aluminium does in fact react quickly with air, but an aluminium oxide coating is produced which is very resistant to further atmospheric attack.

Lead, which has a small electronegativity and would therefore be expected to react, at least with strong

(a)   (b)

Fig. 37.3 (a) Reaction of iron in copper sulphate solution. The copper ions in solution are being replaced by iron ions (lower in table) at the same time as the copper from solution is being deposited as copper metal on the iron sheet. (b) Similarly, the hydrogen in the HCl solution is replaced by aluminium ions and the hydrogen is evolved as gas bubbles

inorganic acids, is in fact used in the production of sulphuric acid (lead-chamber process). In this example an impervious, unreactive layer of lead sulphate is formed on the outside of the lead sheets.

Types of corrosion

The various types of corrosion can be classified by the form in which they manifest themselves. The eight most common types of corrosion are:

1. Uniform attack or general, overall corrosion
2. Galvanic or two-metal corrosion
3. Concentration-cell corrosion
4. Pitting
5. Intergranular corrosion
6. Parting (or dezincification)
7. Stress corrosion
8. Erosion corrosion.

Uniform attack

This is the most common form of corrosion. It is normally an electrochemical reaction in which the anode and cathode move slowly over the surface of the metal. The metal becomes thinner and thinner and eventually

fails, e.g. sheet-iron roof, zinc in acid. Uniform corrosion is the easiest to predict, discover and stop by means of the use of (a) more suitable materials, (b) inhibitors either in the metal or in the product, and (c) protective coatings (paint, plastic etc.).

Galvanic corrosion

This is corrosion between two dissimilar metals (see above). An example could be the case of a concentric pipe heat exchanger in which the main structure is of steel but the heat-exchange pipes are made of copper to improve heat transfer. In domestic central heating systems the commonest situation is to have steel radiators joined by copper piping.

Control of galvanic corrosion   Use only one metal if this is possible. If not:

1. Select combinations of metals as close together as possible in the electrochemical series.
2. Avoid combinations where the area of the more active metal (i.e. the anode) is small, as this increases the anodic reaction rate. It is therefore better to have the more noble metal or alloy for fastenings, bolts etc.

3. Insulate dissimilar metals completely wherever possible.

4. Apply coatings such as paint, bitumen or plastic, but with caution. Small holes in the coating over an anodic region will result in rapid attack. Therefore, it is important to keep the coating in good repair.

5. Add chemical inhibitors to the corrosive solution. The nature of these inhibitors depends on the specific nature of the solution to be inhibited. Particular care must be taken in their selection when the corrosive solution is the pharmaceutical product, or is an intermediate for drug synthesis.

6. Avoid joining metals with threaded connections, as the threads will deteriorate excessively; spilled liquids or condensates can concentrate in thread grooves. Welded joints (using welds of the same alloy) are preferred.

Concentration-cell corrosion

Cells can form because of differences in the environment rather than differences in the metal itself. These are known as concentration (or solution) cells. There are two types, metal-ion cells and oxygen cells.

Metal-ion cells These can form in areas where stagnant liquid collects. Metal-ion concentration cells are caused, as their name suggests, by differences in metal-ion concentration in the corroding solution. A build-up of metal ions can occur in stagnant conditions caused by holes, gaskets, lap joints, surface deposits (scale, dirt) and crevices under bolt heads and rivet heads. They can also be caused by material, such as plastic, rubber etc. lying on the surface of the metal. Figure 37.4 shows the formation of a metal-ion concentration cell at a lap joint.

Oxygen cells These are similar to metal-ion cells in a number of ways, but here the corrosion is caused by differences in the dissolved oxygen content of the solution. The formation of an oxygen concentration cell at a lap joint is shown in Figure 37.5.

Control of concentration-cell corrosion This can be achieved in the following ways:

1. Use welded butt joints instead of riveted or bolted joints in new apparatus.

2. Existing lap joints should be welded, sealed or soldered to close the crevices.

3. Design vessels for complete drainage; avoid sharp corners and stagnant areas.

4. Inspect and clean deposits frequently.

5. Use solid, non-absorbent gaskets, such as Teflon, wherever possible.

6. Use welded pipes rather than the rolled-in type.

Pitting

This is a form of extremely localized attack where the anode remains as one spot. This results in rapid corrosion and deep penetration (small anode area, large cathode). Pits may be isolated or close together, the latter appearing as a rough surface. The pits usually occur at impurities in the metal, grain boundaries, small scratches, rough surfaces etc. Pitting is one of the most destructive forms of corrosion. It is difficult to detect in a laboratory corrosion test because the pits are very small and there will be little loss in weight.

Pitting is responsible for more **unexpected** plant equipment failures than any other form of corrosion. Additionally, the liquid in the pit becomes stagnant, resulting in metal-ion and/or oxygen concentration-cell corrosion. Furthermore, metal ions from the corrosion will accumulate in the pit. The process is therefore self-accelerating.

Control of pitting This is very difficult, but most of the points mentioned under concentration cells will help. If a test material shows the slightest signs of pitting in a laboratory test using microscopy, it must never be used.

Intergranular corrosion

Solid metals consist of a large number of grains (actually metal crystals) and thus have a granular (or polycrystalline) structure. Intergranular corrosion is localized attack at grain boundaries, with relatively little corrosion of the grains themselves. Because of stresses and structural imperfections at the grain boundaries (plus the increased concentration of impurities there), they are usually anodic. As corrosion proceeds the grains fall out and the metal or alloy disintegrates. This type of corrosion occurs in stainless steel, particularly after welding (known as **weld decay**).

Control of intergranular corrosion This can be achieved in the following ways:

1. High-temperature post-weld heat treatment (solution quenching) can be used. This involves heating the metal to about 1000 K and then cooling it rapidly by quenching in water. This reduces the precipitation of carbon at the grain boundaries.

2. Add stabilizers to the metal, such as columbium, tantalum or titanium. These combine strongly

Fig. 37.4 A metal-ion concentration cell at a lap joint.

with free carbon to form carbides, leaving no free carbon at the grain boundaries.

3. Lower the carbon content of the steel to below 0.03%. Below this figure carbon is usually completely soluble.

Parting (or dezincification)

This is a general term referring to selective corrosion of one or more components from a solid solution alloy. The removal of zinc, particularly from brass (a 70/30 copper/zinc alloy), is common.

Control of parting This is not easy. Reduction of the corrosive environment and cathodic protection are suggested. Small amounts of arsenic, antimony or phosphorus can be used as 'inhibitors'. The addi-

tion of 1% tin to brass (to give Admiralty Brass) results in good resistance to seawater.

Stress corrosion

Generally a high stress in a piece of metal tends to make it more anodic. The greater the stress, the greater this effect. There are two main categories.

Stress-accelerated corrosion This is a decrease in corrosion resistance as a result of continuous static stress, such as applied stresses or residual stresses after welding (i.e. as occurs in pressure vessels).

Stress corrosion cracking This is an increase in the tendency of the metal to crack or show brittle fracture. It is usually caused by alternating stresses (i.e. vibrations).

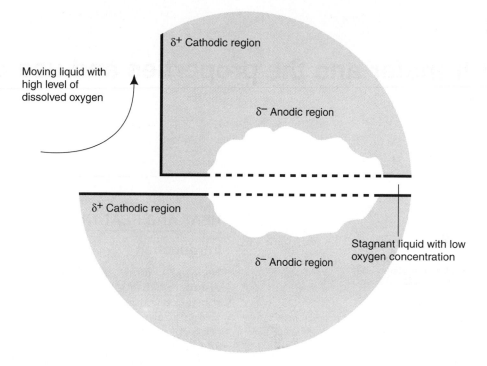

Fig. 37.5 An oxygen concentration cell at a lap joint.

Erosion corrosion

Erosion is a mechanical process, corrosion is electro-chemical. They combine in situations where corrosive products which might have protected metals from further corrosion are eroded by mechanical wear or rapid fluid flow. This maintains a fresh metal surface in contact with the corrosive environment.

BIBLIOGRAPHY

Cole G.C. (1998) *Pharmaceutical Production Facilities – Design and Applications*. 2nd edn., Taylor and Francis. London.

Rules and Guidance for Pharmaceutical Manufacturers, current edition. HMSO 'The Orange Guide.'

38

Heat transfer and the properties and use of steam

Andrew Twitchell

HEAT AND HEAT TRANSFER

Introduction

Heat is a form of energy associated with the disordered/chaotic movement of molecules/ions. A substance will have no heat content only if it is at absolute zero (0 K). Although heat is intangible, it is a form of energy and can be accurately measured and expressed in (preferably) joules (J) or alternatively Nm or kg m^2/s^2. The joule represents a very small quantity of heat; for example, 1 J will raise the temperature of 100 mL of water by only approximately 0.002 °C. A more practically useful quantity is the kilojoule (kJ) or the megajoule (MJ), which denote 1000 and 1 000 000 joules, respectively. It requires about 65 kJ of heat to raise 200 mL of water from room temperature to its boiling point. The temperature of a material is an indication of its internal energy: the greater the molecular motion the greater the internal energy and the higher the temperature. Heat transfer is the exchange or movement of heat energy and will occur spontaneously wherever there is a temperature gradient. The rate of heat transfer indicates how quickly heat is exchanged, and is expressed in J s^{-1} or watts (W).

Many pharmaceutical processes involve the transfer of heat energy. These include:

* melting materials and creating an elevated temperature during cream, suppository or ointment production;
* heating of solvents to hasten dissolution processes, e.g. dissolution of preservatives in the manufacture of solution products;
* sterilization of products, e.g. using steam in autoclaves;
* evaporation of liquids to concentrate products;
* heating or cooling of air in air-conditioning plant;
* drying granules for tablet production;

- heating air to facilitate coating processes;
- controlled cooling during cream manufacture.

It is therefore important to have a basic understanding of how materials may be heated and what influences the rate at which they can be heated (so that the heating or cooling can be controlled). This chapter considers the methods by which heat can be transferred and the factors that influence the rate of heat transfer. Particular emphasis will be given to the properties and use of steam, as heat energy provided by steam is the main source of heating in production processes. It is only intended as an introduction to this complex subject; the reader is referred to texts by Arpaci et al (1999), Long (1999) and Mills (1999) for more detailed information.

Methods of heat transfer

Conduction

Heat transfer by conduction in solids results from the movement of heat energy to adjacent molecules by vibrational energy transfer and the motion of free electrons. The molecule/electron donating the heat energy will subsequently vibrate to a lesser extent and therefore cool down, whereas the molecule receiving the heat energy will vibrate to a greater extent and therefore increase in temperature. No appreciable movement of molecules occurs. Heat transfer due to electron movement is generally a greater effect than that due to vibration of the atomic lattice, therefore metallic solids are good conductors and non-metallic solids are not (as they contain few free electrons).

In *static* fluids (and therefore through boundary layers; see Chapter 4) heat is transferred between molecules as a result of molecular collisions. When a fast-moving molecule from a region of high energy (or temperature) collides with slower-moving molecules from a region of lower energy, energy transfer takes place. Molecules with lower energy gain energy from the high-energy molecules, and the higher-energy molecules lose energy. As a consequence, the temperature of the initially high-energy molecules falls and that of the low-energy molecules rises.

Gases become better conductors at higher temperatures owing to the faster movement of the molecules, whereas most liquids (with the notable exception of water) become poorer conductors at higher temperatures.

Heat transfer by conduction is the main way in which heat is transferred through solids or fluid boundary layers, and is slow compared with heat transfer by convection.

Convection

Heat transfer by convection is due to the movement of molecules and their associated heat energy on a macroscopic scale. It involves the mixing of molecules and occurs within fluids, where the molecules are free to move.

Heat transfer by natural convection occurs when there is a difference in density within the fluid arising from the greater expansion and hence the lower density of the hotter region. Convection currents are set up as the warm, less dense fluid rises and mixes with colder fluid. As the molecules move, heat transfer *between* molecules can occur by conduction.

Heat transfer by forced convection occurs when the fluid is *forced* to move, for example by the movement of a mixer blade, or disruption caused by baffles. Heat transfer usually occurs more quickly by forced convection than by natural convection, owing to the greater intensity of movement and therefore the increased velocity of the fluid. If forced convection also induces turbulent flow (see Chapter 4) then the heat transfer process is aided, as there will be a reduction in the fluid boundary layer thickness.

Radiation

The energy emitted by the sun is transmitted in the form of electromagnetic waves through empty space. These waves can be reflected, transmitted or absorbed. When they are absorbed by a body on which they fall energy reappears as heat and the body increases in temperature. All hot bodies radiate energy in this way, but heat transfer by radiation is only of practical importance to pharmaceutical processing during drying (see Chapter 26).

Heat transfer by conduction and practical heat transfer

Of the three mechanisms of heat transfer described above, the one that will be considered in most detail is heat transfer by conduction. Heat transfer by convection, although important in pharmaceutical processing, is a complex process that is not completely understood and is difficult to define mathematically. More importantly, as far as calculating the rate of heat transfer is concerned, heat transfer by convection is rarely the rate-limiting step in the heat transfer process. If natural convection is inadequate then forced convection can be induced, e.g. by the use of a stirrer.

Many of the principles to be discussed in this chapter can be illustrated by the operation of a laboratory 'water bath', as illustrated in Figure 38.1. Heat energy from the gas burner is transferred through the container wall to the water in the bath, which therefore increases in temperature until its boiling point is reached. The heat gained is referred to as **sensible heat**, as it produces an appreciable rise in temperature and the change can be detected by the senses.

When the boiling point has been reached further heating generates steam without any increase in temperature. This heat gain by the steam is termed **latent heat of evaporation** and is used to change the water from liquid into vapour at constant temperature. The steam produced rises and contacts the dish wall, which initially is at room temperature. The steam condenses on the cool outer surface of the dish and, in doing so, gives up the latent heat it contains, forming a layer of condensate on the dish which runs down over the surface and drops back into the bath. Fresh condensate is continually formed to take its place, so that a layer of condensate will always be present. The latent heat that is liberated passes by conduction through the wall of the dish and into the contents to be heated. Heat is then transferred through the fluid by natural convection and conduction. The term 'water bath' is therefore a misnomer and the equipment is described more accurately as a 'steam bath'.

The steam functions as a heat transfer agent whereby the heat from the gas burner is transferred by the liberation of the latent heat into the liquid in the dish. There are advantages in this indirect heating in that the temperature can never exceed 100°C (at atmospheric pressure), and therefore there is less chance of localized overheating. In addition, because the steam circulates over the whole dish surface, heating is much more uniform than it would be if the dish were heated directly over the gas flame.

The insert in Figure 38.1 shows a section of the dish wall in greater detail. If this is considered to be rotated into a vertical position and straightened slightly it would appear as in Figure 38.2. A temperature drop occurs from the temperature of the condensing steam to the lower temperature of the liquid in the dish. If this liquid is assumed to be of a lower boiling point than water, then eventually it will boil at this lower constant temperature and the temperature gradients would appear as in Figure 38.2. T_S denotes the steam temperature, T_L the temperature of the boiling liquid and T_O and T_I are the temperatures of the outer and inner surfaces of the dish.

In many pharmaceutical processes it is important to know or control the rate at which heat can be transferred, i.e. the quantity of heat transferred in unit time. This must be carefully distinguished from the total quantity of heat that needs to be supplied. Consider heating a beaker of water using a Bunsen burner flame. Under a low flame it might take 20 minutes to boil, whereas using a full flame it may only take 5 minutes. If heat losses to the environment are neglected (i.e. the heat transfer process is assumed to be 100% efficient), and the initial water temperature was the same each time, the total quantity of heat required to boil the water would be the same in each case. The rate of heat transfer, however,

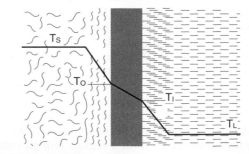

Fig. 38.2 Temperature gradients between steam and a boiling liquid.

Fig. 38.1 Heating a liquid using a steam bath.

would be four times greater over the full flame – i.e. the water will boil in a quarter of the time.

In the heating situation depicted in Figure 38.1 there are three barriers to the flow of heat energy from the steam to the liquid bulk, namely the condensate layer, the dish wall and the liquid side boundary layer adjacent to the dish wall. The origin and nature of this type of boundary layer is discussed in Chapter 4.

The same quantity of heat must pass through each layer in turn at the same rate. Initially we will consider the factors that affect heat transfer through a single layer of material, in this case the dish wall. Conduction is governed by Fourier's law, which states that 'the rate of conduction is proportional to the area measured normal to the direction of heat flow and to the temperature gradient in the direction of heat flow'. The rate of heat transfer, i.e. the quantity of heat transferred (Q, joules) in unit time (t, seconds) will therefore depend on the difference in temperature (ΔT or $T_O - T_I$) between the outer and inner surfaces of the dish (the driving force for the heat transfer process), the dish thickness L_D and the area available for heat transfer, A. The proportionality constant is termed the thermal conductivity of the material and is denoted by the symbol K (K_D in the case of the dish). It gives an indication of the ability of the material to conduct heat: the higher the value the more easily heat is conducted.

Combining all these factors gives:

$$\frac{Q}{t} = \frac{K_D A(T_O - T_I)}{L_D} \qquad (38.1)$$

Equation 38.1 indicates that to increase the heat transfer rate (i.e. conduct heat more quickly) through a layer of material the value of A, ΔT or K may be increased or the value of L decreased.

By rearranging Eqn 38.1 and using appropriate SI units, thermal conductivity can be shown to have units of W/mK. Table 38.1 gives some typical representative thermal conductivity values and shows that metals are the best conductors, followed by non-metallic solids, liquids and gases. It should be noted that the K values will vary with temperature and also with the composition of the material (e.g. from 13 to 19 W/mK in the case of stainless steel).

Illustrative calculation for heat transfer by conduction
Q Calculate the quantity of heat passing in a period of 4 minutes through a stainless steel dish whose effective heating surface area is 25 cm² and whose thickness is 1mm if the temperatures at the outer and inner surfaces of the dish are 90°C and 80°C, respectively.
A The first step is to convert all values into SI units. Thus:

Table 38.1 Thermal conductivity values of some materials encountered during pharmaceutical processing

Material	Thermal conductivity (W/m K)
Copper (pure)	386
Aluminium (pure)	204
Mild steel	43
Stainless steel (typical)	17
Glass	0.86
Water (at 20 °C)	0.60
Water (at 80 °C)	0.67
Boiler scale	0.09–2.3
Glass wool insulation	0.04
Air	0.03

$A = 25$ cm² $= 25 \times 10^{-4}$ m², $L_D = 1$ mm $= 1 \times 10^{-3}$ m, $K = 17$ W/mK (typical value for stainless steel; see Table 38.1), $T_0 - T_I = 10$ K or 10°C (note because it is a temperature **difference** the numerical value is the same whether expressed in K or °C) and Q/t is expressed in watts.

Because $\qquad \dfrac{Q}{t} = \dfrac{K_D A(T_O - T_I)}{L_D}$

then $\qquad \dfrac{Q}{t} = \dfrac{17 \times 25 \times 10^{-4} \times 10}{1 \times 10^{-3}}$

$$= 425 \ W$$

Therefore, 425 J of heat energy will be transferred every second, and in 4 minutes (240 s) the total heat transferred will be 425×240 J $= 102\,000$ J $= 102$ kJ.

Heat transfer through multiple layers

In most practical circumstances heat needs to be transferred through multiple layers (as illustrated in Figure 38.1). In order to calculate the rate of heat transfer through more than one layer the thermal conductivity and thickness values of each layer need to be taken into account. It is not possible, however, to generate a value for the overall conductivity simply by adding the individual K values, as each layer offers a *resistance* to heat transfer. The overall thermal conductivity (K_O) of a system is inversely proportional to the overall thermal resistance (R_O), which in turn is the sum of the thermal resistance of the individual layers.

Thus

$$K_O = 1/R_O$$

and

$$R_O = R_1 + R_2 + R_3 + ... R_N.$$

This situation is analogous to the flow of electricity, where the total resistance to flow needs to be quantified in order to calculate the current flowing at any particular voltage.

To find the thermal resistance of an individual layer, Eqn 38.1 can be rearranged so that it becomes:

$$\frac{Q}{t} = \frac{\Delta T}{L / KA} \qquad (38.2)$$

This represents the general form of an equation for any rate process, where the rate at which the process occurs is expressed as a driving force divided by a resistance. In the case of heat transfer the driving force is the temperature difference across the layer and the group L/KA represents the thermal resistance of that layer. Other rate processes that can be expressed in this form include rate of filtration (see Chapter 22) and rate of dissolution (see Chapter 2).

Film heat-transfer coefficient

Referring back to the situation illustrated in Figure 38.1, it can be seen that heat has to pass three layers (condensate, C, the dish wall, D and the liquid boundary layer, L) in order to reach the liquid to be heated. The total thermal resistance for this heating process can be calculated by adding the thermal resistance of each layer (or film), i.e:

Total thermal resistance $= L_C/K_C A + L_D/K_D A + L_L/K_L A$
$= 1/A \, (L_C/K_C + L_D/K_D + L_L/K_L)$

as the area term is generally the same for each layer. Substituting this back into Eqn 38.2:

$$\frac{Q}{t} = \frac{A\Delta T}{L_C / K_C + L_D / K_D + L_L / K_L} \qquad (38.3)$$

where ΔT is the temperature difference across all the layers, i.e. the difference between the temperature of the steam and that of the boiling liquid.

Overall heat-transfer coefficient

Eqn 38.3 now accounts for the resistance of multiple layers and can be used to calculate the rate of heat transfer through layers of known thickness and thermal conductivity. It is useful for assessing the effect of individual layers on the overall heat transfer process, as indicated below.

The overall conductivity is represented by U, the overall heat transfer coefficient (OHTC), which gives an indication of the ability of a combination of layers to conduct heat. When heat has to be transferred through n layers, U can be calculated as:

$$U = 1/(L_1/K_1 + L_2/K_2 + L_3/K_3 + ... L_n/K_n) \qquad (38.4)$$

and thus for the situation shown in Figure 38.1:

$$U = 1/(L_C/K_C + L_D/K_D + L_L/K_L)$$

Substituting this into Eqn 38.3 gives:

$$Q/t = U A \, \Delta T \qquad (38.5)$$

U has units of W/m²K and is only affected by factors that change the thermal conductivity or thickness of the layers through which heat is transferred; it is not affected by A. The value of the OHTC provides a useful indication of the overall conductivity of a heating system and is obtained using practically obtained data (see calculation number 6 at the end of this chapter), as it is not possible to determine the thermal conductivity and/or thickness of all the layers through which heat has to be transferred.

STEAM AS A HEATING MEDIUM

In pharmaceutical processes at anything other than laboratory scale, the most commonly used heating medium is steam. Steam is also very important as a sterilizing medium. The reasons for the widespread use of steam include:

- The raw material (water) is cheap and plentiful.
- It is easy to generate, distribute and control.
- It is generally cheaper than viable alternative forms of heating, e.g. electricity.
- It is clean, odourless and tasteless, and accidental contamination of the product is less likely to be serious.
- It has a high heat content (in the form of latent heat) and can heat materials very quickly.
- The heat is given up at a constant temperature, which is useful in controlling heating processes and in sterilization.

One disadvantage of the use of steam is that it is used at pressures that are typically two to three times higher than atmospheric, and thus steam presents potential safety problems and necessitates the use of high-strength piping.

To appreciate why steam is used in pharmaceutical processing and the principles of heat transfer using steam it is necessary to consider how the steam is produced, its heat content, and how the heat content varies with pressure and temperature.

Heat content of steam

Consider heating 1 kg of ice-cold water in a closed container at atmospheric pressure. Initially all the heat supplied will be sensible heat, to raise the temperature of the water to the boiling point (100°C in this case). The quantity of heat (Q, joules) required to raise the temperature of a material can be calculated using Eqn 38.6:

$$Q = M S \Delta T \qquad (38.6)$$

where M is the mass heated (kg), S is the specific heat capacity of the material (J/kg K) and ΔT is the change in temperature (K or °C). The specific heat capacity is therefore the quantity of heat (J) required to raise 1 kg by 1°C or 1K.

For water at atmospheric pressure (1.013 bar/ 1.013×10^5 Pa), $S = 4.2$ kJ/kg K, and therefore the quantity of heat required to raise the temperature from 0°C to 100°C = $4200 \times 1 \times 100$ J = 420 000 J (420 kJ).

It should be noted that the value of S for water varies slightly with changes in temperature and pressure.

Once the water has reached boiling point further heat energy input will not raise the temperature of the water but will convert the boiling water at 100°C to vapour at 100°C, i.e. steam at 100°C. Steam at a temperature corresponding to the water boiling point at that pressure (as in this case) is referred to as *saturated steam*.

The energy required to change unit mass from a liquid to a vapour at constant temperature is called the latent heat of vaporization (L, J/kg). For water at atmospheric pressure $L = 2.26 \times 10^6$ J/kg. L is not a constant value and depends on the steam pressure and temperature, e.g. L is 2.20 MJ/kg at 120°C and 2.14 MJ/kg at 140°C. The quantity of heat required to cause vaporization is calculated using the Eqn 38.7:

$$Q = M L \qquad (38.7)$$

where M is the mass vaporized (kg).

To convert 1 kg of water at 100°C to steam at 100°C, $Q = 1 \times 2.26 \times 10^6$ J (2.26 MJ), i.e. the steam now contains 2.26 MJ of latent heat energy. Steam in this state is referred to as *dry saturated steam*, as *all* the water has been converted to steam. This form of steam should ideally be used for heating and sterilization processes, as it contains the maximum latent heat energy and no associated air or water.

If only half the water had been converted to steam the latent heat content would have been $0.5 \times 2.26 \times 10^6$ J = 1.13 MJ. Steam in this state is said to have a *dryness fraction* of 0.5, where dryness fraction is defined as the weight fraction of steam in a steam/water mixture. The dryness fraction is important because it governs the latent heat content of the steam, this being at a maximum when the dryness fraction = 1.

Once all the water has been converted to steam any further heat energy input increases the *steam temperature*, i.e. the steam gains sensible heat. Steam at a temperature above the saturation temperature is called *superheated steam*. It only takes about 50 kJ of heat energy to raise the temperature of steam at 100°C at atmospheric pressure to steam at 200°C at atmospheric pressure.

The changes in the properties of water/steam with increasing heat input at atmospheric pressure are shown in Figure 38.3. The total heat content is measured from a datum at 0°C and is the sum of the sensible heat, latent heat and superheat.

If superheated steam at 200°C (A on Fig. 38.3) is cooled (e.g. if it contacts a colder surface) then it will lose heat energy. First, the steam will decrease in temperature until the small amount of superheat is given up and the steam reaches the saturation temperature. Only when the steam temperature has reduced to 100°C (B on Fig. 38.3) will the steam condense and the latent heat energy be released. When half the steam (0.5 kg) has condensed (C on Fig. 38.3), 1.13 MJ of latent heat energy will have been given up and the saturated steam will have a dryness fraction of 0.5. While there is still steam present, the temperature of the steam and any condensate formed that is in contact with the steam will remain at 100°C. Once all steam has condensed (D

Fig. 38.3 Changes occurring on the addition of heat to ice-cold water at atmospheric pressure.

on Fig. 38.3) the condensate will lose sensible heat and decrease in temperature until the temperature gradient is reduced to zero. If the temperature of the surface in contact with the condensate is at 0°C then point E on Figure 38.3 will be reached.

It is important to note that most of the heat energy of steam (over 80%) is in the form of latent heat, and that when latent heat energy is released there is no drop in temperature. This latter point is important in sterilization processes and in maintaining temperature gradients when heating.

Effect of pressure on steam properties

The temperature at which water boils depends on the pressure exerted on the water surface. If the pressure is above atmospheric water will boil above 100°C, and if it is below atmospheric, for example if a vacuum is applied, water boils at a temperature below 100°C. The saturation temperature (and the temperature at which steam condenses) will also therefore be dependent on pressure. This is utilized in sterilization processes, where adjustment of the pressure allows selection of the temperature at which steam condenses and therefore the temperature at which the articles to be sterilized are exposed. Similarly, in heat transfer processes the desired temperature gradient can be achieved by adjusting the steam pressure. Some examples of how steam temperature changes with increasing pressure are given in Table 38.2.

Steam tables

The values in Table 38.2, along with temperatures at other steam pressures, can be found in **steam tables**, as can values for the sensible and latent heat content at different pressures. It should be noted that there is not a linear relationship between steam pressure and steam temperature, and that the increase in steam temperature becomes less pronounced as the pressure increases.

Table 38.2 Relationship between steam pressure and steam temperature

Steam pressure (10^5 Pa)	Steam saturation temperature (°C)
1.013	100.0
2.000	120.4
3.000	133.7
4.000	143.8

Adverse effects of air in steam

There are two potential ways in which air may contaminate steam. First, water always contains dissolved air, and this air will be driven off when the water is converted to steam. Second, air will be present in equipment in the steam space when the process is started, and the incoming steam may not entirely flush this air out.

Air is a permanent gas which remains when the steam condenses to form a condensate layer, and thus forms an air layer in contact with the condensate.

The adverse effects caused by the contamination of air are twofold:

1. Air is a very poor conductor of heat (see Table 38.1) and forms a formidable barrier to heat flow. A very thin layer of air can markedly reduce the overall heat transfer coefficient (see calculation 4 at the end of this chapter), and the presence of as little as 1% of air in steam can result in a 50% reduction in the OHTC. Because the rate of heat transfer is proportional to the OHTC, there will be a corresponding reduction in the rate of heat transfer and thus an increase in heating-up times, process times and process costs.

2. Air will cause the steam temperature at any measured pressure to be lower than that of air-free steam. Steam containing air will not, therefore, be saturated. This arises from Dalton's law of partial pressures, which states that the total pressure in a system is the sum of the partial pressures of each of the components. Thus in an air/steam mixture the total pressure (P_T) is the sum of the partial pressure of the steam (P_S) and the partial pressure of the air (P_A). Therefore if P_T is 2×10^5 Pa and the steam contains 10% air, then P_A will be 0.2×10^5 Pa and P_S will be 1.8×10^5 Pa. The steam temperature, however, depends solely on the partial pressure exerted by the steam (not the total pressure), and will be 117.3°C (it would be 120.4°C if no air were present and the pressure were 2×10^5 Pa). Thus 10% of air has caused a reduction in the steam temperature at 2×10^5 Pa of 3.1°C. This is important in heating processes, where the temperature gradient will be lower than expected and thus the heating-up rate will be lower. NB: This effect is in addition to that caused by the poor thermal conductivity of air.

Both of the effects described above may also have potentially serious effects if air contaminates steam in autoclaves. Its presence will give rise to an increase in the heating time required for the heating-up phase and the required sterilization temperature will not be reached. Sterilization processes use steam at a specific pressure with the implicit assumption that the steam will be saturated (i.e. no air is present) and will thus be at the saturation temperature. If this does not occur the material may not be exposed to a sufficient temperature for a sufficient time and the material may not be sterilized. Steam pressure alone should therefore never be used as an indirect measure of sterilization temperature.

Steam generation and use

Manufacturing installations for liquid and semisolid products

A diagrammatic representation of a jacketed installation typical of that used for the preparation of liquid and semisolid products is shown in Figure 38.4. This type of installation is available in sizes capable of manufacturing products from development scale (approximately 20 L) up to full production-scale batches of 20 000 L. They are constructed from a suitable grade of stainless steel, as this has acceptable thermal conductivity, is strong and easily fabricated, resists corrosion and is easily cleaned and sterilized (see Chapter 37). The outer surface of the jacket may be suitably lagged with materials having poor thermal conductivity, in order to protect the opera-

Fig. 38.4 Diagrammatic representation of an industrial steam-jacketed vessel. 1. Reducing valve; 2. pressure gauge; 3. temperature gauge; 4. safety valve; 5. control valve; 6. temperature probe; 7. temperature controller; 8. steam trap; 9. air vent; 10. stirrer; 11. homogenizer

tors and reduce heat loss to the environment. In installations used for heating products using steam, the steam is usually generated in a remote boiler house that will supply steam to many different locations and pieces of equipment. The steam is usually generated at high pressures and temperatures (typically $6–8 \times 10^5$ Pa and $160–170°C$), which enables it to be delivered to the equipment where required. Suitably strong pipes are used which need to be well lagged to avoid heat loss and condensation. The ancillary equipment shown in Figure 38.4 is discussed in more detail below.

Most heating installations use steam at about $1.5–3 \times 10^5$ Pa and a temperature of $110–135°C$. This usually gives a sufficient temperature gradient to heat the product at the required rate, but reduces the chances of localized overheating. A *reducing valve* (1 on Fig. 38.4) is used to reduce and control/adjust the pressure to the desired level. This may be operated manually or, on larger equipment, controlled automatically via a *control panel* (7 on Fig. 38.4) and electronic signals from the *pressure gauge* (2 on Fig. 38.4).

A *control valve* (5 on Fig. 38.4) regulates the entry of steam into the jacket. As with the reducing valve, this may be either manually operated, for example on smaller development units, or automatically controlled so that the product is heated to the desired temperature and at the desired rate. An automatically operated system may function by selecting on the control panel the heating-up rate required, e.g. $2°C/min$, and the final product temperature. A temperature probe in contact with the product sends a signal to the control panel, which in turn will cause the control valve to open if the product temperature is below the set value. When the control valve opens steam enters the jacket and the product starts to heat up. The panel will continuously monitor the product temperature, and the extent to which the control valve is opened will be controlled so that the product heats up at the required rate. When the desired temperature is reached a signal from the control panel closes the control valve and so no further steam enters. After a short time the product will start to cool slowly, as it is at a higher temperature than the surrounding environment. The temperature control system will detect this drop and reopen the control valve, so that more steam enters and the process is repeated. Using this type of control system the temperature of the product may be maintained within $\pm 2–3°C$ of the required value. Examples of where this may be used include maintaining a temperature of between 60 and $70°C$ during cream manufacture, or a temperature of $80–90°C$ when preparing solution products where poorly soluble preservatives are employed.

The *pressure* and *temperature gauges* (2 and 3 on Fig. 38.4) allow the monitoring and recording of the steam properties and, as mentioned previously, the latter may be used to control the steam pressure used.

Because steam is generated at high pressures there is the potential to expose the equipment to pressures higher than it can safely withstand. To prevent this, a *safety valve* (4 on Fig. 38.4) is positioned before the control valve and is set to open and direct steam away from the installation if the pressure reaches a value in excess of that of the safe operating pressure of the system.

When steam first enters the jacket surrounding the product it contacts the cooler surface, condenses, and releases latent heat, which is then transferred through the various layers (condensate, vessel wall etc.) to the product. On condensing, steam contracts to a small volume (e.g. at 121°C, 850 mL of steam will condense to approximately 1 mL of condensate), which creates an area of lower pressure within the jacket into which more steam will then flow. Steam will therefore continue to enter the jacket to maintain the desired pressure until the product temperature reaches the steam temperature and no further condensation occurs.

If products are heated to temperatures above 60°C (as is often the case in cream or solution manufacture) then if left to cool naturally they will take a considerable time to cool to ambient temperature. This will be exacerbated as the volume in the vessel increases and if the vessel if efficiently lagged. Some products will need to be cool before volatile components (e.g. flavourings) are added, and to use the manufacturing vessels efficiently the cooling of these products will need to be accelerated. This can be achieved by circulating a cold fluid, e.g. water or 'brine' (a concentrated salt solution), through the vessel jacket. The latter can be at a temperature below 0°C and so will give a greater temperature gradient and faster cooling. If the rate of cooling is important (e.g. to avoid the formation of 'lumps' of higher melting-point components in cream and ointment manufacture) then the inlet and outlet of the cooling fluid can be controlled by a system similar to that used to control the heating rate.

The presence of a *stirrer* (10 in Fig. 38.4) helps ensure the product is evenly heated. The flow created will reduce the thickness of the boundary layer adjacent to the heating surface and thus speed up the heating process, and will mix the components of the product. If more intense mixing is required, as will be the case in the manufacture of emulsion, lotion and cream products, then a homogenizer (see Chapter 13) can be used. This will normally be sited at the bottom of the vessel, as shown in Figure 38.4. Where aqueous and oily phases need to be mixed when they are both at elevated temperatures, two jacketed vessels need to be sited close together and the appropriate phase pumped into the vessel containing the homogenizer.

The presence of a vessel lid protects the product from the operator and environment and vice versa. In addition, if the lid can be sealed then negative or positive pressures can be applied above the product's surface. A negative pressure (vacuum) is useful to minimize the incorporation of air during the manufacture of viscous products, especially when the homogenizer is used. This can avoid the manufacture of a product with an unsightly appearance and can reduce stability problems. A positive pressure can be used to aid emptying of the vessel.

Steam traps To ensure maximum heating efficiency the apparatus should minimize the amount of air and condensate present in the jacket. If the condensate is allowed to build up it will gradually reduce the area over which steam can condense, and therefore progressively slow down the heating process. If the condensate completely fills the jacket then heating will stop. The consequences of not removing the air from the jacket are described above. Fitting a simple drainage pipe to the jacket would be ineffective, as this, as well as removing condensate and air, would also allow steam to escape, which would be both wasteful and potentially dangerous. Condensate and air can be removed and steam retained by using a suitably designed device known as a *steam trap*.

The simplest form of steam trap is a mechanical device, an example of which is shown in Figure 38.5. These devices rely on the fact that condensate is more dense than water and will thus tend to collect at the bottom of the jacket. When sufficient condensate has entered into the trap, the float will rise and

Fig. 38.5 Float-type mechanical steam trap.

open the outlet, allowing the condensate to drain away.

Mechanical traps are robust but have the major disadvantage that they do not allow air to escape, as there will always be condensate in contact with trap outlet. The alternative type of steam traps are referred to as thermostatic devices, and these rely on the fact that condensate can lose sensible heat and thus be at a temperature which is lower than the steam. A common form of thermostatic steam trap is the **balanced pressure thermostatic steam trap** shown diagrammatically in Figure 38.6. This contains a capsule in the form of a bellows, in which is a liquid having a boiling point a few degrees below that of water. Thus, when the capsule is surrounded by steam the liquid in the capsule boils and causes the bellows to expand and close the outlet. When condensate enters the trap it will lose sensible heat and decrease in temperature; the trap is usually constructed of a material with good thermal conductivity, e.g. copper, to hasten this heat loss. The condensate then cools the capsule, the liquid in the capsule ceases to boil (condenses) and the bellows contract, thereby opening the outlet and discharging the condensate. When the condensate is removed steam surrounds the bellows, causing the trap to close again. These traps will operate over a wide pressure range, as any increase in steam pressure not only raises the boiling point of water but, because the same pressure acts on the surface of the bellows, will elevate the boiling point of the liquid in the bellows by a similar amount. Hence the alternative title applied to this type – balanced pressure expansion trap – as it will always operate a few degrees below the saturation temperature of the steam.

Although these devices tend to be less robust than mechanical traps they have one major advantage in

that they will also vent air from the jacket. Because air is more dense than steam, air will tend to collect at the bottom of the jacket and enter the steam trap. Contamination of steam with air will cause the steam temperature to be lower than the water boiling point at any operating pressure (see above), and once sufficient air is in the trap to reduce the steam temperature to below the boiling point of the liquid in the bellows, the bellows will contract and the air-contaminated steam will be removed.

Generally there are at least two traps on a heating installation, one at the bottom of the jacket to remove condensate and air generated during the heating process, and one towards the top of the jacket on the opposite side to which steam enters. This latter trap (which is of the thermostatic type) acts as an air vent and will be open when the equipment is started and therefore help to flush out the air initially present in the jacket. It will close when the temperature of the steam exiting the vent is sufficient to cause the liquid in the bellows to boil.

The condensate released from the jacket will possess significant heat energy and may be fed back to the steam boiler or used for other manufacturing plant, such as air-conditioning systems.

Example calculations involving the use of steam

This chapter concludes with some calculations that illustrate various points raised in the text.

1. **Q** What is the energy requirement to produce 13 kg of dry saturated steam at a pressure of 2×10^5 Pa (2 bar absolute/1 bar gauge) from water at 18.4°C? Assume the specific heat capacity of water is 4.21 kJ/kg K and the latent heat of evaporation is 2.20 J/kg.

   A The saturation temperature at 2×10^5 Pa is 120.4°C. The heat energy required to raise 13 kg of water to 120.4°C = $13 \times 4210 \times 102$ J = 5.582×10^6 J.
   The heat energy required to convert 13 kg of water at 120.4°C to steam at 120.4°C = $13 \times 2.2 \times 10^6$ J = 2.86×10^7 J.
   The total heat energy required therefore = $5.582 \times 10^6 + 2.86 \times 10^7 = 3.418 \times 10^7$ J (34.18 MJ).

2. **Q** What temperature would be reached if the steam produced in Question 1 was used in a steam-jacketed vessel to heat 150 kg of water whose initial temperature was 21.8°C? Assume there are no heat losses to the environment.

Fig. 38.6 Balanced pressure thermostatic steam trap.

A The 2.86×10^7 J of heat energy required to convert water to steam will be released as latent heat when the steam condenses during the heating process.
From $Q = M\,S\,\Delta T$, the increase in temperature of the water = $2.86 \times 10^7 \div (4210 \times 150) = 45.3°C$.
The final water temperature therefore = $45.3 + 21.8°C = 67.1°C$.

3. **Q** If the steam produced in Question 1 was passed through unlagged pipes on its passage to the steam-jacketed vessel and the dryness fraction reduced from 1.0 to 0.94, what temperature would the water reach?

A Because some steam has condensed in the unlagged pipework, the latent heat content of the steam has been reduced and now = $0.94 \times 2.86 \times 10^7$ J = 2.69×10^7 J
The increase in temperature of the water therefore = $2.69 \times 10^7 \div (4210 \times 150) = 42.6°C$ and the final temperature = $64.4°C$.

4. **Q** The data in the table below represent the different layers through which the latent heat from steam has to be conducted in a stainless steel steam-jacketed vessel when scale and air are present and water is heated. What is the overall heat transfer coefficient of the system?

	Thickness (mm)	K (W/m K)
Air film	0.2	0.03
Condensate film	0.1	0.60
Scale	0.2	1.00
Pan wall	3.0	17.0
Water boundary layer	0.4	0.60

A Using Eqn 38.4:

$$U = \cfrac{1}{\left[\dfrac{0.2}{0.03} + \dfrac{0.1}{0.6} + \dfrac{0.2}{1.0} + \dfrac{3.0}{17} + \dfrac{0.4}{0.6}\right]} \times 10^{-3}$$

(The factor 10^{-3} is required to convert from mm to m.)
$U = 127$ W/m^2 K

5. **Q** What would happen if:
(a) the vessel described in Q4 was made of copper ($K = 386$ W/m^2 K)?
(b) the scale was removed?
(c) the air film was halved?
(d) the air film was removed?
(e) the air film was removed, the scale layer eliminated and the water boundary layer halved?

A
(a) $U = 130$ W/m^2 K
Even though copper conducts heat over 20 times more easily than stainless steel, this alone has little effect on the overall conductivity.
(b) $U = 130$ W/m^2 K
Removing the scale alone similarly has little effect.
(c) $U = 220$ W/m^2 K
Removing just 0.1 mm of air gives rise to an approximate 75% increase in thermal conductivity.
(d) $U = 827$ W/m^2 K
If the air film is completely removed there is a huge increase in U, the value being over six times greater than when air was present.
(e) $U = 1478$ W/m^2 K
Reducing the film layers that offer the largest resistance to heat conduction has the greatest effect on increasing heat transfer.

6. **Q** A steam-jacketed vessel of heated area 2.0 m^2, using steam at 2×10^5 Pa, was found to evaporate 11.2 kg of water in a 5-minute period. Assuming the latent heat of vaporization is 2.20×10^6 J/kg, what is the value of U, the overall heat transfer coefficient (OHTC) of the system?

A The heat energy used to evaporate the water = $11.2 \times 2.2 \times 10^6$ J = 2.464×10^7 J.
The rate of heat transfer occurring is 2.464×10^7 J in 300 s = 8.213×10^4 W (82.13 kW).
From Eqn 38.5: $Q/t = U\,A\,\Delta T$
The temperature of steam at 2×10^5 Pa = 120.4°C and therefore the temperature difference between the steam and the boiling water, ΔT = 120.4 − 100°C = 20.4°C.
Therefore, $U = 8.213 \times 10^4 \div (2 \times 20.4) = 2013$ W/m^2 K.

REFERENCES

Arpaci, S.A., Kao S., Selamet, A. (1999) *Introduction to heat transfer*. Prentice Hall, New Jersey.
Long, C.A. (1999) *Essential heat transfer*. Pearson Education, Harlow.
Mills, A.F. (1999) *Basic heat and mass transfer*, 2nd edn. Prentice Hall, New Jersey.

PHARMACEUTICAL MICROBIOLOGY

PART FIVE

PHARMACEUTICAL MICROBIOLOGY

39

Fundamentals of microbiology

Geoff Hanlon

CHAPTER CONTENTS

INTRODUCTION

Microorganisms are ubiquitous in nature and are vital components in the cycle of life. The majority are free-living organisms growing on dead or decaying matter whose prime function is the turnover of organic materials in the environment. Pharmaceutical microbiology, however, is concerned with the relatively small group of biological agents that cause human disease, spoil prepared medicines, or which can be used to produce compounds of medical interest.

In order to understand microorganisms more fully, scientists have grouped together living organisms of similar characteristics into taxonomic units. The most fundamental division is between prokaryotic and eukaryotic cells, which differ in a number of respects (Table 39.1) but particularly in the arrangement of their nuclear material. Eukaryotic cells contain chromosomes, which are separate from the cytoplasm and contained within a limiting nuclear membrane, i.e. they possess a true nucleus. Prokaryotic cells do not possess a true nucleus and their nuclear material is free within the cytoplasm, although it may be aggregated into discrete areas called nuclear bodies. Prokaryotic organisms make up the lower forms of life and include Eubacteria and Archaeobacteria. Eukaryotic cell types embrace all the higher forms of life, of which only the fungi will be dealt with in this chapter.

One characteristic shared by all microorganisms is the fact that they are small; however, it is a philosophical argument whether all infectious agents can be regarded as living. Some are little more than simple chemical entities incapable of any free-living existence. Viroids, for example, are small circular, single-stranded RNA molecules not complexed with protein. One particularly well studied viroid has only 359 nucleotides (one-10th the size of the smallest known virus) and yet causes a disease in potatoes. Prions are small, self-replicating proteins devoid of any nucleic acid. The prion associated with Creutzfeld–Jakob disease in humans, scrapie in sheep and bovine spongiform encephalitis in cattle has only 250 amino acids and is highly resistant to inactivation by normal sterilization procedures.

Viruses are more complex than viroids or prions, possessing both protein and nucleic acid. Despite being among the most dangerous infectious agents known, they are still not regarded as living. Table 39.2 shows the major groups of viruses infecting humans.

VIRUSES

Viruses are obligate intracellular parasites with no intrinsic metabolic activity, being devoid of ribosomes and energy-producing enzyme systems. They are thus incapable of leading an independent existence and cannot be cultivated on cell-free media, no matter how nutritious. The size of human viruses ranges from the largest poxviruses, measuring about 300 nm ($1 \text{ nm} = 10^{-9} \text{ m}$), to the picornaviruses, such as the poliovirus which is approximately 20 nm. When one considers that a bacterial coccus measures 1000 nm in diameter it can be appreciated that only the very largest virus particles may be seen under the light microscope, and electron microscopy is required for visualizing the majority. It will also be apparent that few of these viruses are large enough to be retained on the (0.2 μm) membrane filters used to sterilize thermolabile liquids.

Viruses consist of a core of nucleic acid (either DNA, as in vaccinia virus, or RNA as in poliovirus) surrounded by a protein shell or capsid. Most DNA viruses have linear double-stranded DNA, but in the case of the parvovirus it is single stranded. The majority of RNA-containing viruses contain one molecule of single-stranded RNA, although in reoviruses it is double stranded. The protein capsid comprises 50–90% of the weight of the virus, and as nucleic acid can only synthesize approximately 10% its own weight of protein the capsid must be made up of a number of identical protein molecules. These individual protein units are called capsomeres and are not in themselves symmetrical, but are arranged around the nucleic acid core in characteristic sym-

Table 39.1 Differences between prokaryotic and eukaryotic organisms

Structure	Prokaryotes	Eukaryates
Cell wall structure	Usually contains peptidoglycan	Peptidoglycan absent
Nuclear membrane	Absent	Present. Possess a true nucleus
Nucleolus	Absent	Present
Number of chromosomes	One	More than one
Mitochondria	Absent	Present
Mesosomes	Present	Absent
Ribosomes	70S	80S

Table 39.2 The major groups of viruses that infect humans

Family	Capsid	Nucleic acid	Envelope	Example
Adenoviridae	Icosahedral	dsDNA	No	Human adenovirus
Arenaviridae	Helical	ssRNA	Yes	Lassa fever virus
Flaviviridae	Icosahedral	ssRNA	Yes	Yellow fever virus Hepatitis C virus
Hepadnaviridae	Icosahedral	dsDNA	No	Hepatitis B virus
Herpesviridae	Icosahedral	dsDNA	Yes	Herpes simplex virus Cytomegalovirus Varicella zoster virus
Orthomyxoviridae	Helical	ssRNA	Yes	Influenza virus
Papoviridae	Icosahedral	dsDNA	No	Papillomavirus
Paramyxoviridae	Helical	ssRNA	Yes	Respiratory syncytial virus Measles virus Mumps virus
Picornaviridae	Icosahedral	ssRNA	No	Rhinovirus Poliovirus Coxsackie virus
Poxviridae	Complex	dsDNA	Yes	Molluscum contagiosum Vaccinia virus Variola virus
Reoviridae	Icosahedral	dsRNA	No	Rotavirus Colorado tick fever virus
Retroviridae	Icosahedral	ssRNA	Yes	HIV
Rhabdoviridae	Helical	ssRNA	Yes	Rabies virus
Togaviridae	Icosahedral	ssRNA	Yes	Rubella virus

metrical patterns. Additionally, many of the larger viruses possess a lipoprotein envelope surrounding the capsid arising from the membranes within the host cell. In many instances the membranes are virus modified to produce projections outwards from the envelope, such as haemagglutinins or neuraminidase. The enveloped viruses are often called ether sensitive, as ether and other organic solvents may dissolve the membrane.

The arrangement of the capsomeres can be of a number of types:

- Helical – the classic example is tobacco mosaic virus (TMV), which resembles a hollow tube with capsomeres arranged in a helix around the central nucleic acid core. Other examples include mumps and influenza virus.
- Icosahedral – these often resemble spheres on cursory examination, but when studied more closely they are made up of icosahedra that have 20 triangular faces, each containing an identical number of capsomeres. Examples include the poliovirus and adenovirus.

- Complex – the poxviruses and bacterial viruses (bacteriophages) make up a group whose members have a geometry that is individual and complex.

Reproduction of viruses

Because viruses have no intrinsic metabolic capability they require the functioning of the host cell machinery in order to manufacture and assemble new virus particles. The replication of viruses within host cells can be broken down into a number of stages.

Adsorption to host cell

The first step in the infection process involves virus adsorption on to the host cell. This usually occurs via an interaction between protein or glycoprotein moieties on the virus surface with specific receptors on the host cell outer membrane. Different cells possess receptors for different viruses.

Penetration

Enveloped viruses fuse the viral membrane with the host cell membrane and release the nucleocapsid directly into the cytoplasm. Naked virions generally penetrate the cell by phagocytosis.

Uncoating

In this stage the capsid is removed as a result of attack by cellular proteases, and this releases the nucleic acid into the cytoplasm. These first three stages are similar for both DNA and RNA viruses.

Nucleic acid and protein synthesis

The detailed mechanisms by which DNA- and RNA-containing viruses replicate inside the cell is outside the scope of this chapter and the reader is referred to the bibliography for further information. After nucleic acid replication early viral proteins are produced, the function of which is to switch off host cell metabolic activity and direct the activities of the cell towards the synthesis of proteins necessary for the assembly of new virus particles.

Assembly of new virions

Again, there are differences in the detail of how the viruses are assembled within the host cell, but construction of new virions occurs at this stage and up to 100 new virus particles may be produced per cell.

Release of virus progeny

The newly formed virus particles may be liberated from the cell as a burst, in which case the host cell ruptures and dies. Infection with influenza virus results in a lytic response. Alternatively, the virions may be released gradually from the cell by budding of the host cell plasma membrane. These are often called 'persistent' infections, and an example is hepatitis B.

Latent infections

In some instances a virus may enter a cell but not go through the replicative cycle outlined above and the host cell may be unharmed. The genome of the virus is conserved and may become integrated into the host cell genome, where it may be replicated along with the host DNA during cell division. At some later stage the latent virus may become reactivated and progress through a lytic phase, causing cell damage/death and the release of new virions. Examples of this type of infection are those which occur with the herpes simplex viruses, associated with cold sores, genital herpes and also chicken pox, where the dormant virus may reactivate to give shingles later in life.

Oncogenic viruses

Oncogenic viruses have the capacity to transform the host cell into a cancer cell. In some cases this may lead to relatively harmless, benign growths, such as warts caused by papovavirus, but in other cases more severe, malignant tumours may arise. Cellular transformation may result from viral activation or mutation of normal host genes called proto-oncogenes, or the insertion of viral oncogenes.

Bacteriophages

Bacteriophages (phages) are viruses that attack bacteria but not animal cells. It is generally accepted that the interaction between phage and bacterium is highly specific, and there is probably at least one phage for each species of bacterium. In many cases the infection of a bacterial cell by a phage results in lysis of the bacterium, and such phages are termed virulent. Some phages, however, can infect a bacterium without causing lysis, and in this case the phage DNA becomes incorporated within the bacterial genome. The phage DNA can then be replicated along with the bacterial cell DNA, and this is then termed a prophage. Bacterial cells carrying a prophage are called lysogenic and phages capable of inducing lysogeny are called temperate. Occasionally some of the prophage genes may be expressed, and this will confer on the bacterial cell the ability to produce new proteins. The ability to produce additional proteins as a result of prophage DNA is termed lysogenic conversion.

ARCHAEOBACTERIA

Archaeobacteria are a fascinating group of prokaryotic microorganisms which are frequently found living in hostile environments. They differ in a number of respects from Eubacteria, particularly in the composition of their cell walls. They comprise methane producers, sulphate reducers, halophiles and extreme thermophiles. However, they are of little significance from a pharmaceutical or clinical standpoint and so will not be considered further.

EUBACTERIA

Eubacteria constitute the major group of prokaryotic cells that are of pharmaceutical and clinical significance. They cover a diverse range of microorganisms, from the primitive parasitic rickettsias that share some of the characteristics of viruses, through the more typical free-living bacteria to the branching, filamentous actinomycetes, which at first sight resemble fungi rather than bacteria.

Atypical bacteria

Rickettsiae

The family Rickettsiaceae includes three clinically important genera, *Rickettsia*, *Coxiella* and *Bartonella*. Although these are prokaryotic cells they differ from most other bacteria both in their structure and in the fact that the majority of species lead an obligate intracellular existence. This means that, with a few exceptions, they cannot be grown on cell free media, although unlike many viruses they do possess some independent enzymes. They have a pleomorphic appearance, ranging from coccoid through to rod-shaped cells, and multiplication is by binary fission. Their cell wall composition bears similarities to that of Gram-negative bacteria and in general they stain this way. The genus *Rickettsia* has a number of species that give rise to human diseases, in particular epidemic typhus (*R. prowazekii*), murine typhus (*R. typhi*) and spotted fevers (various species). These are characterized by transmission via bites from insect vectors, particularly ticks, fleas and lice. *Coxiella burnetii* is the only species in the genus *Coxiella* and this gives rise to a disease called Q fever. Although the source of the disease is infected animals, usually no insect vector is involved and the most common route of transmission is by inhalation of infected dust. *Bartonella quintana* is the causative agent of trench fever which, as the name suggests, occurs typically under conditions of war and deprivation. Each of the infections described here can be treated with doxycycline, although the duration of therapy may vary depending upon the nature of the disease and its severity.

Chlamydiae

These are obligate intracellular parasitic bacteria that possess some independent enzymes but lack the ability to generate ATP. Two cellular forms are identified: a small (0.3 μm) highly infectious elementary body which, after infection, enlarges to give rise to the replicative form called the initial or reticulate body (0.8–1.2 μm). These divide by binary fission within membrane-bound vesicles in the cytoplasm of infected cells. Insect vectors are not required for the transmission of infection. Chlamydiae lack peptidoglycan in their cell walls and have weak Gram-negative characteristics. *Chlamydia trachomatis* is the most important member of the group, being responsible for the disease trachoma, characterized by inflammation of the eyelids, which can lead to scarring of the cornea. This is the most common cause of infectious blindness world wide, and it is estimated that 400 million people are infected, with at least 6 million totally blind. The same species is also recognized as one of the major causes of sexually transmitted disease. *C. psittaci* and *C. pneumoniae* are responsible for respiratory tract infections. Chlamydial infections are responsive to treatment by tetracyclines, either topical or systemic as appropriate.

Mycoplasmas

The mycoplasmas are a group of very small (0.3–0.8 μm) prokaryotic microorganisms which are capable of growing on cell-free media but which lack cell walls. The cells are surrounded by a double-layered plasma membrane that contains substantial amounts of phospholipids and sterols. This structure has no rigidity owing to the absence of peptidoglycan, and so the cells are susceptible to osmotic lysis. The lack of peptidoglycan is also the reason for these bacteria being resistant to the effects of cell wall-acting antibiotics such as the penicillins, and also the enzyme lysozyme. Members of this group are pleomorphic, varying in shape from coccoid to filamentous. Most are facultative anaerobes capable of growth at 35°C, and on solid media produce colonies with a characteristic 'fried egg' appearance. They contain a number of genera, of which the most important from a clinical point of view are *Mycoplasma* and *Ureaplasma*. *M. pneumoniae* is a major cause of respiratory tract infections in children and young adults, whereas *U. urealyticum* has been implicated in non-specific genital infections. Despite being resistant to the β-lactam antibiotics, these infections can be effectively treated using either tetracyclines or erythromycin.

Actinomycetes

Many of the macroscopic features of the actinomycetes are those that are more commonly found among the filamentous fungi, but they are indeed prokaryotic cells. They are a diverse group of Gram-positive bacteria morphologically distinguishable from other bacteria because they have a tendency to produce branching filaments and reproductive spores. *Nocardia* contain a number of species that have been shown to be pathogenic to humans, but they occur principally in tropical climates. Reproduction in this genus is by fragmentation of the hyphal strands into individual cells, each of which can form a new mycelium. The genus *Streptomyces* contains no human pathogens, but most species are saprophytic bacteria found in the soil. They are aerobic microorganisms producing a non-fragmenting, branching mycelium that may bear spores. The reason for their pharmaceutical importance is their ability to produce a wide range of therapeutically useful antibiotics, including streptomycin, chloramphenicol, oxytetracycline, erythromycin and neomycin.

Typical bacteria

Shape, size and aggregation

Bacteria occur in a variety of shapes and sizes, determined not only by the nature of the organisms themselves but also by the way in which they are grown (Fig. 39.1). In general, bacterial dimensions lie in the range 0.75–5 μm (1000 μm = 1 mm). The most common shapes are the sphere (coccus) and the rod (bacillus). Some bacteria grow in the form of rods with a distinct curvature, e.g. vibrios are rod-shaped cells with a single curve resembling a comma, whereas a spirillum possesses a partial rigid spiral; spirochaetes are longer and thinner and exhibit a number of turns, and are also more flexible. Rod-shaped cells occasionally grow in the form of chains but this is dependent upon growth conditions rather than a characteristic of the species. Cocci, however, show considerable variation in aggregation, which is characteristic of the species. The plane of cell division and the strength of adhesion of the cells determine the extent to which they aggregate after division. Cocci growing in pairs are called diplococci, those in four tetrads, and in groups of eight sarcina. If a chain of cells is produced resembling a string of beads this is termed a streptococcus, whereas an irregular cluster similar in appearance to a bunch of grapes is called a staphylococcus. In many cases this is sufficiently characteristic to give rise to the name of the bacterial genus, e.g. *Staphylococcus aureus*, *Streptococcus pneumoniae*.

Genus		Approximate dimensions (μm)
Staphylococcus Irregular clusters of spherical cells. Resemble bunch of grapes. Non-motile		0.5–1.5
Streptococcus Spherical or ovoid cells occurring in pairs or in chains. Non-motile		<2.0
Neisseria Small Gram negative cocci. Occur in pairs with adjacent sides flattened. Non-motile		0.6–1.0
Lactobacillus Shape variable between long and slender to short coccobacillus. Non-motile, chain formation common		0.5–0.8 × 2–9
Escherichia Short rods, motile by peritrichous flagella		1.1–1.5 × 2–6
Bacillus Large endospore-forming rods. Motile by lateral flagella (not shown). Gram-positive		0.3–2.2 × 1.2–7.0
Vibrio Short curved or straight rods. Sometimes 'S' shaped. Motile by single polar flagellum		0.5 × 1.5–3.0
Spirochaeta Thin, flexible, helically coiled cells. Motile, possess axial fibrils (not shown)		0.2–0.75 × 5–500
Spirillum Long, slender cells in rigid spirals. Number of turns varies. Motile, bipolar flagellation		0.2–1.7 × 0.5–60
Streptomyces Slender, non-septate branching filaments. Form reproductive spores. Non-motile		0.5–2.0 (diameter)

Fig. 39.1 Morphology of different bacterial genera.

Anatomy

Figure 39.2 is a diagrammatic representation of a typical bacterial cell. The various components are described below.

Capsule Many bacteria produce extracellular polysaccharides, which may take the form of either a

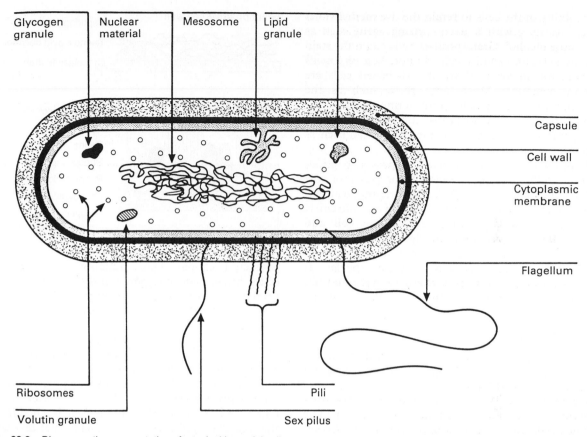

Fig. 39.2 Diagrammatic representation of a typical bacterial cell.

discrete capsule, firmly adhered to the cell, or a more diffuse layer of slime. Not all bacteria produce a capsule, and even those that can will only do so under certain circumstances. Many encapsulated pathogens, when first isolated, give rise to colonies on agar which are smooth (S), but subculturing leads to the formation of rough colonies (R). This S → R transition is due to loss in capsule production. Reinoculation of the R cells into an animal results in the resumption of capsule formation, indicating that the capacity has not been lost irrevocably.

The function of the capsule is generally regarded as protective, as encapsulated cells are more resistant to disinfectants, desiccation and phagocytic attack. In some organisms, however, it serves as an adhesive mechanism, for example *Streptococcus mutans* is an inhabitant of the mouth that metabolizes sucrose to produce a polysaccharide capsule enabling the cell to adhere firmly to the teeth. This is the initial step in the formation of dental plaque, which is a complex array of microorganisms and organic matrix that adheres to the teeth and ultimately leads to decay. The substitution of sucrose by glucose pre-

vents capsule formation and hence eliminates plaque.

A similar picture emerges with *Staph. epidermidis*. This bacterium forms part of the normal microflora of the skin and until recently was thought of as non-pathogenic. With the increased usage of indwelling medical devices coagulase-negative staphylococci, in particular *Staph. epidermidis*, have emerged as the major cause of device-related infections. The normal microbial flora have developed the ability to produce extracellular polysaccharide, which enables the cells to form resistant biofilms attached to the devices. These biofilms are very difficult to eradicate and have profound resistance to antibiotics and disinfectants. It is now apparent that the dominant mode of growth for aquatic bacteria is not planktonic (free swimming) but sessile, i.e. attached to surfaces and covered with protective extracellular polysaccharide or glycocalyx.

Cell wall Bacteria can be divided into two broad groups by the use of the Gram staining procedure (see later for details), which reflects differences in cell wall structure. The classification is based upon the ability of the cells to retain the dye methyl violet after washing with a decolourizing agent such as absolute alcohol. Gram-positive cells retain the stain whereas Gram-negative cells do not. As a *very rough* guide, the majority of small rod-shaped cells are Gram negative. Most large rods, such as the Bacillaceae, lactobacilli and actinomycetes, are Gram positive. Similarly, most cocci are Gram positive, although there are notable exceptions, such as the Neisseriaceae.

Bacteria are unique in that they possess peptidoglycan in their cell walls. This is a complex molecule with repeating units of *N*-acetylmuramic acid and *N*-acetylglucosamine (Fig. 39.3). This extremely long molecule is wound around the cell and crosslinked by polypeptide bridges to form a structure of great rigidity. The degree and nature of crosslinking vary between bacterial species. It imparts to the cell its characteristic shape and has principally a protective function. Peptidoglycan (also called murein or mucopeptide) is the site of action of a number of antibiotics, such as penicillin, bacitracin, vancomycin and cycloserine. The enzyme lysozyme is also capable of hydrolysing the β, 1–4 linkages between *N*-acetylmuramic acid and *N*-acetylglucosamine.

Figure 39.4 shows simplified diagrams of a Gram-positive and a Gram-negative cell wall. The Gram-positive cell wall is much simpler in layout, containing peptidoglycan interspersed with teichoic acid polymers. These latter are highly antigenic but do not provide structural support. Functions attributed to teichoic acids include the regulation of enzyme activity in cell wall synthesis, sequestration

Gram positive cell wall
- Peptidoglycan
- Teichoic acid polymers
- Cytoplasmic membrane

Gram negative cell wall
- Lipopolysaccharide
- Lipoprotein
- Porins
- Phospholipid
- Periplasmic space
- Peptidoglycan
- Cytoplasmic membrane

Fig. 39.4 Structural components of bacterial cell walls.

of essential cations, cellular adhesion, and mediation of the inflammatory response in disease. In general, proteins are not found in Gram-positive cell walls. Gram-negative cell walls are more complex, comprising a much thinner layer of peptidoglycan surrounded by an outer bilayered membrane. This outer membrane acts as a diffusional barrier and is the main reason why many Gram-negative cells are much less susceptible to antimicrobial agents than are Gram-positive cells. The lipopolysaccharide component of the outer membrane can be shed from the wall upon cell death. It is a highly heat-resistant molecule known as endotoxin, which has a number of toxic effects on the human body, including fever and shock. For this reason it is important that solutions for injection or infusion are not just sterile but are also free from endotoxins.

Cytoplasmic membrane The cytoplasmic membranes of most bacteria are very similar and are composed of protein, lipids, phospholipids and a small amount of carbohydrate. The components are arranged into a bilayer structure with a hydrophobic interior and a hydrophilic exterior. The cytoplasmic membrane has a variety of functions:

- It serves as an osmotic barrier.
- It is selectively permeable and is the site of carrier-mediated transport.
- It is the site of ATP generation and cytochrome activity.
- It is the site of cell wall synthesis.
- It provides a site for chromosome attachment.

The cytoplasmic membrane has very little tensile strength and the internal hydrostatic pressure of up to 20 bar forces it firmly against the inside of the cell wall. Treatment of bacterial cells with lysozyme may remove the cell wall and, as long as the conditions are

N-acetyl muramic acid

N-acetyl glucosamine

Lysozyme acts here

Beta lactam antibiotics prevent crosslinking here

- L-alanine
- D-glutamine
- Meso-diaminopimelic acid
- D-alanine

Fig. 39.3 Peptidoglycan

isotonic, the resulting cell will survive. These cells are called protoplasts and, as the cytoplasmic membrane is now the limiting structure, the cell assumes a spherical shape. Protoplasts of Gram-negative bacteria are difficult to obtain because the layer of lipopolysaccharide protects the peptidoglycan from attack. In these cases mixtures of EDTA and lysozyme are used and the resulting cells, which still retain fragments of cell envelope, are termed spheroplasts.

Nuclear material The genetic information necessary for the functioning of the cell is contained within a single circular molecule of double-stranded DNA. When unfolded this would be about 1000 times as long as the cell itself, and so exists within the cytoplasm in a considerably compacted state. It is condensed into discrete areas called chromatin bodies, which are not surrounded by a nuclear membrane. Rapidly dividing cells may contain more than one area of nuclear material, but these are copies of the same chromosome, not different chromosomes, and arise because DNA replication proceeds ahead of cell division.

Mesosomes These are irregular invaginations of the cytoplasmic membrane which are quite prominent in Gram-positive bacteria but less so in Gram-negative bacteria. They are thought to have a variety of functions, including cross-wall synthesis during cell division and furnishing an attachment site for nuclear material, facilitating the separation of segregating chromosomes during cell division. They have also been implicated in enzyme secretions and may act as a site for cell respiration.

Ribosomes The cytoplasm of bacteria is densely populated with ribosomes, which are complexes of RNA and protein in discrete particles 20 nm in diameter. They are the sites of protein synthesis within the cell and the numbers present reflect the degree of metabolic activity of the cell. They are frequently found organized in clusters called polyribosomes or polysomes. Prokaryotic ribosomes have a sedimentation coefficient of 70S, compared to 80S ribosomes of eukaryotic cells. This distinction aids the selective toxicity of a number of antibiotics. The 70S ribosome is made up of RNA and protein and can dissociate into one 30S and one 50S subunit.

Inclusion granules Certain bacteria tend to accumulate reserves of materials after active growth has ceased, and these become incorporated within the cytoplasm in the form of granules. The most common are glycogen granules, volutin granules (containing polymetaphosphate) and lipid granules (containing poly β-hydroxybutyric acid). Other granules, such as sulphur and iron, may also be found in the more primitive bacteria.

Flagella A flagellum is made up of protein called flagellin and it operates by forming a rigid helix that turns rapidly like a propeller. This can propel a motile cell up to 200 times its own length in 1 second. Under the microscope bacteria can be seen to exhibit two kinds of motion, swimming and tumbling. When tumbling the cell stays in one position and spins on its own axis, but when swimming it moves in a straight line. Movement towards or away from a chemical stimulus is referred to as chemotaxis. The flagellum arises from the cytoplasmic membrane and is composed of a basal body, hook and filament. The number and arrangement of flagella depends upon the organisms and varies from a single flagellum (monotrichous) to a complete covering (peritrichous).

Pili (fimbriae) These are smaller than flagella and are not involved in motility. A number of different types of pili have been identified, of which the most important are the common pili and the F-pili. The common pili are found all over the surface of certain bacteria and are believed to be associated with adhesiveness and pathogenicity. They are also antigenic. F-pili are larger and of a different structure to common pili, and are involved in the transfer of genetic information from one cell to another. This is of major importance in the transfer of drug resistance between cell populations.

Endospores Under conditions of specific nutrient deprivation some genera of bacteria, in particular *Bacillus* and *Clostridium*, undergo a differentiation process and change from an actively metabolizing vegetative form to a resting spore form. The process of sporulation is not a reproductive mechanism as found in certain actinomycetes and filamentous fungi, but serves to enable the organism to survive periods of hardship. A single vegetative cell differentiates into a single spore. Subsequent encounter with favourable conditions results in germination of the spore and the resumption of vegetative activities.

Endospores are very much more resistant to heat, disinfectants, desiccation and radiation than are vegetative cells, making them difficult to eradicate from foods and pharmaceutical products. Heating at 80°C for 10 minutes would kill most vegetative bacteria, whereas some spores will resist boiling for several hours. The sterilization procedures now routinely used for pharmaceutical products are thus designed specifically with reference to the destruction of the bacterial spore. The mechanism of this extreme heat resistance was a perplexing issue for many years, and at one time it was thought to be due to the presence of a unique spore component, dipicolinic acid (DPA). This compound is found only in bacterial spores, where it is associated in a complex with calcium ions. The isolation of heat-resistant DPA-less mutants, however, led to the demise of this theory. Spores do not have water content appreciably different from that of vegetative cells, but the distribution within the different compartments is unequal and this is thought to generate the heat resistance. The central core of the spore houses the genetic information necessary for growth after germination, and this becomes dehydrated by expansion of the cortex against the rigid outer protein coats. Water is thus squeezed out of the central core. Osmotic pressure differences also help to maintain this water imbalance.

The sequence of events involved in sporulation is illustrated in Figure 39.5 and is a continuous process, although for convenience it is divided into six stages. The complete process takes about 8 hours, although this may vary depending on the species and the conditions used. Occurring simultaneously with the morphological changes are a number of biochemical events that have been shown to be associated with specific stages and occur in an exact sequence. One important biochemical event is the production of antibiotics. Peptides possessing antimicrobial activity have been isolated from the majority of *Bacillus* species and many of these have found pharmaceutical applications. Examples of

Fig. 39.5 Morphological and biochemical changes during spore formation.

antibiotics include bacitracin, polymyxin and gramicidin. Similarly, the proteases produced by *Bacillus* species during sporulation are used extensively in a wide variety of industries.

Microscopy and staining of bacteria

Bacterial cells contain about 80% water by weight and this results in a very low refractility, i.e. they are transparent when viewed under ordinary transmitted light. Consequently, in order to visualize bacteria under the microscope the cells must be killed and stained with some compound that scatters the light or, if live preparations are required, special adaptations must be made to the microscope. Such adaptations are found in phase-contrast, dark-ground and differential-interference contrast microscopy.

The microscopic examination of fixed and stained preparations is a routine procedure in most laboratories but it must be appreciated that not only are the cells dead, but they may also have been altered morphologically by the often quite drastic staining process. The majority of stains used routinely are basic dyes, i.e. the chromophore has a positive charge and this readily combines with the abundant negative charges present both in the cytoplasm in the form of nucleic acids and on the cell surface. These dyes remain firmly adhered even after washing with water. This type of staining is called simple staining and all bacteria and other biological material are stained the same colour. Differential staining is a much more useful process as different organisms or even different parts of the same cell can be stained distinctive colours.

To prepare a film ready for staining the glass microscope slide must be carefully cleaned to remove all traces of grease and dust. If the culture of bacteria is in liquid form then a loopful of suspension is transferred directly to the slide. Bacteria from solid surfaces require suspension with a small drop of water on the slide to give a faintly turbid film. A common fault with inexperienced workers is to make the film too thick. The films must then be allowed to dry in air. When thoroughly dry the film is fixed by passing the back of the slide through a small Bunsen flame until the area is just too hot to touch on the palm of the hand. The bacteria are killed by this procedure and also stuck on to the slide. Fixing also makes the bacteria more permeable to the stain and inhibits lysis. Chemical fixation is commonly carried out using formalin or methyl alcohol: this causes less damage to the specimen but tends to be used principally for blood films and tissue sections.

Differential stains A large number of differential stains have been developed and the reader is referred to the bibliography for more details. Only a few of those available will be discussed here.

Gram's stain By far the most important in terms of use and application is the Gram stain, developed by Christian Gram in 1884 and subsequently modified. The fixed film of bacteria is flooded initially with a solution of methyl violet. This is followed by a solution of Gram's iodine, which is an iodine–potassium iodine complex acting as a mordant, fixing the dye firmly in certain bacteria and allowing easy removal in others. Decolourization is effected with either alcohol or acetone or mixtures of these. After treatment some bacteria retain the stain and appear a dark purple colour and these are called Gram positive. Others do not retain the stain and appear colourless (Gram negative). The colourless cells may be stained with a counterstain of contrasting colour, such as 0.5% safranin, which is red.

This method, although extremely useful, must be used with caution as the Gram reaction may vary with the age of the cells and the technique of the operator. For this reason, known Gram-positive and Gram-negative controls should be stained alongside the specimen of interest.

Ziehl–Neelsen's acid-fast stain *Mycobacterium tuberculosis* contains within its cell wall a high proportion of lipids, fatty acids and alcohols, which render the bacterium resistant to normal staining procedures. The inclusion of phenol in the dye solution, together with the application of heat, enables the dye (basic fuchsin) to penetrate the cell and, once attached, to resist vigorous decolourization by strong acids, e.g. 20% sulphuric acid. These organisms are therefore called acid fast. Any unstained material can be counterstained with a contrasting colour, e.g. methylene blue.

Fluorescence microscopy Certain materials, when irradiated by short-wave illuminations, e.g. UV light, become excited and emit visible light of a longer wavelength. This phenomenon is termed fluorescence and will persist only for as long as the material is irradiated. A number of dyes have been shown to fluoresce and are useful in that they tend to be specific to various tissues, which can then be demonstrated by UV irradiation and subsequent fluorescence of the attached fluorochrome. Coupling antibodies to the fluorochromes can enhance specificity, and this technique has found wide application in microbiology. As with the staining procedures described above, this technique can only be applied to dead cells. The three following techniques have been developed for the examination of living organisms.

Dark-ground microscopy The usual function of the microscope condenser is to concentrate as much light as possible through the specimen and into the objective. The dark-ground condenser performs the opposite task, producing a cone of light that comes to a focus on the specimen. The rays of light in the cone are at an oblique angle, such that after passing across the specimen they continue without meeting the front lens of the objective, resulting in a dark background. Any objects present at the point of focus scatter the light, which then enters the objective to show up as a bright image against the dark background.

Specimen preparation is more critical, as very dilute bacterial suspensions are required, preferably with all the objects in the same plane of focus. Air bubbles must be absent both from the film and the immersion oil, if used. Dust and grease also scatter light and destroy the uniformly black background required for this technique.

Phase-contrast microscopy This technique allows us to see transparent objects well contrasted from the background in clear detail and is the most widely used image enhancement method used in microbiology. The theory is too complex to explain in detail here, but in essence an annulus of light is produced by the condenser and focused on the back focal plane of the objective. Here a phase plate, comprising a glass disc containing an annular depression, is situated. The direct rays of the light source annulus pass through the annular groove and any diffracted rays pass through the remainder of the disc. Passage of the diffracted light through this thicker glass layer results in retardation of the light, thereby altering its phase relationship to the direct rays and increasing contrast.

Differential-interference contrast microscopy This method uses polarized light and has other applications outside the scope of this chapter, such as detecting surface irregularities in opaque specimens. It offers some advantages over phase-contrast microscopy, notably the elimination of haloes around the object edges, and enables extremely detailed observation of specimens. It does, however, tend to be more difficult to set up.

Electron microscopy The highest magnification available using a light microscope is about 1500 times. This limitation is imposed not by the design of the microscope itself, as much higher magnifications are possible, but by the wavelength of light. An object can only be seen if it causes a ray of light to deflect. If a particle is very small indeed then no deflection is produced and the object is not seen. Visible light has a wavelength between 0.3 and 0.8 μm and objects less than 0.3 μm will not be clearly resolved, i.e. even if the magnification were increased no more detail would be seen. In order to increase the resolution it is necessary to use light of a shorter wavelength, such as UV light. This has been done and resulted in some useful applications but generally, for the purposes of increased definition, electrons are now used and they can be thought of as behaving like very short wavelength light. Transmission electron microscopy requires the preparation of ultrathin (50–60 nm) sections of material mounted on copper grids for support. Because of the severe conditions applied to the specimen during preparation, and the likelihood of artefacts, care must be taken in the interpretation of information from electron micrographs.

Growth and reproduction of bacteria

The growth and multiplication of bacteria can be examined in terms of individual cells or populations of cells. During the cell division cycle a bacterium assimilates nutrients from the surrounding medium and increases in size. When a predetermined size has been reached a cross-wall will be produced, dividing the large cell into two daughter cells. This process is known as binary fission. In a closed environment, such as a culture in a test tube, the rate at which cell division occurs varies according to the conditions, and this manifests itself in characteristic changes in the population concentration. When fresh medium is inoculated with a small number of bacterial cells the number remains static for a short time while the cells undergo a period of metabolic adjustment. This period is called the lag phase (Fig. 39.6) and its length depends on the degree of readjustment necessary. Once the cells are adapted to the environment they begin to divide in the manner described above, and this division occurs at regular intervals. The numbers of bacteria during this period increase in an exponential fashion, i.e. 2, 4, 8, 16, 32, 64, 128 etc., and this is therefore termed the exponential or logarithmic phase. When cell numbers are plotted on a log scale against time a straight line results for this phase.

During exponential growth (Fig. 39.6) the medium undergoes continuous change, as nutrients are consumed and metabolic waste products excreted. The fact that the cells continue to divide exponentially during this period is a tribute to their physiological adaptability. Eventually, the medium becomes so changed due to either substrate exhaustion or excessive concentrations of toxic products, that it is unable to support further growth. At this

Fig. 39.6 Phases of bacterial growth.

stage cell division slows and eventually stops, leading to the stationary phase. During this period some cells lyse and die whereas others sporadically divide, but the cell numbers remain more or less constant. Gradually all the cells lyse and the culture enters the phase of decline.

It should be appreciated that this sequence of events is not a characteristic of the cell but a consequence of the interaction of the organisms with the nutrients in a closed environment, and does not necessarily reflect the way in which the organism would behave in vivo.

Genetic exchange In addition to mutations, bacteria can alter their genetic make-up by transferring information from one cell to another, either as fragments of DNA or in the form of small extrachromosomal elements (plasmids). Transfer can be achieved in three ways: by transformation, transduction or conjugation.

Transformation When bacteria die they lyse and release cell fragments, including DNA, into the environment. Several bacterial genera (*Bacillus*, *Haemophilus*, *Streptococcus* etc.) are able to take up these DNA fragments and incorporate them into their own chromosome, thereby inheriting the characteristics carried on that fragment. Cells able to participate in transformation are called competent, and the development of competence has been shown in some cases to occur synchronously in a culture under the action of specific inducing proteins.

Transduction Some bacteriophages infect a bacterial cell and incorporate their nucleic acid into the host cell chromosome, with the result that the viral genes are replicated along with the bacterial DNA. In many instances this is a dormant lysogenic state for the phage, but sometimes it is triggered into action and lysis of the cell occurs, with liberation of phage particles. These new phage particles may have bacterial DNA incorporated into the viral genome

and this will infect any new host cell. On entering a new lysogenic state the new host cell will replicate the viral nucleic acid in addition to that portion received from the previous host. Bacteria in which this has been shown to occur include *Mycobacterium*, *Salmonella*, *Shigella* and *Staphylococcus*.

Conjugation Gram-negative bacteria such as *Salmonella*, *Shigella* and *Escherichia coli* have been shown to transfer genetic material conferring antibiotic resistance by cellular contact. This process is called conjugation and is controlled by an R-factor plasmid, which is a small circular strand of duplex DNA replicating independently from the bacterial chromosome. R factor comprises a region containing resistance transfer genes that control the formation of sex pili, together with a variety of genes that code for the resistance to drugs. Conjugation is initiated when the resistance transfer genes stimulate the production of a sex pilus and random motion brings about contact with a recipient cell. One strand of the replicating R factor is nicked and passes through the sex pilus into the recipient cell. Upon receipt of this single strand of plasmid DNA the complementary strand is produced and the free ends are joined. For a short time afterwards this cell has the ability to form a sex pilus itself and so transfer the R factor further.

This is by no means an exhaustive discussion of genetic exchange in bacteria and the reader is referred to the bibliography for further information.

Bacterial nutrition Bacteria require certain elements in fairly large quantities for growth and metabolism, including carbon, hydrogen, oxygen and nitrogen. Sulphur and phosphorus are also required but not in such large amounts, and only low concentrations of iron, calcium, potassium, sodium, magnesium and manganese are needed. Some elements, such as cobalt, zinc and copper, are required only in trace amounts and an actual requirement may be difficult to demonstrate.

The metabolic capabilities of bacteria differ considerably and this is reflected in the form in which nutrients may be assimilated. Bacteria can therefore be classified according to their requirements for carbon and energy.

Lithotrophs (synonym: autotrophs) These utilize carbon dioxide as their main source of carbon. Energy is derived from different sources within this group thus:

- Chemolithotrophs (chemosynthetic autotrophs) obtain their energy from the oxidation of inorganic compounds.
- Photolithotrophs (photosynthetic autotrophs) obtain their energy from sunlight.

Organotrophs (synonym: heterotrophs) Organotrophs utilize organic carbon sources and can similarly be divided into:

- Chemoorganotrophs, which obtain their energy from oxidation or fermentation of organic compounds;
- Photo-organotrophs, which utilize light energy.

Oxygen requirements As mentioned above, all bacteria require elemental oxygen in order to build up the complex materials necessary for growth and metabolism, but many organisms also require free oxygen as the final electron acceptor in the breakdown of carbon and energy sources. These organisms are called aerobes. If the organism will only grow in the presence of air it is called a strict aerobe, but most organisms can either grow in its presence or its absence and are called facultative anaerobes. A strict anaerobe cannot grow and may even be killed in the presence of oxygen, because some other compound replaces oxygen as the final electron acceptor in these organisms. A fourth group of microaerophilic organisms has also been recognized which grow best in only trace amounts of free oxygen and usually prefer an increased carbon dioxide concentration.

Influence of environmental factors on the growth of bacteria The rate of growth and metabolic activity of bacteria is the sum of a multitude of enzyme reactions, and so it follows that those environmental factors that influence enzyme activity will also affect growth rate. Such factors include temperature, pH and osmolarity.

Temperature Bacteria can survive wide limits of temperature but each organism will exhibit minimum, optimum and maximum growth temperatures, and on this basis fall into three broad groups:

- Psychrophils: grow best below 20°C but have a minimum about 0°C and a maximum of 30°C. These organisms are responsible for low-temperature spoilage.
- Mesophils: exhibit a minimum growth temperature of 5–10°C and a maximum of 45–50°C. Within this group two populations can be identified: saprophytic mesophils, with an optimum temperature of 20–30°C, and parasitic mesophils with an optimum temperature of 37°C. The vast majority of pathogenic organisms are in this latter group.
- Thermophils: can grow at temperatures up to 70–90°C but have an optimum of 50–55°C and a minimum of 25–40°C.

Organisms kept below their minimum growth temperature will not divide but can remain viable. As a result, very low temperatures (–70°C) are used to preserve cultures of organisms for many years. Temperatures in excess of the maximum growth temperature have a much more injurious effect and will be dealt with in more detail later (see Chapter 41).

pH Most bacteria grow best at around neutrality in the pH range 6.8–7.6. There are, however, exceptions, such as the acidophilic organism lactobacillus, a contaminant of milk products, which grows best at pHs between 5.4 and 6.6. Yeasts and moulds prefer acid conditions with an optimum pH range of 4–6. The difference in pH optima between fungi and bacteria is used as a basis for the design of media permitting the growth of one group of organisms at the expense of others. Sabouraud medium, for example, has a pH of 5.6 and is a fungal medium, whereas nutrient broth, which is used routinely to cultivate bacteria, has a pH of 7.4. The adverse effect of extremes of pH has for many years been used as a means of preserving foods against microbial attack, for example pickling.

Osmotic pressure Bacteria tend to be more resistant to extremes of osmotic pressure than other cells owing to the presence of a very rigid cell wall. The concentration of intracellular solutes gives rise to an osmotic pressure equivalent to between 5 and 20 bar, and most bacteria will thrive in a medium containing around 0.75% w/v sodium chloride. Staphylococci have the ability to survive higher than normal salt concentrations, and this has enabled the formulation of selective media such as mannitol salt agar containing 7.5% w/v sodium chloride, which will support the growth of staphylococci but restrict other bacteria. Halophilic organisms can grow at much higher osmotic pressures, but these are all saprophytic and are non-pathogenic to humans. High osmotic pressures generated by either sodium chloride or sucrose have for a long time been used as preservatives. Syrup BP contains 66.7% w/w sucrose and is of sufficient osmotic pressure to resist microbial attack. This is used as a basis for many oral pharmaceutical preparations.

Handling and storage of microorganisms

Because microorganisms have such a diversity of nutritional requirements there has arisen a bewildering array of media for the cultivation of bacteria, yeasts and moulds. Media are produced either as liquids or solidified with agar. Agar is an extract of seaweed, which at concentrations of between 1 and 2% sets to form a firm gel below 45°C. Unlike gelatin, bacteria cannot use agar as a nutrient and so even after growth the gel remains firm. Liquid media are stored routinely in test tubes or flasks, depending upon the volume, both secured with either loose-fitting caps or plugs of sterile cotton wool. Small amounts of solid media are stored in Petri dishes or slopes (also known as slants), whereas larger volumes may be incorporated in Roux bottles or Carrell flasks.

Bacteria may only be maintained on agar in Petri dishes for a short time (days) before the medium dries out. For longer storage periods the surface of an agar slope is inoculated, and after growth the culture may be stored at 4°C for several weeks. If even longer storage periods are required then the cultures may be stored at low temperatures (−70°C), usually in the presence of a cryoprotectant such as glycerol, or freeze-dried (lyophilized) before being stored at 4°C. Vegetative cells that survive this process may retain their viability for many years in this way.

When a single cell is placed on the surface of an overdried agar plate it becomes immobilized but can still draw nutrients from the substrate, and consequently grows and divides. Eventually the numbers of bacterial cells are high enough to become visible and a colony is formed. Each of the cells in that colony is a descendant from the initial single cell or group of cells, and so the colony is assumed to be a pure culture with each cell having identical characteristics. The formation of single colonies is one of the primary aims of surface inoculation of solid media and allows the isolation of pure cultures from specimens containing mixed flora.

Inoculation of agar surfaces by streaking The agar surface must be smooth and without moisture, which could cause the bacteria to become motile and the colonies to merge together. To dry the surface of the agar the plates are placed in an incubator or drying cabinet until the surface appears wrinkled. An inoculating loop is made of either platinum or nichrome wire twisted along its length to form a loop 2–3 mm in diameter at the end. Nichrome wire is cheaper than platinum but has similar thermal properties. The wire is held in a handle with an insulated grip and the entire length of the wire is heated in a Bunsen flame to red heat to sterilize it. The first few centimetres of the holder are also flamed before the loop is set aside in a rack to cool.

When cool the loop is used to remove a small portion of liquid from a bacterial suspension and this is then drawn across the agar surface from A to B, as indicated in Figure 39.7. The loop is then resterilized

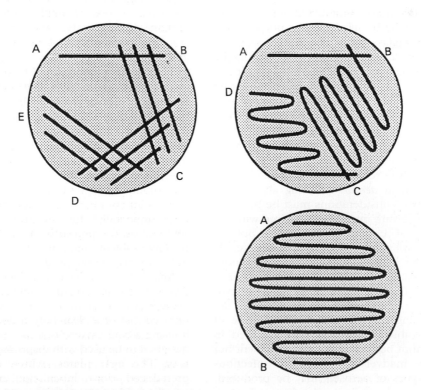

Fig. 39.7 Typical streaking methods for obtaining isolated colonies.

and allowed to cool. At this stage the loop is not reinoculated but streaked over the surface again, ensuring a small area of overlap with the previous streak line. The procedure is repeated as necessary. The pattern of streaking (see other examples in Fig. 39.7) is dictated largely by the concentration of the original bacterial suspension. The object of the exercise is to dilute the culture such that, after incubation, single colonies will arise in the later streak lines where the cells were sufficiently separated. All plates are incubated in an inverted position to prevent condensation from the lid falling on the surface of the medium and spreading the colonies.

Inoculation of slopes A wire needle may be used to transfer single colonies from agar surfaces to the surface of slopes for maintenance purposes. The needle is similar to the loop except that the wire is single and straight, not terminating in a closed end. This is flamed and cooled as before and a portion of a single colony picked off the agar surface. The needle is then drawn upwards along the surface of the slant. Before incubation the screw cap of the bottle should be loosened slightly to prevent oxygen starvation during growth. Some slopes are prepared with a shallower slope and a deeper butt to allow the needle to be stabbed into the agar when testing for gas production.

Transference of liquids Graduated pipettes and Pasteur pipettes may be used for this purpose, the latter being short glass tubes one end of which is drawn into a fine capillary. Both types should be plugged with sterile cotton wool and filled via pipette fillers of appropriate capacity. Mouth pipetting should *never* be permitted. Automatic pipettes have generally replaced glass graduated pipettes in most areas of science for the measurement of small volumes of liquid. Provided they are properly maintained and calibrated they have the advantage of being easy to use and reliable in performance.

Release of infectious aerosols During all of these manipulations two considerations must be borne in mind. First, the culture must be transferred with the minimum risk of contamination from outside sources. To this end all pipettes, tubes, media etc. are sterilized and the manipulations carried out under aseptic conditions. Second, the safety of the operator is paramount. During operations with microorganisms it must be assumed that all organisms are capable of causing disease and that any route of infection is possible. Most infections acquired in laboratories cannot be traced to a given incident but arise from the inadvertent release of infectious aerosols. Two types of aerosols may be produced. The first kind produces large droplets (>5 μm),

containing many organisms, which settle locally and contaminate surfaces in the vicinity of the operator. These may initiate infections if personnel touch the surfaces and subsequently transfer the organisms to eyes, nose or mouth. The second type of aerosol contains droplets less than 5 μm in size, which dry instantly to form droplet nuclei that remain suspended in the air for considerable periods. This allows them to be carried on air currents to situations far removed from the site of initiation. These particles are so small that they are not trapped by the usual filter mechanisms and may be inhaled, giving rise to infections of the lungs. The aerosols just described may be produced by a variety of means, such as heating wire loops, placing hot loops into liquid cultures, splashing during pipetting, rattling loops and pipettes inside test tubes, opening screw-capped tubes and ampoules etc. All microbiologists should have an awareness of the dangers of aerosol production and learn the correct techniques to minimize them.

Cultivation of anaerobes

Anaerobic microbiology is a much-neglected subject owing principally to the practical difficulties involved in growing organisms in the absence of air. However, with the increasing implication of anaerobes in certain disease states and improved cultivation systems the number of workers in this field is growing.

The most common liquid medium for cultivation of anaerobes is thioglycollate medium. In addition to sodium thioglycollate the medium contains methylene blue as a redox indicator, and it permits the growth of aerobes, anaerobes and microaerophilic organisms. When in test tubes the medium may be used after sterilization until not more than one-third of the liquid is oxidized, as indicated by the colour of the methylene blue indicator. Boiling and cooling of the medium just prior to inoculation is recommended for maximum performance. In some cases the presence of methylene blue poses toxicity problems and under these circumstances the indicator may be removed.

Anaerobic jars have considerably improved in recent years, making the cultivation of even strict anaerobes now relatively simple. The most common ones consist of a clear polycarbonate jar with a lid housing a cold catalyst in a mesh container, and are designed to be used with disposable H_2/CO_2 generators. The agar plates, which may need to be prereduced prior to inoculation, are placed in the jar together with a gas generator and an anaerobic indicator. A measured amount of water is added to the gas generator sachet and the lid sealed. Hydrogen and carbon dioxide are evolved and the hydrogen combines with any oxygen present under the action of the cold catalyst to form a light mist of water vapour. Carbon dioxide is produced in sufficient quantities to allow the growth of many fastidious anaerobes, which fail to grow in its absence. The absence of oxygen will be demonstrated by the action of the redox indicator, which in the case of methylene blue will be colourless.

Counting bacteria

Estimates of bacterial numbers in a suspension can be evaluated from a number of standpoints, each equally valid depending upon the circumstances and the information required. In some cases it may be necessary to know the total amount of biomass produced within a culture, irrespective of whether the cells are actively metabolizing. In other instances only an assessment of living bacteria may be required. Bacterial counts can be divided into total counts and viable counts.

Total counts These counts estimate the total number of bacteria present within a culture, both dead and living cells. A variety of methods are available for the determination of total counts and the one chosen will depend largely upon the characteristics of the cells being studied, i.e. whether they aggregate together.

Microscopic methods Microscopic methods employ a haemocytometer counting chamber (Fig. 39.8), which has a platform engraved with a grid of small squares each 0.0025 mm^2 in area. The platform is depressed 0.1 mm and a glass coverslip is placed over the platform, enclosing a space of known dimensions. The volume above each square is 0.00025 mm^3. For motile bacteria the culture is fixed by adding two to three drops of 40% formaldehyde solution per 10 mL of culture to prevent the bacteria from moving across the field of view. A drop of the suspension is then applied to the platform at the edge of the coverslip. The liquid is drawn into the space by capillary action. It is important to ensure that liquid does not enter a trench that surrounds the platform: the liquid must fill the whole space between the coverslip and the platform. This slide is examined using phase-contrast or dark-ground microscopy and, if necessary, the culture is diluted to give 2–10 bacteria per small square. A minimum of 300 bacterial cells should be counted to give statistically significant results.

Fig. 39.8 Counting chamber for microscopic estimation of cell numbers.

Calculation

Assume the mean cell count per small square was 6.
  Each small square

$$= 2.5 \times 10^{-4} \text{ mm}^3$$
$$= 2.5 \times 10^{-7} \text{ cm}^3$$

If the volume above each square contains 6 cells then

$$= \frac{6}{2.5 \times 10^{-7}} \text{ cells/mL}$$
$$= 2.4 \times 10^7 \text{ cells/mL}.$$

Another microscopic technique is Breed's method. A microscope slide is marked with a square of known area (usually 1 cm^2), and 0.01 mL of bacterial suspension is spread evenly over the square. This is allowed to dry, fixed and stained. A squared-eyepiece micrometer is then used to determine the original count, knowing the dilution and the size of each square.

Spectroscopic methods These methods are simple to use and very rapid, but require careful calibration if meaningful results are to be obtained. Either opacity or light scattering may be used, but both methods may only be used for dilute, homogenous suspensions as at higher concentrations the cells obscure each other in the light path and the relationship between optical density and concentration is not linear. Simple colourimeters and nephelometers can be used, but more accurate results are obtained using a spectrophotometer.

Electronic methods A variety of automated methods are available for bacterial cell counting, including electronic particle counting, micro-calorimetry, changes in impedance or conductivity, and radiometric and infrared systems for monitoring CO_2 production.

Other methods If an organism is prone to excessive clumping, or if a measure of biomass is needed rather than numbers, then estimates may be made by performing dry weight or total nitrogen determinations. For dry weight a sample of suspension is centrifuged and the pellet washed free of culture medium by further centrifugation in water. The pellet is collected and dried to a constant weight in a desiccator. Total nitrogen measures the total quantity of nitrogenous material within a cell population. A known volume of suspension is centrifuged and washed as before and the pellet digested using sulphuric acid in the presence of a $CuSO_4$–K_2SO_4–selenium catalyst. This produces ammonia, which is removed using boric acid and estimated either by titration or colourimetrically.

Viable counts These are counts to determine the number of bacteria in a suspension that are capable of division. In all these methods the assumption is made that a colony arises from a single cell, although clearly this is often not the case, as cells frequently clump or grow as aggregates, e.g. *Staphylococcus aureus*. In these cases the count is usually given as colony-forming units (c.f.u.) per mL rather than cells per mL.

Spread plates A known volume, usually 0.2 mL, of a suitably diluted culture is pipetted on to an over-dried agar plate and distributed evenly over the surface using a sterile spreader made of wire or glass capillary. The liquid must all be allowed to soak in before the plates are inverted. A series of tenfold dilutions should be made in a suitable sterile diluent and replicates plated out at each dilution, in order to ensure that countable numbers of colonies (30–300) are obtained per plate.

The viable count is calculated from the average colony count per plate, knowing the dilution and the volume pipetted onto the agar.

Example calculation

Serial dilution scheme

Stock bacterial suspension, 1 mL added to 99 mL of sterile diluent — *call dilution A* (the stock solution has therefore been diluted by a factor of 100 (10^2).

1 mL of dilution A added to 99 mL of sterile diluent — *call dilution B* (dilution B has been diluted by a factor of 10^4).

1 mL of dilution B added to 9 mL of sterile diluent — *call dilution C* (dilution C has been diluted by a factor of 10^5).

1 mL of dilution C added to 9 mL of sterile diluent — *call dilution D* (dilution D has been diluted by a factor of 10^6).

1 mL of dilution D added to 9 mL of sterile diluent — *call dilution E* (dilution E has been diluted by a factor of 10^7).

0.2 mL of each dilution plated in triplicate.

Mean colony counts for each dilution after incubation at 37°C:

Dilution A	too many to count
Dilution B	too many to count
Dilution C	400 colonies
Dilution D	45 colonies
Dilution E	5 colonies.

The result for dilution C is unreliable, as the count is too high. If the colony count exceeds 300 errors arise because the colonies become very small and some may be missed. This is why the colony count for dilution C does not exactly correspond to 10 × that found for dilution D. Similarly, the count for dilution E is unreliable because at counts below about 30 small variations introduce high percentage errors.

The result from dilution D is therefore taken for calculation, as the colony count lies between 30 and 300.

45 colonies in 0.2 mL, therefore
= 45 × 5 colonies per mL
= 225 cfu/mL in dilution D.

This was diluted by a factor of 10^6 ($100 \times 100 \times 10 \times 10$) and so the count in the stock suspension was $225 \times 10^6 = 2.25 \times 10^8$ cfu/mL.

Pour plates A series of dilutions of original culture is prepared as before, ensuring that at least one is in the range 30–300 organisms/mL. One-millilitre quantities are placed into empty sterile Petri dishes and molten agar, cooled to 45°C, is poured on to the suspension and mixed by gentle swirling. After setting the plates are inverted and incubated. Because the colonies are embedded within the agar they do not exhibit the characteristic morphology seen with surface colonies. In general they assume a lens shape and are usually smaller. As the oxygen tension below the surface is reduced this method is not suitable for strict aerobes. Calculations are similar to that given above, except that no correction is necessary for volume placed upon the plate.

Membrane filtration This method is particularly useful when the level of contamination is very low, such as in water supplies. A known volume of sample is passed through a membrane filter, typically made of cellulose acetate/nitrate, of sufficient pore size to retain bacteria (0.2–0.45 μm). The filtrate is discarded and the membrane placed bacteria-uppermost on the surface of an overdried agar plate, avoiding trapped air between membrane and surface. Upon incubation the bacteria draw nutrients through the membrane and form countable colonies.

ATP determination There are sometimes instances when viable counts are required for clumped cultures or for bacteria adhered to surfaces, for example in biofilms. Conventional plate count techniques are not appropriate here and ATP determinations can be used. The method assumes that viable bacteria contain a relatively constant level of ATP, but this falls to zero when the cells die. ATP is extracted from the cells using a strong acid such as trichloroacetic acid, and the extract is then neutralized by dilution with buffer. The ATP assay is based upon the quantitative measurement of a stable level of light produced as a result of an enzyme reaction catalysed by firefly luciferase.

$$\text{ATP} + \text{luciferin} + O_2 \xrightarrow{\text{luciferase}} \text{oxyluciferin} + \text{AMP} + \text{PPi} + CO_2 + \text{Light}$$

The amount of ATP is calculated by reference to light output from known ATP concentrations and the number of bacterial cells is calculated by reference to a previously constructed calibration plot.

Isolation of pure bacterial cultures

Mixed bacterial cultures from pathological specimens or other biological materials are isolated first on solid media to give single colonies, and the resultant pure cultures can then be subjected to identification procedures. The techniques used for isolation depend upon the proportion of the species of interest compared to the background contamination. Direct inoculation can only be used when an organism is found as a pure culture in nature. Examples include bacterial infections of normally sterile fluids such as blood or cerebrospinal fluid.

Streaking is the most common method employed, and if the proportions of bacteria in the mixed culture are roughly equal then streaking on an ordinary nutrient medium should yield single colonies of all microbial types. More usually the organism of interest is present only as a very small fraction of the total microbial population, necessitating the use of selective media.

A selective enrichment broth is initially inoculated with the mixed population of cells and this inhibits the growth of the majority of the background population. At the same time the growth of the organism of interest is encouraged. After incubation in these media the cultures are streaked out on to solid selective media, which frequently contain indicators to further differentiate species on the basis of fermentation of specific sugars.

Classification and identification

Taxonomy is the ordering of living organisms into groups on the basis of their similarities. In this way we can construct a hierarchy of interrelationships such that species with similar characteristics are grouped within the same genus, genera which have similarities are grouped within the same family, families grouped into orders, orders into classes and classes into divisions. The classification of bacteria does pose a problem because a species is defined as a group of closely related organisms that reproduce sexually to produce fertile offspring. Of course, bacteria do not reproduce sexually, and so a bacterial species is simply defined as a population of cells with similar characteristics.

Nomenclature Bergey's Manual of Determinative Bacteriology lists 562 bacterial genera and each of these contains many species. It is therefore extremely important to be sure there is no confusion when describing any one particular bacterial species. Although we are familiar with the use of trivial names in ornithology and botany (we understand what we mean when we describe a sparrow or a daffodil) such an approach could have disastrous consequences in clinical microbiology. For this reason the binomial system of nomenclature is used that Carolus Linnaeus developed in the 18th century. In this system every bacterium is given two names, the first being the genus name and the second the species name. By convention the name is italicized or underlined, and the genus name always begins with a capital letter whereas the species name begins in lower case.

Identification The organization of bacteria into groups of related microorganisms is based upon the similarity of their chromosomal DNA. Although this provides a very accurate indicator of genetic relatedness it is far too cumbersome a tool to use for the identification of an unknown bacterium isolated from a sample. In this instance a series of rapid and simple tests is required that probe the phenotypic characteristics of the microorganism. The tests are conducted in a logical series of steps, the results from each providing information on the next stage of the investigation. An example of such a procedure is given below:

Morphology:	microscopical investigations using a wet mount to determine cell size, shape, formation of spores, aggregation, motility etc.
Staining reactions:	Gram stain, acid-fast stain, spore stain
Cultural reactions:	appearance on solid media (colony formation, shape, size, colour, texture, smell, pigments etc.); aerobic/anaerobic growth, temperature requirements, pH requirements
Biochemical reactions:	enzymatic activities are probed to distinguish between closely related bacteria. Can be performed in traditional mode or using kits.

Biochemical tests   These are designed to examine the enzymatic capabilities of the organism. As there are a large number of biochemical tests that can be performed, the preliminary steps help to narrow down the range to those that will be most discriminatory. Given below are a few examples of commonly used biochemical tests.

Sugar fermentation is very frequently used and examines the ability of the organism to ferment a range of sugars. A number of tubes of peptone water are prepared, each containing a different sugar. An acid–base indicator is incorporated into the medium that also contains a Durham tube (a small inverted tube filled with medium) capable of collecting any gas produced during fermentation. After inoculation and incubation the tubes are examined for acid production, as indicated by a change in the colour of the indicator, and gas production as seen by a bubble of gas collected in the Durham tube.

Proteases are produced by a number of bacteria, e.g. *Bacillus* species and *Pseudomonas*, and they are responsible for the breakdown of protein into smaller units. Gelatin is a protein that can be added to liquid media to produce a stiff gel similar to agar. Unlike agar, which cannot be utilized by bacteria, those organisms producing proteases will destroy the gel structure and liquefy the medium. A medium made of nutrient broth solidified with gelatin is normally incorporated in boiling tubes or small bottles

and inoculated by means of a stab wire. After incubation it is important to refrigerate the gelatin prior to examination, otherwise false positives may be produced. Proteases can also be detected using milk agar, which is opaque. Protease producers form colonies with clear haloes around them where the enzyme has diffused into the medium and digested the casein.

Oxidase is produced by *Neisseria* and *Pseudomonas* and can be detected using 1% tetramethylparaphenylene diamine. The enzyme catalyses the transport of electrons between electron donors in the bacteria and the redox dye. A positive reaction is indicated by a deep purple colour in the reduced dye. The test is carried out by placing the reagent directly on to an isolated colony on an agar surface. Alternatively, a filter paper strip impregnated with the dye is moistened with water and, using a platinum loop, a bacterial colony spread across the surface. If positive, a purple colour will appear within 10 seconds. Note that the use of iron loops may give false positive reactions.

The indole test distinguishes those bacteria capable of decomposing the amino acid tryptophan to indole. Any indole produced can be tested by a colourimetric reaction with *p*-dimethylaminobenzaldehyde. After incubation in peptone water 0.5 mL Kovacs reagent is placed on the surface of the culture, shaken, and a positive reaction is indicated by a red colour. Organisms giving positive indole reactions include *E. coli* and *Proteus vulgaris*.

Catalase is responsible for the breakdown of hydrogen peroxide into oxygen and water. The test may be performed by adding 1 mL of 10-vol hydrogen peroxide directly to the surface of colonies growing on an agar slope. A vigorous frothing of the surface liquid indicates the presence of catalase. *Staphylococcus* and *Micrococcus* are catalase positive, whereas *Streptococcus* is catalase negative.

Urease production enables certain bacteria to break down urea to ammonia and carbon dioxide:

$$NH_2{-}CO{-}NH_2 + H_2O \xrightarrow{\text{urease}} 2NH_3 + CO_2$$

This test is readily carried out by growing the bacteria on a medium containing urea and an acid–base indicator. After incubation the production of ammonia will be shown by the alkaline reaction of the indicator. Examples of urease-negative bacteria include *E. coli* and *Enterococcus faecalis*.

Simmons citrate agar was developed to test for the presence of organisms that could utilize citrate as the sole source of carbon and energy and ammonia as the main source of nitrogen. It is used to differentiate members of the Enterobacteriaceae. The medium, containing bromothymol blue as indicator, is surface inoculated on slopes and citrate utilization demonstrated by an alkaline reaction and a change in the indicator colour from a dull green to a bright blue. *E. coli*, *Shigella*, *Edwardsiella* and *Yersinia* do not utilize citrate, whereas *Serratia*, *Enterobacter*, *Klebsiella* and *Proteus* do and so give a positive result.

The methyl red test is used to distinguish organisms that produce and maintain a high level of acidity from those that initially produce acid but restore neutral conditions with further metabolism. The organism is grown on glucose phosphate medium and, after incubation, a few drops of methyl red are added and the colour immediately recorded. A red colour indicates acid production (positive), whereas a yellow colour indicates alkali (negative).

Some organisms can convert carbohydrates to acetyl methyl carbinol (CH_3–CO–CHOH–CH_3). This may be oxidized to diacetyl (CH_3–CO–CO–CH_3), which will react with guanidine residues in the medium under alkaline conditions to produce a colour. This is the basis of the Voges Proskauer test, which is usually carried out at the same time as the methyl red test. The organism is again grown in glucose phosphate medium and, after incubation, 40% KOH is added together with 5% α-naphthol in ethanol. After mixing, a positive reaction is indicated by a pink colour in 2–5 minutes gradually becoming darker red up to 30 minutes. Organisms giving positive Voges Proskauer reactions usually give negative methyl red reactions, as the production of acetyl-methyl carbinol is accompanied by low acid production. *Klebsiella* species typically give a positive Voges Proskauer reaction.

Rapid identification systems With the increasing demand for quick and accurate identification of bacteria a number of micromethods have been developed combining a variety of biochemical tests selected for their rapidity of reading and high discrimination. The API bacterial identification system is an example of such a micromethod and comprises a plastic tray containing dehydrated substrates in a number of wells. Culture is added to the wells, dissolving the substrate and allowing the fermentation of carbohydrates, or the presence of enzymes similar to those just described, to be demonstrated. In some cases incubation times of 2 hours are sufficient for accurate identification. Kits are available with different reagents, permitting the identification of Enterobacteriaceae, Streptococcaceae, staphylococci, anaerobes, yeasts and moulds. Accurate identification is made by reference to a table of results.

The tests described so far will enable differentiation of an unknown bacterium to species level. However, it is apparent that not all isolates of the same species behave in an identical manner. For example, *E. coli* isolated from the intestines of a healthy person is relatively harmless compared to the well publicized *E. coli* O157.H7, which causes intense food poisoning and haemolytic uraemic syndrome. On occasions it is therefore, necessary to distinguish further between isolates from the same species. This can be performed using, among other things, serological tests and phage typing.

Serological tests Bacteria have antigens associated with their cell envelopes (O-antigens), with their flagella (H-antigens) and with their capsules (K-antigens). When injected into an animal, antibodies will be produced directed specifically towards those antigens and able to react with them. Specific antisera are prepared by immunizing an animal with a killed or attenuated bacterial suspension and taking blood samples. Serum containing the antibodies can then be separated. If a sample of bacterial suspension is placed on a glass slide and mixed with a small amount of specific antiserum, then the bacteria will be seen to clump when examined under the microscope. The test can be made more quantitative by using the tube dilution technique, where a given amount of antigen is mixed with a series of dilutions of specific antisera. The highest dilution at which agglutination occurs is called the agglutination titre.

Phage typing Many bacteria are susceptible to lytic bacteriophages whose action is very specific. Identification may be based on the susceptibility of a culture to a set of such type-specific lytic bacteriophages. This method enables very detailed identification of the organisms to be made, e.g. one serotype of *Salmonella typhi* has been further subdivided into 80 phage types using this technique.

FUNGI

Fungus is a general term used to describe all yeasts and moulds, whereas a mould is a filamentous fungus exhibiting a mycelial form of growth. The study of fungi is called mycology. Yeasts and moulds are eukaryotic microorganisms possessing organized demonstrable nuclei enclosed within an outer membrane, a nucleolus, and chromatin strands that become organized into chromosomes during cell division. Fungal cell walls are composed predominantly of polysaccharide, and in most cases this is chitin mixed with cellulose, glucan and mannan.

Proteins and glycoproteins are also present, but peptidoglycan is absent. The polysaccharide polymers are crosslinked to provide a structure of considerable strength which gives the cell osmotic stability. The fungal membrane contains sterols such as ergosterol and zymosterol not found in mammalian cells, and this provides a useful target for antifungal antibiotics. The role of fungi in nature is predominantly a scavenging one and in this respect they are vital for the decomposition and recycling of organic materials. Of the more than 100 000 species of known fungi fewer than 100 are human pathogens, and most of these are facultative and not obligate parasites.

Fungal morphology

The fungi can be divided into five broad groups on the basis of their morphology.

Yeasts

These are spherical or ovoid unicellular bodies 2–4 μm in diameter which typically reproduce by budding. In liquid cultures and on agar they behave very much like bacteria. Examples include *Saccharomyces cerevisiae*, strains of which are used in baking and in the production of beers and wines. *Cryptococcus neoformans* is the only significant pathogen and this gives rise to a respiratory tract disease called cryptococcosis, which in most cases is relatively mild. However, the microorganism may disseminate, leading to multiorgan disease, including meningitis. Cryptococcosis is of particular significance in immune-compromised patients. If left untreated, 80% of patients with disseminated cryptococcosis will die within 1 year.

Yeast-like fungi

These organisms normally behave like a typical budding yeast but under certain circumstances the buds do not separate and become elongated. The resulting structure resembles a filament and is called a pseudomycelium. It differs from a true mycelium in that there are no interconnecting pores between the cellular compartments comprising the hyphae.

The most important member of this group is *Candida albicans*, which is usually resident in the mouth, intestines and vagina. Under normal conditions *Candida* does not cause problems but if the environmental balance is disturbed then problems can arise. These include vaginal thrush (vaginitis) and oral thrush. Overgrowth of *Candida albicans*

within the gut can lead to symptoms of inexplicable fatigue and malaise, which is difficult to diagnose. Predisposing factors may include poor diet, diabetes, alcoholism and long-term treatment with steroids.

Dimorphic fungi

These grow as yeasts or as filaments depending upon the cultural conditions. At 22°C, either in the soil or in culture media, filamentous mycelial forms and reproductive spores are produced, whereas at 37°C in the body the microorganisms assume a yeast-like appearance. *Histoplasma capsulatum* is an important pathogen that gives rise to respiratory illness. The infectious form is the spore, which is borne on the wind and is inhaled. It has been postulated that a single spore can elicit an infection. On entering the body the spores germinate to give rise to the yeast form. Primary infections are often mild, but progressive disseminated histoplasmosis is a very severe disease that can affect many organs of the body.

Filamentous fungi

This group comprises those multicellular moulds that grow in the form of long, slender filaments 2–10 μm in diameter called hyphae. The branching hyphae, which constitute the vegetative or somatic structure of the mould, intertwine and gradually spread over the entire surface of the available substrate, extracting nutrients and forming a dense mat or mycelium. The hyphae may be non-septate (coenocytic) or septate, but in each case the nutrients and cellular components are freely diffusible along the length of the filament. This is facilitated by the presence of pores within the septa.

Mushrooms and toadstools

This group is characterized by the production of large reproductive fruiting bodies of complex structure. They also possess elaborate propagation mechanisms. Some of these fungi are edible and are used in cooking, but others, such as *Amanita phalloides* (Death Angel), produce potent mycotoxins that may result in death if eaten.

Reproduction of fungi

In the somatic portion of most fungi the nuclei are very small and the mechanism of nuclear division is uncertain. Under the correct environmental conditions the organisms will switch from the somatic or vegetative growth phase to a reproductive form, so that the fungus may propagate the species by producing new mycelia on fresh food substrates. Two types of reproduction are found, asexual and sexual.

Asexual reproduction

Asexual reproduction is in general more important for the propagation of the species and mechanisms include binary fission, budding, hyphal fragmentation and spore formation. Each progeny is an exact replica of the parent and no species variation can occur.

Some yeasts (e.g. *Schizosaccharomyces rouxii*) reproduce by binary fission in the same way as bacteria. The parent cell enlarges, its nucleus divides and, when a cross-wall is produced across the cell, two identical daughter cells form.

Budding occurs in the majority of yeasts and is the production of a small outgrowth or bud from the parent cell. As the bud increases in size the nucleus divides and one of the pair migrates into the bud. The bud eventually breaks off from the parent to form a new individual. A scar is left behind on the parent cell and each parent can produce up to 24 buds.

Fungi growing in a filamentous form may employ hyphal fragmentation as a means of asexual propagation. The hyphal tips break up into component segments (called arthroconidia or arthrospores), each of which can disperse on the wind to other environments and fresh food substrates.

The formation of specialized spore-bearing structures containing reproductive spores is the most common method of asexual reproduction (Fig. 39.9). The spores can be borne in a sporangium, supported on a sporangiophore. A limiting membrane surrounds the sporangium and the spores contained within it are called sporangiospores. The spores are released when the sporangium ruptures. This type of reproduction is found in the lower fungi possessing non-septate hyphae (e.g. *Mucor* and *Rhizopus*). Separate spores produced at the tips of specialized conidiophores are called conidiospores, and a diverse range of structures is found in nature.

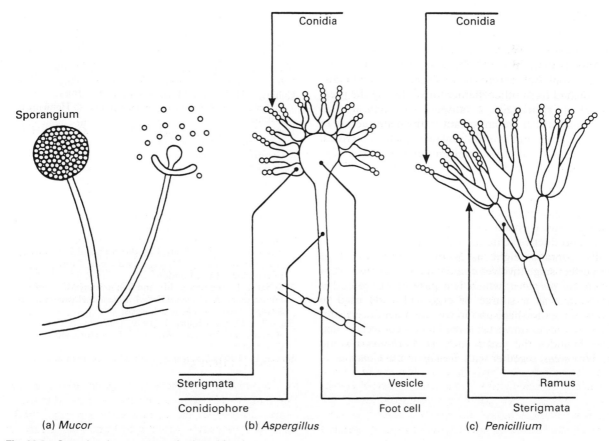

Fig. 39.9 Spore-bearing structures of selected fungi.

Figure 39.9 illustrates some of the different types of asexual spores found in fungi.

Sexual reproduction

Sexual reproduction involves the union of two compatible nuclei and allows variation of the species. Mycology is made much more complex because individual fungi are given different names depending upon whether they are in the sexual or the asexual stage. Not all fungi have been observed to carry out sexual reproduction. Some species produce distinguishable male and female sex organs on the same mycelium and are therefore hermaphroditic, i.e. a single colony can reproduce sexually by itself. Others produce mycelia which are either male or female (called dioecious), and can therefore only reproduce when two dissimilar organisms come together.

Fungal classification

The pharmaceutically important fungi can be found within four main taxonomic classes.

Zygomycetes

These are terrestrial saprophytes possessing non-septate hyphae and are sometimes referred to as the lower fungi. Apart from their hyphae they can be distinguished from other filamentous fungi by the presence of sporangia. Examples are *Mucor* and *Rhizopus*, which are important in the manufacture of organic acids and the biotransformation of steroids. They are also common spoilage organisms.

Ascomycetes

Ascomycetes possess septate hyphae and the sexual or perfect stage is characterized by the presence of a sac-like reproductive structure called an ascus. This typically contains eight ascospores. The asexual or imperfect stage involves conidiospores. An example is *Claviceps purpurea*, which is a parasite of rye and is important as a source of ergot alkaloids used to control haemorrhage and in treating migraine. A subclass of the Ascomycetes is the Hemiascomycetes, and this includes the yeasts such as *Saccharomyces* and *Cryptococcus*, together with *Torulopsis* and *Candida*.

Deuteromycetes

Sometimes called the Fungi Imperfecti this group includes those fungi in which the sexual stage of reproduction has not been observed. *Penicillium* and *Aspergillus* are Ascomycetes but classified among the Deuteromycetes as the perfect stage is apparently absent. *Penicillium chrysogenum* is important in the production of the antibiotic penicillin, whereas *Aspergillus* species have found widespread industrial usage owing to their extensive enzymic capabilities. Some *Aspergillus* species also produce mycotoxins and can cause serious infections in humans. The Deuteromycetes contains most of the human pathogens, such as *Blastomyces, Coccidioides*, and some of the dermatophyte fungi.

Basidiomycetes

This is the most advanced group, containing the mushrooms and toadstools. Sexual reproduction is by basidiospores. The group also includes the rusts (cereal parasites) and smuts.

BIBLIOGRAPHY

Bannister, B.A., Begg, N.T. and Gillespie, S.H. (1996) *Infectious Disease*. Blackwell Science Ltd, Oxford.

Collins, C.H., Lyne, P.M. and Grange, J.M. (1995) *Microbiological Methods*, 7th edn. Butterworth Heinemann, Oxford.

Davies, B.D., Dulbecco, R., Eisen H.N. and Ginsberg H.S. (eds) (1990) *Microbiology* 4th edn. J.B. Lippincott Company, Philadelphia.

Holt, J.G., Krieg, N.R., Sneath, P.H.A., J. Stanley, T. and Williams, S.T. (eds) (1994) *Bergey's Manual of Determinative Bacteriology* 9th edn. Williams and Wilkins, Baltimore.

Hugo, W.B. and Russell, A.D. (1998) *Pharmaceutical Microbiology*, 6th edn. Blackwell Scientific Publications, Oxford.

Mims, C., Playfair, J., Roitt, I., Wakelin D. and R. Williams (eds) (1998) *Medical Microbiology* 2th edn. Mosby International Ltd., London.

Neidhardt, F., Ingraham, J.L. and Schaechter, M. (1990) *Physiology of the Bacterial Cell: A Molecular Approach.* Sinauer Associates, Massachusetts.

Russell, A.D. and Chopra, I. (1990) *Understanding Antibacterial Action and Resistance*. Ellis Horwood, Chichester.

Stryer, L. (1995) *Biochemistry*, 4th edn. Freeman and Co.

40

Pharmaceutical applications of microbiological techniques

Norman Hodges

The purpose of this chapter is to bring together those microbiological methods and procedures that are relevant to the design and production of medicines and medical devices. These are methods used (a) to determine the potency or activity of antimicrobial chemicals, e.g. antibiotics, preservatives and disinfectants; and (b) as part of the microbiological quality control of manufactured sterile and non-sterile products.

There are several areas of biotechnology in which microorganisms or their enzymes are used in the production of medicines. These include antibiotic biosynthesis and 'fermentation'; the production of dextran, asparaginase, streptokinase and other microbial metabolites which have a medicinal application; interconversion of steroid molecules; the detection of mutagenicity by the Ames test; and the toxicity screening of pharmaceutical materials using mammalian cell cultures. Human genes have also been inserted into microorganisms which, as a consequence, are used to produce such materials as insulin, growth hormone and interferons. All of these biotechnological aspects of microbiology are, however, beyond the scope of this book, although they are included in the bibliography.

This chapter describes the experimental procedures which are unique or particularly relevant to pharmacy, rather than those that are common to microbiology as a whole. In the latter category, for example, are procedures used to identify and enumerate microorganisms, and these, together with staining and microscopical techniques, are described in Chapter 39.

Several of the methods and tests discussed in this chapter are the subject of monographs or appendices in the British Pharmacopoeia, or they are described in British Standards or other recognized reference works. It is not the intention to reproduce these official testing procedures in detail here, but rather to explain the principles of the tests, to draw attention to difficult or important aspects, and to indicate the advantages, problems or shortcomings of the various methods.

MEASUREMENT OF ANTIMICROBIAL ACTIVITY

In most of the methods used to assess the activity of antimicrobial chemicals an inoculum of the test organism is added to a solution of the chemical under test, samples are removed over a period of time, the chemical is inactivated and the proportion of cells surviving determined. Alternatively, culture medium is present together with the chemical, and the degree of inhibition of growth of the test organism is measured. In each case it is necessary to standardize and control such factors as the concentration of the test organism, its origin, i.e. the species and strain employed, together with the culture medium in which it was grown, the phase of growth from which the cells were taken, and the temperature and time of incubation of the cells after exposure to the chemical. Because such considerations are common to several of the procedures described here, e.g. antibiotic assays, preservative efficacy (challenge) tests and determinations of minimum inhibitory concentration (MIC), it is appropriate that they should be considered first, both to emphasize their importance and to avoid repetition.

Factors to be controlled in the measurement of antimicrobial activity

Origin of the test organism

Although two cultures may bear the same generic and specific name, i.e. they may both be called *Escherichia coli*, this does not mean that they are identical. Certainly they would normally be similar in many respects, e.g. morphology (appearance), cultural requirements and biochemical characteristics, but they may exhibit slight variations in some of these properties. Such variants are described as strains of *E. coli*, and it is desirable in experimental work to name or describe the strain being used. A variety of strains of a single species may normally be obtained from a culture collection, e.g. the National Collection of Industrial and Marine Bacteria or the National Collection of Type Cultures. Different strains may also occur in hospital pathology laboratories by isolation from swabs taken from infected patients, or by isolation from contaminated food, cosmetic or pharmaceutical products, and from many other sources. Strains obtained in these ways are likely to exhibit variations in resistance to antimicrobial chemicals. Strains from human or animal infections are frequently more resistant to antimicro-

bial chemicals, particularly antibiotics, than those from other sources. Similarly, strains derived from contaminated medicines may be more resistant to preservative chemicals than those obtained from culture collections. Therefore, to achieve results that are reproducible by a variety of laboratories it is necessary to specify the strain of the organism used for the determination.

It is becoming increasingly common, too, for official testing methods to limit the number of times the culture collection specimen may be regrown in fresh medium (called the number of subcultures or passages) before it must be replaced. This is because the characteristics of the organism (including its resistance to antimicrobial chemicals) may progressively change as a result of mutation and natural selection through the many generations that might arise during months or years of laboratory cultivation.

Composition and pH of the culture medium

There are several methods of assessing antimicrobial activity which all have in common the measurement of inhibition of growth of a test organism when the antimicrobial chemical is added to the culture medium. In such cases the composition and pH of the medium may influence the result. The medium may contain substances that antagonize the action of the test compound, e.g. high concentrations of thymidine or para-aminobenzoic acid will interfere with sulphonamide activity.

The antimicrobial activities of several groups of chemical are influenced by the ease with which they cross the cell membrane and interfere with the metabolism of the cell. This, in turn, is influenced by the lipid solubility of the substance, as the membrane contains a high proportion of lipid and tends to permit the passage of lipid-soluble substances. Many antimicrobial chemicals are weak acids or weak bases, which are more lipid soluble in the unionized form. pH therefore affects their degree of ionization, hence their lipid solubility and so, ultimately, their antimicrobial effect. Benzoic acid, for example, is a preservative used in several oral mixtures which has a much greater activity in liquids buffered to an acid pH value than those which are neutral or alkaline. Conversely, weak bases such as the aminoglycoside antibiotics, e.g. streptomycin, neomycin and gentamicin, are more active at slightly alkaline pH values. The presence of organic matter, e.g. blood, pus or serum, is likely to have a marked protective effect on the test organism, and so antimicrobial chemicals may appear less active in the presence of such material.

The activity of several antibiotics, notably tetracyclines and aminoglycosides, is reduced by the presence of high concentrations of di- or trivalent cations in the medium.

Exposure and incubation conditions

The temperature, duration and redox conditions of exposure to the antimicrobial chemical (or incubation of survivors after exposure) may all have a significant effect on its measured activity. Increasing the temperature of exposure of the test organism to the chemical increases the antimicrobial activity by a factor which is quantified by the temperature coefficient (Q_{10} value: the number of -fold increase in activity for a 10°C rise in temperature). Alcohols and phenols, for example, may respectively exhibit Q_{10} values of 3–5 and >10, and so a variation of 5°C in the temperature of exposure (which is permitted by pharmacopoeial preservative efficacy tests, for example) may lead to a markedly different rate of kill of the organism in question.

The period of time for which the test organism is exposed to the antimicrobial chemical may influence the recorded result because it is possible for the organism to adapt and become resistant to the presence of the chemical. In preservative efficacy tests the exposure period is normally 28 days, which is sufficient time for any cells that are not killed during the first 24–48 hours to recover and start to reproduce, so that the final bacterial concentration may be much higher than that at the start. This is illustrated in Figure 40.1, which shows the effect of the quaternary ammonium preservative benzethonium bromide on *Pseudomonas aeruginosa*.

The concentration of bacteria was reduced to approximately 0.01 % of the initial value during the first 6 hours, but the bacteria that survived this early

period recovered to the original level within 2 days. There is the potential for a similar phenomenon to arise in other situations, e.g. in minimum inhibitory concentration (MIC) determinations of bacteristatic agents (those that do not kill, but merely inhibit the growth of the test organism), although it is not common in MICs because the exposure (incubation) time is much shorter than that in preservative testing.

The effect of some antibiotics may be influenced by the redox conditions during their period of contact with the test organism. Aminoglycosides, for example, are far less active, and metronidazole is far more active, under conditions of low oxygen availability. Such effects may even be seen during agar-diffusion antibiotic assays, in which the antibiotic diffuses from a well into an agar gel inoculated with the test organism; the diameter of the zone of growth inhibition that surrounds a well filled with neomycin solution, for example, may be significantly greater at the surface of the agar (where there is abundant oxygen) than at its base, where the oxygen concentration is limited by its poor diffusion through the gel.

Inoculum concentration and physiological state

It is perhaps not surprising that the concentration of the inoculum can markedly affect antimicrobial action, with high inoculum levels tending to result in reduced activity. There are two main reasons for this. First, there is the phenomenon of drug adsorption on to the cell surface or absorption into the interior of the cell. If the number of drug molecules in the test tube is fixed yet the number of cells present is increased, this obviously results in fewer molecules available per cell and consequently the possibility of a diminished effect. In addition to this there is the second, more specialized case, again concerning antibiotics, where it is frequently observed that certain species of bacteria can synthesize antibiotic-inactivating enzymes, the most common of which are the various types of β-lactamase (those destroying penicillin, cephalosporin and related antibiotics). Thus a high inoculum means a high carryover of enzyme with the inoculum cells, or at least a greater potential synthetic capacity.

Perhaps less predictable than the inoculum concentration effect is the possibility of the inoculum history influencing the result. There is a substantial amount of evidence to show that the manner in which the inoculum of the test organism has been grown and prepared can significantly influence its susceptibility to toxic chemicals. Features such as the nature of the culture medium, e.g. nutrient broth or a defined glucose-salts medium, the metal ion

Fig. 40.1 The survival and recovery of *Pseudomonas aeruginosa* exposed to benzethonium chloride during a preservative efficacy test

composition of the medium and hence of the cells themselves and the physiological state of the cells, i.e. 'young' actively growing cells from the logarithmic growth phase or 'old' non-dividing cells from the stationary phase, all have the potential to influence the observed experimental values.

Antibiotic assays

Methods of assaying antibiotics may be broadly divided into three groups:

- Conventional chemical assays, e.g. titrations, spectrophotometry and high-performance liquid chromatography (HPLC);
- Enzyme-based and immunoassays, where the antibiotic is, respectively, the substrate for a specific enzyme or the antigen with which a specific antibody combines;
- Biological assays in which biological activity – in this case bacterial growth inhibition – of the 'test' solution is compared with that of a reference standard.

Biological methods offer the advantage that the parameter being measured in the assay (growth inhibition) is the property for which the drug is used, and so inactive impurities or degradation products will not interfere and lead to an inaccurate result. Biological methods also offer other advantages (Table 40.1), but they have several significant limitations and non-biological methods are now generally preferred.

Enzyme-based and immunoassay kits are used in hospitals, notably for therapeutic monitoring of toxic antibiotics (e.g. aminoglycosides and vancomycin), whereas HPLC tends to be preferred in the pharmaceutical industry, particularly for quality assurance applications. Biological assays are most likely to be used when the alternatives are inappropriate, especially when the active antibiotic cannot readily be separated from inactive impurities, degradation products or interfering substances, or it cannot easily be assayed by HPLC without derivatization to enhance ultraviolet absorption (e.g. aminoglycosides). These situations may arise:

1. when the antibiotic is present in a solution containing a wide variety of complex substances that would interfere with a chemical assay, e.g. fermentation broth, serum or urine;
2. when the antibiotic is present together with significant concentrations of its breakdown products, e.g. during stability studies as part of product development;
3. when it has been extracted from a formulated medicine, for example a cream or linctus, when excipients might cause interference;
4. where the commercially available product is a mixture of isomers that have inherently different antimicrobial activities, which cannot easily be distinguished chemically and which may differ in proportion from batch to batch (e.g. neomycin and gentamicin).

Biological antibiotic assays, or bioassays as they are frequently known, may be of two main types, agar diffusion and turbidimetric. The European Pharmacopoeia (1997) section 2.7.2 describes experimental details for both methods, e.g. test microorganisms, solvents, buffers, culture media and incubation conditions. In each case a reference material of known activity must be available. When antibiotics were in their infancy few could be produced in the pure state free from contaminating material, and specific chemical assays were rarely available. Thus the potency or activity of reference standards was expressed in terms of (international)

Table 40.1 Relative merits of alternative antibiotic assay methods

Assay method	Advantages	Disadvantages
Biological methods	Inactive impurities or degradation properties do not interfere	Slow, usually requiring overnight incubation
	Easily scaled up for multiple samples	Relatively labour-intensive
	Do not require expensive equipment	Relatively inaccurate and imprecise, particularly with inexperienced operators
Non-biological methods	Usually rapid, accurate and precise	May require expensive equipment (e.g. HPLC) or expensive reagents or assay kits (enzyme and immunological methods)
	May be more sensitive than biological assays	
	Enzyme and immunological methods are usually assay kits, which give reliable results with inexperienced operators	HPLC can only assay samples sequentially, so unusually large sample numbers may cause problems

units of activity. There are few antibiotics for which dosage is still normally expressed in units: nystatin and polymyxin are two of the remaining examples. More commonly, potencies are recorded in terms of μg mL^{-1} of solution or μg antibiotic mg^{-1} of salt, with dosages expressed in mg. Antibiotic assay results are usually in the form of a potency ratio of the activity of the unknown or test solution divided by that of the standard.

Agar diffusion assays

In this technique the agar medium in a Petri dish or a larger assay plate is inoculated with the test organism, wells are created in it by removing circular plugs of agar, and these wells are filled with a solution of the chemical under test (Fig. 40.2).

The chemical diffuses through the gel from A towards B and the concentration falls steadily in that direction. The concentration in the region A to X is sufficiently high to prevent growth, i.e. it is an inhibitory concentration. Between X and B the concentration is subinhibitory and growth occurs. The concentration at X at the time the zone edge is formed is known as the critical inhibitory concentration (CIC). After incubation the gel between A and X is clear and that between X and B is opaque as a result of microbial growth which, with the common test organisms, is usually profuse. A zone of inhibition is therefore created, the diameter of which will increase as the concentration of chemical in the well increases.

A graph may be constructed which relates zone diameter to the logarithm of the concentration of the solution in the well (Fig. 40.3). It is normally found to be linear over a small concentration range, but the square of the diameter must be plotted to achieve linearity over a wide range. A plot such as that in Figure 40.3 may, quite correctly, be used to calculate the concentration of a test solution of antibiotic. In practice, however, it is found to be more convenient to obtain reliable mean zone diameters for the standard at just two or three concentrations, rather than somewhat less reliable values for six or seven concentrations. There is no reason why an assay should not be based upon a two- or three-point line, provided that those points are reliable and that preliminary experiments have shown that the plotted relationship over the concentration range in question is linear.

It is not common to conduct antibiotic assays in Petri dishes because too few zones may be accommodated on a standard-sized dish to permit the replication necessary to obtain the required accuracy and precision. Antibiotic assays, when performed on a large scale, are more often conducted using large assay plates 300 mm or more square. The wells are created in a square design and the number that may be accommodated will depend upon the anticipated

Fig. 40.3 Calibration plots for agar diffusion assays.

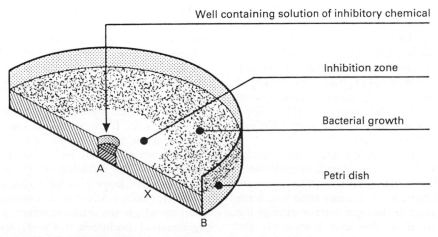

Fig. 40.2 Assessment of antimicrobial activity by agar diffusion.

zone diameters: 36 or 64 wells are common (6×6 or 8×8, respectively). The antibiotic standard material may be used in solution at three known concentrations (frequently referred to as 'doses') and the antibiotic solution of unknown concentration treated likewise; alternatively, each may be employed at two concentrations. A randomization pattern known as a Latin square is used to ensure that there is a suitable distribution of the solutions over the plate, thereby minimizing any errors due to uneven agar thickness.

In the case of an assay based upon standard solutions used at two concentrations, the potency ratio may be calculated directly from the graph (as shown in Fig. 40.4) or by using the formula below:

$$\log X = LDR \times \frac{(UH + UL) - (SH + SL)}{(SH - SL) + (UH - UL)}$$

where X is the potency ratio, LDR is the logarithm of the dose ratio (i.e. ratio of concentrations of standard solutions), UH, UL, SH and SL are the mean zone diameters for the unknown and standard high and low doses. The derivation of this is described in detail by Wardlaw (1999), who deals extensively with the subject of antibiotic assays. The tests for acceptable limits of parallelism between the line joining the standards and that joining the test points, together with confidence limits applicable to the calculated potency ratios, are described in the current EP.

In calculating the potency ratio directly from Figure 40.4 the zone diameters for the standard and unknown high concentrations are plotted at the same abscissa values, and those for the low concentrations similarly. Two zone diameters are considered which are as widely separated on the ordinate as possible while still being covered by the standard and the test lines. The ratio of the concentrations required to achieve the selected diameter is thus an estimate of the potency ratio. The mean of the two estimates taken at the extremes of the range of common zone diameters should be identical to the value by calculation from the formula. Thus, in Figure 40.4, at a zone diameter of 23.75 mm the first estimate of potency ratio is 0.557 (antilog of 0.445 divided by antilog of 0.699); the second is 0.507 (antilog of zero divided by the antilog of 0.295). The mean value of 0.53 indicates the unknown solution to have approximately half the activity of the standard.

Practical aspects of the conduct of agar diffusion assays
The agar may be surface inoculated, or inoculated throughout while in the molten state prior to pouring. In the latter case zones may arise which are different in diameter at the agar surface than at the base of the Petri dish; this may complicate the recording of zone diameters. Zones which are not

Fig. 40.4   Four-point agar diffusion assay of bacitracin.

perfectly circular may be disregarded, although it may be appropriate to record the mean of the long and short axes. Such zones may result from non-circular wells, careless filling, or uneven drying of the agar gel owing to a poorly fitting plate cover. The zones may be read directly with callipers or, more conveniently, after enlargement by projection on to a screen. Automatic zone readers incorporating a series of photocells that detect opacity changes at the zone edge are available, and may be linked to a personal computer which rapidly calculates the result together with the appropriate statistical analyses. The size of the zone is determined by the relative rates of diffusion of the drug molecule and growth of the test organism. If the assay plates are left at room temperature for 1–4 hours prior to incubation, growth is retarded whereas diffusion proceeds. This may result in larger zones and improved precision.

The zone diameter is affected by most of the factors previously stated to influence antimicrobial activity and, in addition, gel strength and the presence of other solutes in the antibiotic solution, e.g. buffer salts. If the antibiotic has been extracted from a formulated medicine, e.g. cream, lotion or mixture, excipients may be simultaneously removed and influence the diffusion of the antibiotic in the gel; sugars are known to have this effect. Because antibiotic assays involve a comparison of two solutions which are similarly affected by changes in experimental conditions, day to day variations in, for example, inoculum concentration will not have a great effect on the accuracy of the potency ratio obtained, but the precision may be affected. The volume of liquid in the well is of minimal importance; it is usually of the order of 0.1 mL and is delivered by semiautomatic pipette. As an alternative to wells the antibiotic may be introduced on to the agar using absorbent paper discs, metal cylinders or 'fish spine' beads (beads having a hole drilled in them which contains the liquid).

For many antibiotics, the test organism is a *Bacillus* species and the inoculum is in the form of a spore suspension, which is easy to prepare, standardize and store. Alternatively, frozen inocula from liquid nitrogen may be used as a means of improving reproducibility.

Careful storage and preparation of the reference standards are essential. The reference antibiotic is usually stored at low temperature in a freeze-dried condition.

Turbidimetric assays

In this case antibiotic standards at several concentrations are incorporated into liquid media and the extent of growth inhibition of the test organism is measured turbidimetrically using a nephelometer or spectrophotometer. The unknown or test antibiotic preparation is run simultaneously, again at several concentrations, and the degree of growth inhibition compared. Such assays are less commonly used than agar diffusion methods because their precision is rather inferior, but they do have the advantage of speed: the result may be available after an incubation period as short as 3–4 hours. They are also more sensitive than diffusion assays and consequently may be applied to low-activity preparations.

The shape and slope of the dose–response plot for a turbidimetric assay may be more variable than that for agar diffusion, and non-linear plots are common. Typical dose–response plots are shown in Hewitt and Vincent (1989). The plotted points are usually the mean turbidity values obtained from replicate tubes, and the assay may be conducted using a Latin square arrangement of tubes incubated in a shaker, which is necessary to ensure adequate aeration and uniform growth throughout the tube.

Practical aspects of the conduct of turbidimetric assays
Incubation time is critical in two respects. First, it is necessary to ensure that the culture in each of the many tubes in the incubator has exactly the same incubation period, because errors of a few minutes become significant in a total of only 3–4 hours' incubation. Care must therefore be taken to ensure that the tubes are inoculated in a precise order, and

that growth is stopped in the same order by the addition of formalin, heating or other means.

The incubation period must be appropriate to the inoculum level so that the cultures do not achieve maximal growth. At the concentrations used for such assays the antibiotics usually reduce growth rate but do not limit total growth. Therefore, if the incubation period is sufficiently long, all of the cultures may achieve the same cell density regardless of the antibiotic concentration.

There are certain other limitations to the use of turbidimetric assays. Because it is the 'cloudiness' of the culture that is measured, standard and test solutions in which the organisms are suspended should, ideally, be clear before inoculation. Cloudy or hazy solutions which may result from the extraction of the antibiotic from a cream, for example, can only be determined after similarly compensating the standards or otherwise eliminating the error. Test organisms that produce pigments during the course of the incubation period should be avoided; so too should those that normally clump in suspension.

The rate of growth of the test organism may vary significantly from one batch of medium to another. Thus it is important to ensure that all the tubes in the assay contain medium from the same batch, and were prepared and sterilized at the same time. Many liquid media become darker brown on prolonged heating, and so samples from the same batch may differ in colour if the sterilizing time is not strictly controlled.

Minimum inhibitory concentration determinations (MICs)

The MIC is the lowest concentration of an antimicrobial chemical found to inhibit the growth of a particular test organism. It is therefore a fundamental measure of the intrinsic antimicrobial activity (potency) of a chemical, which may be an antiseptic, disinfectant, preservative or antibiotic. MIC determinations are applied to chemicals in the pure state, i.e. they are particularly relevant to raw materials rather than to the final formulated medicines; the latter are usually subject to preservative efficacy (challenge) tests to assess their antimicrobial activity. MIC values are usually expressed in terms of μg mL^{-1} or, less commonly, as in the case of some antibiotics, units mL^{-1}. It is important to recognize that the test organism is not necessarily killed at the MIC. Whether or not the cells die or merely cease growing depends upon the mode of action of the antimicrobial agent in question.

An MIC is an absolute value which is not based upon a comparison with a standard/reference preparation, as in the case of antibiotic assays and certain disinfectant tests. For this reason inadequate control of experimental conditions is particularly likely to have an adverse effect on results. Discrepancies in MIC values measured in different laboratories are often attributable to slight variations in such conditions, and care must be taken to standardize all the factors previously stated to influence the result. It is important also to state the experimental details concerning an MIC determination. A statement such as 'the MIC for phenol against *E. coli* is 0.1% w/v' is not, by itself, very useful. It has far more value if the strain of *E. coli*, the inoculum concentration and the culture medium etc. are also stated.

MIC test methods

The most common way to conduct MIC determinations is to incorporate the antimicrobial chemical at a range of concentrations into a liquid medium, the containers of which are then inoculated, incubated and examined for growth.

Test tubes may be used, but microtitre plates (small rectangular plastic trays with, usually, 96 wells each holding approximately 0.2 mL liquid) and other miniaturized systems are common. It is possible to incorporate the chemical into molten agar, which is then poured into Petri dishes and allowed to set. Two advantages of using a series of agar plates are that several organisms can be tested at the same time using a multipoint inoculator, and there is a greater chance of detecting contaminating organisms (as uncharacteristic colonies) on the agar surface than in liquid media. Usually the presence or absence of growth is easier to distinguish on the surface of agar than in liquid media. In tubes showing only faint turbidity it is often difficult to decide whether growth has occurred or not. Regardless of the method used the principle is the same, and the MIC is the lowest concentration at which growth is inhibited.

In addition to the other experimental details that should be described in order to make the measured result meaningful, it is necessary to specify the increment by which the concentration of test chemical changes from one container to the next. The operator could, for example, change the concentration 10-fold from one tube to the next in the rare circumstance where even the likely order of magnitude of the MIC is not known. Far more commonly, however, the concentration changes by a factor of 2, and this is almost invariably the case when antibiotic MIC values are determined; thus, reference is made to 'doubling dilutions' of the antibiotic. If, for example, an MIC was to be measured using test tubes, an aqueous solution of the chemical would normally be mixed with an equal volume of ***double***-strength growth medium in the first tube in the series, then half the contents of the first tube added to an equal volume of ***single***-strength medium in the second, and so on. In this case half the contents of the last tube in the series would have to be discarded prior to inoculation in order to maintain the same volume in each tube. Control tubes may be included to demonstrate (a) that the inoculum culture was viable and that the medium was suitable for its growth (a tube containing medium and inoculum but no test chemical), and (b) that the operator was not contaminating the tubes with other organisms during preparation (a tube with no test chemical or added inoculum). It is possible to use an arithmetic series of concentrations of test chemical, e.g. 0.1, 0.2, 0.3, 0.4 ... rather than 0.1, 0.2, 0.4, 0.8 ... μg mL^{-1}. The potential problem with this approach is that there may be merely a gradation in growth inhibition, rather a sharp point of demarcation, with obvious growth in one tube in the series and no growth in the next.

All the solutions used must be sterilized; it must not be assumed that the test chemical is self-sterilizing. Most disinfectants, antiseptic and preservative chemicals are bactericidal, but they are unlikely to kill bacterial spores. Also, several antibiotics act by inhibiting growth, and so would not necessarily kill vegetative cells with which they might be contaminated. If the experiment is conducted in tubes, all the tube contents must be mixed before inoculation as well as after, otherwise there is the possibility of the inoculum cells being killed by an artificially high concentration of the test chemical towards the top of the tube. If there is any risk of precipitation of the test chemical or the medium components during incubation a turbidity comparison must be available for each concentration (same tube contents without inoculum); alternatively, in the case of bactericidal chemicals the liquid in each tube may be subcultured into pure medium to see whether the inoculum has survived. Each of the tubes in the series may be prepared in duplicate or triplicate if it is considered desirable. This is the case where the incremental change in concentration is small.

Preservative efficacy tests (challenge tests)

These are tests applied to the formulated medicine in its final container to determine whether it is adequately protected against microbial spoilage. Preservative efficacy tests are used for this purpose (rather than chemical assays of preservatives) because it is not normally possible to predict how the activity of a preservative chemical will be influenced by the active ingredients, the excipients and the container itself.

Certain products may contain no added preservative, either because the active ingredients have sufficient antimicrobial activity themselves or because they already contain high concentrations of sugar or salts which restrict the growth of microorganisms. However, such products are rare, and multidose injections or eye drops, the majority of oral mixtures, linctuses and similar preparations, together with creams and lotions, all contain preservatives. They are not normally required in anhydrous products, e.g. ointments, or in single-dose injections.

Again it must not be assumed that products containing antimicrobial agents as the active ingredients are self-sterilizing, It is quite possible for an antibiotic cream, for example, to be active against certain bacteria yet fail to restrict the growth of contaminating yeasts or moulds in the cream itself.

The basic principle of a preservative test is to inoculate separate containers of the product with known concentrations of a variety of test organisms, then remove samples from each container over a period of time and determine the proportion of the inoculum that has survived. When first introduced into national pharmacopoeias, preservative efficacy tests differed to some extent in experimental detail and differed markedly in the required performance criteria for preservatives to be used in different product categories. In the late 1990s moves towards international harmonization of preservative testing procedures in the European, United States and Japanese pharmacopoeias (EP, USP and JP, respectively) meant that many (but not all) of the discrepancies in experimental detail were eliminated. The differences in performance criteria remain, however, with the EP generally requiring a greater degree of microbial inactivation for the preservative to be considered satisfactory than the USP and JP which, in this respect, are very similar.

The EP (2000) recommends the routine use of four test organisms, each at a final concentration of 10^5–10^6 cells mL^{-1} or g^{-1} in the product. Counts are performed on samples removed at 0 h, 6 h, 24 h, 48 h, 7 days, 14 days and 28 days. Various aspects of the test are considered in more detail below.

Choice of test organisms and inoculum concentration

The test organisms used are the bacteria *Staphylococcus aureus*, *Pseudomonas aeruginosa* and *E. coli* (which is used for testing all product types in the USP test but for oral products only in the EP test), together with the yeasts/moulds *Candida albicans* and *Aspergillus niger* (plus the osmophilic *Zygosaccharomyces rouxii* in the EP test for oral syrups). The current EP recommends that the designated organisms be supplemented, where appropriate, by other strains or species that may represent likely contaminants to the preparation. A similar recommendation was contained in all previous versions of the USP preservative test, but this has been deleted from the current test (USP 2000). One problem with adding other organisms (such as those isolated from the manufacturing environment) is that they are not universally available, and so a particular product could be tested at different manufacturing sites of the same company and pass in one location yet fail in another simply because the organisms used locally were not the same. The possibility of using resistant strains isolated from previous batches of spoilt product has been advocated, but this too may pose problems, in that organisms may rapidly lose their preservative resistance unless routinely grown on media supplemented with the preservative in question.

Previous versions of the British Pharmacopoeial test have recommended consideration of extending the sampling period beyond 28-days, and reinoculating the product after the first 28-day sampling period is complete. Both of these practices, however, militate against the development of an international standardized test which is capable of providing reproducible results in different laboratories; consequently, both procedures are no longer part of the current EP or USP tests.

The inoculum concentration of 10^5–10^6 microorganisms mL^{-1} or g^{-1} of the preparation under test has been criticized as being unrealistic, as it is much higher than that which would be acceptable in a freshly manufactured product. It is adopted, however, in order for the 1000-fold fall in microbial concentration that would be required from an effective parenteral or ophthalmic preservative to be easily measured. The test organisms are added separately to different containers rather than as a mixed inoculum.

Inactivation of preservative

It is quite possible for sufficient of the preservative to be contained in, and carried over with, the sample removed from the container to prevent or retard growth of colonies on the Petri dishes. If the inoculum level of the test organism initially is about 10^6 cells mL^{-1} or g^{-1} of product, the problem of carryover may not arise because a dilution factor of 10^3 or 10^4 would be required to achieve a countable number of colonies on a plate; at this dilution most preservatives would no longer be active. When a high proportion of the cells in the product have died, however, little or no such dilution is required, so preservative carryover is a real problem which may artificially depress the count even more. To avoid this, preservative inhibitors or antagonists may be used. There are several of these, common examples being glycine for aldehydes, thioglycollate or cysteine for heavy metals, and mixtures of lecithin and polysorbate-80 with or without Lubrol W for quaternary ammonium compounds, chlorhexidine and parabens. The use of these and other inactivators has been reviewed by Russell (1981).

An alternative method of removing residual preservative is to pass the sample of inoculated product through a bacteria-proof membrane, so that surviving organisms are retained and washed on the surface of the membrane and the preservative is thus physically separated from them. After washing, the membrane is transferred to the surface of a suitable agar medium and colonies of microorganisms develop on it in the normal way. It is necessary to incorporate controls (validate the method) to demonstrate both that the inactivator really works and that it is not, itself, toxic. The former usually involves mixing the inactivator with the concentrations of preservative likely to be carried over, then inoculating and demonstrating no viability loss. Details of these validation procedures and other aspects of the test are described more fully elsewhere (Hodges, 1999).

One further control is a viable count of the inoculum performed by dilution in peptone water to check the actual number of cells introduced into the product. This is necessary because even a 'zero time sample' of the product will contain cells that have been exposed to the preservative for a short period, as it usually takes 15–45 seconds or more to mix the inoculum with the product and then remove the sample. Some of the cells may be killed even in such a short time, and so a viable count of the inoculum culture will reflect this.

Interpretation of results

The extent of microbial killing required at the various sampling times for a preservative to be considered acceptable for use in parenteral or ophthalmic products is greater than that required for a preservative to be used in topical products, which

in turn exceeds that for an oral product preservative (Table 40.2).

In the case of the first two product categories the EP specifies two alternative performance criteria, designated A and B. The A criteria express the recommended efficacy to be achieved, whereas the B criteria must be satisfied in justified cases where the A criteria cannot be attained, for example because of an increased risk of adverse reactions. The baseline used as the reference point to assess the extent of killing is the concentration of microorganisms expected to arise in the product after addition and mixing of the inoculum, *as calculated from a viable count performed on the concentrated inoculum suspension prior to its addition to the product*. The viable count on the time-zero sample removed from the inoculated product is not the baseline.

Disinfectant evaluation

A variety of tests have been described over many years for the assessment of disinfectant activity. Those developed during the early part of the 20th century, e.g. the Rideal–Walker and Chick–Martin tests, were primarily intended for testing phenolic disinfectants against pathogenic organisms such as *Salmonella typhi*. Such phenol coefficient tests are now rather outmoded because *S. typhi* is no longer endemic in Britain and phenolics are no longer preeminent; in a recent survey, phenolics represented only 26% of the total biocides used for floor disinfection in aseptic dispensing areas in British hospital pharmacies (Murtough et al 2000).

In the second half of the 20th century several other testing procedures were described for use in the UK which reduced the sampling or other problems associated with the early phenol coefficient tests; these included the Berry and Bean method, the British Standard 3286 test for quaternary ammonium compounds and the Kelsey–Sykes test. Other countries adopted procedures that were similar in concept but which differed in experimental detail, e.g. the American Association of Official Analytical Chemists (1990) described a collection of methods applicable to a variety of situations. These and other tests used in the UK, Europe and the USA are described by Reybrouck (1999). At present there is no internationally applicable and officially recommended disinfectant testing procedure, although a measure of uniformity has emerged in Europe with the establishment by the European Committee for Standardization in 1990 of Technical Committee (TC) 216, which has a responsibility for chemical

Table 40.2 Log reductions required in viable counts of microorganisms used in EP (2000) preservative efficacy tests

Product type	Microorganism	Criteria	6 h	24 h	48 h	7 d	14 d	28 d
Parenteral and ophthalmic	Bacteria	A	2	3				NR
	Pseudomonas aeruginosa	B		1		3		NI
	Staphylococcus aureus							
	*Escherichia coli**							
	Fungi	A					2	NI
	Aspergillus niger	B					1	NI
	Candida albicans							
Topical	Bacteria	A			2	3		NI
		B					3	NI
	Fungi	A					2	NI
		B					1	NI
Oral	Bacteria						3	NI
	Fungi						1	NI
Ear Preparations	Bacteria		2	3				NR
BP (1998) only	Fungi					2		NI

* In oral products only.
NR, no recovery;
NI, no increase (see text).

disinfectants and antiseptics. The European Standard BS EN 1276 (1997) was the first result of the work of TC 216; this deals with assessment of bactericidal activity of disinfectants on bacteria in aqueous suspension. Other procedures applicable to more specialized situations, e.g. disinfection of solid surfaces, are currently under development by TC 216.

A confusing variety of methods for describing and categorizing test procedures are in use. Thus, some schemes classify tests according to the organisms to be killed (bactericidal, fungicidal, virucidal etc.), but classification based upon test design is more common, e.g. suspension tests; capacity tests which measure the extent to which the disinfectant can withstand repeated additions of test organisms; carrier tests, where the organism is loaded or dried on to a carrier; and in-use tests, which are intended to simulate actual conditions of use as closely as possible.

Although most suspension tests of disinfectants have in common the addition of a defined concentration of test organism to the disinfectant solution at a specified temperature, followed by assessment of viability in samples removed after suitable time periods, there are four aspects of disinfectant testing that merit special note:

1. Because disinfectants are normally used in circumstances where there is a significant amount of organic 'dirt' present, modern testing procedures invariably attempt to take this into consideration. Thus, yeast, albumin or other material is added in known concentration to the disinfectant/microorganism mixture.

2. Regardless of the method by which the antimicrobial activity is assessed (see below), it is a fundamental principle of disinfectant testing, just as it is with preservative efficacy tests, that the antimicrobial activity of the disinfectant must be halted (also referred to as neutralized, inactivated or quenched) in the sample when it is removed from the disinfectant/organism mixture. Clearly, meaningful results cannot be obtained if it is impossible to distinguish what fraction of the microbial killing occurred during the timed period of exposure to the disinfectant from that arising due to carryover of disinfectant into the incubation step that follows exposure. Verification that the disinfectant inactivation method is effective and that any chemical neutralizers used are, themselves, non-toxic to the test organisms, is an integral part of the test.

3. It is in viability assessment that there is a fundamental difference of approach between recently developed tests (exemplified by BS EN 1276) and many of the tests that originated before the 1980s. The simplest method of viability assessment, which was employed in the

Rideal–Walker and Kelsey–Sykes tests, for example, is to transfer the sample from the disinfectant/microorganism mixture to a known volume of neutralizing broth, incubate and examine for growth (manifest as turbidity). This procedure contains the inherent defect that any growth in the tubes of broth may result from the transfer of very few surviving cells, or from many. Thus, it is possible for the disinfectant to kill a high proportion of the inoculum within a short period yet fail to kill a small fraction of the cells, possibly mutants, which have atypically high resistance. In this case there is the risk that the disinfectant may be dismissed as insufficiently active despite the fact that it achieved a rapid and extensive initial kill. For this reason it has become common for disinfectant and preservative efficacy tests to be very similar in design, in that both employ viable counting methods to assess microorganism survival, but the former utilize a sampling period of minutes or hours, whereas the latter use a 28-day period.

4. When viable counting is used to assess the survival of test organisms the adoption of disinfection performance criteria based upon a required reduction in the number of surviving organisms is a logical strategy, just as it is in preservative testing. Thus, the so-called 5-5-5 testing principle has found much favour. Here, five test organisms are (separately) exposed for 5 minutes to the disinfectant, which is considered satisfactory if a 5-log reduction in viable numbers (a 10^5 fall in viable cells mL^{-1}) is recorded in each case. This principle is adopted in the BS EN 1276, although only four bacterial strains are recommended for routine use; there is, however, the option to supplement the standard organisms with others more relevant to the intended use of the disinfectant in question.

MICROBIOLOGICAL QUALITY OF PHARMACEUTICAL MATERIALS

Non-sterile products

Non-sterile pharmaceutical products obviously differ from sterile products in that they are permitted to contain some microorganisms, but the European Pharmacopoeia (1997) specifies in section 5.1.4 the maximum concentrations acceptable in different types of product and the species of organism that are not permitted at all (Table 40.3). Similar specifications arise in the U S and other pharmacopoeias.

The required microbiological quality of the manufactured medicine cannot be achieved by the application of an antimicrobial process (heating, radiation etc.) as the final production step for two reasons: first, an approach that uses poor-quality raw materials and manufacturing procedures and then attempts to 'clean up' the product at the end is not acceptable to the licensing authorities; and secondly, some products would not withstand such antimicrobial treatment, e.g. heating an emulsion may cause cracking or creaming. Thus, the most reliable approach to ensure that the manufactured medicine complies with the pharmacopoeial specification is to ensure that the raw materials are of good quality and that the manufacturing procedures conform to the standards laid down in the *Rules and Guidance for Pharmaceutical Manufacturers and Distributors (1997)*.

Implicit in these standards is the principle that the extent of product contamination originating from the manufacturing environment and production personnel should be subject to regular monitoring and control.

Environmental monitoring

Environmental monitoring is normally taken to mean regular monitoring of the levels of microbial contamination of the atmosphere, of solid surfaces and, less frequently, of the personnel in the production areas. Water used to clean floors, benches and equipment (as distinct from water incorporated in the product) may be considered as part of environmental monitoring, but will not be considered here as the procedures for counting microorganisms in water are described below.

Atmospheric monitoring is most commonly undertaken by means of settle plates, which are simply Petri dishes containing media suitable for the growth of bacteria and/or yeasts and moulds, e.g. tryptone soya agar, which are exposed to the atmosphere for periods of, typically, 1–4 hours. Microorganisms in the air may exist as single cells, e.g. mould spores, but more commonly they are attached to dust particles, so that any organisms in the latter category (for which the culture medium is suitable) will grow into visible colonies during incubation after dust particles have settled on the agar surface. The colony counts recorded on the plates are obviously influenced by:

· the duration of exposure;
· the degree of air turbulence, which determines the volume of air passing over the plate;

Table 40.3 European Pharmacopoeia (2000) specifications for the microbiological quality of pharmaceutical products*		
Product Category	Quantitative specification	Organisms which must be absent
Topical and non-sterile respiratory products	• Not more than 10^2 aerobic bacteria and fungi per g or mL • Not more than 10^1 enterobacteria and certain other Gram-negative bacteria per g or mL	• *Pseudomonas aeruginosa* • *Staphylococcus aureus*
Oral and rectal products	• Not more than 10^3 aerobic bacteria per g or mL • Not more than 10^2 fungi per g or mL	• *Escherichia coli*
Oral products containing raw materials of natural origin for which antimicrobial pretreatment is not feasible	• Not more than 10^4 aerobic bacteria and not more than 10^2 fungi per g or mL • Not more than 10^2 enterobacteria and certain other Gram-negative bacteria per g or mL	• *Salmonella* • *Escherichia coli* • *Staphylococcus aureus*
Herbal remedies made with boiling water	• Not more than 10^7 aerobic bacteria and not more than 10^5 fungi per g or mL • Not more than 10^2 *Escherichia coli* per g or mL	
Other herbal remedies	• Not more than 10^5 aerobic bacteria and not more than 10^4 fungi per g or mL • Not more than 10^3 enterobacteria and certain other Gram-negative bacteria per g or mL	• *Escherichia coli* • *Salmonella*

* Excluding transdermal patches.

• the intrinsic level of atmospheric contamination (microorganisms per litre of air), which in turn is often a reflection of the number and activity level of the operating personnel, as skin scales shed by the operators are usually the most potent source of atmospheric contaminants.

The disadvantage of settle plates is that it is not possible to relate colony counts directly to air volume. This limitation is overcome in active sampling methods, whereby a known volume of air is drawn over, or caused to impact upon, the agar surface. These methods and the equipment available for active sampling have been reviewed recently by Baird (2000).

Surface and equipment sampling is most frequently undertaken by swabbing or the use of contact plates (also known as RODAC – replicate organism detection and counting – plates). Swabbing a known area of bench, floor or equipment with a culture medium-soaked swab is convenient for irregular surfaces. The organisms on the swab may be counted after they have been dispersed, by agitation, into a fixed volume of suspending medium, but it is not easy to quantify either the proportion of total organisms removed from the swabbed surface or the proportion dispersed in the diluent. This second limitation is overcome using contact plates, which are simply specially designed Petri dishes slightly overfilled with molten agar which, on setting,

presents a convex surface that projects above the rim of the plate. When the plate is inverted on to the surface to be sampled, microorganisms are transferred directly on to the agar.

Sampling of manufacturing personnel usually consists of sampling clothing, face masks or, more commonly, gloves. 'Finger dabs' is the phrase used to describe the process whereby an operator rolls the gloved surface of each finger over a suitable solid medium in a manner similar to that in which fingerprints are taken. Operator sampling by any means other than finger dabs is rare, particularly outside aseptic manufacturing areas.

Counting of microorganisms in pharmaceutical products

Most pharmaceutical raw materials are contaminated with microorganisms. The levels of contamination are often a reflection of the source of the raw material in question, with 'natural' products derived from vegetable or animal sources, or mined minerals such as kaolin and talc, being more heavily contaminated than synthetic materials whose microbial burden has been reduced by heat, extremes of pH or organic solvents during the course of manufacture. Determining the bioburden in these materials is often straightforward, utilizing without modification the viable counting procedures described in Chapter 41. Occasionally the physical nature of the raw material makes this difficult or impossible, and this is often found to be the case with the finished manufactured medicine, where problems of dispersibility, sedimentation or viscosity cause complications. As a consequence, modifications to the standard viable counting procedures are necessary to reduce errors. Some of modifications and the circumstances that necessitate them are considered below.

Very low concentrations of microorganisms in aqueous solutions   The reliability of calculated viable cell concentrations becomes much reduced when they are based upon colony counts much lower than about 10–15 per Petri dish. Using a surface-spread method it is rarely possible to place more than about 0.5 mL of liquid on to the agar surface in a standard Petri dish because it will not easily soak in. By a pour-plate method 1 mL or more may be used, but a point is reached where the volume of sample significantly dilutes the agar and nutrients. Thus using a conventional plating technique the lowest concentration conveniently detectable is of the order of 10–50 cells mL^{-1}. When the cell concentration is below this value it is necessary to pass a known quantity of the liquid – 10–100 mL or more – through a filter membrane having a pore size sufficiently small to retain bacteria. The membrane is then placed with the organisms uppermost on to the agar surface in a Petri dish, which is incubated without inversion. As a result of diffusion of nutrients through the membrane colonies grow on the surface in the normal way. Diffusion may be assisted by the inclusion of a medium-soaked pad between the membrane and the agar. It is important to ensure that all of the membrane is in contact with the pad or agar, otherwise elevated areas may become dry and no colonies will appear upon them.

Insoluble solids   It is necessary to suspend an insoluble solid in a medium that will permit uniform dispersion and adequate wetting of the suspended material. Nutrient broth, peptone water or a buffered salt solution are frequently used and a low concentration of a surfactant incorporated to promote wetting, e.g. polysorbate 80 (0.01–0.05%). Suspension in distilled water alone carries the risk of osmotic damage to sensitive cells, with a consequently low count; for this reason it is best avoided. Having obtained the suspension, there are two options available depending upon the nature and concentration of the suspended material.

The first is to remove a sample of the mixed suspension, dilute if necessary, and plate in or on a suitable medium using a pour- or spread-plate method. If the concentration of suspended material is low it may still be possible to see clearly the developing colonies. High concentrations may obscure the colonies and make counting impossible. The alternative is to dislodge the microbial cells from the solid to which they are attached, allow the solid to sediment out and then sample the supernatant. Methods of removal include vigorous manual shaking, use of a vortex mixer, or instruments designed for the purpose, e.g. the Colworth 'stomacher', in which the aqueous suspension is placed in a sealed sterile bag which is repeatedly agitated by reciprocating paddles. The use of ultrasonics to dislodge the cells carries the risk of damage to or lysis of the cells themselves.

Assuming the suspended material has no antimicrobial activity, plating the 'whole suspension' is probably the easiest and most reliable method. The alternative strategy of sampling the supernatant involves the assumption that all the cells have been removed from the solid, but this would have to be confirmed by control (validation) experiments in which a known quantity of similar organisms were artificially dried on to sterile samples of the material. The second method also relies upon the solid sedimenting sufficiently rapidly for it to be separated from the bacteria in aqueous suspension above. If all or part of the sample has a particle size similar to that of bacteria, yeasts or mould spores, i.e. approximately 1–5 μm, then a separation cannot easily be achieved.

Oils and hydrophobic ointments   These materials are usually not heavily contaminated because they are anhydrous and microorganisms will not multiply without water. Thus the microorganisms contained in oily products have usually arisen by contamination from the atmosphere, equipment used for manufacture, and from storage vessels. To perform a viable count the oil sample must be emulsified or solubilized without the aid of excessive heat or any other agent that might kill the cells.

An oil-in-water emulsion must be produced using a suitable surfactant; non-ionic emulsifiers generally have little antimicrobial activity. The proportion of surfactant to use must be determined experimentally and validation experiments conducted to confirm that the surfactant is not, itself, toxic to the species that typically arise as contaminants of the sample in question; Millar (2000) has described the use of up to 5.0 g of polysorbate-80 added to a 10.0 g sample. Such an emulsion may be diluted in water or buffered salts solution if necessary, and aliquots placed on or in the agar medium in the usual way. Alternatively, the oil may be dissolved in a sterile non-toxic solvent and passed through a membrane filter. Isopropyl myristate, for example, is recommended in pharmacopoeial sterility testing procedures as a solvent for anhydrous materials, but it may kill a significant fraction of the cells of some sensitive species, even during an exposure period of only a few minutes.

Creams and lotions   Oil-in-water emulsions do not usually represent a problem because they are miscible with water and thus easily diluted. Water-in-oil creams, however, are not miscible and cannot be plated directly because bacteria may remain trapped in a water droplet suspended in a layer of oil on the agar surface. Such bacteria are unlikely to form colonies because the diffusion of nutrients through the oil would be inadequate. These creams are best diluted, dispersed in an aqueous medium and membrane filtered, or converted to an oil-in-water type and then counted by normal plating methods.

Dilution and emulsification of the cream in broth containing Lubrol W, polysorbate-80 or Triton X 100 is probably the best procedure, although the addition of approximately 0.1 g of the w/o emulsion sample to 25 g of isopropyl myristate followed by membrane filtration may be satisfactory.

Detection of specific hazardous organisms

In addition to placing limits on the maximum concentration of microorganisms that is acceptable in different materials, pharmacopoeias usually specify certain organisms that must not be present at all. In practice, this means that detection methods which are described in the pharmacopoeia must be applied to a known weight of material (typically 1–50 g), and the sample passes the test if no organisms arise on the culture plates that conform to the standard textbook descriptions of those to be excluded. Typically the pharmacopoeial methods involve preliminary stages using selective liquid culture media; these are designed to increase the concentration of the organism that is the subject of the test ('target' organism) and so render it more readily detectable. There are, too, supplementary biochemical tests used to **confirm** the identity of any isolates having the typical appearance of the target organisms.

Both the EP (2000) and the USP (2000) describe detection tests for *Staphylococcus aureus*, *Pseudomonas aeruginosa*, *Escherichia coli* and salmonellae; in addition, the EP describes a test for clostridia, but this is unlikely to be applied to any material other than mined minerals, e.g. talc and bentonite. The four organisms common to both pharmacopoeias are the subject of these tests primarily because of their potential to cause infections, but they may also represent common contaminants of the products to which the tests are applied, or their presence may be indicative of the quality of the raw material or finished manufactured product. *E. coli*, for example, is a natural inhabitant of mammalian intestines and so its presence in a material such as gelatin (which originates in the slaughterhouse) would indicate unacceptable quality. The most likely source of *Staphylococcus aureus* in a manufactured medicine is the production personnel, so that if this origin were confirmed it would indicate the need for higher manufacturing standards. In general the tests are applied to pharmaceutical raw materials of 'natural' origin, e.g. carbohydrates, cellulose derivatives, gums and vegetable drugs. In addition, there is a requirement that topical products should be free of both *Pseudomonas aeruginosa* and *Staphylococcus aureus*. Table 40.4 summarises the EP (2000) testing schemes for the four principal organisms of interest. These schemes are described in more detail elsewhere, together with photographs of the typical appearance of the organisms in question (Hodges 2000).

Microbiological assays of B-group vitamins

Microbiological assays of B-group vitamins employ similar techniques to turbidimetric assays of antibiotics (see earlier in this chapter). A culture medium is used which is suitable for the assay organism, except for the omission of the vitamin in question. The extent of bacterial growth in the medium is thus directly proportional to the amount of reference standard or test vitamin added. It is important to select an assay organism that has an absolute requirement for the substance in question and is unable to obtain it by metabolism of other medium components; species of *Lactobacillus* are often used for this purpose. 'Carryover' of the vitamin with the inoculum culture must be avoided because this results in some growth even when none of the test material has been added. Growth may be determined turbidimetrically or by acid production from sugars.

Just as HPLC has become the favoured method of antibiotic assay, so too has it become the method of choice for assaying B-group vitamins. Turbidimetric assays *are* still used, however, for example when insurmountable problems arise in resolving the many peaks that might arise on an HPLC chromatogram from a multivitamin product (which might contain 10 or more active ingredients plus excipients, all of which may cause assay interference). Further details of vitamin assays are provided by Hewitt and Vincent (1989).

Table 40.4 Procedures recommended by the EP (2000) in tests for specified microorganisms

Medium	Organism				
	Escherichia coli	Salmonellae		*Pseudomonas aeruginosa*	*Staphylococcus aureus*
Liquid enrichment	MacConkey broth	Tetrathionate bile brilliant green broth		Casein soya bean digest broth (tryptone soya broth)	Casein soya bean digest broth (tryptone soya broth)
			Appearance		
Agar media (primary test)	MacConkey agar (appearance: pink colonies with precipitation of bile due to acid production)	Deoxycholate citrate agar, Xylose lysine deoxycholate (XLD) agar and Brilliant green agar	Yellow colonies with grey or black centre Red colonies with black centres Pink colonies	Growth on cetrimide agar	Baird-Parker agar (black colonies immediately surrounded by zones of opacity beyond which are zones of clearing)
Result(s) of secondary tests which confirm the presence of organism in question	Production of indole at 44°C	Reactions characteristic of *Salmonella* on triple sugar iron agar and other biochemical or serological tests	Black precipitate of iron sulphide Yellow (acid) butt (i.e. subsurface), with pink (alkaline) slope (i.e. surface)	Absence of growth at 41–43°C	Positive coagulase or deoxyribonuclease tests

Sterile products

Sterile products must, by definition, be free of microorganisms, and it is important to understand that this is an absolute requirement. Thus, the presence of one single surviving microbial cell is sufficient to render the product non-sterile; there is not a level of survivors which is so small as to be regarded as negligible and therefore acceptable.

The principal component of microbiological quality assurance which has traditionally been applied to sterile products is, of course, the test for sterility itself. In essence, this is quite simple: a sample of the material to be tested is added to culture medium which is incubated and then examined for signs of microbial growth. If growth occurs the assumption is made that the contamination arose from the sample, which consequently fails the test. However, the limitations of this simplistic approach became more widely recognized throughout the second half of the 20th century, and there was an increasing awareness of the fact that contaminated products could pass the test and sterile ones apparently fail it (because of contamination introduced during the testing procedure itself). For these reasons the sterility test alone could no longer be relied upon to provide an assurance of sterility, and that assurance is now derived from a strict adherence to high-quality standards throughout the manufacturing process. These encompass:

1. The adoption of the highest possible specifications for the microbiological quality of the raw materials. The rationale here is that sterilization processes are more likely to be effective when the levels of microorganisms to be killed or removed (bioburdens) are as low as possible to begin with. Procedures used to determine bioburdens are described in Chapter 39 and earlier in this chapter.

2. The rigorous application of environmental monitoring procedures (as described above) during the course of manufacture, with more stringent limits for acceptable levels of microorganisms than those applicable during the manufacture of non-sterile products.

3. Comprehensive validation procedures when sterilization processes are designed, together with regular in-process monitoring when those processes are in operation for product manufacture. Initial validation seeks to demonstrate that adequate sterilizing conditions are achieved throughout the load, and entails extensive testing with thermocouples, radiation dosimeters and biological indicators (see below) as appropriate.

The pharmacopoeias and regulatory authorities require a sterility assurance level for terminally sterilized products of 10^{-6} or better. This means that the probability of non-sterility in an item selected at random from a batch should be no more than 1 in 1 million. This sterility assurance level (SAL) may be demonstrated in the case of some terminally sterilized products simply by reference to data derived from bioburdens, environmental monitoring and in-process monitoring of the sterilization procedure itself. In this case the sterility test is unnecessary and omitted; the term 'parametric release' is used to describe the release of products for sale or use under these circumstances.

Sterilization monitoring

Sterilization processes may be monitored physically, chemically or biologically. Physical methods are exemplified by thermocouples, which are routinely incorporated at different locations within an auto-clave load, whereas chemical indicators usually exhibit a colour change after exposure to a heat sterilization process. Biological indicators consist of preparations of spores of the *Bacillus* species that exhibits the greatest degree of resistance to the sterilizing agent in question. The principle of their use is simply that if such spores are exposed to the sterilization process and fail to survive it can be assumed that all other common organisms will also have been killed and the process is safe. Spores of *Bacillus stearothermophilus* are used to monitor autoclaves and gaseous hydrogen peroxide or per-acetic acid sterilization processes, whereas *Bacillus subtilis* var *niger* is the organism normally employed for dry heat, ethylene oxide and low-temperature steam–formaldehyde methods; *Bacillus pumilus* is used in radiation sterilization procedures.

Such biological indicators are regularly employed for validation of a sterilization process which is under development for a new product, or when a new autoclave is being commissioned; they are less commonly used for routine monitoring during product manufacture. Spores possess the advantage that they are relatively easy to produce, purify and dry on to an inert carrier, which is frequently an absorbent paper strip or disc, or a plastic or metal support. Spore resistance to the sterilizing agent must be carefully controlled, and so rigorous standardization of production processes followed by observance of correct storage conditions and expiry dates is essential.

Tests for sterility

It is sufficient here to repeat that the test is really one of the absence of gross contamination with readily grown microorganisms, and is not capable of affording a guarantee of sterility in any sample that passes.

The experimental details of these procedures are described in the European Pharmacopoeia (2000). This section is therefore restricted to an account of the major features of the test and a more detailed consideration of those practical aspects that are important or problematical.

It is obviously important that materials to be tested for sterility are not subject to contamination from the operator or the environment during the course of the test. For this reason it is essential that sterility tests are conducted in adequate laboratory facilities by competent and experienced personnel. Clearly, the consequences of recording an incorrect sterility result may be very severe. If a material which was *really* sterile were to fail the test it would need to be resterilized or, more probably, discarded, with significant cost implications. If, on the other hand, a contaminated batch were to pass a test for sterility and be released for use this would obviously represent a significant health hazard. For these reasons sterility testing procedures have improved significantly in recent years and failures are now viewed very seriously by the regulatory authorities. If a product does fail, it means either that the item in question was *really* contaminated, in which case the manufacturing procedures are seriously inadequate, or it means that the item was in fact sterile but the testing procedure was at fault. Either way, it is not possible to dismiss a failure lightly.

Sterility tests may be conducted in clean rooms or laminar flow cabinets which provide a grade A atmosphere as defined by the *Rules and Guidance for Pharmaceutical Manufacturers and Distributors* (1997). However, it is becoming increasingly common for testing to be undertaken in an isolator, which physically separates the operator from the test materials and so reduces the incidence of false positive test results due to extraneous contamination introduced during the test itself. Such isolators are similar in principle to a glove box, and typically consist of a cabinet (supported on legs or a frame) which is sufficiently large for the operator, who is covered by a transparent hood of moulded flexible plastic forming the cabinet base, to sit or stand within it.

A sterility test may be conducted in two ways. The direct inoculation method involves the removal of samples from the product under test and their transfer to a range of culture media that might be expected to support the growth of contaminating organisms. After incubation the media are examined for evidence of growth which, if present, is taken to indicate that the product may not be sterile. It is not certain that the product is contaminated because the organisms responsible for the growth may have arisen from the operator or have been already present in the media to which the samples were transferred, i.e. the media used for the test were not themselves sterile. Thus, in conducting a sterility test it is necessary to include controls that indicate the likelihood of the contaminants arising from these sources. The size and number of the samples to be taken are described in the EP (2000).

Again it is necessary to inactivate any antimicrobial substances contained in the sample. These may be the active drug, e.g. antibiotic, or a preservative in an eye drop or multidose injection. Suitable in activators may be added to the liquid test media to neutralize any antimicrobial substances, but in the case of antibiotics particularly, no such specific inactivators are available (with the exception of β-lactamases which hydrolyse penicillins and cephalosporins). This problem may be overcome using a membrane filtration technique. This alternative method of conducting sterility tests is obviously only applicable to aqueous or oily solutions that will pass through a membrane having a pore size sufficiently small to retain bacteria. The membrane, and hence the bacteria retained on it, is washed with isotonic salts solution, which should remove any last traces of antimicrobial substances. It is then placed in a suitable liquid culture medium. This method is certainly to be preferred to direct inoculation because there is a greater chance of effective neutralization of antimicrobial substances.

Solids may be dissolved in an appropriate solvent; almost invariably water is used because most other common solvents have antimicrobial activity. If no suitable solvent can be found the broth dilution method is the only one available. If there is no specific inactivator available for antimicrobial substances that may be present in the solid then their dilution to an ineffective concentration by use of a large volume of medium is the only course remaining.

The controls associated with a sterility test are particularly important because incomplete control of the test may lead to erroneous results. Failure to neutralize a preservative completely may lead to contaminants in the batch going undetected and subsequently initiating an infection when the product is introduced into the body.

The EP (2000) recommends four controls be incorporated. The so-called growth promotion test simply involves the addition of low inocula (10–100 cells or spores per container) of suitable test organisms into the media used in the test to show that they do support the growth of the common contaminants for which they are intended. *Staphylococcus aureus,* *Bacillus subtilis* and *Pseudomonas aeruginosa* are the three aerobic bacteria used, *Clostridium sporogenes* the anaerobic bacterium and *Candida albicans* and *Aspergillus niger* the fungi. Organisms having particular nutritional requirements, such as blood, milk or serum, are not included; therefore they, in addition to the more obvious omissions such as viruses, may not be detected in a routine sterility test because suitable cultural conditions are not provided. On the other hand, it is impossible to design an all-purpose medium, and sterilization processes that kill the spore-forming bacteria and other common contaminants are likely also to eradicate the more fastidious pathogens such as streptococci and *Haemophilus* species, which would be more readily detected on blood-containing media. This argument does not, however, cover the possibility of such pathogens entering the product, perhaps via defective seals or packaging, after the sterilization process itself and then going undetected in the sterility test.

The second control (validation test) is intended to demonstrate that any preservative or antimicrobial substance has been effectively neutralized. This requires the addition of test organisms to containers of the various media as before, but in addition, samples of the material under test must also be added to give the same concentrations as those arising in the test itself. For the sterility test as a whole to be valid growth must occur in each of the containers in these controls.

It is necessary also to incubate several tubes of the various media just as they are received by the operator. If the tubes are not opened but show signs of growth after incubation this is a clear indication that the medium is, itself, contaminated. This should be an extremely rare occurrence, but in view of the small additional cost or effort the inclusion of such a control is worthwhile.

A control to check the likelihood of contamination being introduced during the test may be included in the programme of regular monitoring of test facilities. The European Pharmacopoeia 2000 recommends the use of 'preparations known to be sterile', which may be employed to check the adequacy of facilities and operator technique. These items, identical to the sample to be tested, are manipulated in exactly the same way as the test samples. If, after incubation, there are signs of microbial growth in the media containing these 'known steriles', the conclusion is drawn that the contamination arose during the testing process itself.

Some items present particular difficulties in sterility testing because of their shape or size, e.g. surgical dressings and medical devices. These problems are most conveniently overcome simply by testing the whole sample rather than attempting to withdraw a portion of it. So, for example, large clear plastic bags which have been radiation sterilized may be used to hold the entire medical device or complete roll or pack of dressings, which would then be totally immersed in culture medium. This method would only be valid if the culture medium gained access to the entire sample; otherwise the possibility exists, for example, of aerobic bacterial spores trapped within it failing to grow owing to insufficient diffusion of oxygen. This approach has the advantage of imposing a more rigorous test because a much larger sample is used. In the case of dressings, it may also reduce the risk of operator-induced contamination compared to the alternative approach, which would require the withdrawal of representative samples for testing from different areas of the roll or pack.

The final aspect of the test which is worthy of comment is the interpretation of results. If there is evidence that any of the test samples is contaminated the batch fails the test. If, however, there is convincing evidence that the test was invalid because the testing facility, procedure or media were inadequate, a single retest is permitted; this contrasts with earlier pharmacopoeial protocols, which under certain circumstances permitted two retests.

Endotoxin and pyrogen testing

This is an aspect of microbial contamination of medicines which is not normally considered part of microbiology but is discussed here because pyrogens are normally the products of microbial growth. A pyrogen is a material which when injected into a patient will cause a rise in body temperature (pyrexia). The lipopolysaccharides that comprise a major part of the cell wall of Gram-negative bacteria are called endotoxins, and it is these that are the most commonly encountered pyrogens (although any other substance that causes a rise in body temperature may be classified under the same heading). Bacterial cells may be pyrogenic even when they are dead and when they are fragmented, and so a solution or material that passes a test for sterility will not necessarily pass a pyrogen test. It follows from this that the more heavily contaminated with bacteria an aqueous injection becomes during manufacture, the more pyrogenic it is likely to be at the end of the process.

Two main procedures are used for the detection of pyrogens. The traditional method requires the administration of the sample to laboratory rabbits, whose body temperature is monitored for a period of time thereafter. The alternative procedure, which is now by far the most common, is to use the Limulus Amoebocyte Lysate Test (LAL), in which the pyrogen-containing sample causes gel formation in the lysis product of amoebocyte cells of the giant horseshoe crab *Limulus polyphemus*. A detailed account of endotoxin testing is outside the scope of this chapter but the review by Weary (1996) describes both LAL and rabbit testing.

REFERENCES

AOAC (Association of Official Analytical Chemists) (1990) Disinfectants. In: *Official Methods of Analysis*. AOAC Inc. Arlington. Ch 6, 133–146.

Baird, R.M. (2000) Sampling. In: Baird R M, Hodges N A, Denyer S.P. *Handbook of Microbiological Quality Assurance*. Taylor & Francis, London, 22–37.

BS EN 1276 (1997) Quantitative suspension test for the evaluation of bactericidal activity of chemical disinfectants and antiseptics used in food, industrial, domestic and institutional areas. British Standards Institute, London.

European Pharmacopoeia (2000) 3rd edn. Council of Europe, Strasbourg, pp. 259–260.

Hewitt, W., Vincent, S. (1989) *Theory and Application of Microbiological Assay*, Academic Press, London.

Hodges, N.A. (2000) Pharmacopoeial methods for the detection of specified microorganisms In: Baird, R.M., Hodges, N.A., Denyer, S.P. *Handbook of Microbiological Quality Assurance*. Taylor & Francis, London, 86–106.

Hodges, N.A. (1999) Assessment of preservative activity during stability studies. In: Mazzo D J (ed) *International Stability Testing*. Interpharm Press, Buffalo Grove, US 161–192.

Millar, R. (2000) Enumeration In: Baird, R.M., Hodges, N.A., Denyer, S.P. *Handbook of Microbiological Quality Assurance*. Taylor & Francis, London, 54–68.

Murtough, S.M., Hiom, S.J., Palmer, M., Russell, A.D. (2000) A survey of disinfectant use in hospital pharmacy aseptic preparation areas. *Pharm. J.* **264**, 446–448.

Reybrouck, G. (1999) Evaluation of the antibacterial and antifungal activity of disinfectants. In: Russell, A.D., Hugo, W.B. and Ayliffe, G.A.J. (eds) *Principles and Practice of Disinfection, Preservation and Sterilization*, 3rd edn. Blackwell Science, Oxford, 124–144.

Rules and Guidance for Pharmaceutical Manufacturers and Distributors (1997) HMSO, London.

Russell, A.D. (1981) Neutralization procedures in the evaluation of bacterial activity. In: Collins, C.H., Allwood, M.C., Bloomfield, S.F., Fox, A. (eds) *Disinfectants: their use and Evaluation of Effectiveness*. Society for Applied Bacteriology, Technical Series No. 16, Academic Press, London.

United States Pharmacopoeia (2000) 24th edn. US Pharmacopoeial Convention Inc. 2000 Rockville, US 1809–1811.

Wardlaw, A.C. (1999) *Practical Statistics for Experimental Biologists*, 2nd edn. Wiley, Chichester.

Weary (1996) Pyrogens and pyrogen testing In: Swarbrick, J., Boylan, J.C. *Encyclopedia of Pharmaceutical Technology*, Vol 13. Marcel Dekker, New York, 179–206.

BIBLIOGRAPHY

Freshney, R.I. (1994) *Culture of Animal Cells: a Manual of Basic Technique*. Wiley-Liss, New York.

Glazer, A.N., Nikaido, H. (1995) *Microbial Biotechnology*. Freeman, New York.

41

The action of physical and chemical agents on microorganisms

Geoff Hanlon, Norman Hodges

The subject of this chapter is of importance to pharmaceutical scientists because they have a responsibility for:

1. the production of medicines having as their prime function the destruction of microorganisms, e.g. antiseptic liquids and antibiotic formulations;
2. the production of sterile medicaments having no living microorganisms, e.g. injections and eye drops;
3. the production of a wide range of medicines which must be effectively protected against microbial spoilage.

Thus the major pharmaceutical interest in microorganisms is that of killing them, or at least preventing their growth. Consequently it is necessary to have both an understanding of the physical processes, e.g. heating and irradiation, that are used to kill microorganisms and a knowledge of the more diverse subject of antimicrobial chemicals.

This background knowledge must therefore include an understanding of the kinetics of cell inactivation, the calculation of parameters by which microbial destruction or growth inhibition are measured, and an appreciation of the factors that influence the efficiency of the physical and chemical processes used. These aspects, together with a synopsis of the major groups of antimicrobial chemicals, are the subject of this chapter.

THE KINETICS OF CELL INACTIVATION

The death of a population of cells exposed to heat or radiation is often found to follow or approximate to first-order kinetics. In this sense it is similar to bacterial growth during the logarithmic phase of the cycle, the graphs representing these processes being similar but of opposite slope. Assuming first-order kinetics (the exceptions will be considered later), an initial population of N_o cells per mL will, after a time t minutes, be reduced to N_t cells per mL, according to the following equations in which k is the inactivation rate constant;

$$N_t = N_o\, e^{-kt} \qquad (41.1)$$

$$\ln N_t = \ln N_o - kt \qquad (41.2)$$

$$\log_{10} N_t = \log_{10} N_o \frac{-kt}{2.303} \qquad (41.3)$$

Thus the data in Table 41.1 may be used to produce a plot of logarithm of cell concentration against exposure time (Fig. 41.1), where the intercept is log N_o and the slope is $-k/2.303$. This may be plotted with the logarithm of the percentage of survivors as the ordinate; thus the largest numerical value on this axis is 2.0. An important feature of Figure 41.1 is the fact that there is no lower end-point to the ordinate scale – it continues indefinitely. If the initial population was 1000 cells mL^{-1} the logarithmic value would be 3.0; at 100 cells mL^{-1} the value would be 2.0; at 10 cells mL^{-1} 1.0, and at 1 cell mL^{-1} zero. The next incremental point on the logarithmic scale would be -1, which corresponds to

0.1 cells mL^{-1}. It is clearly nonsense to talk of a fraction of a viable cell per mL, but this value corresponds to one whole cell in 10 mL of liquid. The next point, -2.0, corresponds to one cell in 100 mL, and so on. Sterility is the complete absence of life, i.e. zero cells mL^{-1}, which has a log value of $-\infty$. **Guaranteed** sterility would therefore require an infinite exposure time.

D value, or decimal reduction time

It is characteristic of first-order kinetics that the same percentage change in concentration occurs in successive time intervals. Thus in Figure 41.1 it can be seen that the viable population falls to 10% of its initial value after 7.5 minutes; in the next 7.5-minute period the population again falls to 10% of its value at the start of that period. This time period for a 90% reduction in count is related to the slope of the line and is one of the more useful parameters by which the death rate may be indicated. It is known as the decimal reduction time, or D value, and usually has a subscript showing the temperature at which it was measured, e.g. D_{121} or D_{134}. It is quite possible to indicate the rate of destruction by the inactivation rate constant calculated from the slope of the line, but the significance of this value cannot be as readily appreciated during conversation as that of a D value, and so the former is rarely used.

Z values

When designing steam sterilization processes it is necessary to know both the D value, which is a measure of the effectiveness of heat at any given temperature, and the extent to which a particular increase in temperature will reduce the D value, i.e. it is necessary to have a measure of the effect of temperature change on death rate. One such measure is the Z value, which is defined as the number of degrees temperature change required to achieve a tenfold change in D value, e.g. if the D value for *Bacillus stearothermophilus* spores at 110°C is 20 minutes and they have a Z value of 9°C, this means that at 119°C the D value would be 2.0 minutes and at 128°C the D value would be 0.20 minutes. The relationship between D and Z values is shown in Figure 41.2. The Z value is one of several parameters that relate change in temperature to change in death rate, and is probably the most commonly used and readily understood. The activation energy obtained from an Arrhenius plot (see Chapter 7) or a temperature coefficient, a Q_{10} value (change in rate for a 10°C change in temperature), does the same but is less commonly used.

Table 41.1 Death of *B. megaterium* spores in pH 7.0 buffer at 95°C			
Time (minutes)	Viable cell concentration mL^{-1}	Percent survivors	Log$_{10}$ % survivors
0	2.50×10^6	100	2.000
5	5.20×10^5	20.8	1.318
10	1.23×10^5	4.92	0.692
15	1.95×10^4	0.78	-0.108
20	4.60×10^3	0.18	-0.745
25	1.21×10^3	0.048	-1.319
30	1.68×10^2	0.0067	-2.174

Fig. 41.1 Heat inactivation of *B. megaterium* spores at 95 °C.

Fig. 41.2 Relationship between logarithm of *D* value and exposure temperature for heated *B. megaterium* spores. Individual *D* values (minutes) are shown in parentheses.

Alternative survivor plots

It was stated earlier that bacterial death often approximates to first-order kinetics, although exceptions do arise. Some of the more common are illustrated in Figure 41.3. The plot labelled A is that conforming to first-order kinetics, which has already been described. A shoulder on the curve, as in case B, is not uncommon and various explanations have been offered. Cell aggregation or clumping may be responsible for such a shoulder, because it would be necessary to apply sufficient heat to kill all of the cells in the clump, not merely the most sensitive, before a fall is observed in the number of colonies

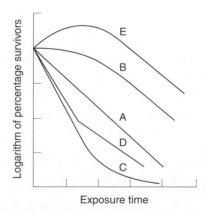

Fig. 41.3 Alternative survivor plots for cells exposed to lethal agents.

appearing on the agar. Under normal circumstances one single colony could arise both from one cell alone or, say, from 100 cells aggregated together. In the latter case, if sufficient heat was applied to kill only the 99 most sensitive cells in the clump the colony count would be unaltered. Clumping is not the only explanation, because substantial shoulders may arise using suspensions where the vast majority of cells exist individually.

Tailing of survivor curves, as in plot C, is often observed if the initial cell concentration is high. This has been attributed to the presence of mutants that are exceptionally resistant to the lethal agent. If the proportion of mutants was 1 in 10^6 cells and the initial concentration only 10^5 cells mL^{-1} the mutant would not be detected, but an initial population of 10^9 cells mL^{-1} would permit easy detection if the inactivation plot were continued down to low levels of survivors. Again there are alternative explanations, one of the most common being that the cells dying during the early exposure period release chemicals which help to protect those that are still alive.

A sharp break in the line, as in D, usually indicates that there are two distinct populations of cells present which have markedly different resistances. Contamination of a cell suspension or culture is a possible explanation, or it may be that a mutant has arisen naturally and the cultural conditions are such that it has a selective advantage and its numbers have increased until it is a substantial proportion of the population.

Plot E is uncommon and is usually only seen as a result of 'heat activation' of bacterial spores. This is a situation in which a significant proportion of a population of spores (usually a thermophil) remain dormant and fail to germinate and produce colonies under 'normal' conditions. If the suspension receives a heat stimulus or shock which is insufficient to kill the spores, some or all of those that would otherwise remain dormant become activated, germinate, and thus produce a rise in the colony count.

Killing of microorganisms by chemicals results in first-order kinetics less commonly than heat- or radiation-induced killing. This is because the chemical must interact with a target molecule within the cell, and the concentration of both the chemical and the intracellular target might influence death rate and so result in second-order kinetics. In practice, however, the antimicrobial chemical is often present in such a high concentration that the proportion of it that is 'used up' by interaction with the cell is negligible; this means its concentration is effectively constant, and pseudo-first order kinetics result.

ANTIMICROBIAL EFFECTS OF MOIST AND DRY HEAT

Moist heat (steam) and dry heat (hot air) both have the potential to kill microorganisms but their efficiencies and their mechanisms of action differ. In autoclaves dry, saturated steam, i.e. 100% water vapour with no liquid water present, is used at temperatures between 121 and 135°C, at which it rapidly kills microorganisms. An advantage of using steam is that it possesses latent heat of vaporization, which it transfers to any object upon which it condenses (see Chapter 38). It is essential to use dry saturated steam if maximal autoclaving efficiency is to be achieved. If the steam is wet, i.e. contains liquid water, penetration of vapour-phase steam into dressings may be retarded. If the steam is superheated, i.e. its temperature has been raised while the pressure remained constant, or the pressure fell while the temperature remained constant, it contains less moisture and latent heat than dry saturated steam at the same temperature. In this case the effect is similar to using a steam–air mixture at that temperature. The process by which steam kills cells is hydrolysis of essential proteins (enzymes) and nucleic acids. In contrast, dry heat causes cell death by oxidative processes, although again it is the proteins and nucleic acids that are the vulnerable targets. Dry heat is much less effective at killing microorganisms than steam at the same temperature. Exposures of not less than 2 hours at 160°C (or an equivalent temperature/time combination) are recommended in the BP for sterilization by dry heat methods. The state of hydration of a cell is thus an important factor determining its resistance to heat.

Resistance of microorganisms to moist and dry heat

Numerous factors influence the observed heat resistance of microbial cells and it is difficult to make comparisons between populations unless these factors are controlled. Not surprisingly, marked differences in resistance exist between different genera, species and strains, and between the spore and vegetative cell forms of the same organism. The resistance may be influenced, sometimes extensively, by the age of the cell, i.e. lag, exponential or stationary phase; its chemical composition, which in turn is influenced by the medium in which the cell is grown; and by the composition and pH of the fluid in which the cell is heated. It is difficult to obtain strictly comparable heat resistance data for grossly dissimilar organisms, but the values quoted in Table 41.2 indicate the relative order of heat resistance of the

Table 41.2   A 'league table' of heat resistances of different microorganisms and infectious agents

Organism or agent	Heat resistance (values are for fully hydrated organisms unless otherwise stated)
Prions	The most heat-resistant infectious agent. May survive steam sterilization at 134–138°C for 1 hour
Bacterial spores (endospores)	Little or no inactivation at <80°C. Some species survive boiling for several hours
Fungal spores	Ascospores of *Byssochlamys* species may survive 88°C for 60 minutes but most fungal spores are less resistant
Actinomycete spores	Spores of *Nocardia sebivorans* reported to survive for 10 minutes at 90°C, but the majority of species are less resistant
Mycobacterium tuberculosis	May survive for 30 minutes at 100°C in the dry state but when hydrated is killed by pasteurization (63°C for 30 minutes or 72°C for 15 seconds)
Yeasts	Ascospores and vegetative cells show little difference in resistance. Survival for 20 minutes at 60°C is typical
Most non-sporing bacteria of pharmaceutical or medical importance	D_{60} of 1–5 minutes is typical of staphylococci and many Gram-negative enteric organisms. Enterococci may be more resistant, and pneumococci may survive for 30 minutes at 110°C when dry
Fungi and actinomycetes	Vegetative mycelia exhibit similar resistance to that of non-sporing bacteria described above
Viruses	Rarely survive for > 30 minutes at 55–60°C except perhaps in blood or tissues, but papovaviruses and hepatitis viruses are more resistant
Protozoa and algae	Most are no more resistant than mammalian cells and survive only a few hours at 40–45°C, but cysts of *Acanthamoeba* species are more resistant

various microbial groups. Tabulation of D values at a designated temperature is perhaps the most convenient way of comparing resistance, but this is only suitable for first-order kinetics. Alternative methods of comparison include the time to achieve a particular percentage kill or the time required to achieve no survivors; the latter is, of course, dependent upon the initial population level.

The most heat-resistant infectious agents (as distinct from microbial cells) are prions, which are proteins rather than living cells and the cause of spongiform encephalopathies e.g. Creutzfeldt–Jakob disease (CJD) and bovine spongiform encephalopathy (BSE, or 'mad cow disease'). Prion proteins are so resistant to heat inactivation that an autoclave cycle of 134–138°C has been recommended for the decontamination of prion-contaminated materials, and the efficacy of even this extreme heat treatment has been questioned.

Bacterial endospores are invariably found to be the most heat resistant *cell* type, and those of certain species may survive boiling water for many hours. (The term endospores refers to the spores produced by *Bacillus* and *Clostridium* species and is not to be confused with the spores produced by other bacteria, such as actinomycetes, which do not develop within the vegetative cell.) The majority of *Bacillus* and *Clostridium* species normally form spores which survive in water for 15–30 minutes at 80°C without significant damage or loss of viability. Because endospores are more resistant than other cells they have been the subject of a considerable amount of research in the food and pharmaceutical industry over the last 50 years, and much of the earlier work has been reviewed by Russell (1999).

Mould spores and those of yeasts and actinomycetes usually exhibit a degree of moist heat resistance intermediate between endospores and vegetative cell forms; survival at 60°C for several hours but death at 80°C or higher would be typical of such cells. Bacterial and yeast vegetative cells and mould mycelia all vary significantly in heat resistance: mycobacteria, which possess a high proportion of lipid in their cell wall, tend to be more resistant than others. Protozoa and algae are, by comparison, susceptible to heat and, when in the vegetative (uncysted) state, like mammalian cells they rapidly die at temperatures much in excess of 40°C. Information on the heat resistance of viruses is limited, but the available data suggest that they may vary significantly between types. The majority of viruses are no more heat resistant than vegetative bacteria, but hepatitis viruses have been reported to be less susceptible than others.

Resistance to dry heat by different groups of infectious agents and microorganisms usually follows a pattern similar to that in aqueous environments. Again, prions head the 'league table' by exhibiting extreme heat resistance, and endospores are substantially more resilient than other cell types, with those of *B. stearothermophilus* and *B. subtilis* usually more resistant than other species. Exposures of 2 hours at 160°C are required by the European Pharmacopoeia (1997) to achieve an acceptable level of sterility assurance for materials sterilized by dry heat.

Cells of pneumococci have been reported to survive dry heat at 110°C for 30 minutes, but this represents exceptional resistance for vegetative cells, most of which may be expected to die after a few minutes, heating at 100°C or less.

Valid comparisons of dry heat resistance among dissimilar organisms are even less common than those for aqueous environments because there is the additional problem of distinguishing the effects of drying from those of heat. For many cells desiccation is itself a potentially lethal process, even at room temperature, so that experiments in which the moisture content of the cells is uncontrolled may produce results that are misleading or difficult to interpret. This is particularly so when the cells are heated under conditions where their moisture content is changing and they become progressively drier during the experiment.

Factors affecting heat resistance and its measurement

The major factors affecting heat resistance are listed in the previous section and will be considered in some detail here. The subject has been extensively studied, and again many of the experimental data and consequently many of the examples quoted in this section come from the field of spore research.

The measurement of heat resistance in fully hydrated cells, i.e. those suspended in aqueous solutions or exposed to dry saturated steam, does not normally represent a problem when conducted at temperatures less than 100°C, but errors may occasionally arise when spore heat resistance is measured at higher temperatures. In these circumstances it is necessary to heat suspensions sealed in glass ampoules immersed in glycerol or oil baths or to expose the spores to steam in a modified autoclave. Monitoring and control of heat-up and cool-down times become important, and failure to pay adequate attention to these aspects may lead to apparent differences in resistance, which may be due simply to factors such as variations in the thickness of glass in two batches of ampoules.

Species and strain differences

Variations in heat resistance between the species within a genus are very common, although it is difficult to identify from the published reports the precise magnitude of these differences because different species may require different growth media and incubation conditions which, together with other factors, might influence the results. Murrell and Warth (1965), for example, described a 700-fold variation in spore heat resistance within 13 *Bacillus* species, but to produce the spore crops for testing they necessarily had to use eight culture media, three incubation temperatures and six procedures for cleaning the spores. Differences between strains of a single species are, not surprisingly, more limited; D_{90} values ranging from 4.5 to 120 minutes have been reported for five strains of *Clostridium perfringens* spores.

Cell form

Whether or not the heated cells exist in the vegetative or the spore form may in some cases be related to the age of the culture or the cell population being heated. In cultures of *Bacillus* and *Clostridium* species the proportion of spores usually increases as the incubation period is extended and the culture ages. This may be due to more and more of the vegetative cells producing spores, in which case the spore count increases. Alternatively, the spore count may remain unchanged but the vegetative cell count falls as a result of the action of lytic enzymes produced by the cells themselves. Among the common mesophilic *Bacillus* species spore formation is largely complete 6–10 hours after the end of exponential growth under optimal cultural conditions. The degree of heat resistance and the concentration of spores would not be expected to rise much after this time. Conducting heat-resistance studies on a mixture of spores and vegetative cells is undesirable because the likely result is a rapid initial fall in count due to killing of the vegetative cells, and a subsequent slower rate due to death of spores. If necessary the vegetative cells can usually be removed by addition of the enzymes lysozyme and trypsin.

The degree of heat resistance shown by vegetative cells may also be influenced by the stage of growth from which the cells were taken. It is normally found that stationary-phase cells are more heat resistant than those taken from the logarithmic phase of growth, although several exceptions have been reported.

Cultural conditions

The conditions under which the cells are grown is another factor that can markedly affect heat resistance. Insufficient attention has been paid to this potential source of variation in a substantial part of the research conducted during the first half of the 20th century, and the same criticism might even be made of some of that reported more recently. Not infrequently, insufficient details of the cultivation procedures are described in the scientific reports, or materials of variable composition, e.g. tap water or soil extracts, were used in media without regard to the possible differences that might have arisen between successive batches or populations of cells.

Factors such as growth temperature, medium pH and buffering capacity, oxygen availability and concentrations of culture medium components may all affect resistance.

Thermophilic organisms are generally more heat resistant than mesophils, which in turn tend to be more resistant than psychrophils. If a 'league table' of spore heat resistance were constructed it is probable that *B. stearothermophilus*, *B. coagulans* and *Cl. thermosaccharolyticum* would head the list; all three have growth optima of 50–60°C. Variable results have arisen when single species have been grown at a variety of temperatures. *Escherichia coli* and *Streptococcus faecalis* have both been the subject of conflicting reports on the influence of growth temperature on heat resistance, whereas spores of *B. cereus* produced at temperatures between 20 and 41°C showed maximal resistance at 30°C.

The effects of medium pH, buffering capacity, oxygen availability and the concentrations of culture medium components are often complex and interrelated. An unsuitable pH, inadequate buffer or insufficient aeration may all limit the extent of growth, with the result that the cells that do grow each have available to them a higher concentration of nutrients than would be the case if a higher cell density had been achieved. The levels of intracellular storage materials and metal ions may therefore differ and so influence resistance to heat and other lethal agents. Cells existing in or recently isolated from their 'natural' environment, e.g. water, soil, dust or pharmaceutical raw materials, have often been reported to have a greater heat resistance than their progeny, which have been repeatedly subcultured in the laboratory and then tested under similar conditions.

pH and composition of heating menstruum

It is frequently found that cells survive heating more readily when they are at neutrality (or their optimum pH for growth, if this differs from neutrality). The combination of heat and an unfavourable pH may be additive or even synergistic in killing effects; thus

B. stearothermophilus spores survive better at 110°C in dilute pH 7.0 phosphate buffer than at 85°C in pH 4.0 acetate buffer. Differences in heat resistance may also result merely from the presence of the buffer, regardless of the pH it confers. Usually an apparent increase in resistance occurs when cells are heated in buffer rather than in water alone. A similar increase is often found to occur on the addition of other dissolved or suspended solids, particularly those of a colloidal or proteinaceous nature, e.g. milk, nutrient broth, serum. Because dissolved solids can have such a marked effect on heat resistance, great care must be taken in attempting to use experimental data from simple solutions to predict the likely heat treatment required to kill the same cells in a complex formulated medicine or food material. An extreme case of protection of cells from a lethal agent is the occlusion of cells within crystals. When spores of *B. subtilis* var. *niger* were occluded within crystals of calcium carbonate their resistances to inactivation were approximately 900 times and 9 times higher than for unoccluded spores when subjected to steam and dry heat, respectively; an exposure period of 2.5 hours at 121°C (moist heat) was required to eliminate survivors within the crystals. It is to minimize the risk of such situations arising that there is a requirement in the *Guide to Good Manufacturing Practice* that medicines be prepared in clean conditions.

The solute concentrations normally encountered in dilute buffer solutions used as suspending media for heat-resistance experiments cause no significant reduction in the vapour pressure of the solution relative to that of pure water, i.e. they do not reduce the water activity, A_w, of the solution (which has a value of 1.0 for water). If high solute concentrations are used or the cells are heated in a 'semi-dry' state the A_w is significantly lower and the resistance is increased, e.g. a 1000-fold increase in D value has been reported for *B. megaterium* spores when the water activity was reduced from 1.0 to between 0.2 and 0.4.

Recovery of heat-treated cells

The recovery conditions available to cells after exposure to heat may influence the proportion of cells that produce colonies. A heat-damaged cell may require an incubation time longer than normal to achieve a colony of any given size, and the optimum incubation temperature may be several degrees lower. The composition of the medium may also affect the colony count, with nutritionally rich media giving a greater percentage survival than a 'standard' medium, whereas little or no difference can be detected between the two when unheated cells are used. Adsorbents such as charcoal and starch have been found to have beneficial effects in this context.

IONIZING RADIATIONS

Ionizing radiations can be divided into electromagnetic and particulate (corpuscular) types. Electromagnetic radiations include γ-rays and X-rays, whereas particulate radiation includes α and β particles, positrons and neutrons.

Particulate radiation

The nuclear disintegration of radioactive elements results in the production of charged particles. α particles are heavy and positively charged, being equivalent to the nuclei of helium atoms. They travel relatively slowly in air, and although they cause a great deal of ionization along their paths they have very little penetrating power, their range being just a few centimetres in air. α particles have no application in this aspect of pharmacy and will not be considered further. β particles are negatively charged and have the same mass as an electron. In air the penetrating power of these particles is a few metres, but they will be stopped by a thin sheet of aluminium. β particles resulting from radioactive decay are therefore not sufficiently penetrative for use in sterilization processes, but the production of accelerated electrons from man made machines (cathode rays) results in particles of great energy with enhanced penetrating power.

Electromagnetic radiation

γ radiation results when the nucleus still has too much energy even after the emission of α or β particles. This energy is dissipated in the form of very short wavelength radiation which, as it has no mass or charge, travels with the speed of light, penetrating even sheets of lead. Although travelling in a wave form γ radiation behaves as if composed of discrete packets of energy called quanta (photons). A ^{60}Co source emits γ-rays with photons of 1.17 and 1.33 MeV, and the source has a half-life of 5.2 years. X-rays are generated when a heavy metal target is bombarded with fast electrons, and they have similar properties to γ-rays despite originating from a shift in electron energy rather than from the nucleus.

Units of radioactivity

The unit of activity is the becquerel (Bq), which is equal to one nuclear transformation per second. This replaces the term curie (Ci), and 3.7×10^{10} becquerels = 1 curie. The unit of absorbed dose according to the SI system is the gray (Gy), which is equal to one joule per kilogram. However, the term rad is still widely used and is equivalent to 100 ergs per gram of irradiated material.

$$1 \text{ gray} = 100 \text{ rads}$$

The energy of radiation is measured in electron volts (eV) or millions of electron volts (MeV). An electron volt is the energy acquired by an electron falling through a potential difference of 1 volt.

Effect of ionizing radiations on materials

Ionizing radiations are absorbed by materials in a variety of ways, depending upon the energy of the incident photons.

1. *Photoelectric effect*: low-energy radiation (< 0.1 MeV) is absorbed by the atom of the material, resulting in the ejection or excitation of an electron.
2. *Compton effect*: incident photons of medium energy 'collide' with atoms and a portion of the energy is absorbed with the ejection of an electron. The remaining energy carries on impacting with further atoms and emitting further electrons until all the energy is scattered.
3. *Pair production*: radiations of very high energy are converted on impact into negatively charged electrons and positively charged particles called positrons. The positron has an extremely short life and quickly annihilates itself by colliding with an orbital electron.

The ionization caused by the primary radiation results in the formation of free radicals, excited atoms etc. along a discrete track through the material. However, if secondary electrons contain sufficient energy they may cause excitation and ionization of adjacent atoms, thereby effectively widening the track. (Accelerated electrons used in electron beam sterilizers are essentially equivalent to the secondary electrons arising from γ irradiation – they cause direct ionization of molecules within materials.) Temperature rise during irradiation is very small and even high-energy radiation resulting in pair production is only accompanied by an increase of approximately 2°C, but nevertheless the chemical changes that occur in irradiated materials are very widespread. Of particular significance here are the deleterious changes that may occur in packaging materials at normal dosage levels. Such effects may include changes in tensile strength, colour, odour and gas formation. Polymers most affected include acetal, FEP, PTFE and PVA. Total absorbed energy determines the extent of physical and chemical reactions that occur, and so damage is cumulative. For sterilization purposes exposure times can be long, but the process is predictable and delivers a reproducible level of lethality.

The lethal effect of irradiation on microorganisms can occur in two ways.

1. *Direct effect* In this case the ionizing radiation is directly responsible for the damage by causing a direct hit on a sensitive target molecule. It is generally accepted that cellular DNA is the principal target for inactivation, and that the ability to survive irradiation is attributable to the organism's ability to repair damaged DNA rather than to any intrinsic resistance of the structure. Further damage may be caused by free radicals produced within the cell but not directly associated with DNA. These radicals can diffuse to a sensitive site and react with it, causing damage.
2. *Indirect effect* The passage of ionizing radiation through water causes ionization along and immediately next to the track and the formation of free radicals and peroxides. These peroxides and free radicals are highly reactive and destructive and are responsible for both killing capability and the ability to modify the properties of polymers.

Some of the possible reactions are as follows:

$$\overset{\text{radiation}}{H_2O \rightarrow H_2O^+ + e^-}$$

$$H_2O^+ \rightarrow \cdot OH + H^+$$

$$e^- + H_2O \rightarrow OH^- + H\cdot$$

$$2H\cdot \rightarrow H_2$$

$$2\cdot OH \rightarrow H_2O_2$$

The presence of oxygen has a significant effect on the destructive properties of ionizing radiation owing to the formation of hydroperoxyl radicals.

$$H\cdot + O_2 \rightarrow \cdot HO_2$$

Peroxides and free radicals can act as both oxidizing and reducing agents according to the conditions.

Factors affecting the radiation resistance of microorganisms

Across the spectrum of microorganisms viruses are the most resistant forms to the effects of radiation, followed by bacterial endospores, then Gram-positive cells and finally, Gram-negative cells. Resistance to radiation is genetically determined and a particularly resistant bacterium called *Deinococcus radiodurans* can withstand a radiation dose up to three times that which would kill a normal bacterium. Fortunately, this organism does not have any clinical significance. It is worth noting that microbial products such as endotoxins will not be inactivated by normal doses of ionizing radiations, and so it is important to ensure that initial bioburden levels are low.

Oxygen has already been mentioned as having a significant effect on radiation resistance as the increased levels of hydroperoxyl radicals lead to marked increases in sensitivity. Vegetative cells such as *E. coli* and *Pseudomonas aeruginosa* are three to four times more sensitive in the presence of oxygen than in its absence. The presence of moisture will influence sensitivity, and dehydration increases resistance owing to an indirect effect on the formation and mobility of free radicals. Freezing also increases radiation resistance owing to the reduction of mobility of free radicals in the menstruum, preventing them from diffusing to sites of action at the cell membrane. Above the freezing point there is very little effect of temperature.

A variety of organic materials provide a protective environment for microorganisms, and comparison of radiation resistance is greatly complicated by different complexities of the media used. Sulphydryl groups, such as may be found in amino acids and proteins, have a protective effect on microorganisms owing to their interaction with free radicals. In contrast, compounds that combine with -SH groups, such as halogenated acetates, tend to increase sensitivity. Some naturally occurring materials, particularly foods, may have a profound protective effect on contaminant bacteria, and this is of concern to the food processing industry.

ULTRAVIOLET RADIATION

Although UV radiation has a range of wavelength from approximately 15 nm to 330 nm its range of maximum bactericidal activity is much narrower (220–280 nm), with an optimum of about 265 nm. Whereas ionizing radiations cause electrons to be ejected from atoms in their path, UV radiation does not possess sufficient energy for this and merely causes the electrons to become excited. It has much less penetrating power than ionizing radiations and tends to be used for the destruction of microorganisms in air and on surfaces.

The bactericidal effect of UV light is due to the formation of linkages between adjacent pyrimidine bases in the DNA molecule to form dimers. These are usually thymine dimers, although other types have been identified. The presence of thymine dimers alters the structural integrity of the DNA chain, thereby hindering chromosome replication. Certain cells can repair damaged DNA in a variety of ways, enhancing their radiation resistance.

Exposure of UV-damaged cells to visible light (photoreactivation) enables a light-dependent photoreactivating enzyme to split the thymine dimers into monomers. A second mechanism is not light dependent and is called dark recovery. In this case the thymine dimers are removed by a specific endonuclease enzyme that nicks the damaged DNA strand either side of the dimer. DNA polymerase then replaces the missing nucleotides and the ends are joined by a ligase enzyme.

Factors affecting resistance to UV light

As already mentioned, UV light has very little penetrating power and anything that acts as a shield around the cells will afford a degree of protection. The formation of aggregates of cells will result in those cells at the centre of the aggregate surviving an otherwise lethal dose of radiation. Similarly, microorganisms suspended in water withstand considerably higher doses of radiation than in the dry state owing to lack of penetration of the radiation. Suspension of bacteria in broth containing organic matter such as proteins increases the resistance of the cells still further. The stage of growth of the culture will affect the sensitivity of the cells, with maximum sensitivity being shown during the logarithmic phase.

Other factors shown to influence radiation resistance include pH, temperature and humidity, although the effect of the last parameter is still somewhat confused.

GASES

The use of gases as antimicrobial agents has been documented for centuries, although it is only recently that their mechanisms of action and factors affecting activity have been elucidated. A wide variety of gaseous agents have been used for their antimicrobial properties, but owing to the constraints of space only a few of the major ones will be dealt with here.

Ethylene oxide

Ethylene oxide is a gas at room temperature (with a boiling point at 10.7°C) which readily permeates a variety of materials (plastics, cardboard, cloth etc.) but not crystals. Its odour is reported as being rather pleasant, although the levels at which it is detected in the atmosphere (700 ppm) greatly exceed the 5 ppm maximum safety limit for humans. Toxicity problems include burns and blistering if the material comes into contact with the skin, whereas inhalation results in lachrymation, headache, dizziness and vomiting. Great care must be taken to ensure the removal of ethylene oxide from treated products (e.g. rubber gloves) to avoid the risk of skin reactions. Explosive mixtures are formed when ethylene oxide is mixed with air at any concentration above 3%, and this is especially dangerous if the gas mixture is confined. The addition of carbon dioxide or fluorinated hydrocarbons will eliminate this risk, and for sterilization purposes gas mixtures of 10% ethylene oxide/90% carbon dioxide are typically used.

Ethylene oxide is extremely effective at killing microorganisms and its activity is related to its action as an alkylating agent. Reactive hydrogen atoms on hydroxyl, carboxyl, sulphydryl and amino groups can all be replaced with hydroxyethyl groups, thereby interfering with a wide range of metabolic activities. Ethylene oxide inactivates the complete spectrum of microorganisms, including endospores and viruses. The difference in resistance between endospore-forming bacteria and vegetative cells is only of the order of five to ten times, compared to several thousandfold differences with other physical and chemical processes. In addition, no microorganism of genetically determined high resistance has been found. Spores of *B. subtilis* var. *niger* are among the most resistant to the effect of ethylene oxide. The moist heat-resistant spore-former *B. stearothermophilus* and spores of *Clos. sporogenes* are no more resistant than a number of vegetative organisms, such as *Staph. aureus* and *Micrococcus luteus*. Fungal spores exhibit the same order of resistance as vegetative cells.

Factors affecting the activity of ethylene oxide

The bactericidal activity of ethylene oxide is proportional to the partial pressure of gas in the reaction chamber, time of exposure, temperature of treatment and level and type of contamination. At room temperature the time taken to reduce the initial concentration of cells by 90% can be very slow, and for this reason elevated temperatures of 50–60°C are recommended, which results in greatly increased rates of kill. Concentrations of ethylene oxide between 500 and 1000 mg L^{-1} are usually employed. Relative humidity has a most pronounced effect, as at very high humidities ethylene oxide may be hydrolysed to the much less active ethylene glycol, and this is borne out by the observation that the gas is 10 times more active at 30% RH than at 97% RH. The optimum value for activity appears to be between 28 and 33%. Below 28% the alkylating action of ethylene oxide is inhibited due to lack of water. The degree of dehydration of cells greatly influences activity and it may not be possible to rehydrate very dry organisms simply by exposure to increased RH. In practice the RH value chosen is usually between 40 and 70%.

Microorganisms may be protected from the action of ethylene oxide by occlusion within crystalline material or when coated with organic matter or salts. *B. subtilis* var. *niger* spores dried from salt-water solutions are much more resistant to the gas than are suspensions dried from distilled water.

Biological indicators used to test the efficacy of ethylene oxide treatment employ spores of *B. subtilis* dried on to suitable carriers, such as pieces of aluminium foil.

Formaldehyde

Formaldehyde (H.CHO) in its pure form is a gas at room temperature, with a boiling point of −19°C, but readily polymerizes at temperatures below 80°C to form a white solid. The vapour, which is extremely irritating to the eyes, nose and throat, can be generated either from solid polymers such as paraformaldehyde or from a solution of 37% formaldehyde in water (formalin). Formalin usually contains about 10% methanol to prevent polymerization. As with ethylene oxide, formaldehyde is a very reactive molecule and there is only a small differential in resistance between bacterial spores and vegetative cells. Its bactericidal powers are superior to those of ethylene oxide (concentrations of 3–10 mg L^{-1} are effective) but it has weak penetrating power and is really only a surface bactericide. It is also more readily inactivated by organic matter. Adsorbed gas is very difficult to remove and long airing times are required. Its mechanism of action is thought to involve the production of intramolecular crosslinks between proteins, together with interactions with RNA and DNA. It acts as a mutagenic agent and an alkylating agent, reacting with carbonyl, thiol and hydroxyl groups. In order to be effective the gas must dissolve in a film of moisture surrounding the bacteria, and for this reason relative humidities in the order of 75% are required. Formaldehyde used in conjunction with low-temperature steam is a very effective sterilization medium.

β-Propiolactone

$$H—CH—CH—H$$
$$C—O$$
$$O$$

This is a colourless liquid at room temperature, with a pungent odour and a boiling point of 162°C. It has a wide spectrum of activity, the vapour being bactericidal to both Gram-positive and Gram-negative bacteria, viruses, rickettsiae, fungi and also *Mycobacterium* species. It is less active against bacterial spores. It is faster acting than formaldehyde and does not give problems with polymerization, but it has feeble penetrating powers. In order to sterilize enclosed spaces concentrations between 2 and 5 mg L^{-1} of air are necessary at a relative humidity of 80%, and these conditions must be maintained for 2 hours at 24°C.

Unfortunately, the use of β-propiolactone has been limited by doubts about its safety, as there is evidence showing it to be carcinogenic in animals. Acute short-term inhalation exposure causes severe irritation of the eyes, nose, throat and respiratory tract. Acute dermal exposure may cause irritation of the skin, blistering or burns. It has been used in liquid form for the sterilization of rabies vaccine and of various graft tissues.

Propylene oxide

Propylene oxide is a liquid (boiling point = 34°C) at room temperature which requires heating to volatilize. It is inflammable between 2.1 and 21.5% by volume in air, but this can be reduced by mixing with CO_2. Its mechanism of action is similar to that of ethylene oxide and involves the esterification of carbonyl, hydroxyl, amino and sulphydryl groups present on protein molecules. It is, however, less effective than ethylene oxide in terms of its antimicrobial activity and its ability to penetrate materials. Whereas ethylene oxide breaks down to give ethylene glycol or ethylene chlorohydrin, both of which are toxic, propylene oxide breaks down to propylene glycol, which is much less so.

Methyl bromide

Methyl bromide boils at 3.46°C and is a gas at room temperature. It is used as a disinfectant and a fumigant at concentrations of 3.5 mg L^{-1} with a relative humidity between 30 and 60%. It has inferior antimicrobial properties compared to the previous compounds but has good penetrating power.

Gas plasmas

A plasma is formed by applying energy to a gas or vapour under vacuum. Natural examples are lightning and sunlight, but plasmas can also be generated under low energy such as in fluorescent strip lights. Within a plasma, positive and negative ions, electrons and neutral molecules collide to produce free radicals. The destructive power of these entities has already been described, and so plasmas can be used as biocidal agents in a variety of applications. This type of system can be produced at temperatures below 50°C using vapours generated from hydrogen peroxide or peracetic acid.

ANTIMICROBIAL EFFECTS OF CHEMICAL AGENTS

Chemical agents have been used since very early times to combat such effects of microbial proliferation as spoilage of foods and materials, infection of wounds and decay of bodies. Thus, long before the role of microorganisms in disease and decay was recognized salt and sugar were used in food preservation, a variety of oils and resins were applied to wounds and employed for embalming, and sulphur was burned to fumigate sick rooms.

The classic researches of Pasteur, which established microorganisms as causative agents of disease and spoilage, paved the way for the development and rational use of chemical agents in their control. Traditionally, two definitions have been established describing the antimicrobial use of chemical agents. Those used to destroy microorganisms on inanimate objects are described as *disinfectants*, and those used to treat living tissues, as in wound irrigation, cleansing of burns or eye washes, are called *antiseptics*. Other definitions have been introduced to give more precise limits of meaning, namely, *bactericide* and *fungicide* for chemical agents that kill bacteria and fungi, respectively; and *bacteriostat* and *fungistat* for those that prevent the growth of a bacterial or fungal population. The validity of drawing a rigid demarcation line between those compounds that kill and those that inhibit growth without killing is doubtful. In many instances concentration and time of contact are the critical factors. The term *preservative* describes those antimicrobial agents used to protect medicines, pharmaceutical formulations, cosmetics, foods and general materials against microbial spoilage, and **biocide** is a general term for antimicrobial chemicals, but it excludes antibiotics and other agents used for systemic treatment of infections.

The mechanisms whereby biocides exert their effects have been intensively investigated and the principal sites of their attack upon microbial cells identified. These are the cell wall, the cytoplasmic membrane and the cytoplasm. Chemical agents may weaken the cell wall, thereby allowing the extrusion of cell contents, distortion of cell shape, filament formation or complete lysis. The cytoplasmic membrane, controlling as it does permeability, and being a site of vital enzyme activity, is vulnerable to a wide range of substances that interfere with reactive groups or can disrupt its phospholipid layers. Chemical and electrical gradients exist across the cell membrane and these represent a proton-motive force which drives such essential processes as oxidative phosphorylation, adenosine triphosphate (ATP) synthesis and active transport; several agents act by reducing the proton-motive force. The cytoplasm, site of genetic control and protein synthesis, presents a target for those chemical agents that disrupt ribosomes, react with nucleic acids or generally coagulate protoplasm.

Principal factors affecting activity

The factors most easily quantified are temperature and concentration. In general an increase in temperature increases the rate of kill for a given concentration of agent and inoculum size. The commonly used nomenclature is Q_{10} (temperature coefficient), which is the change in activity of the agent per 10°C rise in temperature (e.g. Q_{10} phenol = 4).

The effect of change in concentration of a chemical agent upon the rate of kill can be expressed as:

$$\eta = \frac{\log t_2 - \log t_1}{\log C_1 - \log C_2}$$

where C_1 and C_2 represent the concentrations of agent required to kill a standard inoculum in times t_1 and t_2. The concentration exponent η represents the slope of the line when log death time (t) is plotted against log concentration (C).

When values of η are greater than 1, changes of concentration will have a pronounced effect. Thus, in the case of phenol, when $\eta = 6$, halving the concentration will decrease its activity by a factor of 2^6

(64-fold), whereas for a mercurial compound, $\eta = 1$, the same dilution would only reduce activity twofold (2^1). Further details and tabulations of both temperature coefficients and concentration exponents may be found in Denyer and Wallhaeusser (1990).

The range of chemical agents

The broad categories of antibacterial chemical compounds have remained surprisingly constant over the years, with phenolics and hypochlorites comprising the major disinfectants and quaternary ammonium compounds widely used as antiseptics. The compounds capable of use as preservatives in preparations for oral, parenteral or ophthalmic administration are obviously strictly limited by toxicity requirements. As concerns over toxicity have intensified the range of available preservatives has diminished: mercury-containing compounds, for example, are now very little used for the preservation of parenteral and ophthalmic products, and the high cost of research and testing coupled with the poor prospects for an adequate financial return militate against the introduction of new agents. For this reason there is a tendency towards the use of existing preservatives in combination, with a view to achieving one or more of the following benefits: synergy; a broader antimicrobial spectrum; or reduced human toxicity resulting from the use of lower concentrations. The subjects of preservative toxicity and their potentiation and synergy are reviewed by Denyer and Wallhaeusser (1990), and Hugo and Russell (1999) have described in detail characteristics of the commonly used biocides.

Phenolics

Various phenolic compounds are shown in Figure 41.4.

Various distillation fractions of coal tar yield phenolic compounds, including cresols, xylenols and phenol itself, all of which are toxic and caustic to skin and tissues. Disinfectant formulations traditionally described as 'black fluids' and 'white fluids' are prepared from higher-boiling coal tar fractions. The former make use of soaps to solubilize the tar fractions in the form of stable homogenous solutions, whereas the latter are emulsions of the tar products and unstable on dilution.

Remarkable success has been achieved in modifying the phenol molecule by the introduction of chlorine and methyl groups, as in chlorocresol and chloroxylenol. This has the dual effect of eliminating toxic and corrosive properties while at the same time enhancing and prolonging antimicrobial activity.

Fig. 41.4 Chemical structures of a range of phenols.

Thus, chlorocresol is used as a bactericide in injections and to preserve oil-in-water creams, whereas chloroxylenol is employed as a household and hospital antiseptic. Phenol may itself be rendered less caustic by dilution to 1% w/v or less for lotions and gargles, or by dissolving in glycerol for use as ear drops. Bisphenols, such as hexachlorophane and triclosan (Irgasan), share the low solubility and enhanced activity of the other phenol derivatives described, but have a substantive effect which makes them particularly useful as skin antiseptics. Formulated as creams, cleansing lotions or soaps, they have proved valuable in reducing postoperative and cross-infection. Again toxicity concerns have emerged, and so, for example, hexachlorophane is restricted in the UK both in respect of the concentrations that may be employed and the type of product in which it may be used.

Phenols generally are active against vegetative bacteria and fungi, are readily inactivated by dilution and organic matter, and are most effective in acid conditions. Depending on concentration, phenols may cause cell lysis at low concentrations, or general coagulation of cell contents at higher concentrations.

Alcohols, aldehydes, acids and esters

Ethyl alcohol has long been used, usually as 'surgical spirit' for rapid cleansing of preoperative areas of skin before injection, and is most effective at concentrations of 60–70%. It is rapidly lethal to bacterial vegetative cells and fungi, but has no activity against bacterial endospores and little effect on viruses. The effect of aromatic substitution is to produce a range of compounds which are less volatile and less rapidly active and find general use as preservatives, e.g. phenylethanol for eye drops and contact lens solutions, benzyl alcohol in injections, Bronopol (2-bromo-2-nitropropane-1,3-diol) in shampoos and other toiletries. Phenoxyethanol, which has good activity against *Ps. aeruginosa*, has been used as an antiseptic. In general the alcohols act by disrupting the bacterial cytoplasmic membrane and can also interfere with the functioning of specific enzyme systems contained within the membrane.

Formaldehyde and glutaraldehyde are both powerful disinfectants, denaturing protein and destroying vegetative cells and spores. Formaldehyde is used in sterilization procedures both as a gas and as a solution in ethyl alcohol. Glutaraldehyde solutions are also used to sterilize surgical instruments.

The organic acids, sorbic and benzoic and their esters, because of their low toxicity, are well established as preservatives for food products and medicines (see Chapter 42). The exact mode of action of these agents on microorganisms is still uncertain, but they have been shown to influence the pH gradient across the cell membrane, and at higher concentrations the parabens induce leakage of intracellular constituents.

Quaternary ammonium compounds

The chemical formula for quaternary ammonium compounds is shown in Figure 41.5.

These cationic surface-active compounds are, as their name implies, derivatives of an ammonium halide in which the hydrogen atoms are substituted by at least one lipophilic group, a long-chain alkyl or aryl-alkyl radical containing C_8–C_{18} carbon atoms. In marked contrast to phenol and the cresols these compounds are mild in use and active at such high dilutions as to be virtually non-toxic. Their surface-active properties make them powerful cleansing agents, a useful adjunct to their common use as skin antiseptics and preservatives in contact lens cleansing and soaking solutions. They are also safe for formulating into eye drops and injections, and are widely used in gynaecology and general surgery. Active as cations, ambient pH is important, as is interference caused by anions. Thus, alkaline conditions promote activity and it is important that all traces of soap, which is anion active, are removed from the skin prior to treatment with a quaternary ammonium compound. Foreign organic matter and grease also cause inactivation.

One effect of the detergent properties of these compounds is to interfere with cell permeability such that susceptible bacteria – mainly the Gram-positive groups – leak their contents and eventually undergo lysis. Gram-negative bacteria are less susceptible and, to widen the spectrum to include these, mixtures of quaternary ammonium compounds with other antimicrobial agents such as phenoxyethanol or chlorhexidine are used.

Biguanides and amidines

Chlorhexidine is a widely used biocide which has activity against Gram-positive and Gram-negative bacteria but has little activity against endospores or viruses (Fig. 41.6). It is widely used in general surgery, both alone and in combination with cetrim-

Cetrimide BP
$R_1 R_2 R_3$—CH_3
R_4—mainly $C_{14}H_{29}$
X—Br
Benzalkonium Chloride BP
$R_1 R_2$ — CH_3
R_3 — $C_6H_5CH_2$
R_4 — mainly $C_{13}H_{27}$
X — Cl

Fig. 41.5 Chemical structure of centrimide and benzalkonium chloride.

ide, and can also be used as a preservative in eye drops. Polyhexamethylene biguanide (PHMB) is a polymeric biguanide used widely in the food, brewing and dairy industries, and has also found application as a disinfectant in contact lens cleaning solutions. The biguanides act on the cytoplasmic membrane, causing leakage of intracellular constituents.

The aromatic diamidines, propamidine and dibromopropamidine, are non-toxic antiseptics mainly active against Gram-positive bacteria and fungi. However, resistance to these agents can develop quickly during use.

The halogens and their compounds

Chlorine gas is a powerful disinfectant used in the municipal treatment of drinking water and in swimming baths. Solutions of chlorine in water may be made powerful enough for use as general household bleach, and disinfectant and dilute solutions are

Cl—⬡—NH—C(=NH)—NH—C(=NH)—NH—$(CH_2)_6$—NH—C(=NH)—NH—C(=NH)—HN—⬡—Cl

Chlorhexidine

Fig. 41.6 Chemical structure of chlorhexidine.

used for domestic hygiene. Unionized hypochlorous acid (HOCl) is an extremely potent and widely used bactericidal agent which acts as a non-selective oxidant, reacting readily with a variety of cellular targets. Well-known pharmaceutical formulations containing chlorine are Eusol (Chlorinated Lime and Boric Acid Solution BPC 1973) and Dakin's Solution (Surgical Chlorinated Soda Solution BPC 1973), both of which are designed to provide slow release of chlorine.

An alternative method of obtaining more prolonged release of chlorine is by the use of organic chlorine compounds such as Chloramine T (sodium *p*-toluene-sulphonchloramide) and Halazone BPC 1973 (*p*-sulphondichloramide benzoic acid), the former used as a skin antiseptic and the latter for treating contaminated drinking water. The high chemical reactivity of chlorine renders it lethal to bacteria, fungi and viruses, and to some extent spores and this activity is optimal at acid pH levels around 5.0.

Iodine, like chlorine a highly reactive element, denatures cell proteins and essential enzymes by its powerful oxidative effects. Traditionally it has been used in alcoholic solutions such as Tincture of Iodine (BP 1973) or complexed with potassium iodide to form an aqueous solution (Lugol's Iodine BP 1973). The staining and irritant properties of iodine have resulted in the development of iodophores, mixtures of iodine with surface-active agents, which hold the iodine in micellar combination from which it is released slowly. Such a preparation is Betadine (polyvinylpyrrolidone-iodine), used as a non-staining, non-irritant antiseptic.

Metals

Many metallic ions are toxic to essential enzyme systems, particularly those utilizing thiol (–SH) groups, but those used medically are restricted to mercury, silver and aluminium. The extreme toxicity of mercury has rendered its use obsolete apart from in organic combination. The organic compounds that still have a limited use in pharmacy are phenylmercuric nitrate (and acetate) as a bactericide in eye drops and injections, and thiomersal (sodium ethylmercurithiosalicylate) as a preservative in biological products and certain eye drops.

Silver, in the form of the nitrate, has been used to treat infections of the eyes, as have silver protein solutions. Aluminium foil has been used as a wound covering in the treatment of burns and venous ulcers, and has been shown to adsorb micro-organisms and inhibit their growth.

The acridines

This group of compounds interferes specifically with nucleic acid function and has some ideal antiseptic properties, thus aminacrine hydrochloride is non-toxic, non-irritant, non-staining and active against Gram-positive and Gram-negative bacteria even in the presence of serum.

This brief survey has given some indication of the variety of antimicrobial compounds available. Each of these has a defined spectrum of utility and in the correct conditions of use can substantially contribute to the control of microbial proliferation and infection.

REFERENCES

Denyer, S.P., Wallhaeusser, K.H. (1990) Antimicrobial preservatives and their properties. In: Denyer, S.P., Baird, R. (eds) *Guide to Microbiological Control in Pharmaceuticals*. Ellis Horwood, Chichester, pp. 251–273.

European Pharmacopoeia (2000) 3rd edn. Strasbourg: Council of Europe, p 284.

Hugo, W.B., Russell, A.D. (1999) Types of antimicrobial agents. In: Russell, A.D., Hugo, W.B., Ayliffe, G.A.J. (eds) *Principles and Practice of Disinfection Preservation and Sterilisation*, 3rd edn. Blackwell Science. Oxford, pp. 5–94.

Russell, A.D. (1999) Destruction of bacterial spores by thermal methods. In: Russell, A.D., Hugo, W.B., Ayliffe, G.A.J. (eds) *Principles and Practice of Disinfection, Preservation and Sterilisation*, 3rd edn. Blackwell Science. Oxford, pp. 640–656.

BIBLIOGRAPHY

Brinston, R.M., Norton, J.L. (1994) Cobalt 60: the heart of gamma radiation sterilization. *Med. Dev. Tech.*, May 1994, 14–16.

Hugo, W.B., Russell, A.D. (1998) *Pharmaceutical Microbiology* 6th edn. Blackwell Science, Oxford.

Pelczar M.J., Chan E.C.S., Krieg N.R. (1993) *Microbiology – concepts and applications*. McGraw-Hill, New York.

Rules and Guidance for Pharmaceutical Manufacturers and Distributors (1997) HMSO, London.

Russell, A.D., Chopra, I. (1990) *Understanding antibacterial action and resistance*. Ellis Horwood Ltd, Chichester.

42

Microbiological contamination and preservation of pharmaceutical products

Malcolm Parker (updated by Norman Hodges)

SOURCES AND INCIDENCE OF CONTAMINATION

Microorganisms form an integral part of our environment. They are present in the air that we breathe, the food that we eat and the water that we drink. Some microorganisms indigenous to the body are present in considerable numbers: they constitute up to one-third of the dry weight of faeces. In this situation it is apparent that both raw materials and final medicines will contain microorganisms unless specific measures are adopted to exclude them. The preparation of sterile medicaments is a skilled and expensive procedure demanding sophisticated equipment, skilled personnel and a controlled working environment. To produce all medicines to such a standard would require clear arguments to justify the considerable costs involved and the consequent expense to consumers. Factors to be considered are: the sources and incidence of microorganisms in drugs and medical preparations, the consequences of such contamination both for the stability of medicines and for the health of the patient and, arising from these, the levels and types of microorganism that might be tolerated.

As indicated in Table 42.1 and Fig. 42.1, many factors potentially contribute to the microbial load carried by a pharmaceutical preparation at every stage of manufacture, from assembling the raw materials to packaging the final product.

There have been many reports, particularly in the 1960s and 1970s, of pathogenic organisms isolated, sometimes in large numbers, from pharmaceutical raw materials and manufactured products. These reports, reviewed by Bloomfield (1990) and, more recently, by Spooner (1996), drew attention to the need for better control of the microbiological quality of both raw materials and manufacturing processes. As a consequence, the frequency with which high concentrations or hazardous species are isolated has been reduced in recent years, although the problem has by no means

Table 42.1   Sources of microbial contaminants

Water	Low-demand Gram-negative groups: *Pseudomonas, Xanthamonas, Flavobacterium, Achromobacter*
Air	Mould spores: *Penicillium, Mucor, Aspergillus* Bacterial spores: *Bacillus* spp. Yeasts Micrococci
Raw materials Earths	Anaerobic spore formers: *Clostridium* spp.
Pigments	*Salmonella*
Starches	Coliforms
Gums	*Achnomyces*
Animal products	*Salmonella* Coliforms
Personnel	Coliforms Staphylococci Streptococci Corynebacteria

Table 40.3) and the relatively high levels of contamination of natural products is reflected in these limits.

The usual waterborne organisms found are the *Pseudomonas–Achromobacter–Alcaligenes* types, including occasionally *Ps. aeruginosa*. Purified water has proved to be a typical source of microorganisms in that, during use, the ion-exchange column may become contaminated from the water passing through and the entrapped organisms rapidly multiply to produce high counts in the outflowing water.

Water produced by reverse osmosis might also represent a problem if the osmosis membrane is not disinfected at regular intervals. Even distilled water, which is free of microorganisms on leaving the still, may be a significant source of contamination after storage. This is because the chlorine that protects tap water is lost on distillation, and Gram-negative bacteria may grow to concentrations as high as 10^5-10^6 mL^{-1} within a few days at ambient temperature. These bacteria usually gain access to distilled water by way of poor-quality rubber or plastic connection tubing or inadequate closure of storage containers.

Some manufactured medicines possess antimicrobial activity, by virtue of unfavourable pH, for example, so it is not inevitable that medicines made from contaminated raw materials will, themselves, be contaminated, although this is normally the case. Further, it is important to realize that in some cases the initial bacterial count in a freshly prepared

been eliminated. It is well established that major sources of microbial contamination of medicines are water – the most common raw material – and raw materials of natural origin, including vegetable drugs and mined minerals such as talc, kaolin and bentonite. The European Pharmacopoeia (2000) specifies limits for microorganisms in different product types (see

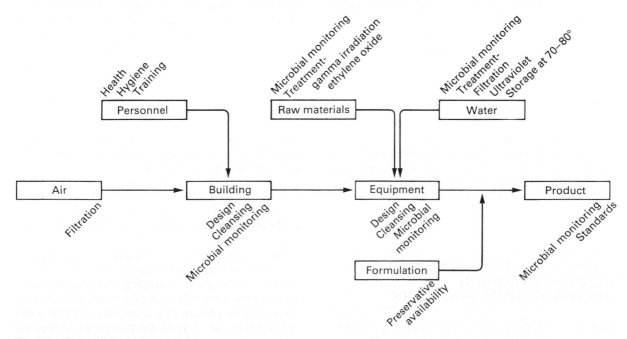

Fig. 42.1   Factors in hygienic manufacture

mixture can increase substantially during storage, particularly in those cases in which the formulation contains no preservative.

A major potential source of microbial contamination is that represented by the personnel preparing medicines and the patients using them (Table 42.1). In the environment generally it is people who generate most of the airborne bacteria. Body movements, exhaling, speaking and, of course, coughing and sneezing, represent significant sources of contamination. The microorganisms that can be disseminated in this way include staphylococci, present on the skin and in the nostrils of healthy persons, streptococci, sometimes present in the throat, and a variety of *Enterobacteriaceae*, including salmonellae and coliforms present in the intestines. Other microflora that may be found as contaminants of medicines, and which are not normally associated with humans, are the airborne spores of both bacteria and moulds, including several wild yeasts, anaerobic inhabitants of soil and earths such as the clostridia and low-demand water-borne bacteria, usually Gram-negative forms.

There is considerable potential for microorganisms to enter medicines during both manufacture and use, and in this situation it is not surprising that whenever non-sterile preparations and their ingredients are screened for microbial contamination, organisms are detected. As has been discussed, the incidence of microflora in medicines as issued from the dispensary or manufacturers is dictated very much by the nature of the ingredients, i.e. whether natural or synthetic, the quality of the vehicle, and the care and attitude of personnel involved.

The situation is very different for sterile preparations in that detection of any microorganisms represents an unacceptable situation usually indicative of a breakdown in the sterilization process. Thus when in 1972 infusion fluids used in a Plymouth hospital were found to be contaminated, the Secretary of State required the Medicines Commission to 'review measures which should be taken in the course of the production, distribution, storage and use of medicinal products to prevent their becoming vehicles of infection'. It is indicative of the rarity of such incidents that an inquiry was deemed to be necessary.

GROWTH AND MULTIPLICATION OF MICROORGANISMS IN PHARMACEUTICAL PRODUCTS

Most raw materials, and consequently the pharmaceutical preparations containing them, will support some form of microorganism. Although this ability varies considerably according to the nutritive properties and moisture content of the materials concerned, it is unwise to assume that, for instance, a dry powder or a tablet is safe from microbial spoilage. The problem can be appreciated by considering the range of habitats of microorganisms, encompassing as they do volcanic regions to the Antarctic wastes and nutrient sources as unlikely as glass and concrete. The majority of medicines present a ready source of nutrients and moisture and there are many reports of the effects of microbial proliferation within them, with attendant odours and visible spoilage. Troublesome and expensive as this obvious deterioration may be, a more serious problem is the development of microorganisms without obvious signs or involving delayed effects. For this reason it is important to have a knowledge of the microbial content of all drugs and medicines, rather than restrict attention to those required to be sterile and those shown to be particularly spoilage prone. A study of the interaction of microorganisms in foods such as milk or meat products has shown how pioneer forms can prepare the way for later invaders by degrading complex nutrients, altering pH levels, or making more moisture available until the final spoilage population is established. The initial invaders, in either foods or medicines, can reach high levels without visible effects, and furthermore, when the finally spoiled product is investigated, they may have been completely displaced by a final spoilage form. Unless this chain reaction of spoilage is appreciated harmful effects of apparently stable medicines can be unresolved and the importance of some contaminants not realized. Thus, syrup or mixtures rich in sugar may become initially contaminated by osmophilic yeasts which can thrive at high sugar concentrations and, by utilizing the sugars create conditions that allow secondary, less specialized organisms to become established. When such syrups are examined there may be little evidence of the yeasts that initiated the spoilage process, and so their role may be overlooked.

CONSEQUENCES OF CONTAMINATION

It is now realized that the presence of microorganisms in a pharmaceutical preparation may have a variety of consequences, ranging from the negligible to the very serious. For example, spores of the mould *Mucor* may be present in a dormant form and never produce spoilage or harm the patient who takes the medicine. In complete contrast to this would be the presence of *Salmonella* in a medicine which, although causing little or no visible spoilage, would represent a serious health hazard.

The instances in which there have been serious consequences attending contaminations have been, in the main, concerned with those preparations which are required to be supplied sterile. This might be anticipated, as sterile preparations are usually administered parenterally or into the eyes, and in these circumstances extraneous microorganisms present a particular danger. Intravenous infusion fluids are recognized as a potential area for concern, particularly because of their implication in the case previously mentioned, where contaminated fluid resulted in the death of several patients. The established practice of adding drugs to infusions, often at patient level in hospital wards, can present an additional microbiological hazard unless closely supervised by skilled staff. Preparations for ophthalmic use, including contact lens solutions, have been responsible for serious infections of the eye, some resulting in blindness, as a result of microbial contamination.

Considered against the background of the high volume of medicinal products used annually by the public, the serious consequences of contamination are very few. Where they do occur, however, the public is justifiably worried and the implications for the profession are grave.

Apart from possible infection of patients the other important effect of contamination of medicines is that of general spoilage. This may result in obvious changes, such as discolouration, breakdown of emulsions and the production of gas and various odours. Such comparatively dramatic effects of deterioration do have the virtue of directing the consumer's attention to the problem and, hopefully, discouraging their use of the medicine. In other cases, however, active ingredients may be utilized by invading microorganisms without overt visible signs of spoilage. Thus, salicylates (including aspirin), paracetamol, atropine, chloramphenicol, prednisolone and hydrocortisone can be degraded to a variety of therapeutically inactive products. Preservatives, intended to protect formulations against microorganisms, can themselves present a ready source of microbial nutrition, particularly if their levels become depleted and if they are aromatic in structure.

Bacteria can produce various toxic substances which are a potential danger in contaminated products, even when a sterilization procedure has been applied and only dead cells or their residues remain. In parenteral preparations endotoxins, which are lipopolysaccharide components of Gram-negative

bacteria, may cause fever following injection (see Chapter 40). Moulds produce mycotoxins, which from early times have been implicated in illnesses such as ergotism, and more recently with gastroenteritis, both caused by using contaminated grain. The involvement of mycotoxins, particularly aflatoxin, in cancer has added an urgency to our study of them.

SCREENING FOR CONTAMINATION

A consideration of Figure 42.1 will show that if contamination is to be minimized then a knowledge of the microbial levels associated with all aspects of the production of a medicine is required. Thus, examining prepared medicines for their contamination will not, in itself, further our efforts to reduce this unless parallel screening is done upon the manufacturing process and environment, including air, equipment, personnel and raw materials.

Methods for the detection, enumeration and identification of microorganisms have been described in Chapters 39 and 40. Some of these can be applied to determine the number and type of microorganisms present at any stage in the preparation or manufacture of a medicine. The most relevant are discussed below and are considered also in Chapter 40).

Air sampling

The usual methods for sampling from air are by free fall or settling, forced air flow and filtration.

Free fall or settling

As the name implies, this involves the sampling of organisms deposited naturally from the atmosphere. This is typically carried out by exposing plates of suitable nutrient medium for selected periods in the locations to be sampled. The procedure is empirical, with the counts obtained depending upon time of exposure, the nature of any activity in the area and the siting of the plates in relation to such activity.

Forced air flow

Forced air flow samplers allow a measured volume of air to be examined by directing it on to a solid agar surface or drawing it through sterile saline or nutrient broth from which plate counts can be made. A variety of commercially available apparatus may be used to apply this method.

Filtration

Filtration involves the drawing of air through a membrane filter which is then aseptically removed, placed upon suitable nutrient agar and incubated.

Care must be taken in interpreting results obtained by these various methods and thought given to location and timing of sampling, period of exposure or volume of air examined and movement of personnel. In general, if contamination problems are likely to be due to particles settling from the air, then free-fall methods are adequate. If, however, contaminating particles tend to remain airborne some form of forced air sampling is essential. The actual timing of sampling will provide information on conditions during typical busy working periods and the efficiency of any air filtration system in coping at peak times.

Sampling of surfaces and equipment

Simple techniques can be used to assess the level of contamination of surfaces, such as swabbing with sterile cotton-tipped sticks, which can be transferred to suitable recovery media, or by placing a sterile agar surface in contact with the area to be sampled and, after removal, incubating. It is easier to use swabs for flexible and uneven surfaces and agar contact methods for firm flat surfaces.

Measuring contamination levels in raw materials and final preparations

The nature of raw material and final preparations will determine the method used to detect microbial contamination. Water, water-miscible liquids or soluble solids present no difficulties for conventional plate counting or filter membrane methods. Insoluble or oily materials and preparations need to be suitably dispersed and homogenized if contaminating microorganisms are to be isolated. In every instance any antimicrobial activity of the sample under examination must be neutralized. Methods of counting microorganisms and the inherent errors are described briefly in Chapter 40 and in more detail in standard bacteriological textbooks.

There is increasing interest in methods for the rapid detection of microorganisms in food and drugs which can be automated and should remove much of the drudgery of traditional counting techniques. These methods are based upon the measurement of some metabolic activity or other feature of organisms, and include adenosine triphosphate (ATP) assays, direct epifluorescence techniques and imped-

ance techniques; the pharmaceutical applications of these and other methods are reviewed by Newby (2000), and the instrumentation is described by Collins et al (1995). In the case of sterile production, the entire system can be monitored by processing a sterile nutrient medium (for liquid preparations) or soluble sterile powder (for solids) and examining final preparations for contamination, together with samples taken at various intermediate stages.

CONTROL OF MICROBIAL CONTAMINATION

There are essentially two strategies to be adopted in the preparation of microbiologically acceptable pharmaceutical preparations. The first and most important is to minimize the access of microorganisms from the sources summarized in Figure 42.1 and Table 42.1, and the second is to formulate the final product so as to be hostile to microorganisms, normally by the addition of preservatives.

For sterile preparations there is either a terminal sterilization process or a closely controlled aseptic manufacturing procedure. In every case the final pack should be designed to protect the product during storage and minimize in-use contamination. The *Rules and Guidance for Pharmaceutical Manufacturers and Distributors (1997)* or 'Orange Guide' provides guidance on premises, equipment, raw materials, packaging, storage and the training of personnel.

Premises and equipment

Premises need to be purpose-built to provide a logical workflow, with separation of areas of different grades of cleanliness, appropriate air supplies, and construction materials which are resistant to dirt and easy to keep clean. The equipment should be as simple as possible for the purposes required, with a minimum of junctions, valves and pumps to allow cleaning in place by the circulation of detergents or other chemical antimicrobial agents such as hypochlorites, followed by steam or hot-water flushing. The degree of air treatment required will depend upon the type of product involved, with aseptic manipulation demanding filtration efficient enough to remove particles down to 0.1 μm. For aseptic preparation and filling a grade A clean room is required; this requires an atmosphere containing no more than 3500 particles m^{-3} in the 0.5–5μm range when the room is not in operation. The

Fig. 42.2 Preservative availability.

Table 42.2 Examples of preservatives commonly used in pharmaceutical formulations

Product type	Preservative	Concentration (%w/v)	% of USP formulations in which preservative used*
Parenteral	Benzyl alcohol	0.1–3.0	31.0
	Methyl/propyl paraben	0.08–0.1/0.001–0.023	13.8
	Phenol	0.2–0.5	7.9
	Methyl paraben (alone)	0.1	6.6
	Chlorbutanol	0.25–0.5	5.3
	Sodium metabisulphite	0.025–0.66	5.3
	Sodium bisulphite	0.13–0.2	2.6
			Total 69.9
Ophthalmic	Benzalkonium chloride	0.0025–0.0133	50.0
	Thiomersal	0.001–0.5	19.8
	Methyl/propyl paraben	0.05/0.01	6.6
	Benzalkonium chloride plus EDTA	0.01/0.1	3.3
			Total 79.7
Oral	Sodium benzoate	NA	34.4
	Methyl/propyl paraben	NA	18.3
	Methyl paraben (alone)	0.1	9.7
	Methyl paraben plus sodium benzoate	NA	7.5
			Total 69.9
Creams	Benzyl alcohol	1.0–2.0	25.4
	Methyl/propyl paraben	NA	18.6
	Methyl paraben (alone)	0.1–0.3	11.9
	Benzoic acid	0.2	8.5
	Sorbic acid	0.1	8.5
	Chlorocresol	0.05	6.8
			Total 79.7

NA, not available.
* Only the most commonly used agents are listed, so the percentages in each product category do not total 100%.
After Dabbah (1996)

'Orange Guide' gives advice upon basic environmental standards, with allowance made for people present in working areas.

Raw materials

Raw materials, particularly those of natural origin, and water are a potentially rich source of microorganisms and may require treatment to reduce or eliminate them. Potable (tap) water may be used for the manufacture of some pharmaceuticals, but as the microbial load in potable water may vary with geographical region and season of the year it is more common to use deionized water. Provided the deionizing bed (ion-exchange resin) is regenerated on a regular basis, an acceptable microbiological standard can be maintained for deionized water. Water may be treated by UV treatment units or filtration and stored at elevated temperature (65–80°C) to discourage microbial growth.

For raw materials generally, any treatment applied to remove or reduce the microbial load must be such that the materials are not adversely affected. A variety of processing procedures are available, including ionizing radiations, microwaves, gassing and, of course, heat. In every case close monitoring for possible deleterious effects is essential.

Personnel

There is little doubt that however comprehensive the procedures adopted to control contamination, they will be of little avail unless the personnel involved understand and appreciate the problems and significance of microbial contamination. This requires education in hygiene to minimize the introduction of microorganisms by staff and to underline the importance of appropriate protective measures. The approach will, of course, differ depending upon the level of education of the people involved, but it cannot be overemphasized that all personnel and visitors, however senior, must be required to comply with regimens of hygiene and protective clothing. A full range of appropriate clothing is commercially available which, for the manufacturer of sterile preparations, completely shields the product from body surfaces with, for instance, hood, mask, overall, protective gloves and boots. For other manufacturing areas good-quality overalls, overshoes and head cover represent a minimal requirement. General dispensing requires careful attention to hygiene, the provision of suitable overalls and a ban on food consumption and smoking in the dispensary.

THE PRESERVATION OF PHARMACEUTICAL PREPARATIONS

With an understanding of the many factors involved in the microbial contamination of medicines and application of the procedures described, a range of products can be obtained which, if required, are sterile or have an acceptable level of organisms present. This in itself is not sufficient without further steps being taken to minimize contamination and spoilage of the medicines during use. Well designed containers, usually single-dose in the case of sterile preparations, and sensible storage contribute a great deal to this end, but whenever acceptable an added safeguard is to incorporate an antimicrobial substance or preservative into the formulation.

The correct approach to preservation has as its foundation two important principles. The first is that a preservative must not be added to a product to mask any deficiencies in the manufacturing procedures, and the second is that the preservative should be an integral part of the formulation, chosen to afford protection in that particular environment. The increasing care now being given to the hygienic preparation of pharmaceutical products has removed the need for preservatives to cope with high initial microbial loads, but the problem remains of protecting against spoilage resulting from in-use contamination. If a preservative is to prevent such spoilage the factors affecting its efficacy must be appreciated.

Factors in preservative efficacy

The range of antimicrobial agents available is apparently very wide (see Chapter 41 and Table 42.2) until the particular requirements of a preservative for a formulated medicine are considered. A review of the United States Pharmacopoeia formulae (Dabbah 1996) showed that 38 different preservatives were in use, together with 42 different preservative combinations. However, an analysis of the most commonly used agents revealed that the same few were regularly employed in 70% or more of the products in each of the various categories (Table 42.2). When this table is compared with the corresponding one in the first edition of this book it is apparent that no new preservatives have entered into common use during the intervening period; indeed some, e.g. the phenylmercury salts, have become less popular because of toxicity concerns, so the range of available preservatives is diminishing not expanding.

To state that the preservative must be non-toxic, odourless, stable and compatible with other formulation components while exerting its effect against the wide range of potential microbial contaminants is an oversimplification. Toxicity alone debars many antimicrobial compounds from use in preparations for parenteral, ophthalmic or oral use, and the increased sophistication of some modern formulations makes it difficult to avoid preservative–ingredient interactions. Any organisms that do enter a preparation will multiply in the aqueous phase or immediate interface, and so it is the prime function of the preservative to attain a protective concentration in this phase. As shown in Figure 42.2, the major reasons for a preservative not attaining an effective concentration in the aqueous phase are its possible solubility in oil, interaction with emulgents, hydrocolloids and suspended solids, its interaction with the container or its volatility. In addition, the ambient pH of the formulation can have a marked influence upon preservative effectiveness.

Oil/water partition

In a simple two-phase system of oil and water a preservative will partition until:

$$\frac{C_o}{C_w} = K_w^o$$

where C_o is the concentration of preservative in oil at equilibrium, C_w is the concentration of preservative in water at equilibrium and K_w^o is the oil/water partition coefficient at the given temperature. Oil solubility is an important parameter in preserving formulations containing vegetable oils such as arachis or soya; and for such preparations the esters of parahydroxybenzoic acid (parabens) are unsuitable owing to their high oil/water partition coefficients ($K^o = 0.02$ for methyl paraben in mineral oil and 7.5 in vegetable oil: for propyl paraben $K^o = 0.5$ in mineral oil and 80.0 in vegetable oil). Faced with this problem it is necessary to change the preservative or alter the formulation and, given the restricted choice of preservatives, the formulation becomes all important. Thus, it was found that by substituting liquid paraffin (mineral oil) for arachis oil (vegetable oil) in formulations of Calamine Cream, a preservative such as chlorocresol would afford better protection ($K_w^o = 117$ (arachis oil): 1.5 (liquid paraffin)). The further step of using a less oil-soluble preservative such as phenoxyethanol ($K_w^o = 0.12$ liquid paraffin) further improved the system.

Emulsions

Many emulgents are used in pharmaceutical preparations to produce elegant applications or palatable medicines (see Chapter 23). A variety of interactions will occur between preservatives and the emulsified oil phase and with emulgent molecules or micelles. Attempts have been made to quantify such interactions by measuring the proportion of free preservative in emulsions in a variety of ways, including dialysis and dissolution techniques. The use of predictive data can greatly assist in the formulation, provided that the different behaviour of different emulgents, effects of temperature and influence of oil:water ratio are appreciated. A simple mathematical model has been developed:

$$C_w = C \frac{\phi + 1}{K_w^o \phi + 1}$$

where C_w is the concentration of preservative in the aqueous phase, C is the total concentration of preservative and ϕ is the oil:water ratio. In the presence of an emulgent the amount of free preservative can be measured and the ratio expressed as the factor R:

$$\text{where } R = \frac{\text{total preservative}}{\text{free preservative}}$$

The equation then becomes:

$$C_w = C \frac{\phi + 1}{K_w^o \phi + R}$$

where C_w is now the free concentration in the water.

Using this model it can be calculated, for instance, that to attain the required protective concentration of 0.2% w/v methyl paraben in a liquid paraffin/water emulsion containing 5% polysorbate-80 and 50% oil, a total concentration of some 0.5% must be used. Alterations in the type and concentration of emulgent, nature of oil and oil:water ratio will all influence the concentration of preservative needed to protect the system.

Interaction with other formulation components

Many of the hydrocolloids used as dispersants or thickeners, such as methylcellulose, alginates, polyvinylpyrrolidone and tragacanth, can interact to some degree with preservatives and diminish their activity. In some cases this is a direct incompatibility, as between alginates, which are anionic, and cation-active preservatives, whereas in other cases a variety of physicochemical interactions operate.

Therapeutically active ingredients in the form of suspended solids in mixtures, such as magnesium trisilicate and kaolin, have been shown to deplete preservative concentrations, probably by adsorption. Similarly, fillers and disintegrants cause problems in tablet preservation owing to their interaction with added preservatives such as methylhydroxybenzoate.

Effects of containers

Preparations packed in traditional glass containers can be expected to retain their preservative content provided the closure is suitably airtight. The greatly increased use of plastics in packaging has brought with it a number of difficulties, ranging from permeation of preservatives through the container to interaction with it. There is a great deal of published work describing the losses of preservative to plastic medicine bottles, contact lenses and their containers and plastic syringes. Given the complexity of modern plastics, with their differences in thickness, surface characteristics, filler and plasticizer content, it is necessary to choose the material for the pack of a preserved formulation on the basis of adequate trials.

Although rubber reacts with many preservatives it still finds use for teats and closures. These are required to be pretreated with the preservatives they are to be in contact with, in order to minimize subsequent uptake during storage.

Influence of pH

An appreciation of the many obstacles that may prevent a preservative attaining an adequate protective concentration in a given preparation must be complemented by some understanding of the interaction between that preservative and any microorganisms present as contaminants. Thus, not only must free preservative be available in a formulation, but it must be present in an active form. This is particularly important when activity is related to degree of ionization, as is the case with both anion- and cation-active antimicrobial agents. An example is that of a weak acid preservative such as benzoic acid, which requires to be predominantly in the undissociated form in order to exert antimicrobial activity. Since this acid has a pK_a value of 4.2, an ambient pH below this is needed for efficient preservative activity.

The relationship between degree of dissociation and pH is given by:

$$\text{Fraction of undissociated preservative} = \frac{1}{1 + \text{antilog}\left(\text{pH} - pK_a\right)}$$

In most cases more than one factor is involved, as for example when benzoic acid is used to preserve kaolin mixtures. The dual problem here is that the adsorption of the benzoic acid by the light kaolin diminishes at pH values above 5, whereas the acid preservative is most efficient at lower values. In this situation the formulator faces opposing choices, opting for an alternative preservative or using a mixture of preservatives. Kaolin mixture has the added interest that in order to render it attractive to children, raspberry syrup flavouring is used and so the pH is reduced to 3.5, at which value about 83% of benzoic acid is present in the biologically active undissociated form but adsorption on to the kaolin is favoured.

The majority of preservatives are less dependent upon pH, although cationic active quaternary ammonium compounds are more active at high pH values.

Preservatives in combination

The use of a single preservative to protect a pharmaceutical preparation may be unrealistic. Increasing attention has been focused on the use of mixtures of preservatives and the addition of various potentiators to achieve better results. The justification for using mixtures of antimicrobial compounds must reside in an increased spectrum of antimicrobial activity, a synergistic effect enabling decreased levels of component preservatives to be used, an attendant decrease in toxicity, and a reduction in the emergence of resistant forms. One of the oldest examples of a preservative mixture used in pharmacy is the former vehicle for eye drops, 'Solution for Eyedrops', which contained a mixture of methyl and propyl esters of p-hydroxybenzoic acid designed to exert antibacterial and antifungal effects. Modern formulations for eye drops and contact lens solutions include phenylethyl alcohol and phenoxetol, in conjuction with benzalkonium chloride to widen the antimicrobial spectrum and aid access to susceptible sites on the microorganisms. The chelating agent ethylenediamine tetra-acetate (EDTA) has also been used with preservatives other than those yielding metallic ions, to enhance activity by interfering with vital metal ion balance and associated permeability. A rather different mechanism is to increase the availability of lipophilic preservatives by reducing their loss to emulgents in the formulation, as with the addition of propylene glycol to emulsions preserved with parabens to reduce loss to micelles.

A correctly designed preservative system is the appropriate complement to hygienic manufacture. Both demand a rational approach based on an appreciation of interacting factors. Thus, just as there is little justification in providing a high-quality manufacturing environment and introducing poor-quality raw materials, there is equally little point in an ad hoc addition of preservatives to preparations without investigation of formulation interactions involved.

MICROBIAL STANDARDS FOR PHARMACEUTICAL PREPARATIONS

The design of microbial standards for pharmaceutical preparations must be realistic in that they relate to the intended use of the preparation and can be applied without ambiguity. The types of standard used to monitor microbial content are twofold, namely, an absolute exclusion of all microorganisms or named organisms, and a numerical limit upon all organisms or named organisms. The first type, or exclusion standard in its most severe form, is that requiring sterility, and is applied to solutions for injection, ophthalmic preparations and certain other fluids for body irrigation. In these cases no organisms can be tolerated and the role of any preservative is to maintain the sterility of the sterilized preparation during use. Although such an absolute standard is not required for medicines for oral or topical use, nevertheless certain bacteria can represent a hazard and be indicative of poor manufacturing practice and should be excluded. The US Pharmacopoeia suggests an exclusion standard for *E. coli* to all solutions for oral use and for *Staph. aureus* and *Ps. aeruginosa* in topical preparations. In addition, both the British and US pharmacopoeias apply exclusion standards for named organisms from certain raw materials and final preparations (Table 40.3).

Compliance with these standards can only be assured by strict control of manufacture from raw materials to final preparation (Fig. 42.1). The incorporation of a product-designed preservative system is an additional safeguard.

The application of the various standards described depends in the last analysis upon the reliability of the techniques available for detection and enumeration of microorganisms in raw materials and final preparations. The established methods of the microbiologist are time-consuming and have the errors of any biological measurements. As indicated earlier, a range of methods of detection and quantification based upon other physiological or metabolic characteristics are well established in the food industry and their adoption in the pharmaceutical industry should add a new dimension to the use of microbial standards.

Challenge testing

The methods and philosophy of challenge testing are dealt with in Chapter 40. In the particular case of preserved preparations the test must be designed to provide a realistic measure of the ability of the formulation to cope with normal use. Many arguments have been made for the choice of challenge organisms, their use at various concentrations, the number of challenges made and so on. The current BP test specifies all of these parameters for parenteral, ophthalmic, topical and oral liquid preparations, together with the end-point required. In this respect it provides general guidelines, but in addition most manufacturers apply their own challenge tests based on their experience with the particular product.

CONCLUSION

As with many areas of study that of the microbial contamination of pharmaceuticals began with an awareness that a problem existed. The consequences of this problem extended both to economy of production and to the safety of the patient. The skills of the microbiologist, chemist, engineer and pharmacist have been combined to enable medicines to be prepared which are microbiologically safe. The maintaining of this situation depends upon constant vigilance over every aspect of manufacture and formulation.

REFERENCES

Bloomfield, S.F. (1990) Microbial contamination: spoilage and hazard. In: Denyer, S., Baird, R. (eds) *Guide to Microbiological Control in Pharmaceuticals*. Ellis Horwood, London, pp 29–52.

Collins, C.H., Lyne, P.M., Grange, J.M. (1995) Automated methods. In: *Microbiological Methods*. Butterworth-Heinemann, Oxford, pp 121–136.

Dabbah, R. (1996) The use of preservatives in compendial articles. *Pharm. Forum*. **22(4)**, 2696–2704.

European Pharmacopoeia (2000) 3rd edn. Strasbourg, Council of Europe, pp 259–260.

Newby, P. (2000) Rapid methods for enumeration and identification in microbiology. In: Baird, R.M., Hodges, N.A., Denyer, S.P. (eds) *Handbook of Microbiological Quality Assurance*. Taylor & Francis, London, 107–119.

Rules and Guidance for Pharmaceutical Manufacturers and Distributors (1997) HMSO London.

Spooner, D.F. (1996) Hazards associated with the microbiological contamination of cosmetics, toiletries and non-sterile pharmaceuticals. In: Baird, R.M., Bloomfield, S.F. (eds) *Microbial Quality Assurance in Cosmetics, Toiletries and Non-sterile Pharmaceuticals*. Taylor & Francis, London, pp 9–30.

Index